The CliniBook

CLINICAL GENE TRANSFER:
STATE-OF-THE-ART

Éditions EDK/Groupe EDP Sciences
25, rue Daviel
75013 Paris, France
Tél. : 01 58 10 19 05
Fax : 01 43 29 32 62
edk@edk.fr
www.edk.fr

EDP Sciences
17, avenue du Hoggar
PA de Courtabœuf
91944 Les Ulis Cedex A, France
www.edpsciences.org

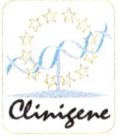

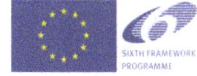

The CliniBook

CLINICAL GENE TRANSFER:
STATE-OF-THE-ART

Edited by
ODILE COHEN-HAGUENAUER

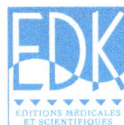

EDK ÉDITIONS MÉDICALES ET SCIENTIFIQUES

edp sciences

« Hope lies in dreams, in imagination and in the courage
of those who dare to make dreams into reality »
Jonas Salk, 1914-1995

« The joys of science lie in the work itself;
the ultimate reward being the progress of mankind »
Rosalind Elsie Franklin, 1920-1958

*« The utmost limitations in science and discovery are not
at the frontiers and complexity of research but in people's minds:
it's all about keeping the faith … »*

à Julien, Antoine et Paul

CliniGene Partners and Boards

CliniGene Acting Partners

• Academic partners

ALESSANDRO AIUTI (and EUGENIO MONTINI), *FCSR-TIGET, San Raffaele Telethon Institute for Gene Therapy, Milan, Italy; Medical Genetics, Department of Pediatrics, "Federico II" University, Naples, Italy.*

ROBIN R. ALI, *Institute of Opthalmology, UCL, London, England.*

ALBERTO AURICCHIO, *Telethon Institute of Genetics and Medicine, FTELE-IGM, Napoli, Italy.*

SÉGOLÈNE AYMÉ, *Orphanet, Inserm SC11, Plate-forme Maladies Rares, Paris, France.*

CHRISTOPHER BAUM (and TONI CATHOMEN[1]), *Medizinische Hochschule Hannover, MHH, Hannover, Germany.*

FATIMA BOSCH, *CBATEG-UAB, Universitat Autonòma de Barcelona, Barcelona, Spain.*

JAN BUBENIK - MILAN REINIS, *Institute of Molecular Genetics, IMG CAS, Prague, Czech Republic.*

NATHALIE CARTIER, *Inserm UMR 745, University Paris-Descartes, Sorbonne Paris-Cité, Paris, France.*

KLAUS CICHUTEK (and MATTHIAS SCHWEIZER), *Paul-Ehrlich-Institut, PEI, Langen, Germany.*

MANUEL J.T. CARRONDO (and PEDRO E. CRUZ), *Instituto de Biologia Experimental e Tecnologica, IBET-ITBQ, Oeiras, Portugal.*

NICOLE DÉGLON, *MIRCEN, Commissariat à l'Énergie Atomique-CEA, Saclay, France.[2]*

GEORGES DICKSON (and RAFAEL J. YÁÑEZ-MUÑOZ), *School of Biological Sciences, Royal Holloway-University of London (RHUL), Egham, Surrey, United Kingdom*

MARK FEDERSPIEL - STEPHEN J. RUSSELL, *Gene Therapy Program, Mayo Clinic College of Medicine, Rochester, USA.*

GÖSTA GAHRTON, *Department of Medicine, Karolinska Institutet-KI, Stockholm, Sweden.*

BERND GÄNSBACHER, *Institute of Experimental Oncology and Therapy Research, Klinikum rechts der Isar der Technischen Universität München, Munich, Germany.*

MAURO GIACCA, *International Centre for Genetic Engineering and Biotechnology, ICGEB, Trieste, Italy.[3]*

---

[1]*Now at Laboratory of Cell and Gene Therapy, University Medical Center Freiburg, Engesserstr. 4, D-79108 Freiburg, Germany.*
[2]*Now at Laboratory of Cellular and Molecular Neurotherapies, Lausanne University Medical School (CHUV), Lausanne, Switzerland.*
[3]*A CliniGene-SAB member until 2010.*

HANSJÖRG HAUSER (and DAGMAR WIRTH), *The Helmholtz Centre for Infection Research-HZI, Braunschweig, Germany.*

ZSUZSANNA IZSVAK, *Max Delbrück Center for Molecular Medicine, MDC, Berlin, Germany.*

ANDREAS H. JACOBS, *Laboratory for Gene Therapy and Molecular Imaging at the Max Planck Institute for Neurological Research with Klaus-Joachim-Zülch-Laboratories of the Max Planck Society and the Faculty of Medicine of the University of Cologne, Cologne, Germany; European Institute for Molecular Imaging (EIMI), University of Münster (WWU) Münster, Germany; Department of Geriatric Medicine, Johanniter Hospital, Bonn, Germany. ahjacobs@uni-muenster.de*

CHRISTOF VON KALLE (and MANFRED SCHMIDT), *National Center for Tumor Diseases, NCT and German Cancer Research Center, DKFZ, Heidelberg, Germany.*

DAVID KLATZMANN, *Immunologie-Immunopathologie-Immunothérapie, Assistance Publique-Hopitaux de Paris (APHP), CNRS UMR7211 and Inserm U959, CERVI, Hôpital Pitié-Salpêtrière, Paris, France.*

STEFAN KOCHANEK, *University of Ulm, Ulm, Germany.*

OTTO-WILHELM MERTEN - FULVIO MAVILIO *(CSO)* **- FRÉDÉRIC REVAH** *(CEO), Généthon, Évry, France.*[4,5]

NICOLAS MERMOD, *Institut de Biotechnologie, UNIL, Lausanne, Switzerland.*

LLUIS MIR, *UMR 8121 CNRS, Institut Gustave-Roussy, Villejuif, France.*

PHILIPPE MOULLIER, *CHU de Nantes, Laboratoire de Thérapie Génique, Inserm UMR649, Faculté de Médecine et Université, Nantes, France.*[4]

AMOS PANET, *Institute for Medical Research, Hebrew University, Hadassah Medical School-HUJI, Jerusalem, Israel.*

MARC PESCHANSKI, *I-STEM, Inserm UEVE 861, AFM, 5, rue Henri-Desbruères, 91030 Évry Cedex, France.*

DANIEL SCHERMAN, *Inserm U1022, CNRS UMR 8151, Faculté de Pharmacie, Université Paris Descartes, Sorbonne Paris-Cité, Paris, France; Chimie Paris Tech, Paris, F-75005, France.*

THIERRY VANDENDRIESCHE, *Division of Gene Therapy and Regenerative Medicine, Free University of Brussels-VUB, Brussels, Belgium.*

SEPPO YLÄ-HERTTUALA, *A.I. Virtanen Institute, University of Eastern Finland, Kuopio, Finland*

and ODILE COHEN-HAGUENAUER, *CliniGene-NoE coordinator, École Normale Supérieure de Cachan, CNRS UMR 8113; and Oncogenetics, Department of Clinical Oncology, Hôpital Saint-Louis AP-HP; Faculté de Médecine, Université Paris-Diderot, Sorbonne Paris-Cité, 75475 Paris Cedex 10, France.*

[4] *Anne-Marie Masquelier was CEO of Généthon from 2005 to 2008.*
[5] *Philippe Moullier was CSO of Généthon from 2009 to 2011.*

PITER BOSMA, *Gaubius Institute for Cardiovascular Research of TNO, Leiden, The Netherlands.*

MARY COLLINS, *University College of London, London, United Kingdom.*

OLIVIER DANOS, *Necker Hospital CNRS and UCL-UK (now, NYC, USA).*

JEAN-LUC DARLIX, *École Normale Supérieure de Lyon, Lyon, France.*

JANE FARRAR, *University College Cork, Cork, Ireland.*

JÜRGEN KLEINSCHMIDT, *DKFZ, Heidelberg, Germany.*

BERNARD MASSIE, *University of Montreal, Montreal, Canada.*

AMIT NATHWANI, *Haematology, Cancer, University College London Hospitals, London, United Kingdom.*

MARC SITBON, *IGMM, CNRS-Inserm, Université de Montpellier 2, Montpellier, France.*

MICHAEL THEMIS, *Imperial College London, London, United Kingdom.*

WITH THE EDITOR'S SPECIAL THANKS TO:

■ *Fernand Sauer and Octavi Quintana-Trias, for their thrilling vision of the European research area and advancement of progress in Human Health,*

■ *Mario Capecchi and Bob Weinberg for triggering deep inspiration and perseverance,*

■ *Paul Janiaud for sharing his magical views and unlimited enthusiasm,*

■ *Wonderful colleagues of the Euregenethy EC-DG research network [Fatima Bosch, Pedro Cruz, Manuel Carrondo, Klaus Cichutek, Nicole Déglon, George Dickson, Bernd Gänsbacher, Gösta Gahrton, Luigi Naldini, Felicia Rosenthal, Seppo Ylä-Herttuala], together with Christian Auclair, Stephen J. Russell, Lucio Luzzatto, Inder Verma, Gabriel Mergui, Pierre Tambourin, Ted Friedmann and our late friend Ketty Schwartz who placed trust in the initiation of the CliniGene-NoE,*

■ *Fatiha Sadallah, Arnd Hoeveler, Brigitte Sambain, Jean-Emmanuel Faure, Gérard Rivières and Jacques Demotes,*

■ *Jacqueline Corrigan-Curay and Allan Shipp for fruitful interaction,*

■ *Celia Tunc and Nicolas Creff, the two main CliniGene managers who gave graceful everyday life to our endeavour with special dedication and to Michel Profeta,*

■ *The amazingly gifted young trainees - acting as professionals - of the NSIGMA (ENSIMAG, Grenoble, 2006) and ESCP Europe Conseil (ESCP-Europe, Paris, 2010) junior enterprises who produced our dedicated CliniSoft scientific and strategic software and the CliniGene Strategic-Business Plan, respectively,*

■ *Caroline Duros, Alexandre Artus for shared jubilation and high fidelity,*

■ *Dr Marc Espié, for his patience, generosity, humanism and faithful support,*

■ *The whole administrative staff of the École Normale Supérieure de Cachan and its former President, Jean-Yves Mérindol,*

■ *Late Sabrina Tafuro-Ayuso for initiating the CliniGene training courses with Fatima Bosch,*

■ *Marc Sitbon and Jean-Michel Heard for pivotal initial training,*

■ *Isabelle Benoit and Christian Grenaudier, for sharing style with science,*

■ *EDK Publisher, in particular the lovely and smart Martine Krief and François Flori, acting as a magician,*

■ *Enlightened Cloro who gave me birth twice and took us to have faith in whatever would be done, should be for love.*

It's all about keeping the faith, hope and turning dreams into reality
O.C.H.

List of authors

ALESSANDRO AIUTI

San Raffaele Telethon Institute for Gene Therapy, Milan, Italy; Department of Pediatrics, University of Rome Tor Vergata, Children's Hospital Bambino Gesù, Rome, Italy. a.aiuti@hsr.it

ROBIN R. ALI

UCL Institute of Ophthalmology, Department of Genetics, 11-43 Bath Street, London EC1V 9EL, United Kingdom. r.ali@ucl.ac.uk

EVREN ALICI

Cell and gene therapy center, department of medicine, divison of hematology, Karolinska Institutet, Karolinska University Hospital, Huddinge, Sweden.

PER ALMQVIST

Department of Clinical Neuroscience, Karolinska Institutet, Stockholm, Sweden; Department of Neurosurgery, Karolinska University Hospital, Stockholm, Sweden.

PATRIZIA ANNUNZIATA

Telethon Institute of Genetics and Medicine (TIGEM), Naples, Italy; Medical Genetics, Department of Pediatrics, Federico II University, Naples, Italy.

MARTINA ANTON

Institute of Experimental Oncology and Therapy Research, Klinikum rechts der Isar der Technischen Universität München, Munich, Germany.

ALEXANDRE ARTUS

CNRS UMR 8113 and CliniGene, École Normale Supérieure de Cachan, 94235 Cachan, France.

TAKIS ATHANASOPOULOS

School of Biological Sciences, Royal Holloway, University of London, Egham Hill, Egham, Surrey, TW20 0EX, United Kingdom.

PATRICK AUBOURG

Inserm UMR 745, University Paris Descartes, Sorbonne Paris-Cité, 75279, Paris, France; Department of Pediatric Endocrinology and Neurology, Hôpital de Bicêtre, 94275 Le Kremlin-Bicêtre, France.

GWENNAELLE AUREGAN

CEA, Institute of Biomedical Imaging (I2BM) and Molecular Imaging Research Center (MIRCen), Fontenay-aux-Roses, France; CNRS-CEA URA2210, Fontenay-aux-Roses, France.

ALBERTO AURICCHIO

Telethon Institute of Genetics and Medicine (TIGEM), Naples, Italy; Medical Genetics, Department of Pediatrics, "Federico II" University, Naples, Italy. auricchio@tigem.it

EDUARD AYUSO

Center of Animal Biotechnology and Gene Therapy and Department of Biochemistry and Molecular Biology, School of Veterinary Medicine, Universitat Autònoma de Barcelona, 08193 Bellaterra, Spain. CIBER de Diabetes y Enfermedades Metabólicas Asociadas (CIBERDEM), Spain. eduard.ayuso@uab.es

VANESSA BANDEIRA

IBET, Apartado 12, 2781-901 Oeiras, Portugal.

RITA N. BÁRCIA

ECBio, S.A., R. Henrique Paiva Couceiro, 27, 2700-451 Amadora, Portugal.

CYNTHIA C. BARTHOLOMAE

National Center for Tumor Diseases and German Cancer Research Center, 69120 Heidelberg, Germany.

CHRISTOPHER BAUM

Hannover Medical School (MHH) Institute of Experimental Haematology, Carl-Neuberg-Str. 1, D-30625 Hannover, Germany. baum.christopher@mh-hannover.de

ÉMILIE BAYART

CNRS UMR 8113 and CliniGene, École Normale Supérieure de Cachan, 94235 Cachan, France.

CHRISTIEN BEDNARSKI

Laboratory of Cell and Gene Therapy, Center for Chronic Immunodeficiency, University Medical Center Freiburg, Engesserstr. 4, D-79108 Freiburg, Germany.

BERTRAND BELLIER

UPMC Université Paris 06, CNRS, UMR 7211, Inserm, U959, Bâtiment CERVI, Hôpital Pitié-Salpêtrière, 83, boulevard de l'Hôpital, F-75013 Paris, France.

LUCA BIASCO

San Raffaele Telethon Institute for Gene Therapy, Milano, Italy; Università Vita-Salute San Raffaele, Milano, Italy.

PASCAL BIGEY

CNRS, UMR8151, Inserm, U1022, Université Paris Descartes, Sorbonne Paris Cité, Faculté de Pharmacie, Chemical and Genetic Pharmacology and Imaging Laboratory, Paris, F-75270 France; École Nationale Supérieure de Chimie de Paris, Chimie ParisTech, Paris, F-75005 France.

VÉRONIQUE BLOUIN

CHU de Nantes, Faculté de Médecine, Université de Nantes, Nantes, France.

JUERGEN BODE

Hannover Medical School (MHH), Institute of Experimental Haematology, OE 6960, D-30625 Hannover, Germany. bode.juergen@mh-hannover.de

GILLES BONVENTO

CEA, Institute of Biomedical Imaging (I2BM) and Molecular Imaging Research Center (MIRCen), Fontenay-aux-Roses, France; CNRS-CEA URA2210, Fontenay-aux-Roses, France.

FATIMA BOSCH

Center of Animal Biotechnology and Gene Therapy and Department of Biochemistry and Molecular Biology, School of Veterinary Medicine, Universitat Autònoma de Barcelona, 08193 Bellaterra, Spain. CIBER de Diabetes y Enfermedades Metabólicas Asociadas (CIBERDEM), Spain. fatima.bosch@uab.es

PIERRE BOUGNÈRES

Department of Pediatric Endocrinology and Neurology, Hôpital de Bicêtre, 94275 Le Kremlin-Bicêtre, France.

IMMACOLATA BRIGIDA

San Raffaele Telethon Institute for Gene Therapy, Milan, Italy.

SANDRA BROLL

Helmholtz Centre for Infection Research (HZI), Department Mol Biotech, Braunschweig, Germany.

CHRISTIAN J. BUCHHOLZ

Division of Medical Biotechnology, Paul-Ehrlich-Institut, Langen, Germany.

MICHEL-FRANCIS BUREAU

CNRS, UMR8151, Paris, F-75006 France; Inserm, U1022, Université Paris Descartes, Sorbonne Paris-Cité, Faculté de Pharmacie, Chemical and Genetic Pharmacology and Imaging Laboratory, Paris, F-75270 France; École Nationale Supérieure de Chimie de Paris, Chimie ParisTech, Paris, F-75005 France.

DAVID CALLEJAS

Center of Animal Biotechnology and Gene Therapy and Department of Biochemistry and Molecular Biology, School of Veterinary Medicine, Universitat Autònoma de Barcelona, 08193-Bellaterra, and CIBER de Diabetes y Enfermedades Metabólicas Asociadas (CIBERDEM), Spain.

MANUEL J.T. CARRONDO

Instituto de Tecnologia Química e Biológica-Universidade Nova de Lisboa/Instituto de Biologia Experimental e Tecnológica (ITQB-UNL/IBET), P-2781-901 Oeiras, Portugal; Faculdade de Ciências e Tecnologia/Universidade Nova de Lisboa (FCT/UNL), P-2825 Monte da Caparica, Portugal.

NATHALIE CARTIER

Inserm U745, Faculty of Pharmaceutical Sciences, Paris Descartes University, Sorbonne Paris-Cité, 4, avenue de l'Observatoire, 75006, Paris, France; Department of Pediatric Endocrinology and Neurology, Hôpital de Bicêtre, 94275 Le Kremlin-Bicêtre, France. nathalie.cartier@inserm.fr

TONI CATHOMEN

Laboratory of Cell and Gene Therapy, Center for Chronic Immunodeficiency, University Medical Center Freiburg, Engesserstr. 4, D-79108 Freiburg, Germany. toni.cathomen@uniklinik-freiburg.de

MARINA CAVAZZANA-CALVO

Department of Biotherapy, Hôpital Necker-Enfants Malades, 75743 Paris, France; Inserm UMR768, University Paris-Descartes, Sorbonne Paris-Cité, 75743 Paris, France; Clinical Investigation Center in Biotherapy, Groupe Hospitalier Universitaire Ouest, 75743 Paris, France.

MARINEE K.L. CHUAH

Department of Gene Therapy and Regenerative Medicine, Free University of Brussels (VUB), Faculty of Medicine and Pharmacy, University Medical Center - Jette, Laarbeeklaan 103, B-1090 Brussels, Belgium; Department of Molecular Cardiovascular Medicine, University of Leuven, University Hospital Campus Gasthuisberg, Belgium. marinee.chuah@vub.ac.be

KLAUS CICHUTEK

President, Paul-Ehrlich-Institut, Paul-Ehrlich-Straße 51-59, 63225 Langen, Germany. cickl@pei.de

ODILE COHEN-HAGUENAUER

École Normale Supérieure de Cachan, CliniGene, CNRS UMR 8113, 94235 Cachan; and Department of Medical Oncology, Hôpital Saint-Louis AP-HP; Faculté de Médecine, University Paris7-Diderot, Sorbonne-Paris-Cité, 75475 Paris Cedex 10, France. odile.cohen@lbpa.ens-cachan.fr

ANGÉLIQUE COLIN

CEA, Institute of Biomedical Imaging (I2BM) and Molecular Imaging Research Center (MIRCen), Fontenay-aux-Roses, France; CNRS-CEA URA2210, Fontenay-aux-Roses, France.

GONZALO CORDOVA

CNRS, UMR8151, Paris, F-75006 France; Inserm, U1022, Université Paris Descartes, Sorbonne Paris-Cité, Faculté de Pharmacie, Chemical and Genetic Pharmacology and Imaging Laboratory, Paris, F-75270 France; École Nationale Supérieure de Chimie de Paris, Chimie ParisTech, Paris, F-75005 France.

ANA SOFIA COROADINHA

Instituto de Tecnologia Química e Biológica-Universidade Nova de Lisboa/Instituto de Biologia Experimental e Tecnológica (ITQB-UNL/IBET), P-2781-901 Oeiras, Portugal. avalente@itqb.unl.pt

FRANÇOIS-LOÏC COSSET

École Normale Supérieure de Lyon; Inserm, U758, Human Virology laboratory, EVIR Team; University of Lyon, UCB-Lyon1, Lyon, F-69007, France. flcosset@ens-lyon.fr

GABRIELLA COTUGNO

Telethon Institute of Genetics and Medicine (TIGEM), Naples, Italy; Medical Genetics, Department of Pediatrics, "Federico II" University, Naples, Italy.

PEDRO E. CRUZ

Instituto de Tecnologia Química e Biológica-Universidade Nova de Lisboa/Instituto de Biologia Experimental e Tecnológica (ITQB-UNL/IBET), P-2781-901 Oeiras, Portugal; ECBio, S.A., P-2700-451 Amadora, Portugal. pcruz@itqb.unl.pt

HELDER J.S. CRUZ

ECBio, S.A., R. Henrique Paiva Couceiro, 27, 2700-451 Amadora, Portugal.

CHRISTOPHE DARMON

CHU de Nantes, Faculté de Médecine, Université de Nantes, Nantes, France; EFS-Atlantic Bio GMP, Saint-Herblain, France.

ANDREW M. DAVIDOFF

Department of Surgery, St. Jude Children's Research Hospital, Memphis, TN, USA.

NICOLE DÉGLON

CEA, Institute of Biomedical Imaging (I2BM) and Molecular Imaging Research Center (MIRCen), Fontenay-aux-Roses, France; CNRS-CEA URA2210, Fontenay-aux-Roses, France; **Present address:** Centre Hospitalier Universitaire Vaudois (CHUV), Département des Neurosciences Cliniques, Laboratoire de Neurothérapies Cellulaires et Moléculaires, Pavillon 3, Avenue de Beaumont, 1011 Lausanne, Suisse. nicole.deglon@chuv.ch

GEORGE DICKSON

School of Biological Sciences, Royal Holloway, University of London, Egham Hill, Egham, Surrey, TW20 0EX, United Kingdom. g.dickson@rhul.ac.uk

KURT E.J. DITTMAR

Department of Gene Regulation and Differentiation, Helmholtz Centre for Infection Research (HZI), Inhoffenstr. 7, D-38124 Braunschweig, Germany.

RUXANDRA DRAGHIA-AKLI

MD, PhD, RTD-Director Health, Research and Innovation DG European Commission, B - 1049 Brussels, Belgium. ruxandra.draghia-akli@ec.europa.eu

NOËLLE DUFOUR

CEA, Institute of Biomedical Imaging (I2BM) and Molecular Imaging Research Center (MIRCen), Fontenay-aux-Roses, France; CNRS-CEA URA2210, Fontenay-aux-Roses, France.

LYDIA DÜRNER

Pharma Research and Early Development, Roche Glycart AG, CH-8952 Schlieren, Switzerland.

CAROLINE DUROS

CNRS UMR 8113 and CliniGene, École Normale Supérieure de Cachan, 94235 Cachan, France.

MARIA ERIKSDOTTER-JÖNHAGEN

Department of Neurobiology, Caring Sciences and Society, Division of Clinical Geriatrics, Karolinska Institutet and Karolinska University Hospital, Huddinge, Novum, Plan 5, SE-141 86, Stockholm, Sweden; Department of Geriatrics, Karolinska University Hospital, Stockholm, Sweden. maria.eriksdotter.jonhagen@ki.se

CAROLE ESCARTIN

CEA, Institute of Biomedical Imaging (I2BM) and Molecular Imaging Research Center (MIRCen), Fontenay-aux-Roses, France; CNRS-CEA URA2210, Fontenay-aux-Roses, France.

VIRGINIE ESCRIOU

CNRS, UMR8151, Paris, F-75006 France; Inserm, U1022, Université Paris Descartes, Sorbonne Paris Cité, Faculté de Pharmacie, Chemical and Genetic Pharmacology and Imaging Laboratory, Paris, F-75270 France; École Nationale Supérieure de Chimie de Paris, Chimie ParisTech, Paris, F-75005 France.

HELGA EYJOLFSDOTTIR

Department of Neurobiology, Caring Sciences and Society, Division of Clinical Geriatrics, Karolinska Institutet, Sweden; Department of Geriatrics, Karolinska University Hospital, Stockholm, Sweden.

MATHILDE FAIDEAU

CEA, Institute of Biomedical Imaging (I2BM) and Molecular Imaging Research Center (MIRCen), Fontenay-aux-Roses, France; CNRS-CEA URA2210, Fontenay-aux-Roses, France.

HELEN FOSTER

School of Biological Sciences, Royal Holloway, University of London, Egham Hill, Egham, Surrey, TW20 0EX, United Kingdom.

KEITH FOSTER

School of Biological Sciences, Royal Holloway, University of London, Egham Hill, Egham, Surrey, TW20 0EX, United Kingdom.

ALAIN FISCHER

Inserm UMR768, University Paris-Descartes, Sorbonne Paris-Cité et Service d'Immuno-Hématologie, Hôpital Necker-Enfants Malades, 75743 Paris, France.

GÖSTA GAHRTON

Karolinska Institutet, Department of Medicine, Karolinska University Hospital, Huddinge, SE 14186 Stockholm, Sweden. gosta.gahrton@ki.se

MELANIE GALLA

Hannover Medical School (MHH) Institute of Experimental Haematology, Carl-Neuberg-Str. 1, D-30625 Hannover, Germany.

ANNE GALY

Inserm U951 and Généthon, 1, rue de l'Internationale, BP60, F-91002 Évry Cedex, France.

LEONOR GAMA-NORTON

Instituto de Tecnologia Química e Biológica-Universidade Nova de Lisboa/Instituto de Biologia Experimental e Tecnológica (ITQB-UNL/IBET), P-2781-901 Oeiras, Portugal; Helmholtz Centre for Infection Research, D-38124 Braunschweig, Germany.

BERND GÄNSBACHER

Institute of Experimental Oncology and Therapy Research, Klinikum rechts der Isar der Technischen Universität München, Munich, Germany. bernd.gansbacher@lrz.tum.de

HENK S.P. GARRITSEN

Institute for Clinical Transfusion Medicine, Städtisches Klinikum Braunschweig gGmbH, Braunschweig, Germany.

ANASTASIOS GEORGIADIS

UCL Institute of Ophthalmology, Department of Genetics, 11-43 Bath Street, London EC1V 9EL, United Kingdom.

MAURO GIACCA

Molecular Medicine Laboratory, International Centre for Genetic Engineering and Biotechnology (ICGEB), Padriciano, 99, 34149 Trieste, Italy. giacca@icgeb.org

MARI GILLJAM

Cell and gene therapy center, department of medicine, divison of hematology, Karolinska Institutet, Karolinska University Hospital, Huddinge, Sweden.

SALIMA HACEIN-BEY-ABINA

Department of Biotherapy, Hôpital Necker-Enfants Malades, 75743 Paris, France; Inserm UMR768, University Paris-Descartes, Sorbonne Paris-Cité, 75743 Paris, France; Clinical Investigation Center in Biotherapy, Groupe Hospitalier Universitaire Ouest, 75743 Paris, France.

EVA-MARIA HÄNDEL

Institute of Experimental Hematology, Hannover Medical School, Carl-Neuberg-Strasse 1, D-30625 Hannover, Germany.

PHILIPPE HANTRAYE

CEA, Institute of Biomedical Imaging (I2BM) and Molecular Imaging Research Center (MIRCen), Fontenay-aux-Roses, France; CNRS-CEA URA2210, Fontenay-aux-Roses, France.

MARK HASKINS

Departments of Patho- biology and Clinical Studies, School of Veterinary Medicine, University of Pennsylvania, Philadelphia, PA, USA.

RAYMONDE HASSIG

CEA, Institute of Biomedical Imaging (I2BM) and Molecular Imaging Research Center (MIRCen), Fontenay-aux-Roses, France; CNRS-CEA URA2210, Fontenay-aux-Roses, France.

HANSJÖRG HAUSER

Department of Gene Regulation and Differentiation, Helmholtz-Zentrum für Infektionsforschung, Inhoffenstr. 7, D-38124 Braunschweig, Germany. hha@helmholtz.de

NIELS HEINZ

Hannover Medical School (MHH), Institute of Experimental Haematology, OE 6960, D-30625 Hannover, Germany.

ZOLTÁN IVICS

Max Delbrück Centrum for Molecular Medicine, Robert Rossle Strasse 10, Berlin D-13122, Germany

ZSUZSANNA IZSVÁK

Max Delbrück Centrum for Molecular Medicine, Robert Rossle Strasse 10, Berlin D-13122, Germany. zizsvak@mdc-berlin.de

ANDREAS H. JACOBS

[1] Laboratory for Gene Therapy and Molecular Imaging at the Max Planck Institute for Neurological Research with Klaus-Joachim-Zülch-Laboratories of the Max Planck Society and the Faculty of Medicine of the University of Cologne, Cologne, Germany; [2] European Institute for Molecular Imaging (EIMI), University of Münster (WWU), Münster, Germany; [3] Department of Geriatric Medicine, Johanniter Hospital, Bonn, Germany. ahjacobs@uni-muenster.de

SUSAN JARMIN

School of Biological Sciences, Royal Holloway, University of London, Egham Hill, Egham, Surrey, TW20 0EX, United Kingdom.

VERONICA JIMENEZ

Center of Animal Biotechnology and Gene Therapy and Department of Biochemistry and Molecular Biology, School of Veterinary Medicine, Universitat Autònoma de Barcelona, 08193-Bellaterra, and CIBER de Diabetes y Enfermedades Metabólicas Asociadas (CIBERDEM), Spain.

CHRISTOF VON KALLE

National Center for Tumor Diseases NCT and German Cancer Research Center DKFZ, 69120 Heidelberg, Germany.

JAGJEET KANG

School of Biological Sciences, Royal Holloway, University of London, Egham Hill, Egham, Surrey, TW20 0EX, United Kingdom.

ALASTAIR KENT

Genetic Alliance UK, Unit 4D, Leroy House, 436 Essex Road, London N1 3QP, United Kingdom.

ABED KHALAILEH

Departments of Biochemistry and Surgery, the Hebrew University-Hadassah Medical School, IMRIC, Jerusalem, Israel.

ANTOINE KICHLER

CNRS, UMR8151, Paris, F-75006 France; Inserm, U1022, Université Paris Descartes, Sorbonne Paris Cité, Faculté de Pharmacie, Chemical and Genetic Pharmacology and Imaging Laboratory, Paris, F-75270 France; École Nationale Supérieure de Chimie de Paris, Chimie ParisTech, Paris, F-75005, France.

NANCY M.P. KING

JD, Professor, Department of Social Sciences and Health Policy, Wake Forest University School of Medicine, Co-Director, WFU Center for Bioethics, Health, and Society, Wells Fargo 14, Medical Center Boulevard, Winston-Salem, NC 27157, USA.

DAVID KLATZMANN

UPMC Université Paris 06, CNRS, UMR 7211, Inserm, U959, Bâtiment CERVI, Hôpital Pitié-Salpêtrière, 83, boulevard de l'Hôpital, F-75013 Paris, France. david.klatzmann@upmc.fr

STEFAN KOCHANEK

Department of Gene Therapy, University of Ulm, Helmholtz Str. 8/1, 89081 Ulm, Germany. stefan.kochanek@uni-ulm.de

DROR KOLODKIN-GAL

Departments of Biochemistry and Surgery, the Hebrew University-Hadassah Medical School, IMRIC, Jerusalem, Israel.

TAEYOUNG KOO

School of Biological Sciences, Royal Holloway, University of London, Egham Hill, Egham, Surrey, TW20 0EX, United Kingdom.

NIKOLAI KUNICHER

Departments of Biochemistry and Surgery, the Hebrew University-Hadassah Medical School, IMRIC, Jerusalem, Israel.

KRISTINA LACHMANN

Fraunhofer-Institut für Schicht- und Oberflächentechnik (IST), Braunschweig, Germany.

STEPHANIE LAUFS

Department of Translational Oncology, National Center for Tumor Diseases NCT and German Cancer Research Center (DKFZ), Heidelberg, Germany.

STÉPHANIE LEMAIRE

CNRS UMR 8113 and CliniGene, École Normale Supérieure de Cachan, 94235 Cachan, France.

FRANÇOIS LEMOINE

Université Pierre et Marie Curie, UPMC Université Paris 06, CNRS UMR7211, Inserm U959, Clinical Investigation Center in Biotherapy, AP-HP, Hôpital Pitié-Salpêtrière, F-75651, Paris 13, France.

GÖRAN LIND

Department of Clinical Neuroscience, Karolinska Institutet, Stockholm, Sweden; Department of Neurosurgery, Karolinska University Hospital, Stockholm, Sweden.

WERNER LINDENMAIER

Department of Gene Regulation and Differentiation, Helmholtz Centre for Infection Research (HZI), Inhoffenstr. 7, D-38124 Braunschweig, Germany. werner.lindenmaier@helmholtz-hzi.de

BENGT LINDEROTH

Department of Clinical Neuroscience, Karolinska Institutet, Stockholm, Sweden; Department of Neurosurgery, Karolinska University Hospital, Stockholm, Sweden.

MARTIN LOCK

Gene Therapy Program, Department of Pathology and Laboratory Medicine, University of Pennsylvania, Philadelphia, USA.

TANJA LUCAS

Department of Gene Therapy, University of Ulm, Helmholtz Str. 8/1, 89081 Ulm, Germany.

LUCIO LUZZATTO

Honorary Professor of Haematology, University of Firenze; Scientific Director, Istituto Toscano Tumori, Via Taddeo Alderotti 26N, 50139 Firenze, Italy.
lucio.luzzatto@ittumori.it

LARS MACKE

Department of Molecular Biotechnology, Helmholtz Centre for Infection Research (HZI), Inhoffenstr. 7, Institute for Clinical Transfusion Medicine, Städtisches Klinikum Braunschweig gGmbH, D-38124 Braunschweig, Germany.

TOBIAS MAETZIG

Hannover Medical School (MHH) Institute of Experimental Haematology, Carl-Neuberg-Str. 1, D-30625 Hannover, Germany.

THOMAS MALDINEY

Unité de Pharmacologie Chimique et Génétique et d'Imagerie; CNRS, UMR 8151, Inserm, U 1022, Université Paris Descartes, Sorbonne Paris-Cité, Faculté des Sciences Pharmaceutiques et Biologiques, Paris, F-75270 cedex France; ENSCP, Paris, F-75231 Cedex France. thomas.maldiney@parisdescartes.fr

ALBERTO MALERBA

School of Biological Sciences, Royal Holloway, University of London, Egham Hill, Egham, Surrey, TW20 0EX, United Kingdom.

CHRISTOPHER MANN

Center of Animal Biotechnology and Gene Therapy and Department of Biochemistry and Molecular Biology, School of Veterinary Medicine, Universitat Autònoma de Barcelona, 08193-Bellaterra, Spain.

CORINNE MARIE

UPCGI, Inserm U1022 - CNRS UMR8151, Faculté des Sciences Pharmaceutiques et Biologiques, 4, avenue de l'Observatoire, 75270 Paris Cedex 06, France.
corinne.marie@parisdescartes.fr

PAULA MARQUES ALVES

Instituto de Tecnologia Química e Biológica-Universidade Nova de Lisboa/Instituto de Biologia Experimental e Tecnológica (ITQB-UNL/IBET), P-2781-901 Oeiras, Portugal.

OTTO-WILHELM MERTEN

Généthon, 1, rue de l'Internationale, BP60, F-91000 Évry Cedex, France.

WILHELM MEYRING

Department of Molecular Biotechnology, Helmholtz Centre for Infection Research (HZI), Inhoffenstr. 7, Institute for Clinical Transfusion Medicine, Städtisches Klinikum Braunschweig gGmbH, D-38124 Braunschweig, Germany.

NATHALIE MIGNET

CNRS, UMR8151, Inserm, U1022, Université Paris Descartes, Sorbonne Paris-Cité, Faculté de Pharmacie, Chemical and Genetic Pharmacology and Imaging Laboratory, Paris, F-75270 France; École Nationale Supérieure de Chimie de Paris, Chimie ParisTech, Paris, F-75005 France.

FEDERICO MINGOZZI

Center for Cellular and Molecular Therapeutics, Children's Hospital of Philadelphia, Philadelphia, PA, USA. mingozzi@email.chop.edu

KYRIACOS MITROPHANOUS

Oxford BioMedica plc, The Oxford Science Park, Medawar Centre, Oxford OX4 4GA, United Kingdom.

UTE MODLICH

Hannover Medical School (MHH) Institute of Experimental Haematology, Carl-Neuberg-Str. 1, D-30625 Hannover, Germany.

PARISA MONFARED

[1] Laboratory for Gene Therapy and Molecular Imaging at the Max Planck Institute for Neurological Research with Klaus-Joachim-Zülch-Laboratories of the Max Planck Society and the Faculty of Medicine of the University of Cologne, Cologne, Germany; [2] European Institute for Molecular Imaging (EIMI), University of Münster (WWU), Münster, Germany.

EUGENIO MONTINI

San Raffaele Telethon Institute for Gene Therapy, Milano, Italy.

PHILIPPE MOULLIER

Department of Molecular Genetics and Microbiology, College of Medicine, University of Florida, Gainesville, FL, USA; Laboratoire de Thérapie Génique, Inserm UMR649, CHU de Nantes, IRT UN, 30 boulevard Jean Monnet, F-44035 Nantes Cedex 1, France; Généthon, Évry, France. moullier@ufl.edu

LUIGI NALDINI

San Raffaele Telethon Institute for Gene Therapy, Department of Regenerative Medicine, Stem Cells and Gene Therapy, San Raffaele Institute Milan, Via Olgettina-58, 20132 Milan, Italy.

AMIT C. NATHWANI

Department of Haematology, UCL Cancer Institute; Katharine Dormandy Haemophilia Centre and Thrombosis Unit, Royal Free NHS Trust, United Kingdom; National Health Services Blood and Transplant, United Kingdom. amit.nathwani@ucl.ac.uk

ARTHUR W. NIENHUIS

Department of Hematology, St. Jude Children's Research Hospital, Memphis, TN, USA.

STÉPHANE PALFI

Service de neurochirurgie Hôpital Henri Mondor, 51, avenue du Maréchal de Lattre de Tassigny, UPEC, Faculté de Médecine, 94010 Créteil Cedex, France. stephane.palfi@hmn.aphp.fr

AMOS PANET

Departments of Biochemistry and Surgery, the Hebrew University-Hadassah Medical School, IMRIC, Jerusalem, Israel. paneta@cc.huji.ac.il

FRÉDÉRIC PÂQUES

Cellectis S.A. 8, rue de la Croix Jarry, 75013 Paris, France.

CRISTINA PEIXOTO

IBET, Apartado 12, 2781-901 Oeiras, Portugal.

SUSANNE POHL

Helmholtz-Centre for Infection Research, Inhoffenstr. 7, D-38124 Braunschweig, Germany.

LINDA POPPLEWELL

School of Biological Sciences, Royal Holloway, University of London, Egham Hill, Egham, Surrey, TW20 0EX, United Kingdom.

DEEPAK RAJ

Department of Haematology, UCL Cancer Institute; National Health Services Blood and Transplant, United Kingdom.

R. SCOTT RALPH

Oxford BioMedica plc, The Oxford Science Park, Medawar Centre, Oxford OX4 4GA, United Kingdom.

ULRIKE REISS

Department of Hematology, St. Jude Children's Research Hospital, Memphis, TN, USA.

CYRILLE RICHARD

Unité de Pharmacologie Chimique et Génétique et d'Imagerie; CNRS, UMR 8151, Inserm, U 1022, Université Paris Descartes, Sorbonne Paris-Cité, Faculté des Sciences Pharmaceutiques et Biologiques, Paris, F-75270 cedex France; ENSCP, Paris, F-75231 Cedex, France. cyrille.richard@parisdescartes.fr

ANJA RISCHMÜLLER

PlasmidFactory GmbH and Co. KG, Meisenstrasse 96, D-33607 Bielefeld, Germany.

ANA F. RODRIGUES

Instituto de Tecnologia Química e Biológica-Universidade Nova de Lisboa/Instituto de Biologia Experimental e Tecnológica (ITQB-UNL/IBET), P-2781-901 Oeiras, Portugal.

MICHELLE ROSENZWAJG

Université Pierre et Marie Curie, UPMC Université Paris 06, CNRS UMR7211, Inserm U959, Hôpital Pitié-Salpêtrière, 83, boulevard de l'Hôpital, 75013 Paris, France; Clinical Investigation Center in Biotherapy, AP-HP, Hôpital Pitié-Salpêtrière, F-75651, Paris 13, France.

JORGE M. SANTOS

ECBio, S.A., R. Henrique Paiva Couceiro, 27, 2700-451 Amadora, Portugal.

SONJA SCHÄFERS

European Institute for Molecular Imaging (EIMI), University of Münster (WWU), Münster, Germany.

AXEL SCHAMBACH

Hannover Medical School (MHH) Institute of Experimental Haematology, Carl-Neuberg-Str. 1, D-30625 Hannover, Germany.

THOMAS SCHASER

Miltenyi Biotec GmbH, Bergisch Gladbach, Germany.

DANIEL SCHERMAN

UPCGI, CNRS, UMR8151, Inserm, U1022, Université Paris Descartes, Sorbonne Paris-Cité, Faculté de Pharmacie, Chemical and Genetic Pharmacology and Imaging Laboratory, F-75270, Paris Cedex 06, France; École Nationale Supérieure de Chimie de Paris, Chimie ParisTech, Paris, F-75005 France. daniel.scherman@parisdescartes.fr

MARTIN SCHLEEF

PlasmidFactory GmbH and Co. KG, Meisenstrasse 96, D-33607 Bielefeld, Germany. martin.schleef@plasmidfactory.com

MARCO SCHMEER

PlasmidFactory GmbH and Co. KG, Meisenstrasse 96, D-33607 Bielefeld, Germany.

MANFRED SCHMIDT

Department of Translational Oncology, National Center for Tumor Diseases NCT and German Cancer Research Center (DKFZ), 69120 Heidelberg, Germany.

MATTHIAS SCHWEIZER

Paul-Ehrlich-Institut, Paul-Ehrlich-Straße 51-59, 63225 Langen, Germany. matthias.schweizer@pei.de

ÅKE SEIGER

Department of Neurobiology, Caring Sciences and Society, Division of Clinical Geriatrics, Karolinska Institutet, Sweden; Department of Geriatrics, Karolinska University Hospital, Stockholm, Sweden.

ANA CARINA SILVA

IBET, Apartado 12, 2781-901 Oeiras, Portugal; ITQB-UNL, Apartado 12, 2781-901 Oeiras, Portugal.

DANIEL SIMÃO

IBET, Apartado 12, 2781-901 Oeiras, Portugal.

ADRIEN SIX

UPMC Université Paris 06, CNRS, UMR 7211, Inserm, U959, Bâtiment CERVI, Hôpital Pitié-Salpêtrière, 83, boulevard de l'Hôpital, F-75013 Paris, France.

JULIANNE SMITH

Cellectis Therapeutics, 8, rue de la Croix Jarry, 75013 Paris, France. smith@cellectis.com

ALEXANDER J. SMITH

UCL Institute of Ophthalmology, Department of Genetics, 11-43 Bath Street, London EC1V 9EL, United Kingdom.

RICHARD O. SNYDER

Department of Molecular Genetics and Microbiology, College of Medicine, University of Florida, Gainesville, FL, USA; Laboratoire de Thérapie Génique, Inserm UMR649, IRT UN, Nantes, France; Department of Pediatrics, College of Medicine, University of Florida, FL, USA.

MARCOS F.Q. SOUSA

IBET, Apartado 12, 2781-901 Oeiras, Portugal.

JULIA D. SUERTH

Hannover Medical School (MHH) Institute of Experimental Haematology, Carl-Neuberg-Str. 1, D-30625 Hannover, Germany.

ERIK SUNDSTRÖM

Department of Neurobiology, Caring Sciences and Society, Division of Clinical Geriatrics, Karolinska Institutet, Sweden; Stockholms Sjukhem, Stockholm, Sweden.

SHAY TAYEB

Departments of Biochemistry and Surgery, the Hebrew University-Hadassah Medical School, IMRIC, Jerusalem, Israel.

MICHAEL THOMAS

Fraunhofer-Institut für Schicht- und Oberflächentechnik (IST), Braunschweig, Germany.

VÉRONIQUE THOMAS-VASLIN

UPMC Université Paris 06, CNRS, UMR 7211, Inserm, U959, Bâtiment CERVI, Hôpital Pitié-Salpêtrière, 83, boulevard de l'Hôpital, F-75013 Paris, France.

EDWARD G.D. TUDDENHAM

Department of Haematology, UCL Cancer Institute; Katharine Dormandy Haemophilia Centre and Thrombosis Unit, Royal Free NHS Trust, United Kingdom.

THIERRY VANDENDRIESSCHE

Department of Gene Therapy and Regenerative Medicine, Free University of Brussels (VUB), Faculty of Medicine and Pharmacy, University Medical Center - Jette, Laarbeeklaan 103, B-1090 Brussels, Belgium; Department of Molecular Cardiovascular Medicine, University of Leuven, University Hospital Campus Gasthuisberg, Belgium. thierry.vandendriessche@vub.ac.be

ELS VERHOEYEN

Inserm, EVIR, U758, Human Virology Department, École Normale Supérieure de Lyon, Université Lyon 1, F-69007, Lyon, France. els.verhoeyen@ens-lyon.fr

INDER M. VERMA

Irwin and Joan Jacobs Chair in Exemplary Life Science, American Cancer Society Professor of Molecular Biology, Laboratory of Genetics, The Salk Institute, 10010 North Torrey Pines Road, La Jolla, CA 92037, USA. verma@salk.edu

THOMAS VIEL

[1] Laboratory for Gene Therapy and Molecular Imaging at the Max Planck Institute for Neurological Research with Klaus-Joachim-Zülch-Laboratories of the Max Planck Society and the Faculty of Medicine of the University of Cologne, Cologne, Germany; [2] European Institute for Molecular Imaging (EIMI), University of Münster (WWU), Münster, Germany.

YANNIC WAERZEGGERS

[1] Laboratory for Gene Therapy and Molecular Imaging at the Max Planck Institute for Neurological Research with Klaus-Joachim-Zülch-Laboratories of the Max Planck Society and the Faculty of Medicine of the University of Cologne, Cologne, Germany; [2] European Institute for Molecular Imaging (EIMI), University of Münster (WWU), Münster, Germany.

LARS WAHLBERG

Department of Neurobiology, Caring Sciences and Society, Division of Clinical Geriatrics, Karolinska Institutet, Sweden; NsGene A/S, Ballerup, Denmark.

ALEXANDRA WINKELER

[1] Laboratory for Gene Therapy and Molecular Imaging at the Max Planck Institute for Neurological Research with Klaus-Joachim-Zülch-Laboratories of the Max Planck Society and the Faculty of Medicine of the University of Cologne, Cologne, Germany; [2] Laboratory for Experimental Molecular Imaging, Inserm U1023, University Paris Sud, Paris, France.

DAGMAR WIRTH

Model Systems for Infection (MSYS), Helmholtz-Zentrum für Infektionsforschung, Inhoffenstr. 7, D-38124 Braunschweig, Germany. dkl@helmholtz-hzi.de

SEPPO YLÄ-HERTTUALA

A.I. Virtanen Institute, University of Eastern Finland, P.O. Box 1627, FI-70211 Kuopio, Finland. seppo.ylarherttuala@uef.f

SERENA ZACCHIGNA

Molecular Medicine Laboratory, International Centre for Genetic Engineering and Biotechnology (ICGEB), Padriciano, 99, 34149 Trieste, Italy.

GIDI ZAMIR

Departments of Biochemistry and Surgery, the Hebrew University-Hadassah Medical School, IMRIC, Jerusalem, Israel.

Contents

TECHNOLOGIES - Retrovirus mediated gene transfer state-of-the-art

TECHNOLOGIES - Highlights on lentivirus mediated gene transfer

TECHNOLOGIES - Non-viral based gene transfer: a new era

TECHNOLOGIES - Highlights on emerging technologies, iPS induction and genetic stability

PRE-CLINICAL STUDIES, BIOSAFETY AND ANIMAL MODELS - Preclinical assessment tools

PRE-CLINICAL STUDIES, BIOSAFETY AND ANIMAL MODELS - General biosafety: immune responses, immunotoxicity and genotoxicity

PART II: CLINICAL TRIALS AND REGULATORY ISSUES

CLINICAL TRIALS

INTRODUCTION

The CliniBook: Clinical gene transfer
Edited by Odile Cohen-Haguenauer – EDK, Paris © 2012, pp. 3-7

In-1
Foreword

LUCIO LUZZATTO*
Chair of the CliniGene Scientific Advisory Board, University of Firenze, Scientific Director, Istituto Toscano Tumori, Firenze, Italy.
lucio.luzzatto@ittumori.it

INDER M. VERMA*
Chair of the CliniGene International Board, Laboratory of Genetics, The Salk Institute, La Jolla, CA, USA.
verma@salk.edu
* Corresponding authors

We are delighted to write a foreword for this *CliniBook*, a wonderful accumulation of articles on the trials, tribulations and tiny triumphs of gene therapy. Some three decades ago the first promises of gene therapy to cure many human ills began to glitter with limitless enthusiasm and, in hindsight, with a bit of naivety not free of hubris. Since then the field has experienced many ups and downs, but its practitioners have remained steadfast in generating better delivery systems, demystifying the immune problems, solving production issues and undertaking clinical trails. Having believed since its beginning in *gene transfer for the ultimate purpose of gene therapy* [1, 2], the most gratifying fact for us to record is that today gene therapy exists. There are now five diseases in which gene therapy has had a clinical impact in at least one case [3-7]; and in one of these diseases gene therapy can be regarded as the standard of care, at least if a bone marrow donor is not available [8]. Thus, there has been success in treating children with near fatal immunodeficiencies, in improving the outlook and quality of life of patients with a variety of blood disorders, restore some vision to someone nearly blind. There are also encouraging developments with respect to debilitating degenerative diseases, and glimmers of hope for major scourges like coronary artery disease, cancer, and HIV infection. For years one might have wondered whether it was wise, before any patient had had any benefit from gene therapy, to publish gene therapy journals; but now the stand of their editors – including one of us – has been vindicated.

Yet, the obvious question is: could we or should we do better? Detractors might argue that it has taken too long from recombinant DNA to clinical gene therapy: but we think that is not a valid criticism, if we consider that it has taken more than three centuries from William Harvey's *"De Motu Cordis"* (otherwise known as *"On the Motion of the Heart and Blood"*) to the first heart transplant. We also shudder at the idea that somebody may like to indulge in calculating the cost in research dollars (or euros) for each patient who has received successful gene therapy: but again, what about the 2008 *Tufts Center for the Study of Drug Development* report, stating that the cost incurred to make a chemical into a drug available in the pharmacy averages about $1.3 billion (http://futurememes.blogspot.com/2008/09/cost-of-each-new-drug-13-billion.html)? And with gene therapy we are not talking of a chemical, but of an entirely new modality of treating serious disease conditions [9].

So let us not talk about the past, but about the future. There are three major threads well woven in this book: (a) the vector, (b) the target cell or tissue, (c) ectopic integration *versus* homologous recombination; and the three threads are indeed interwoven. With respect to the first two items, a glaring fact is that gene therapy has succeeded when gene transfer has been carried out with retro/lentiviral vectors into hematopoietic stem cells (HSC) or into cells that are close relatives of HSCs. These viruses, judging from their structure and from the imprints they have left in their host genomes, are professional genetic engineers: therefore it is fortunate – and certainly not a trivial coincidence – that we have been able to harness them to the cause of medicine. Since HSCs must give progeny in order to fulfill their physiological role, that the transferred gene becomes part of the host cell genome is exactly what we want. There is no conceptual reason why this could not be done with AAV-based vectors: and AAV has just come to prominence with the successful treatment of hemophilia B [7]; but so far lentiviruses have delivered more, and it may prove difficult to beat a gene vehicle that has been shaped by evolution.

It is natural that we want to take maximum advantage from what we have learnt already from blood diseases; but the biology of each individual tissue is paramount, and therefore we cannot extrapolate uncritically. In this respect one might have thought that, for example, in the liver or in the CNS where, unlike in the hematopoietic tissue, cell turnover is limited or non-existent, we ought to obtain gene expression in existing cells, which would make vector integration unnecessary. However, it has transpired gradually that organ-specific stem cells may be present in many organs, and even in the adult. The identification of neural stem cells that can make neurons or glial cells is some 20 years old [10]; but now we know of liver stem cells that can make hepatocytes or bile duct cells [11], of mammary stem cells that can make acinar, myoepithelial, and ductal cells [12], of cardiac stem cells that can make cardiomyocytes, smooth muscle cells and endothelial cells [13]: in all of these cases it may be possible to target those cells rather than terminally differentiated cells. We have quoted these examples because the stem cells involved satisfy both cardinal criteria that define stem cells, *i.e.* self-renewal and multi-lineage differentiation. Of the two the latter is the more stringent one: thus, lentiviral vector technology that has proven successful with HSCs could be immediately tested with these other organ-specific stem cells. Of course there may be many examples of cells that are competent for self-renewal but do not have multi-lineage potential: they have been called uni-lineage stem cells and they may be otherwise biologically analogous to *bona fide* stem cells. Partly for this reason (and partly to cover uncertainty!) the term *progenitor cells* is often added to the term stem cells, with a comma or with a slash in between. In the mouse, stem cells/progenitor cells with a life span ranging from 1 month to 1 year have been characterized from no less than 15 organs or tissues [14]; it is not impossible that in humans for at least some of these cells the life span may be of years or decades. From the point of view of gene therapy we must be probably very pragmatic: if cells have extensive renewal potential it may not be critical to decide whether they are true stem cells or 'just' progenitor cells: it will be more important to test for each one of these cell types whether they share with HSCs the ability to be transduced by appropriately pseudotyped lentiviral vectors, and to find out for how long they can support the production of terminally differentiated cells in the diseased organ. For instance, epidermal "stem cells" from an adult patient affected by LAM5-beta3 (LAMB3)-deficient *junctional epidermolysis bullosa* (JEB), after transduction with a retroviral vector expressing LAMB3 cDNA, were used successfully to make autografts, resulting in the development of a firmly adherent epidermis that remained stable [15]: in principle JEB can be treated by this approach. Coming to the third issue, random integration *versus* homologous recombination, the latter has been established for a quarter of a century [16] in mouse embryonic stem cells (ESC); it is known to be feasible with human ESCs [17], but it seemed out or reach for gene therapy simply because we never had enough adult stem cells. The situation changed suddenly since human induced pluripotent stem cells (iPSCs) were obtained from normal tissues of adults [18]; and this was quickly followed by achieving correction of the mutation of the archetypal molecular disease, sickle cell anemia, not only in mouse iPSCs [19], but also in human iPSCs [20, 21]. Since this approach can produce gene correction precise to the nucleotide ("a labour of love" [2]) rather than gene insertion, it has the added advantage of being immediately applicable to dominant as well as to recessive diseases. Of course nothing in human therapy can be presumed safe until proven to be safe: and safety issues arise even for homologous recombination, in view of the manipulations required in order to obtain iPSCs; and those required in order to remove the genes that have been introduced for this purpose, as well as remnants, if any [20], of the targeting vector [22]. Thus, at the moment we should keep an open mind as to whether it may be better to select "safe harbor" clones after random integration [23], or to increase the efficiency of gene correction by combining zinc finger nucleases with *piggyBac* technology [24], which also makes it possible to clean away all non-human sequences from the cells that will be finally transferred back to the patient.

Finally, we think it is most appropriate that this book deals not only with regulatory issues, but with ethical issues as well. Some of these have bedevilled the area of gene therapy since the untimely and rather reckless attempt to throw a plasmid into a bone marrow cavity of two patients with thalassemia (see *The Washington Post*, 8th October 1980: the experiment has never been otherwise published). Gene therapy was again unpleasantly in the news in September 1999, when a young man with ornithine transcarbamylase deficiency died after injection of an adenoviral vector. This experiment has been fully published [25], and has made it clear how important it is not only that there should be no conflict of interest, but that any remote suspicion of it be pre-empted. An entirely different issue was the most unfortunate development of leukemia in children with immune deficiency treated with gene therapy [26]: this was an example of the fact that there is no previously unexplored therapeutic procedure that may not carry unpredicted risks; and we note that higher rates of fatalities and of complications have been accepted in previously introduced innovative therapeutic procedures, including the early days of bone marrow transplantation and of organ transplantation.

The Clinibook will be a living testimonial to *CliniGene*, a lighthouse which for several years has helped the navigation of Gene Therapy sailors from Europe and from elsewhere. The waters have been stormy at times, and we have no delusions that they may never be choppy again also in the future. But this is a good time to take stock; and in doing that, we are not surprised to discover that the role of the *CliniGene* Director and Editor of this book, Odile Cohen-Haguenauer, emerges as a key figure. Under her relentless devotion *CliniGene* has provided resources, and a format to bring diverse scientists to work on the common goal of achieving success in approaches to gene therapy. All chapters in this book are a testimony to what has been achieved under the aegis of *CliniGene*, a group characterised by a lively spirit of cooperation and sharing among various stake holders: a wonderful model to build upon for future collaborative projects. We like to pay tribute to Odile for her unflinching determination and ever collegial spirit; and for her vision, perseverance and passion to make gene therapy a successful cutting edge instrument of contemporary medicine. We are convinced that in the next decade patients with several more human diseases will be cured by gene therapy.

REFERENCES

1. Miller AD, Eckner RJ, Jolly DJ, Friedmann T, Verma IM. Expression of a retrovirus encoding human HPRT in mice. *Science* 1984; 225: 630-2.

2. Luzzatto L. Concluding remarks. In: Cohen-Haguenauer O, Boiron M, eds. *Human gene transfer.* London: John Libbey, 1991: 340-6.

3. Aiuti A, Vai S, Mortellaro A, Casorati G, Ficara F, Andolfi G, *et al.* Immune reconstitution in ADA-SCID after PBL gene therapy and discontinuation of enzyme replacement. *Nat Med* 2002; 8: 423-5.

4. Hacein-Bey-Abina S, Le Deist F, Carlier F, Bouneaud C, Hue C, De Villartay JP, *et al.* Sustained correction of X-linked severe combined immunodeficiency by *ex vivo* gene therapy. *N Engl J Med* 2002; 346: 1185-93.

5. Cavazzana-Calvo M, Payen E, Negre O, Wang G, Hehir K, Fusil F, *et al.* Transfusion independence and HMGA2 activation after gene therapy of human beta-thalassaemia. *Nature* 2010; 467: 318-22.

6. Cartier N, Hacein-Bey-Abina S, Bartholomae CC, Veres G, Schmidt M, Kutschera I, *et al.* Hematopoietic stem cell gene therapy with a lentiviral vector in X-linked adrenoleukodystrophy. *Science* 2009; 326: 818-23.

7. Nathwani AC, Tuddenham EG, Rangarajan S, Rosales C, McIntosh J, Linch DC, *et al.* Adenovirus-associated virus vector-mediated gene transfer in hemophilia B. *N Engl J Med* 2011; 365: 2357-65.

8. Aiuti A, Roncarolo MG. Ten years of gene therapy for primary immune deficiencies. *Hematology Am Soc Hematol Educ Program* 2009; 682-9.

9. Verma IM, Weitzman MD. Gene therapy: twenty-first century medicine. *Annu Rev Biochem* 2005; 74: 711-38.

10. Reynolds BA, Weiss S. Generation of neurons and astrocytes from isolated cells of the adult mammalian central nervous system. *Science* 1992; 255: 1707-10.

11. Cardinale V, Wang Y, Carpino G, Cui CB, Gatto M, Rossi M, *et al.* Multipotent stem/progenitor cells in human biliary tree give rise to hepatocytes, cholangiocytes and pancreatic islets. *Hepatology* 2011; 54: 2159-72.

12. Smith GH, Chepko G. Mammary epithelial stem cells. *Microsc Res Tech* 2001; 52: 190-203.

13. Bearzi C, Rota M, Hosoda T, Tillmanns J, Nascimbene A, De Angelis A, *et al.* Human cardiac stem cells. *Proc Natl Acad Sci USA* 2007; 104: 14068-73.

14. Snippert HJ, Clevers H. Tracking adult stem cells. *EMBO Rep* 2011; 12: 113-22.

15. Mavilio F, Pellegrini G, Ferrari S, Di Nunzio F, Di Iorio E, Recchia A, *et al.* Correction of junctional epidermolysis bullosa by transplantation of genetically modified epidermal stem cells. *Nat Med* 2006; 12: 1397-402.

16. Thomas KR, Capecchi MR. Introduction of homologous DNA sequences into mammalian cells induces mutations in the cognate gene. *Nature* 1986; 324: 34-8.

17. Zwaka TP, Thomson JA. Homologous recombination in human embryonic stem cells. *Nat Biotechnol* 2003; 21: 319-21.

18. Takahashi K, Tanabe K, Ohnuki M, Narita M, Ichisaka T, Tomoda K, Yamanaka S. Induction of pluripotent stem cells from adult human fibroblasts by defined factors. *Cell* 2007; 131: 861-72.

19. Hanna J, Wernig M, Markoulaki S, Sun CW, Meissner A, Cassady JP, *et al.* Treatment of sickle cell anemia mouse model with iPS cells generated from autologous skin. *Science* 2007; 318: 1920-3.

20. Zou J, Mali P, Huang X, Dowey SN, Cheng L. Site-specific gene correction of a point mutation in human iPS cells derived from an adult patient with sickle cell disease. *Blood* 2011; 118: 4599-608.

21. Sebastiano V, Maeder ML, Angstman JF, Haddad B, Khayter C, Yeo DT, *et al. In situ* genetic correction of the sickle cell anemia mutation in human induced pluripotent stem cells using engineered zinc finger nucleases. *Stem Cells* 2011; 29: 1717-26.

22. Tenzen T, Zembowicz F, Cowan CA. Genome modification in human embryonic stem cells. *J Cell Physiol* 2010; 222: 278-81.

23. Papapetrou EP, Lee G, Malani N, Setty M, Riviere I, Tirunagari LM, *et al.* Genomic safe harbors permit high beta-globin transgene expression in thalassemia induced pluripotent stem cells. *Nat Biotechnol* 2011; 29: 73-8.

24. Yusa K, Rashid ST, Strick-Marchand H, Varela I, Liu PQ, Paschon DE, *et al.* Targeted gene correction of alpha1-antitrypsin deficiency in induced pluripotent stem cells. *Nature* 2011; 478: 391-4.

25. Raper SE, Chirmule N, Lee FS, Wivel NA, Bagg A, Gao GP, *et al.* Fatal systemic inflammatory response syndrome in a ornithine transcarbamylase deficient patient following adenoviral gene transfer. *Mol Genet Metab* 2003; 80: 148-58.

26. Cavazzana-Calvo M, Fischer A. Gene therapy for severe combined immunodeficiency: are we there yet? *J Clin Invest* 2007; 117: 1456-65.

The CliniBook: Clinical gene transfer
Edited by Odile Cohen-Haguenauer – EDK, Paris © 2012, pp. 8-25

In-2
Main achievements and prospects downstream of the CliniGene-NoE

Odile Cohen-Haguenauer

*MD-PhD, NoE coordinator on behalf of CliniGene partners and Boards
(www.clinigene.eu).
École Normale Supérieure de Cachan, CliniGene, CNRS UMR 8113, 94235 Cachan and
Department of Medical Oncology, Hôpital Saint-Louis and Université Paris-Diderot,
PRES Sorbonne-Paris-Cité, 75475 Paris Cedex 10, France.
odile.cohen@lbpa.ens-cachan.fr*

The role of the European Network for the Advancement of Clinical Gene Transfer and Therapy (CLINIGENE) has been to mobilise efficiently all interested parties, mostly involving academic research and production centers together with companies, patients' groups and regulatory bodies. Our main goal was to integrate multidisciplinary research in order to decipher the key elements which can lead to improved safety and clinical efficacy of gene transfer/therapy medicinal products, *i.e.* for clinical applications. Control and test methods may be applied as platforms for particular gene transfer products. Besides quality control, safety is of germane concern since in the event where the treatment would be proven safe, it could be administered early enough in the course of the disease to achieve genuine cure, so that clinical gene transfer may be called therapy.

The general objectives of CLINIGENE thus were the following:
1. To foster interaction between all stakeholders: regulators, pre-clinical and clinical investigators, scientists, companies (otherwise competitors), patients' groups, in order to streamline integration of multidisciplinary expertise.
2. To establish quality, safety, efficacy and morally acceptable standards for clinical gene transfer products.
3. To identify the "critical path" to accelerate the transit phase from preclinical to clinical phase by integrating expertise and generating new knowledge.
4. To improve European competitiveness by spreading of excellence and disseminating knowledge.
5. To obtain clinically significant improvement in the treatment of some human diseases by gene therapy.

The European Network for the Advancement of Clinical Gene Transfer and Therapy, the CliniGene Network of Excellence has been funded by the European Commission's 6th Framework programme. It has created both critical mass and momentum towards high quality gene transfer and cell therapy research at the level of basic science and its translation into well-designed clinical trials. After successfully achieving EU-wide integration, plans are underway to create a sustainable not-for-profit structure. It should preserve and further develop the expertise that CliniGene has created and master the momentum underpinning gene transfer and cell therapy (GCT) research and its safe, effective clinical applications.

THE NoE ACHIEVEMENTS AFTER RUNNING FIVE YEARS

While encompassing a broad range of technologies and their potential applications, the NoE has succeeded in establishing intensive networking which crosses the boundaries between the technology-platforms including emerging technologies and a human iPS platform, from April 1st 2010 on. This challenge has been successfully fulfilled with the NoE achieving integration and translating into the multiplication of clinical trial initiatives. The participating laboratories and clinical centers of excellence have rallied around this common overarching goal, in adding to shared expertise, their own skills and lines of research, as study cases developed and accompanied by the NoE.

The added value of CliniGene are the following:
1. Integration of EU-wide research and facilities: accelerating the pace at which scientific issues are being taken up and eventually solved.
2. Scientific progress and breakthrough overcoming most scientific bottlenecks that were initially identified and targeted by the seven technology platforms which have extensively interacted instead of working in parallel: by December 2011, 795 papers with CliniGene affiliation had been published among which 20 in outstanding journals and 116 involving two or more partners.
3. Central to these successes and their acceleration is the flexibility funds for internal collaborative and exchange programme (*see Figure 4*), with over 90 projects funded targeting novelty and international collaborations between 45 laboratories and companies, *e.g.*:
   i. Creation of new improved producer cells, development of highly efficient production and purification for most important vectors: AAV, AdV, γRV LVs and NV vectors (minicircles in particular).
   ii. Standard materials: CliniGene initiating the generation of AAV8 reference material (AAV8RSS) and active participation to AAV2RSS characterization.
4. Implementation of a reliable and validated "Vector Biosafety Platform" focusing on the translational and clinical aspects addressing safety and efficiency of current and newly developed systems *in vitro* and *in vivo*. This platform is aiming at comprehensiveness so as to not leave out newest developments.
5. An important Ethical, Legal and Regulatory component which makes CliniGene a central European Medicines Agency stake-holder with expert advisory potential.
6. Facilitation of clinical trials, with as many as 17 ongoing clinical trials and 12 about to begin while the initial target was in the 10 range at most. First clinical successes have been reported in: ADA-SCIDs, Leber congenital amaurosis, Parkinson's disease and X-linked adrenoleukodystrophy with the first clinical use of lentivectors in the EU (*Table I*).
7. High-level training and technology transfer to Industry.
8. Integration of the private sector to the EU-effort towards advancement of clinical GCT.

The CliniGene outreach
1. CliniGene web-site displaying unique information and recently displaying a video tutorial on gene therapy;
2. Patients'associations: meetings and publications;
3. Bridging with a broad community of external expert scientists at the International

level; in particular, CliniGene has been acting as the main partner and support of the Learned Society, ESGCT (www.esgct.eu) over the past six years (the CliniGene coordinator acted as the Founder of the Society, back in 1992).

4. CliniGene public international conference in April 2011: Clinical gene transfer: state-of-the-art and e-ChiPS: European conference on human iPS.

5. Publication of two books: (i) The CliniBook: Clinical gene transfer: state-of-the-art, (*ibid*. fall 2012) and (ii) Special December 2010 issue of *Current Gene Therapy* Journal on the manufacture of gene transfer vectors intended for clinical translation.

THE FUTURE PROSPECTS OF CLINIGENE

To effectively address the unmet complexity of this field, specific expertise is needed which can only be found at the European level. These unique challenges have been actively taken up in the past six years by CliniGene: a strong community has built up to foster European integration in this field and thus overcoming European fragmentation (*Figures 1 and 2*). As a result, the formation of a non-profit "European Foundation for Clinical Gene and Cell Therapy" is expected. The non-profit Initiative would be well positioned to respond quickly to the changing demands of our rapidly developing area of science. This would provide the opportunity not only to incorporate novel scientific and technical possibilities, but also to create the appropriate ethical, regulatory and public communication frameworks necessary to secure public endorsement to legitimate clinical gene transfer and cell therapy research. Key components of the Foundation work might be as follows:

1. Education, policy development, advisory ethical review, information-sharing through conferences, publications, and public education that combines ethics and science and involves all relevant stakeholders in a comprehensive advisory role, complementing that of the responsible regulatory authorities.

2. Administering and awarding Flexi-funds, in order to provide rapidly responsive pilot funding to help investigators develop Gene and Cell Therapy Medicinal Products (GCTMPs) and the materials on which their development depends (assays, vectors, etc.). Requests for proposals will be open to a broader EU gene therapy community, so that the spirit of innovation and flexibility fostered by CliniGene can be expanded. A criteria of application for Flexi-funds will still be cross-country collaboration.

3. Facilitating the establishment of contacts between the investigator and the private sector interested in supporting phase I/II clinical trials.

Because of the CliniGene programme and actions, the necessity of the creation of a Pan-European ressource for gene transfer vectors towards clinical application has also emerged. The objectives are the following: structuring a distributed infrastructure: integrated governance, coordinated services, one-stop-shop access to services: (i) To built up a Pan-European infrastructure of vector engineering facilities providing state-of-the art gene transfer vectors towards pre-clinical developments of GT and stem cells engineering; (ii) To serve a community of users in providing advice on the best system and accompany their project in providing prototypes and material; (iii) To develop efficient and safer emerging technologies relying on multidisciplinary expertise, in a coordinated manner; (iv) To provide access to complementary skills, in order to answer the needs of the scientific community addressing a wide scope of applications and conditions. This infrastructure could help harmonise practices and quality in the production of GMP vector lots and GM-cells. Such a "Tool-box" would be instrumental in facilitating a number of clinical trials that are going to be funded, *e.g.* by DG-research. Application to a specific line of call in the forecoming EC-infrastructure programme is pivotal (Cohen-Haguenauer *et al.*, 2010, in special December 2010 issue of *Current Gene Therapy* Journal).

Table I. Selected clinical trials leading to the structuration of the 7 technology-platforms and their integration into the: "European Platform for Clinical development in Gene Therapy".

Programmes in the clinic		
RVV (& cells)	ADA-deficiency	FCSR-TIGET
AdV	Suicide in Glioblastoma	Multicentric Phase III/UEF & Ark[*1]
AAV	Inherited degenerative retinopathy (Leber)	UCL
AAV	Inherited degenerative retinopathy (Leber)	FTELE-IGM
Lentis (EIAV)-ProSavin	Parkinson's disease	OBM - APHP
Lentis (& cells)	Childhood cerebral adrenoleukodystrophy.	INSERM - APHP
Lentis (& cells)	Wiskott Aldrich Syndrome	Genethon, UCL
Lentis (& cells)	Wiskott Aldrich Syndrome	FCSR-TIGET, Molmed
Non-viral	Treatment with nerve growth factior (NGF) in Alzheimer's disease	KI
Non-viral – morpholinos	Antisense for DMD (Exon-skipping)	RHUL[*2]
AdenoV	Ad-VEGF-D into ischemic myocardium	UEF
Treg cells	Immunotherapy of cancer	APHP - INSERM
Measles-Oncolytic virus	Ovarian Cancer (IP) & Myeloma (IV)	Mayo Clinic
HPV Vaccine	Early stage of cervical carcinoma	Transgene
AAV	Gamma-sarcoglycan muscular disorder	GENETHON – APHP (pilot ended)
HSV-1	Glioblastoma	On-hold KUK
Allo-cell tumour vaccine	Prostate cancer	TUM (pending: phase 2 funding)
Programmes close to the clinic		
Cell-therapy	NK cells for cancer treatment (Myeloma)	KI[*3]
AAV	CNTF in Huntington chorea	CEA
AAV	Inherited degenerative retinopathy (Leber)	CHU-Nantes – INSERM - EFS
Sin RVV (& cells)	X-SCIDs	MHH[*4], UCL, APHP
Lentis (& cells)	Bêta-thalassemia	FCSR-TIGET
Non-viral	Melanoma	CNRS & BioAlliance
Cells (dendritic)	Melanoma	HZI – Braunschweig hospital
AdenoV	YB-1 dep oncolytic AdV in Cancer	TUM, BioReliance
AAV	Diabetes mellitus	CBATEG
AAV	Limb-ischemia	UEF
AAV	AILP1 deficiency (retinopathy)	UCL
AAV	MPS VI (lysosomal sotrage disease)	FTELE-IGM
Progress expected during the next years		
AdenoV	Oncolytic viruses in cancer	ULM
Electro-transfer/Stem-cells	Diabetes mellitus	CBATEG
Insulated SIN RVV (& cells)	Fanconi's aneamia	ENSC - APHP
Cell & CK therapy	Optimised treatment of HPV16-tumours with gene-modified cellular vaccines	IMG-CAS
LentiV	Inherited hypercholesterolemia	UEF
Oncolytic	Cancer	UEF
LentiV (& cells)	SCID-Zap deficiency	APHP –INSERM - ENSC
Combination: Oncolytic & Immuno-modulation	Breast & colon cancers including Inherited	Task Force leader: ENSC/AP-HP

[*1] *Initiated at UEF-Kuopio & continued as multicentric, industry driven by Ark-Therapeutics.*
[*2] *In collaboration with UK MDEX Consortium.*

*³ Infusion of autologous expanded NK cells, for the treatment of recurrent malignant disease after autologous hematopoietic stem cell transplantation. A phase I-II pilot trial.
*⁴ Clinical trial conducted by the Institute of Child Health, University College London, UK, Necker APHP, Paris FR, vector development by MHH.

The CliniGene-NoE added value lies in the quality of its integration of valuable multi-disciplinary expertise which require a European level (*Figure 3*). In including two important components, the General Biosafety and the Ethical and Regulatory platforms, the NoE is adding to specialised facilities and technology, synergies which operate under its umbrella. External scientists and companies with which an active exchange programme has developed over years, are considering the CliniGene-NoE as an international reference (*Tables II* and *III*). Therefore, the consortium prospects are aiming, with EC-support under different and complementary programmes at the establishment of both:
• a "European Foundation for Clinical Gene and Cell Therapy".
• Pan-European resource for gene transfer vectors towards clinical translation under as a EU-research Infrastructure.

MAIN FEATURES OF THE CLINIGENE OUTCOME

I. Technology development, emerging technologies towards clinical translation

A special attention has been brought to the field of emerging technologies, translating into new collaborations funded through flexi-funds as a start-up mechanism intended for feasibility studies. In fact, the opportunity for joint applications between two (or more) labs and competition for flexifunds, has resulted in a huge number of high-quality original programmes. 90 collaborative projects have now been successfully funded following a stringent review process. Altogether, with this internal collaborative flexi-funds programme, an emerging vector platform has build up addressing the bottleneck problem of translational gene therapy research towards improved safety/efficacy (*Figure 1*). In order to streamline the clinical translation of the most advanced technologies, the Joint Research Programme has developed and concentrated on four main directions:
(i)   Pre-clinical evaluation of new generation of safer and more efficacious gene transfer vectors which have been developed. Besides the NoE has integrated new partners in order to address transposons derived non-viral integrating vectors and compare them to available technologies.
(ii) Safety and efficacy improved integrating vectors (viral or non-viral such as transposons-based) since predicting or even controlling the fate of transgenes integration is a major priority in the field. Progress in this regard is likely to pave the way to the treatment of numerous conditions, noticeably accessible by *ex-vivo* gene-manipulation of stem cells, whether intended at repairing the cell defect like with hemoglobinopathies, Wiskott-Aldrich syndrome or Fanconi's anemia, or with view to enzyme replacement therapy like with adrenoleukodystrophy or ADA-deficiency.
(iii) Improvement of the therapeutic index of viral and non-viral vectors noticeably *via* direct *in vivo* administration routes is another key issue in gene therapy related to the immune responses directed at vector particles, transduced cells and/or therapeutic proteins themselves, that can curtail long-term gene expression. The risk of inadvertent immune responses can be minimised in avoiding vector uptake and gene expression in antigen-presenting cells, including modified administration routes. This can also be based on targeting of cell-entry and tight transcription regulation taking advantage of miRNAs. In addition, the NoE has attracted new partners developing *in vivo* selected miRNAs libraries, cloned into AAV shuttles (ICGEB).

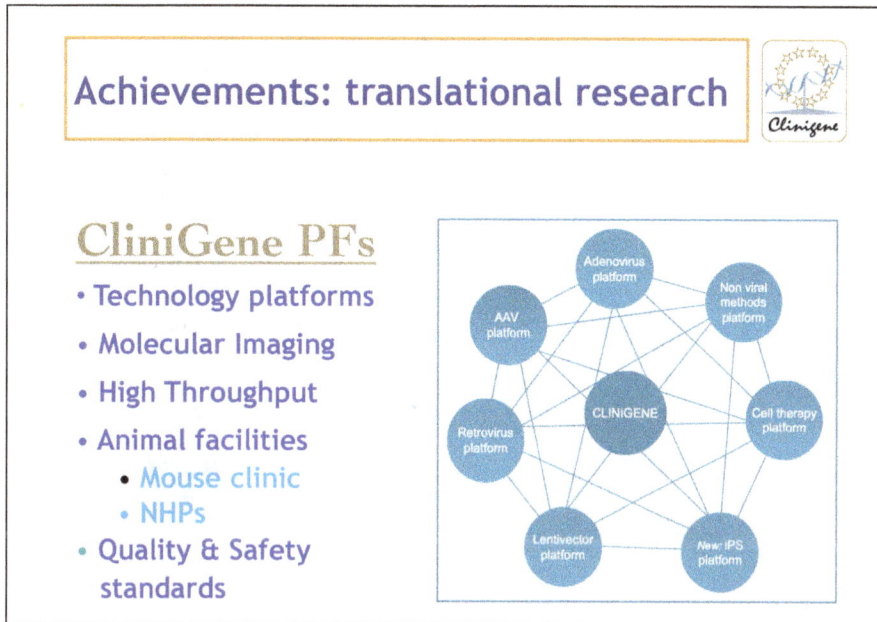

Figure 1. Achievements - translational research.

(iv) A new iPS technology platform (WP4.7) has been created in the fourth year of the programme. This WP adressed gene transfer technologies towards induction of iPS together with characterisation and differentiation. Experimental research and flexi-funded collaborations included regenerative medicine related projects with stem cells expansion and genetic modification.

Finally, the paramount issue of vector production and manufacture has translated into a vision for the building of a Pan-European Vector infrastructure the description of which appears above. In fact, one key bottleneck of translating innovative technologies from bench-to-bedside is related to the production scale-up of the retargeted cell-type specific vectors or alternative serotypes. As high-titre vector preparation strongly depends on the capsid or envelope, the production efficiency substantially varies in between different vector types and according to the design of the transgene cassette. The ability to produce high-titer vectors that are capable of achieving increased gene transfer efficiency and expression in the desired target cells while preventing expression in non-target cells and genotoxicity, are measurable outcomes and addresses a current unmet need in the field.

II. Scientific platforms: approach and methodology

The CliniGene-NoE has elected to accompany the development of novel protocols using cutting edge technology, rather than investigate already closed protocols in retrospect.

As mentioned, a strong integration plan has been inforced and a stepwise implementation adopted. All partners in the seven technology platforms initiated work according to accurate plans matching and adapting to the specific requirements of each technology under consideration (*Figure 2*).

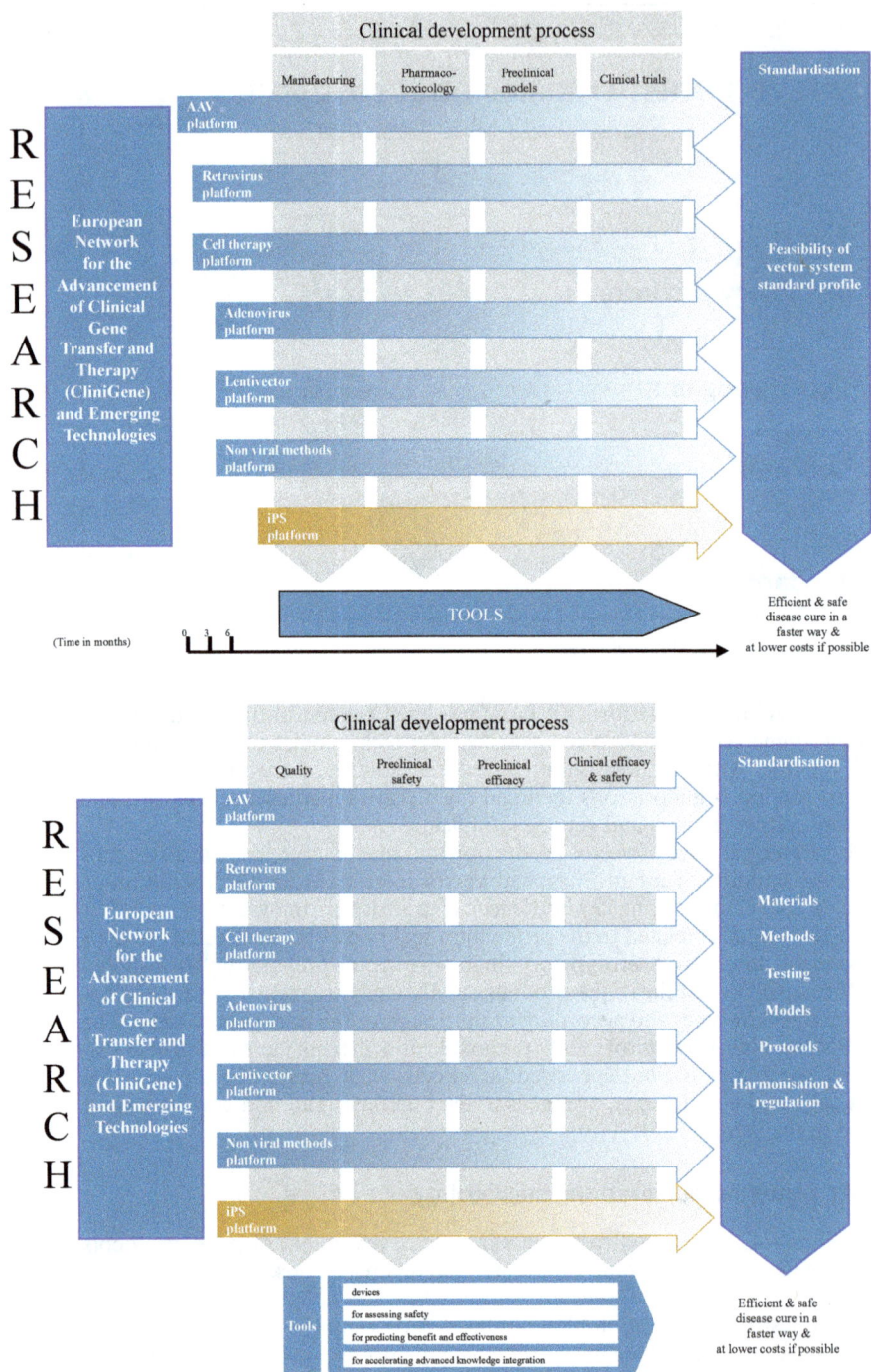

Figure 2. The CliniGene network of excellence structure and outcome.

The integration of the seven CliniGene technology platforms within a core-structure including emerging technologies, biosafety and immunotoxicology task-forces is represented as follows (*Figure 3*). This cartoon reflects on the high level of exchanges, indicative of a high added value from one technology to the next. In fact, during the two first annual meetings, task-forces presented work and exchanged in parallel sessions. This organisation was discontinued following partners' request to learn from the others. Indeed, this has increased networking during the course of the programme as materialised by the level of international interaction supported by the CliniGene-flexifunds (*Figure 4*).

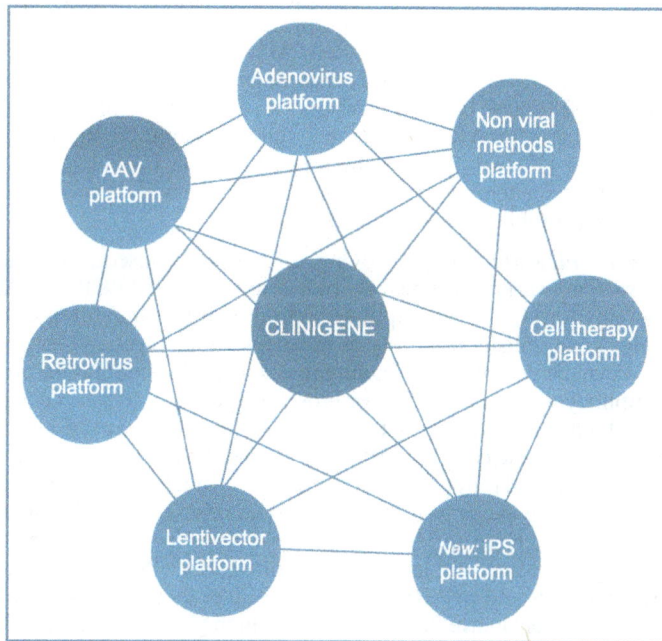

Figure 3. Core structure of the CliniGene-NoE.

Safety has been considered from both the pharmaco-toxicology, immunotoxicology and the virus safety sides. Whatever the technology, viral safety assessement includes a series of common checkpoints to consider which need to be standardised. An important safety issue relates to vector integration with a concurrent risk of insertional mutagenesis. The Network addressed potential improvement using a variety of experimental approaches, as mentioned in the joint programme and emerging technologies section. In order to establish quality, common standards of reference have to be shared. The latter must be tested, broad consensus be reached and then agreed upon by both academic centers and companies specialising in the manufacture of gene transfer vectors for the purpose of human gene therapy. During the course of our programme, the need and specification of such standards have been identified from one vector system to the next since with distinct technologies, the requirements are diverse. Because of CliniGene successful networking, the need for a specific programme has emerged in order to work out these consensus standards and methods (planned as part of the infrastructure project or PEVI).

III. Overview of emerging technology projects initiated through flexifunds

A majority of the groups assembled in CliniGene have addressed these issues and both collaborative programmes and exchanges of personnel have developed under the umbrella of competitive calls for flexibillity funds (*Figure 4*). International exchanges have been developed along five main topics, as follows:

1. *Development of a new generation of safer and more efficacious gene transfer vectors:* Coordinated expression of multiple genes has been achieved both in the adenoviral and the lentiviral context; New and genetically stable insulated retrovirus vectors (both gammas and lentis) have been engineered; Successful elucidation of the possibility to transduce quiescent cells with HIV-1 or MLV vectors by providing the SIVsmmPBj Vpx protein; Transposon-based technology has been developed both with Sleeping Beauty (SB) and Piggy-Bag; Design and engineering of a new class of AAV8 vectors harbouring SMAR elements to enhance episomal replication and retention; Generation of HD-Ad plasmids by recombination; novel class of oncolytic adenoviral vectors; Generation of an immuno-gene therapy vector for auto-activation of human natural killer cells.

2. *It's all about transgene integration:* (i) Improving analysis and consequences of integration: A non-restricted variant of linear amplification-mediated PCR (nrLAM-PCR) has been developed; High-throughput screening of integrome for assessing and predicting vector/gene transfer biosafety of novel insulated retro- and lenti-vectors; Genetic and epigenetic determinants leading to a cell-specific integration profile of RV vector in lymphocytes and HSCs; Vector biosafety studies in first clinical gene therapy using HIV-1 based SIN-vectors for the treatment of X-linked cerebral Adrenoleukodystrophy; Murine cells immortalisation genotoxicity assays to detect the consequences of insertional mutagenesis in primary murine hematopoietic cells; cancer-prone mice models in order to decipher the oncogenesis potential of integrating vectors; (ii) Emphasis has also been put on non-integrating vectors as emerging technologies: Integration-deficient lentivirus vectors (IDLV); Non-viral vectors, with emphasis on minicircles and pFAR: minicircle modules (among these an optimized 733 bp S/MAR element) have been combined which generate a highly characterized superhelical minicircle (MC) with expression features clearly superior to any parental plasmid; Development of protein-transfer vectors for iPS induction or targeting antigen-presenting cells; (iii) Targeted Integration: development of Zinc finger nucleases for targeted gene repair, based on either lentivirus or AAV technology and further developing meganucleases or TALENS-based technology; integration targeting of insulated lentivectors to the heterochromatin.

3. *Direct* **in vivo** *gene transfer: off-the shelf gene therapy:* Cell-targeting of lentiviral vectors in designing and generating chimeric pseudotypes; Down-regulation of expression in primary cell cultures using siRNA lentiviral vectors; Adenovirus vector design and development such as PEGylated vectors to overcome extra-cellular barriers and HD-Ad delivery to the pancreas: controlled expression under pancreatic promoters; Development of new transcription-targeted oncolytic retrovectors restricting the expression of the transgene to tumour cells; The entire AAV platform is developing *in vivo* approaches for the treatment of a broad variety of disorders such as: Retinopathies, Diabetes mellitus, Neurological disorders, Mucopolysaccharidosis IIA, cardio-vascular disorders, Muscular dystrophy in which interesting data have been gathered with Systemic/Loco-regional AAV Vector Gene Therapy in the GRMD Muscular Dystrophy Dog;

4. *Prospects for Regenerative Medicine:* stem cells expansion and genetic modification: Conditional expansion of human umbilical vein derived endothelial cells; Development of 3D-strategies for improved stem cells (SC) expansion and differentiation *in vitro*, exploiting the potential of bioreactor technology; Transduction of mesenchymal stem cells in a closed bag system aiming at fine-tuning GVHD and anti-tumor activity in blood stem cells transplantation; Evaluation of *ex vivo* expansion of murine hematopoietic stem cells by novel cytokine combinations; Development of iPS models for DMD; Spinal muscular atrophy; Fanconi's anaemia; Studying the genetic stability of human iPSC lines applying SB transposon- and evaluation of the risk of genomic destabilization of resulting iPSC lines; Transduction, expansion and differentiation into neural and mesenchymal lineages of iPS cells transduced with insulated lentivectors; High-throughput AAV-mediated selection of secreted proteins and miRNAs which protect from retinal degeneration and contribute to establishing accurate conditions for the regeneration of pancreatic β-cell mass in diabetes mellitus.

5. *Vector Production:* non-viral: Large scale production of pilot-pharmaceutical grade pFARs: biosafe plasmids devoid of antibiotic reference markers; viral: Evaluation of a recently generated amniocyte-derived cell line allowing production of E1-deleted Ad vectors; Mechanisms by which oncogenes regulate Lentiviral vector production and packaging; Feasibility study of lentivector production scale-up using chimeric integrases which target insulated vectors insertion to the heterochromatin;

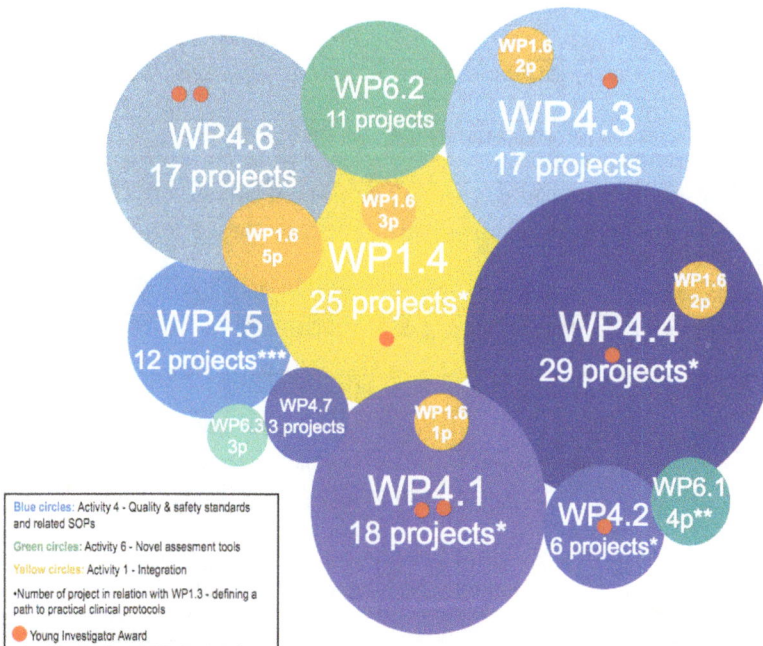

Figure 4. Integration of emerging technologies: international collaborative programmes through flexifunds.

IV. Integrating Ethics and Regulation with Science and Clinical translation: the CliniGene-NoE experience

Education, policy development, advisory ethical review, information-sharing through conferences, publications, and public education that combines ethics and science and involves all relevant stakeholders in a comprehensive advisory role, as developed in CliniGene, holds a potential for complementing that of the regulatory authorities: this is to ensure early dialogue, robust accountability, high levels of transparency, open, clear, and timely flow of communications, and clarity of decision making roles, all of which represent key values for safe clinical trials and, ultimately, effective Gene and Cell Therapy Medicinal Products (GCTMPs). Indeed, research on GCTMPs must be translational – that is, coordinated across the development of technologies, assays and materials, and from preclinical through clinical trials, rather than simply focusing on research with human subjects.

Table II. List of EU-centralised guidelines commented by CliniGene from March 2009 on.

Oncolytic viruses	EMEA/CHMP/GTWP/607698
Quality, non-clinical and clinical issues relating specifically to recombinant AAV	EMEA/CHMP/GTWP/587488/2007
Scientific recommendation on classification of ATMPs in accordance with article 17 of regulation (EC) N°1394/2007	EMEA/99623/2009
The EMEA Transparency policy	EMEA/232037/2009
General principles to address virus and vector shedding	EMEA/CHMP/ICH/449035/2009
Scientific Guideline on the minimum quality and non-clinical data for ATMPs certification	EMEA/CAT/486831/2008
Information on benefit-risk of medicines: patients', consumers' and healthcare professionals expectations	EMA/40926/2009
Assessment of the "Clinical Trials Directive" 2001/20/EC	ENTR/F/2/SF D(2009) 32674
Concept paper on the revision of the NfG on the quality, pre-clinical and clinical aspects of GT medicinal products	EMA/CHMP/GTWP/BWP/234523/2009
Questions and Answers document on Gene therapy	EMA/CHMP/GTWP/212377/2008
Concept paper on the development of a guideline on the risk-based approach: Annex I, Part IV of Dir. 2001/83/EC	EMA/CHMP/CPWP/708420/ 2009
Draft paper for the strategic development of EMA for 5 years	EMA/299895/2009
Detailed guidelines on GCP specific to ATMPs	ENTR/F/2/SF/dn D(2009) 35810
Reflection paper on stem cell-based medicinal products	EMA/CAT/571134/2009
Guideline on quality, non-clinical and clinical aspects of medicinal products containing genetically modified cells	EMA/CHMP/ GTWP/ 671639/2008
Concept paper submitted for public consultation: The European Commission is planning to put forward, in 2012, a legislative proposal to revise the Clinical Trials Directive 2001/20/EC	Clinical trials directive 2001/20/ec (SANCO/C/8/PB/SF D(2011) 143488)

Integration of clinical trials: The consortium has integrated its effort and skills in order to: (i) progress from gene discovery, through pre-clinical research to clinical approaches and (ii) decipher the key elements which could be drivers to clinical success so that reference standards and requisites implementing relevant good practices can be established, if possible. In order to foster safe and high quality clinical gene transfer treatments, the European Network for the advancement of gene transfer and therapy approached the definition of key-criteria resulting from interesting pre-clinical results which enable the decision as to whether it is a "go" or a "no go to the clinic" with a reasonable enough margin of confidence towards foreseable success. The Clinigene-NoE has aimed to: (i) avoid the reproduction of Phase I trials asking the same questions and (ii) to prevent predictable failures to enter the clinical phase, which besides the deleterious consequences on the patients entering the study, would also penalise the field; (iii) deliver practical results opening new opportunities for funding research and clinical development in this field, and thereby favour the expansion of the high-tech industry sector. Altogether, over 20 clinical trials have been accompanied by CliniGene.

Ethical Issues: Ethics has been envisioned as a Network priority: all CliniGene meetings have included Ethics sessions or workshops, and during each ESGCT meeting, where CliniGene has organised and supported the session mobilising over 200 participants in every instance. After the international Think Tank "The ethics of human clinical gene transfer, which took place in April 2007, an important publication has appeared in the March 2008 issue of Molecular Therapy: "En route to ethical recommendations for gene transfer clinical trials". In March 2009, a joint workshop was organised with patients' group at the Abbaye de Royaumont: "Gene Transfer Clinical trials CliniGene Workshop: A Patients group driven initiative. The related publication *Towards a proportionate regulatory framework for gene transfer clinical trials* has been issued in the February 2011 issue of *Human Gene Therapy* Journal. Bridging at the International level and in particular with NIH-OBA RAC has been attempted in each CliniGene driven initiative and successfully materialised into a joint NIH-OBA RAC CliniGene workshop "Safety Symposium: Retroviral/ Lentiviral Vector Insertional Oncogenesis in Human Gene Transfer Research" which took place on December 9-10, 2010, in Bethesda. The RAC and CliniGene convened this symposium with the major goal of increasing awareness in the scientific community and the public by providing comprehensive updates of: (i) Retro/lentivirus integration and insertional mutagenesis research, including non-enhancer mediated mechanisms; (ii) Safety modifications for retro/lentiviral vectors; (iii) Appropriate *in vitro* and animal models to predict safety of human gene transfer; (iv) Clinical and ethical considerations for review of human GT research. A report has been published in the June 2012 issue of *Molecular Therapy*.

An important ethical, legal and regulatory component makes CliniGene a central European Medicines Agency (EMA) stake-holder with expert advisory potential (*Table II*): the quality of interaction which has been established with Regulatory Authorities would not be possible at the level of individual institutions. CliniGene has provided a forum where regulatory compliance issues can be discussed, and scientifically-based solutions are proposed, thereby facilitating the dialogue with the regulatory authorities and streamlining the development of centralized procedures. In addition, several parameters that address vector quality and safety are being actively investigated in pre-clinical models inside the Network, contributing useful and sometimes unique expertise. Gene and cell therapy medicinal products are new and innovative medicinal products. They are biological medicinal products according to Regulation (EC) No 1394/2007 within the meaning of Annex I to Directive 2001/83/EC. The Committee for Advanced Therapies (CAT) was created and entered into force on January 1st, 2010, which is responsible for preparing draft opinions on the quality, safety and efficacy of each advanced therapy medicinal product (ATMP) for final approval by EMA. In addition, Part IV, Annex I to Directive 2001/83/EC was revised as regard to the specificity of ATMPs. Now is a pivotal time point for sustaining interaction with the regulatory bodies, due to the:

1. Foreseen revision of the "Clinical Trials Directive", a subject which has been open for public comments to DG-Enterprise; CliniGene contributed some. A new revised concept paper had been submitted for public consultation until May 2011, RE: SANCO/C/8/PB/SF D(2011) 143488 (See chapter C2-2, *ibid.*).
2. Revision of The Note For Guidance On The Quality, Pre-Clinical And Clinical Aspects Of Gene Transfer Medicinal Products (GT-NfG), a unique consolidated reference document as it is by far the most mature in the EU gene therapy field and internationally recognised as such. The revision-process is interesting since the original guideline was drafted over a decade ago; its revised version will take into account the new framework implementing the CAT. So far, there has been no essential issue found to be missing in this GT-NfG when proceeding with side to side comparison with many newer but minor and redundant guidelines. The user needs to refer to a comprehensive, adequately organised and cross-indexed document which makes it both accurate and user-friendly.
3. Entering into force of the EMA-CAT Implementation of the ATMPs regulation.
   • Prospect for Vector profiles generic DB and IMPD dossier: these vector profiles generic data-base will consist of a compilation of safety and quality issues, biodistribution profiles and pharmacotoxicology, building up "master files", which will need constant update as data will show. Information gathered and access to it will vary according to the vector system. Lentivectors are being used for both *ex-vivo* transduction of gene-manipulated cells and *via* direct *in-vivo* administration routes while AAV-derived vectors are mostly used *in vivo*. Nevertheless the data-set which need to be assembled prior to clinical authorisation follow rigorous common frames (See chapter C2-3, *ibid.*).
   • Altogether, CliniGene has contributed to create a flexible, responsive, and sustainable platform for coordination and collaboration involving a full range of stakeholders (scientists, clinicians, patients groups, regulators, policy decision-makers, industry and ethicists), to promote effective partnerships, regulatory harmonisation, equitable access to GCTMPs, and public confidence in GCT research and its products. Utmost recently, the first Gene Therapy Product was granted a marketing authorisation by EMA.

V. Dissemination *(Table III)*

The CliniBook: Clinical Gene Transfer State-of-the-art
This is a major deliverable/achievement of the Network of Excellence. The goal is for the CliniGene-Noe to report on past developments in the last 15 years and present enthusiastic prospects to come next. This book is intended to provide a reference for state-of-the-art gene transfer technology and the different aspects of its clinical translation in Europe. As examples of successful outcomes, recent clinical trials are presented together with ethical and safety issues which are discussed. Undergraduates, postgraduates, scientists, clinicians, regulators and patients' advocacy groups looking for state-of-the-art information as well as emerging prospective in clinical gene transfer will find here a comprehensive update of the field.

Special issue of Current Gene Therapy *Journal*

A Special issue of *Current Gene Therapy* Journal has been coordinated by Manuel Carrondo and Pedro Cruz on the manufacture of gene transfer vectors intended for clinical translation, which appeared on December 2010.

Table III. Communication and disseminating knowledge inforced.

1. Knowledge Integration: media
• Sharing Facilities; GMP-production whether Academic or PCO
• Public Web-site: www.clinigene.eu
• Quaterly newsletter: CliniNews
• − Link between partners & their own networks
• − Club of Interest: R&D; Policy; Patients' groups
• E-communication: CliniSoft; videoconferences
• Gene Therapy Video available from the CliniGene website

2. Dissemination & Outreach
• The CliniBook: Clinical Gene Transfer, state-of-the-art
• Organisation of Meetings & Trainings sessions
− CliniGene as main partner and support of the European Society for Gene and Cell Therapy (ESGCT) over six years
• International cooperation and International Board
• Public website: www.clinigene.eu
− Publicly available interactive data-base
− EU Inventory of clinical trials http://141.39.175.7/eutrials/
− Adverse Events
− Current Gene Therapy Weekly
• Ethics: Geneva Think Tank & Publications (*Mol Ther*, 2008; *Hum Gene Ther*, 2011; *Mol Ther*, 2012 & "the CliniBook")

3. The CliniGene Clubs of Interest
• Industry Club of Interest CliniGene
− Streamlining interaction between the private and the academic sectors, an objective identified as a CliniGene priority
− Joint platform between Industry & Centers of Excellence: A Clinigene satellite workshop at annual ESGCT meetings from October 2007 on
• High-level external scientists (CliniGene Associate Partners)
• Interaction with Regulators
• Patients' concerns: Royaumont meeting (*Hum Gene Ther*, 2011)
• Public awareness: understanding of clinical trials
• Decision-makers: EU-level & member-states

The CliniGene public website

The CliniGene website is accessible at the following address: http://www.clinigene.eu. As an EC-NoE, CliniGene was aimed at increasing synergies and fostering faster accumulation of new data: the appropriate collation, production, validation, dissemination and exploitation of new knowledge standing as a primary objective. CliniGene activities aimed at making key information available to all relevant players in a transparent and free-accessible manner through the CliniGene public website, scientific publications, presentations, workshops and conferences *(Figure 5)*.

The CliniGene public website displays a broad range of accurate web-links and includes:
• 3 searchable interactive data-bases:
  – Gene Transfer and Therapy References DB.
  – Published Human Gene Therapy Clinical Trials DB.
  – The European clinical trials DB.

- EU and International Regulation.
- Serious Adverse events reports and publications.
- An interactive box to submit a request for the manufacture of a GMP-GT product among CliniGene partners' institutions, companies or Club of Interest.
- Links to main Gene Therapy related events: conferences, meetings and trainings.
- Links to the EC DG research directorate, to the European Medicines Agency and to the DG-Sanco.
- Programmes and Powerpoint presentations (when authorised by the speakers) of the past events organised by CliniGene.
- 20' Video explaining the main purpose of Gene Therapy dedicated to non-scientists or young scientist is display on the CliniGene Web.
- CliniGene Current Gene Therapy Weekly collated PubMed abstracts of gene therapy related papers which have appeared in peer-review scientific journals during the past week. A service interrupted at the end of 2011.

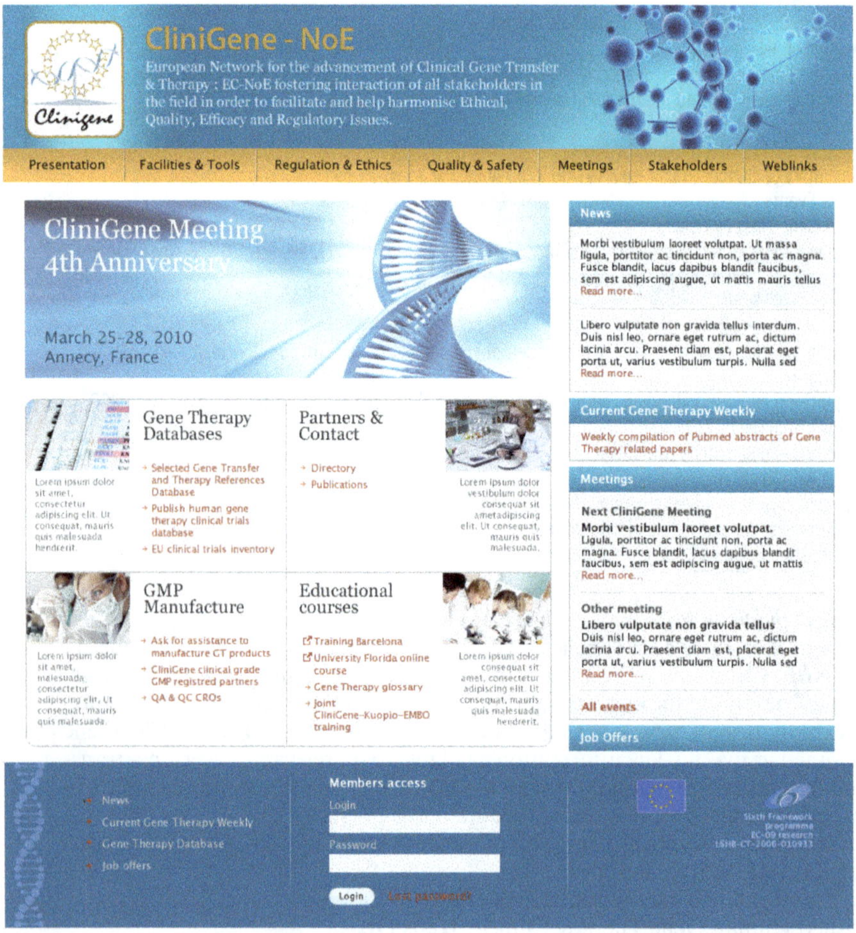

Figure 5. CliniGene web-site: www.clinigene.eu.

Current Gene Therapy Weekly

The CliniGene Current Gene Therapy Weekly (CGTW), created in April 2006, has been released every week up until the end of 2011. Each release included the PubMed abstracts of gene therapy related papers which have appeared in peer-review scientific journals during the past week.

CliniNews

The CliniNews, the internal quarterly electronic newsletter of CliniGene, was produced under a coloured two-columns print-ready format. The first CliniNews has been issued in February 2007. It provided all partners and Board Members with a media to contribute and share information and news which are are important to the field or their facility.

Public Video on Gene Therapy on line on the CliniGene Website

During the last period a 20' video has been produced at CBATEG (UAB, Barcelona) which is available on-line on the CliniGene website and addresses young scientists and a broader public in general. The aim of this video is to explain the basics of what is gene therapy and its goals. During the 2011 ESGCT Brighton meeting the video was shown and appreciated by young scientists; it has further received very good appraisal from Patients' groups. The video can be seen from the following link: http://www.clinigene.eu/video-intro-gene-therapy.html

IN CONCLUSION, A SUSTAINABLE ROLE FOR THE CLINIGENE CONSORTIUM

The CliniGene Network of Excellence, funded by the European Commission's 6th Framework programme, has created both critical mass and momentum towards high quality gene transfer research at the level of basic science and its translation into well-designed clinical trials. Like all EU funded NoEs, it is time-limited, and was terminated in its present contractual format at the end of 2011. However, plans are underway to create a sustainable not-for profit structure that will preserve the expertise that CliniGene has created and master the momentum underpinning gene transfer research and its safe, effective clinical applications. This would result in the eventual formation of a non-profit "European Foundation for Clinical Gene and Cell Therapy" to promote good practice and develop standards in gene transfer research. This initiative could contribute to implement and streamline European and international exchange of information and experience, the organisation of workshops, seminars, conferences, trainings and summer schools and sustain the promotion of publications in any form, submission of expert advisory opinions, and cooperation with European and international public and non-government organisations.

The objectives of such an initiative should focus on the facilitation, development, and implementation of the full range of professional activity of gene transfer and cell therapy researchers (*Tables IVa* and *IVb*). It would be well positioned to undertake the role of an Expert EU-Platform in a dynamic framework able to respond quickly to the changing demands of a rapidly developing area of science. This would provide the opportunity not only to incorporate novel scientific and technical possibilities, but also to create the appropriate Ethical, Regulatory and Public communication frameworks necessary to secure public endorsement and legitimisation for gene transfer research. During the past six years, research on gene and cell therapy has made enormous progress, owing in large part to the integration of research in Europe with EC support. Initiatives such as the CliniGene-NoE have been key catalysts serving this purpose. As a result, several GCT small-scale trials – all investigator-driven and based on new vector technologies matching improved efficacy and safety requirements – are currently in search of the means and sponsors to undertake full-fledged clinical trials. There is currently an urgent need to streamline cooperation and interoperability among GMP facilities. Complex technical challenges require existing production facilities to adapt to emerging technologies in a coordinated manner.

There is likewise an urgent need to fund and support the collaborative cultivation of human skills in GCTMP development, in order to promote high-quality innovative GCT science. These investments can dramatically enhance academic-led "first-in-human" gene transfer research. The not-for-profit business framework proposed for the Foundation would ensure that its efforts are focussed on the needs of stakeholders rather than on financial returns. Once proof of efficacy is gathered, technology can be transferred to the private sector, which is best placed to then take over further phases of development.

Table IV a. Patients' views for future prospects: a platform for progress. A genuinely contributory platform for progress should operate independently from regulatory bodies, ideally at a pan-European level, since accurate expertise can be found at this level only.

The elements of a platform for progress might include:
• A mentoring framework for researchers, including regulatory support and advice.
• Clinical trial support.
• Data and sample collection frameworks that create common access to information, avoid duplication and allow "second generation" studies to start farther along the road to GCTMP development through utilisation of relevant data (e.g. on vector safety issues) created by others.
• The establishment of dedicated CROs for gene transfer clinical trials, including some specialising in supporting not-for-profit organisations.
• Funding streams that are sustained for the duration of the medicinal product development process.
• A Pan-European infrastructure for vectors engineering and General Biosafety.
• Periodic evaluation criteria and examination of the public impact of Platform outcomes.
• Support for pricing and reimbursement (including help on issues such as benefit sharing and commercialisation for medicinal products developed with private donations or taxpayer funding).

Table IV b. Objectives of the CliniGene-sustainability as an European Foundation for Clinical Gene and Cell therapy.

Focus on the facilitation, development, and implementation of professional activity:
1. To facilitate the development and implementation of Phase I/II and pilot gene and cell therapy clinical trials, through provision of flexible pilot funding so that investigators may later seek trial sponsorship from industry or academia;
2. To facilitate access to essential knowledge and infrastructure, including GLP, in pre-clinical development;
3. To facilitate access to GMP manufacture of GCTMPs for Phase I/II trials and rare diseases;
4. To facilitate the establishment and sharing of processes, procedures and standards in gene and cell therapy in order to advance existing and emerging technologies;
5. to actively contribute to progress in Ethical, Safety and Regulatory issues, and to foster relevant interaction with the scientific community and the stakeholders;
6. To contribute to training in gene and cell therapy and to dissemination of scientific innovation, knowledge, and standards in this field;
7. To raise funds and to manage activities designed to achieve these objectives, including expenses for personnel, meetings, e-communication, supplies & equipment without aiming at economic profit.

Tables IVa and IVb reproduced from Kent et al., 2011.

ACKNOWLEDGMENTS

This work has been performed with the support of the EC-DG research through the FP6-Network of Excellence, CLINIGENE: LSHB-CT-2006-018933.

REFERENCES

Cohen-Haguenauer O, Creff N, Cruz P, *et al*. Relevance of an academic GMP Pan-European vector infra-structure (PEVI). *Curr Gene Ther* 2010; 10: 414-22.

The CliniBook. *Clinical Gene Transfer: state-of-the-art*. Cohen-Haguenauer O, ed. Paris: EDK, 2012.

Luzzatto L, Verma I. Foreword. In: *The CliniBook, Clinical Gene Transfer: state-of-the-art*. Cohen-Haguenauer O, ed. Paris: EDK, 2012.

King NMP, Cohen-Haguenauer O. En route for ethical recommandations for gene transfer clinical trials. *Mol Ther* 2008; 16: 432-8.

Kent A, King NMP, Cohen-Haguenauer O. Toward a proportionate regulatory framework for gene transfer: a patient group-led initiative. *Hum Gene Ther* 2011; 2: 126-34.

Corrigan-Curay J, Cohen-Haguenauer O, O'Reilly M, *et al*. Challenges in vector and trial design using retroviral vectors for long term gene correction in hematopoietic stem cell gene therapy: summary of a symposium sponsored by the NIH office of biotechnology activities and the EC DG-research NoE for the advancement of clinical gene transfer and therapy. *Mol Ther* 2012; 20: 1084-94.

PART I

Technologies and pre-clinical studies

Highlights on AAV mediated gene transfer

COORDINATED BY
FATIMA BOSCH
AND
PHILIPPE MOULLIER

The CliniBook: Clinical gene transfer
Edited by Odile Cohen-Haguenauer – EDK, Paris © 2012, pp. 31-34

A1-1
Highlights on AAV mediated gene transfer: introduction

Eduard Ayuso[1,2], Fatima Bosch[1,2]*

[1]Center of Animal Biotechnology and Gene Therapy and Department of Biochemistry and Molecular Biology, School of Veterinary Medicine, Universitat Autònoma de Barcelona, 08193 Bellaterra, Spain.
[2]CIBER de Diabetes y Enfermedades Metabólicas Asociadas (CIBERDEM), Spain.
fatima.bosch@uab.es
* Corresponding author

Adeno-associated viruses (AAVs) are members of the parvoviridae family of viruses and are characterized by a small protein capsid of 20nm containing a single stranded DNA genome of about 4.7kb. AAVs are nonpathogenic and require a helper virus for replication and completion of their life cycle. The genome of AAV vectors contains only two genes: rep, which is responsible for viral DNA replication, and cap, which packages the viral genome [1]. Wild-type AAV has the ability to integrate into a specific region of chromosome 19 in the human genome [2, 3], a process requiring rep gene. Recombinant AAV particles (rAAV) can be generated by removing all viral genes, but leaving the inverted terminal repeats (ITRs) as the only viral sequences. The ITRs sequences are located at the ends of the AAV genome and contain all the *cis* sequence information necessary for vector DNA replication and encapsidation [4, 5]. Compared to other viruses, rAAV vectors have shown high transduction efficiency *in vivo* and are able of transducing both dividing and non-dividing cells. The ability to integrate into the host genome is not maintained in rAAV because of the substitution of the viral genome with the transgene expression cassette. Therefore, upon transduction, rAAV genomes remains almost exclusively in episomal forms, in concatameric structures [6]; thereby considerably reducing the risk of insertional mutagenesis [7, 8].

Despite many advantages of rAAV, the limited cloning capacity (<4.7kb) may preclude its use for gene therapy diseases that require a large transgene, such as Duchenne muscular dystrophy (DMD). To solve this issue several approaches have been explored, such as the construction of a minigene or a *trans*-splicing rAAV system. A minigene consists of selected deletions within the coding region and removal of the untranslated sequences. Therefore, the encoded protein is necessarily a truncated form of the wild-type protein, but designed in such a way that it retains its main functionality (see chapter A1-4 on DMD in this section). The *trans*-splicing approach allows the reconstitution of a functional gene from two vectors encoding the 5' and the 3' portions of the gene. The presence of donor and acceptor splice sites in appropriate locations, allows the production of a complete mRNA [9]. Converting the single-strand DNA (ssDNA) rAAV genome into double-stranded DNA (dsDNA) prior to gene expression has been identified as a rate-limiting steps for efficient transduction. This critical step can be effectively bypassed through the use of self-complementary AAV (scAAV) vectors, which package an inverted repeat genome that can fold into dsDNA without the requirement for DNA synthesis or base-pairing between multiple vector genomes. Nevertheless, there is a negative consequence to this: the reduction by half of the coding capacity of the vector (~2.3 kb). The increases in efficiency gained with scAAV vectors have ranged from modest to stunning, depending on the tissue, cell type, and route of administration [10].

Most of the early studies on the biology of AAV focused on the first serotype isolated, the human-derived AAV serotype 2. Since then, hundreds of AAV with variant capsids have been isolated from tissues of non-human primates and humans by molecular techniques [11], but only a few have been incorporated into vectors and studied in animals. Improved vectors have also been obtained by experimentally modifying the capsid sequence [12-15]. Capsid proteins are largely responsible for the specificity and transduction efficacy of the vector. Hence, the use of non-type 2 AAV capsids to deliver transgenes to target cells might offer two important advantages over conventional AAV2 vectors: an overall broader host range, and an escape from anti-AAV2 immune responses that are highly frequent in humans ([16, 17], also see chapter B2-1, *ibid*).

Production of recombinant AAV vectors with high purity and potency to support pre-clinical and clinical studies remains a critical task for the field; this is reflected in the large number of novel technologies developed for AAV production and purification [18]. Depending on the target tissue, the AAV amounts needed for performing clinical trials can vary considerably; being, for example, extremely high for the systemic delivery of AAV for the treatment of neuro-muscular diseases. Consequently, highly efficient large scale manufacturing process, GMP compatible, is needed for producing high vector quantities for advanced clinical trials. Here, pros and cons of several approaches for large scale production of rAAV vectors are reviewed (see chapter A1-7). Despite the progress in the field, there is a lack of standarization to characterize rAAV preparations made by different laboratories and/or produced by different methodologies. Indeed, hundreds of preclinical experiments based on AAV-mediated gene transfer have been published with excellent results, but no comparisons are usually performed between studies. The same is true for reported clinical trials. To be able to share and compare these data, the AAV community initiated a worldwide project to generate AAV reference standard materials (RSM). In this chapter, the generation of the AAV serotype 2 and AAV serotype 8 RSM is reported and the anticipated uses of such standards are discussed.

Due to their safety profile and low immunogenicity rAAV is becoming the vector of choice for many gene therapy approaches. Pre-clinical studies have shown that AAV vector-mediated gene transfer results in long-term gene expression in small and large animal models of disease [19]. In past years, these preclinical data have been translated into humans with encouraging results for treating several disorders ([19, 20]; also see chapters C1-1 and C1-6, *ibid*). Monogenic recessive disorders are particularly amenable to treatment by gene replacement therapy through the delivery of normal copies of the defective gene. Conversely, the selection of the candidate gene is not trivial for polygenic/environmental diseases, such as diabetes and heart failure. Nonetheless, several AAV-mediated gene therapy approaches are under development. This chapter will cover *in vivo* applications of AAV vectors to treat monogenic disorders like Duchenne muscular dystrophy, mucopolysaccharidosis type VI and inherited retinal dystrophies. Novel strategies to treat diabetes mellitus and cardiovascular disorders with gene therapy are also discussed.

ACKNOWLEDGMENTS

This work has been performed with the support of the EC-DG research through the FP6-Network of Excellence, CLINIGENE: LSHB-CT-2006-018933.

REFERENCES

1. Srivastava A, Lusby EW, Berns KI. Nucleotide sequence and organization of the adeno-associated virus 2 genome. *J Virol* 1983; 45: 555-64.

2. Kotin RM, Siniscalco M, Samulski RJ, Zhu XD, Hunter L, Laughlin CA, *et al*. Site-specific integration by adeno-associated virus. *Proc Natl Acad Sci USA* 1990; 87: 2211-5.

3. Samulski RJ, Zhu X, Xiao X, Brook JD, Housman DE, Epstein N, Hunter LA. Targeted integration of adeno-associated virus (AAV) into human chromosome 19. *EMBO J* 1991; 10: 3941-50.

4. McLaughlin SK, Collis P, Hermonat PL, Muzyczka N. Adeno-associated virus general transduction vectors: analysis of proviral structures. *J Virol* 1988; 62: 1963-73.

5. Samulski RJ, Chang LS, Shenk T. Helper-free stocks of recombinant adeno-associated viruses: normal integration does not require viral gene expression. *J Virol* 1989; 63: 3822-8.

6. Penaud-Budloo M, Le Guiner C, Nowrouzi A, Toromanoff A, Cherel Y, Chenuaud P, *et al*. Adeno-associated virus vector genomes persist as episomal chromatin in primate muscle. *J Virol* 2008; 82: 7875-85.

7. Li H, Malani N, Hamilton SR, Schlachterman A, Bussadori G, Edmonson SE, *et al*. Assessing the potential for AAV vector genotoxicity in a murine model. *Blood* 2011; 117: 3311-9.

8. Nakai H, Montini E, Fuess S, Storm TA, Grompe M, Kay, MA. AAV serotype 2 vectors preferentially integrate into active genes in mice. *Nat Genet* 2003; 34: 297-302.

9. Lai Y, Yue Y, Liu M, Ghosh A, Engelhardt JF, Chamberlain JS, Duan D. Efficient *in vivo* gene expression by trans-splicing adeno-associated viral vectors. *Nat Biotechnol* 2005; 23: 1435-9.

10. McCarty DM. Self-complementary AAV vectors; advances and applications. *Mol Ther* 2008; 16: 1648-56.

11. Gao G, Vandenberghe LH, Wilson JM. New recombinant serotypes of AAV vectors. *Curr Gene Ther* 2005; 5: 285-97.

12. Choi VW, McCarty DM, Samulski RJ. AAV hybrid serotypes: improved vectors for gene delivery. *Curr Gene Ther* 2005; 5: 299-310.

13. Zhong L, Li B, Mah CS, Govindasamy L, Agbandje-McKenna M, Cooper M, *et al*. Next generation of adeno-associated virus 2 vectors: point mutations in tyrosines lead to high-efficiency transduction at lower doses. *Proc Natl Acad Sci USA* 2008; 105: 7827-32.

14. Li W, Asokan A, Wu Z, Van Dyke T, DiPrimio N, Johnson JS, *et al*. Engineering and selection of shuffled AAV genomes: a new strategy for producing targeted biological nanoparticles. *Mol Ther* 2008; 16: 1252-60.

15. Grimm D, Lee JS, Wang L, Desai T, Akache B, Storm TA, Kay MA. *In vitro* and *in vivo* gene therapy vector evolution via multispecies interbreeding and retargeting of adeno-associated viruses. *J Virol* 2008; 82: 5887-911.

16. Calcedo R, Vandenberghe LH, Gao G, Lin J, Wilson JM. Worldwide epidemiology of neutralizing antibodies to adeno-associated viruses. *J Infect Dis* 2009; 199: 381-90.

17. Boutin S, Monteilhet V, Veron P, Leborgne C, Benveniste O, Montus MF, Masurier C. Prevalence of serum IgG and neutralizing factors against adeno-associated virus (AAV) types 1, 2, 5, 6, 8, and 9 in the healthy population: implications for gene therapy using AAV vectors. *Hum Gene Ther* 2010; 21: 704-12.

18. Ayuso E, Mingozzi F, Bosch F. Production, purification and characterization of adeno-associated vectors. *Curr Gene Ther* 2010; 10: 423-36.

19. Mingozzi F, High KA. Therapeutic *in vivo* gene transfer for genetic disease using AAV: progress and challenges. *Nat Rev Genet* 2011; 12: 341-55.

20. Mueller C, Flotte TR. Clinical gene therapy using recombinant adeno-associated virus vectors. *Gene Ther* 2008; 15: 858-63.

The CliniBook: Clinical gene transfer
Edited by Odile Cohen-Haguenauer – EDK, Paris © 2012, pp. 35-40

A1-2
Preclinical studies of AAV gene therapy for inherited retinal dystrophies

ALEXANDER J. SMITH, ANASTASIOS GEORGIADIS, ROBIN R. ALI*

UCL Institute of Ophthalmology, Department of Genetics, 11-43 Bath Street, London EC1V 9EL, United Kingdom.
r.ali@ucl.ac.uk
* Corresponding author

GENE THERAPY AND OCULAR DISEASE

A variety of monogenic recessive disorders may eventually be amenable to treatment by gene replacement therapy through the delivery of normal copies of the defective gene *via* replication-deficient viral vectors. Over the past decade, there has been a substantial effort to develop gene therapy for inherited retinal degeneration - of which there are many forms - culminating in the recent initiation of clinical trials. The eye has several features that make it particularly suitable as a target organ for gene therapy. The transparent nature of ocular tissues enables the visualisation of vector delivery and the subsequent non-invasive imaging of transduced tissues. It is a relatively small, compartmentalised and enclosed organ, enabling the delivery of small quantities of viral vector to particular subsets of ocular cell types with minimal risk of vector dissemination to the rest of the body. The blood-retinal barrier and blood-aqueous barrier maintain a degree of protection from immune responses directed against vector antigens that might otherwise cause inflammation and limit transgene expression. Finally, retinal function can be assessed using a variety of electrophysiological and psychophysical tests commonly used in the clinic [1].

Inherited retinal degeneration is diverse group of disorders that includes conditions such as retinitis pigmentosa (RP), Leber congenital amaurosis (LCA) and cone dystrophy. It can be caused by mutations in any of >100 genes and it affects ~1/3000 people (see: http://www.sph.uth.tmc.edu/Retnet/). Retinal degeneration is characterised by progressive apoptotic loss of photoreceptor cells and increasing visual impairment. Substantial variation exists with respect to the onset, rate of vision loss and the primary cell type affected [2]. The most severe forms of inherited retinal degeneration are the various types of LCA, in which there is severe visual impairment from birth and often complete loss of vision during the first two decades [3]. Although the primary cell type most commonly affected in retinal degeneration is the photoreceptor cell, defects in other cell types such as the retinal pigment epithelium (RPE) and the Müller cells can lead to reduced photoreceptor function and their subsequent loss [1]. An example of an inherited retinal degeneration due to a defect in the RPE is a form of LCA caused by defects in the enzyme RPE65. Its absence results in the disruption of the visual cycle leading to absent rod function and consequently to photoreceptor degeneration. The successful treatment of the RPE65-deficient dogs [4-6] and mice [7, 8], using AAV-mediated gene replacement has been the inspiration for three clinical trials, the first trials to use gene replacement therapy in the eye [9-11]. These trials are described in more detail elsewhere in this book.

GENE THERAPY FOR FORMS OF SEVERE EARLY ONSET RETINAL DEGENERATION

AIPL1 is a chaperone protein responsible for the folding and/or translocation of phosphodiesterase (PDE) to the outer segment. The *AIPL1* gene is mutated in LCA type 4, which comprises approximately 5% of all LCA [3]. Several murine models of this disease exist, which have varying rates of photoreceptor cell loss. *Aipl1* knockout mice are fully deficient in AIPL1 activity and they lose all photoreceptor cells within a month, making it the most rapidly degenerating mouse model of LCA. However, the very rapid degeneration in the *Aipl1*[-/-] mice can be successfully treated by subretinal injection of a relatively novel AAV serotype, AAV2/8, carrying *Aipl1*. Gene therapy with AAV2/8-hAIPL1 at postnatal day 10 results in increased expression of *Aipl1*, restoration of PDE to the outer segment and prolonged survival and function of the photoreceptors for up to 5 months [12, 13].

Recently, we reported the use of AAV2/8 for the treatment of GC1-deficiency in *Gucy2e*[-/-] mice, a model for LCA1, the most common form of LCA. After subretinal administration of an AAV2/8 based vector carrying the human *GUCY2D* gene or the murine equivalent, we obtained a 65% rescue of cone ERG, and a similar improvement in cone mediated vision. Longitudinal assessment of cone function and cone survival showed that the treatment of the cones lasted for at least six months. In addition to a rescue of the cones, we could detect a 35% rescue of rod function [14]. In contrast, using an AAV5 construct, Boye *et al.* showed a 45% recovery of cone photoreceptor ERG, an improvement in cones vision as well as partial preservation of cone cells, lasting at least three months [15]. However, this treatment did not lead to an improvement in rod ERG. Besides the difference in AAV serotype used, there are a number of variables that could have contributed to the difference in efficacy, including the age at which the animals were treated, the promoter driving *GUCY2D* expression and the vector titre administered. It is important that, before a clinical trial for GC1-deficiency is considered, the relative contribution of these factors is resolved, to achieve the best chance of a positive outcome.

GENE THERAPY FOR PRIMARY CONE DEGENERATIONS

Although the focus of much research has been on the development of gene therapy for retinal dystrophies caused by rod defects, it is the cone photoreceptor cells that are required for visual acuity. Whilst cone loss, the main debilitating factor in retinal dystrophy, can be a consequence of rod photoreceptor degeneration, it is the primary (and possibly sole) outcome in cone and cone-rod dystrophies. In view of the importance of cone vision on patients' quality of life, development of gene therapy for cone disease is an important focus of our work.

Stationary disorders are attractive targets for the development of gene therapy, as their slowly progressing nature creates a large window of opportunity for intervention. A second advantage to treating a stationary condition is the fact that the treatment need only restore the function of the photoreceptor cells without prolonging their survival to have a large impact on the course of the disease. The impact of stationary night blindness on patients' wellbeing is probably not sufficiently severe to consider treating this disorder with gene therapy, especially while the technique is still in its infancy. Achromatopsia, on the other hand, is a very debilitating condition and patients could benefit substantially from the development of successful gene therapy protocols.

Table I. Overview of retinal disease genes treated successfully using AAV-mediated gene supplementation therapy.

Disease	Gene	Outcome of pre-clinical treatment studies
RP	PDE6B	AAV2/5-mediated rescue of rod function and survival in hypomorphic mutant (rd10) mice, no convincing rescue in null mutant (rd1) mice with various vectors
	PRPH2	AAV2-mediated rescue of rod structure and function, no effect on progression of cell loss
	RHO	AAV2/5-mediated gene transfer leads to improved rod structure and function for at least 3 months in mice
Cone dystrophy	CNGA3	AAV5-mediated gene transfer improves cone function cone-mediated vision and cone survival in mice
	CNGB3	Gene transfer by AAV5 or AAV2/8 in dogs and mice leads to long term improvements in cone function, survival and vision
	GNAT2	Improved cone function and vision for 7 months in mice post treatment with AAV2 gene transfer
LCA	ABCA4	AAV2/5-mediated rescue of PRC function and survival in mice. The suitability of the vector for clinical application is in doubt.
	GUCY2D	AAV5 and AAV2/8-mediated rescue of cone and rod function, vision and survival for at least 6 months in mice
	LRAT	Improved rod function after AAV2 gene transfer in mice
	MERTK	Gene transfer using AAV2 rescues RPE function and PRC survival for up to 3 months in rats
	RPE65	AAV2-mediated improved rod and cone function in mice and dogs, improved retinal sensitivity and vision in clinical trials
	RPGRIP1	AAV2-mediated rescue of rod function and prolongation of rod survival for at least 5 months in mice
Syndromic disease	BBS4	scAAV5 gene transfer in mice corrects Rho mislocalisation and slows PRC loss for at least 3 months in mice
	USH2D	AAV5-mediated gene transfer restored USH2 complex formation in rods; no assessment of PRC survival
Albinism	GPR143	Improvement of RPE structure and partial rescue of PRC function using AAV2/1 gene transfer in adult mice
	TYR	AAV2/1-mediated melanosome synthesis improves retinal function and preserves PRCs from light damage
Others	ABCA4	Stargardt Disease – AAV2/5-mediated rescue of PRC function and survival in mice. The suitability of the vector for clinical application is in doubt
	NP4	Leber hereditary optic neuropathy – AAV2-mediated allotropic expression rescues RGC and optic nerve in rat model of disease created using AAV2 carrying a mutated NP4
	RS1	Retinoschisis – Improvement in retinal function and integrity after intravitreal administration of an AAV8 vector

We have successfully treated an animal model of achromatopsia using AAV-mediated gene supplementation therapy. The cone-specific cyclic nucleotide gated (CNG) channel, which is an essential component of the phototransduction cascade, consists of two subunits encoded by the *CNGA3* and *CNGB3* genes respectively. Mutations in these genes are known to cause the two most prevalent forms of achromatopsia [16, 17]. AAV-mediated transfer of the *CNGB3* gene to the retina of a murine model of CNGB3-deficiency resulted in the restoration of both A and B subunits of the channel to the outer segments of the cones. This subsequently led to a almost complete rescue of the light-adapted ERG, which is absent in these animals and a stable improvement in bright light vision for at least one year in the mice (*Table I*) [18].

Macular dystrophies affect the central cone-rich part of the retina leading to loss of visual acuity with progressive loss of peripheral vision later in life. Patients with macular dystrophies caused by dominant mutations are usually diagnosed between the third and fifth decade of life. The majority of dominant mutations in the *PRPH2* (also known as *RDS*) gene cause macular dystrophy and to date no effective treatment exists [19]. While progress has been made in the treatment of recessive retinopathies using gene therapy, there have been few pre-clinical studies and no clinical studies focusing on dominant retinopathies. There are various potential methods to correct a dominant mutation using gene therapy, but the most efficient in our hands appears to be miRNA-template based RNA interference. We have shown that AAV2/8 vectors carrying miRNA-based hairpins can successfully silence the *Prph2* gene expression in mice. Using non-specific miRNA cassettes against the Prph2 mRNA we could efficiently target the endogenous messenger RNA, resulting in an 80% reduction of Prph2 mRNA and a concomitant decrease in Peripherin protein [20]. Following on from this study, we aim to develop AAV2/8 vectors that will specifically silence a dominant Prph2 mutation commonly present in the British population. AAV delivery of an miRNA that is able to discriminate between the mutated and the wild-type allele should allow the amelioration of the dominant macular dystrophy phenotype.

CONCLUDING REMARKS

Over the past years, there has been major progress in development of gene replacement therapy for inherited retinal dystrophies. The technical advances in vector technology, particularly for AAV based vectors, and a better understanding of potential difficulties surrounding gene transfer to the retinal cells, have allowed us to achieve substantial rescue of retinal degeneration in various animal models. Following our recent clinical trial demonstrating proof of principle for gene replacement therapy for inherited retinal dystrophy due to defects in RPE65, the preclinical work described here is likely to enable us to initiate clinical trials for these retinal disorders in the next few years.

ACKNOWLEDGMENTS

This work has been performed with the support of the EC-DG research through the FP6-Network of Excellence, CLINIGENE: LSHB-CT-2006-018933.

REFERENCES

1. Buch PK, Bainbridge JW, Ali RR. AAV-mediated gene therapy for retinal disorders: from mouse to man. *Gene Ther* 2008; 15: 849-57.

2. Bok D. Contributions of genetics to our understanding of inherited monogenic retinal diseases and age-related macular degeneration. *Arch Ophthalmol* 2007; 125: 160-4.

3. Den Hollander AI, Roepman R, Koenekoop RK, Cremers FP. Leber congenital amaurosis: genes, proteins and disease mechanisms. *Prog Retin Eye Res* 2008; 27: 391-419.

4. Acland GM, Aguirre GD, Ray J, Zhang Q, Aleman TS, Cideciyan AV, *et al.* Gene therapy restores vision in a canine model of childhood blindness. *Nat Genet* 2001; 28: 92-5.

5. Narfstrom K, Katz ML, Bragadottir R, Seeliger M, Boulanger A, Redmond TM, *et al.* Functional and structural recovery of the retina after gene therapy in the RPE65 null mutation dog. *Invest Ophthalmol Vis Sci* 2003; 44: 1663-72.

6. Le Meur G, Stieger K, Smith AJ, Weber M, Deschamps JY, Nivard D, *et al.* Restoration of vision in RPE65-deficient Briard dogs using an AAV serotype 4 vector that specifically targets the retinal pigmented epithelium. *Gene Ther* 2006; 14: 292-303.

7. Roman AJ, Boye SL, Aleman TS, Pang JJ, McDowell JH, Boye SE, *et al.* Electroretinographic analyses of Rpe65-mutant rd12 mice: developing an in vivo bioassay for human gene therapy trials of Leber congenital amaurosis. *Mol Vis* 2007; 13: 1701-10.

8. Bennicelli J, Wright JF, Komaromy A, Jacobs JB, Hauck B, Zelenaia O, *et al.* Reversal of blindness in animal models of Leber congenital amaurosis using optimized AAV2-mediated gene transfer. *Mol Ther* 2008; 16: 458-65.

9. Bainbridge JWB, Smith AJ, Barker SS, Robbie S, Henderson R, Balaggan K, *et al.* Effect of gene therapy on visual function in Leber's congenital amaurosis. *N Engl J Med* 2008; 358: 2231-9.

10. Maguire AM, Simonelli F, Pierce EA, Pugh EN Jr, Mingozzi F, Bennicelli J, *et al.* Safety and efficacy of gene transfer for Leber's congenital amaurosis. *N Engl J Med* 2008; 358: 2240-8.

11. Hauswirth W, Aleman TS, Kaushal S, Cideciyan AV, Schwartz SB, Wang L, *et al.* Phase I trial of Leber congenital amaurosis due to RPE65 mutations by ocular subretinal injection of adeno-associated virus gene vector: short-term results. *Hum Gene Ther* 2008; 19: 979-90.

12. Tan MH, Smith AJ, Pawlyk B, Xu X, Liu X, Bainbridge JB, *et al.* Gene therapy for retinitis pigmentosa and Leber congenital amaurosis caused by defects in AIPL1: effective rescue of mouse models of partial and complete Aipl1 deficiency using AAV2/2 and AAV2/8 vectors. *Hum Mol Genet* 2009; 18: 2099-114.

13. Sun X, Pawlyk B, Xu X, Liu X, Bulgakov OV, Adamian M, *et al.* Gene therapy with a promoter targeting both rods and cones rescues retinal degeneration caused by AIPL1 mutations. *Gene Ther* 2010; 17: 117-31.

14. Mihelec M, Pearson RA, Robbie SJ, Buch PK, Azam SA, Bainbridge JW, *et al.* Long-term preservation of cones and improvement in visual function following gene therapy in a mouse model of leber congenital amaurosis caused by guanylate cyclase-1 deficiency. *Hum Gene Ther* 2011; 22: 1179-90.

15. Boye SE, Boye SL, Pang J, Ryals R, Everhart D, Umino Y, *et al.* Functional and behavioral restoration of vision by gene therapy in the guanylate cyclase-1 (GC1) knockout mouse. *PLoS One* 2010; 5: e11306.

16. Kohl S, Varsanyi B, Antunes GA, Baumann B, Hoyng CB, Jagle H, *et al.* CNGB3 mutations account for 50% of all cases with autosomal recessive achromatopsia. *Eur J Hum Genet* 2005; 13: 302-8.

17. Kohl S, Baumann B, Broghammer M, Jagle H, Sieving P, Kellner U, *et al.* Mutations in the CNGB3 gene encoding the beta-subunit of the cone photoreceptor cGMP-gated channel are responsible for achromatopsia (ACHM3) linked to chromosome 8q21. *Hum Mol Genet* 2000; 9: 2107-16.

18. Carvalho LS, Xu J, Pearson RA, Smith AJ, Bainbridge JW, Morries LM, *et al*. Long-term and age-dependent restoration of visual function in a mouse model of CNGB3-associated achromatopsia following gene therapy. *Hum Mol Genet* 2011; 20: 3161-75.

19. Boon CJ, den Hollander AI, Hoyng CB, Cremers FP, Klevering BJ, Keunen JE. The spectrum of retinal dystrophies caused by mutations in the peripherin/RDS gene. *Prog Retin Eye Res* 2008; 27: 213-35.

20. Georgiadis A, Tschernutter M, Bainbridge JW, Robbie SJ, McIntosh J, Nathwani AC, *et al*. AAV-mediated knockdown of peripherin-2 *in vivo* using miRNA-based hairpins. *Gene Ther* 2010; 17: 486-93.

The CliniBook: Clinical gene transfer
Edited by Odile Cohen-Haguenauer – EDK, Paris © 2012, pp. 41-45

A1-3
AAV-mediated gene therapy for MPS VI

GABRIELLA COTUGNO[1,2], PATRIZIA ANNUNZIATA[1,2], MARK HASKINS[3], ALBERTO AURICCHIO[1,2]*

[1]*Telethon Institute of Genetics and Medicine (TIGEM), Naples, Italy;* [2]*Medical Genetics, Department of Pediatrics, "Federico II" University, Naples, Italy,* [3]*Departments of Pathobiology and Clinical Studies, School of Veterinary Medicine, University of Pennsylvania, Philadelphia, PA, USA.*
auricchio@tigem.it
* *Corresponding author*

MUCOPOLYSACCHARIDOSIS VI

Mucopolysaccharidosis VI (MPS VI; OMIM #253200) is an autosomal recessive lysosomal storage disorder (LSD), belonging to the group of mucopolysaccharidoses (MPS). The MPS are caused by defects in lysosomal enzymes resulting in widespread intra- and extra-cellular accumulation of glycosaminoglycans (GAGs). MPS VI, also known as Maroteaux-Lamy syndrome, is caused by deficiency of the enzyme arylsulfatase B (ARSB, N-acetylgalactosamine-4-sulfatase) required for the lysosomal degradation of the glycosaminoglycans dermatan sulfate (DS) [1]. Deficiency of ARSB results in the intralysosomal storage and urinary excretion of this partially degraded GAGs.

The clinical manifestations of MPS VI include communicating hydrocephalus, spinal cord compression, corneal clouding and visual impairment, hearing loss, coarse facial features, macroglossia, heart valve disease, cardiomyopathy, respiratory insufficiency, hepatosplenomegaly, inguinal and abdominal hernias, dwarfism/growth retardation, skeletal dysplasia, and joint stiffness [1]. The rate of clinical progression in MPS VI patients varies considerably, generating a spectrum of clinical presentation ranging from rapidly to slowly progressive disease [1]. Nevertheless, all patients within this spectrum will eventually experience significant morbidity and in most cases early mortality. Mental development is usually normal in MPS VI patients, although physical and visual impairment affects psychomotor performance [1].

The biochemical diagnosis of MPS VI is based on the detection of elevations in urinary GAGs and reduced ARSB activity measured in white blood cells or cultured skin fibroblasts (below the 10% of the lower limit of normal range) with the presence of clinical findings consistent with MPS VI [1].

Mutational analysis in MPS VI patients has led to the identification of 128 different ARSB mutations (Human Gene Mutation Database; http://www.hgmd.cf.ac.uk/ac/index.php).

Most of these are missense mutations (approximately 83%), thus predicted to result in the presence of a cross reactive immunological material (CRIM) and variable levels of residual ARSB activity [1].

LIMITATIONS OF ENZYME REPLACEMENT THERAPY FOR MPS VI

Advances in the understanding of the biochemical and molecular bases of LSDs have led to the development of specific treatment regimens, relying on the ability of lysosomal enzymes, including ARSB, to be secreted by producing cells and taken-up by most cells *via* the mannose-6-phosphate receptor pathway [2].

Enzyme replacement therapy (ERT) with recombinant human ARSB (rhARSB or galsulphase, Naglazyme; BioMarin Pharmaceutical Inc, Novato, CA) has been approved by the Food and Drug Administration (FDA) and the European Medicines Agency (EMA) and is available in the United States, Europe, and Australia. ERT is the current standard of care for MPS VI [1].

Clinical ERT studies show that weekly infusions of 1mg/kg of rhARSB are well tolerated and result in long term (97-260 weeks) reduction in urinary GAG levels and visceromegaly, and great improvement in endurance on a 12-minute walk test (12-MWT). Patients treated with ERT also show improvement in the 3-minute stair climb test (3MSC) [1]. However, ERT has several limitations. First, rhARSB has a short half-life requiring weekly intravenous infusions that carry a risk of immune-mediated anaphylactoid reactions [3] and often require a central venous access which carries risks of sepsis. Second, some organs and tissues are not corrected, likely because of limited biodistribution of rhARSB. For example, in MPS VI patients, ERT failed to ameliorate cardiac function, visual impairment, and bone density while inconsistent improvements have been shown in lung volumes (FEV1 and FVC), obstructive apnea parameters, joint range of motion and stiffness [3]. Third, the cost of ERT is extremely high thus representing a significant burden for the health system or preventing the access to therapy to patients from less developed countries. Thus, there is high need to develop more effective therapeutic strategies.

AAV-MEDIATED LIVER ARSB GENE TRANSFER FOR MPS VI

Gene therapy holds a great potential for the treatment on MPS VI. A selected target tissue can be converted *via* ARSB gene transfer, in a "factory" for production and systemic release of stable and high levels of ARSB enzyme. Uptake of the enzyme from circulation by affected cells can then allow cross-correction of multiple tissues. Notably, the absence of central nervous system involvement in MPS VI has the potential to fully rescue the disease phenotype by this approach.

The liver represents an ideal target for expression of therapeutic ARSB through somatic gene transfer since hepatocytes are highly accessible *via* the blood-stream and are physiologically tasked with the synthesis and secretion of numerous biological molecules [4]. Gene therapy vectors based on the adeno-associated virus serotype 8 (AAV2/8) are able to efficiently transduce the liver resulting in long term expression of therapeutic transgenes after a single systemic administration [4, 5]. Importantly, preliminary results from an ongoing clinical trial using AAV2/8 in hemophilia B patients suggest that systemic AAV2/8 administration is safe and efficient in humans [4]. Thus, we have developed an AAV2/8-based liver-directed ARSB gene transfer approach for the treatment of MPS VI [6]. We selected a liver specific promoter (thyroxine-binding globulin, TBG) to drive ARSB expression specifically in hepatocytes and we produced AAV2/8-TBG-ARSB vectors [6].

MPS VI animal models are critical tools for the investigation of experimental therapies. Two spontaneous animal models of MPS VI are available, which closely mimic the human disease: a rat with a frameshift null mutation resulting in the absence of the ARSB protein [6] and a cat bearing a missense mutation resulting in retention of the ARSB protein in the endoplasmic reticulum [6]. In both models, we showed that AAV2/8-TBG-mediated ARSB gene expression in the liver provides a source of enzyme for systemic distribution resulting in biochemical, pathological, skeletal, and functional improvements [6-8].

AAV2/8-MEDIATED ARSB GENE TRANSFER IN MPS VI RATS

In newborn MPS VI rats, ARSB gene delivery to liver, through intravascular injections of AAV2/8-TBG-ARSB at a dose of 4.1×10^{13} genome copies/kilogram (gc/kg), resulted in long term expression of the enzyme which is secreted in the bloodstream thereby achieving systemic therapeutic levels and amelioration of the disease phenotype [6]. We observed skeletal improvement and reduction in GAG storage, inflammation, and apoptosis. However MPS VI rats which bear the null ARSB mutation, developed a neutralizing immune response to the transgene, resulting in below normal levels of circulating ARSB [6]. To confirm this and to obtain high levels of circulating enzyme, we co-administered AAV (4×10^{13} gc/kg) with immunosuppressive drugs (IS) [7] to newborn or juvenile MPS VI rats. Co-administration of IS with AAV resulted in variably high levels of circulating ARSB, associated with decreased levels of anti-ARSB antibodies, thus confirming that the neutralizing response elicited by gene delivery was otherwise limiting liver transduction efficiency. We then assessed the impact of different ARSB serum levels following AAV delivery on the various disease manifestations, in newborn or juvenile MPS VI rats (*Figure 1*).

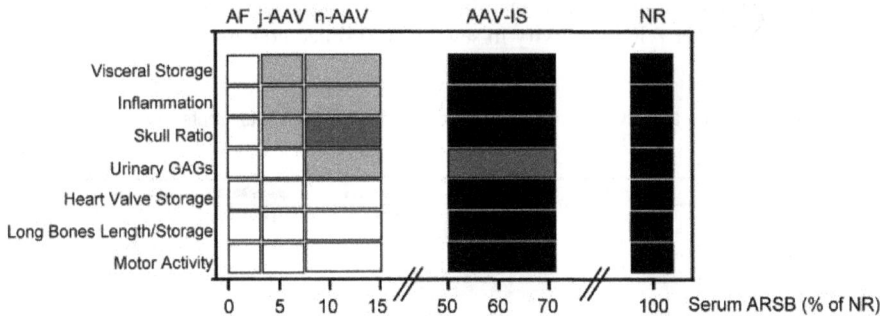

Figure 1. Different serum ARSB levels are required to improve different MPS VI phenotypic aspects. The graph shows is the correlation between improvement of the various MPS VI systemic features observed and the ARSB serum levels in control and treated MPS VI rats. The different pathological aspects analyzed are reported on the left and serum ARSB levels are reported at the bottom, as a percentage of normal (NR) levels. Affected (AF), NR, and MPS VI rats receiving either AAV alone at birth (n-AAV) and on postnatal day 30 (j-AAV) or receiving AAV with various IS drugs (AAV-IS) are depicted at the top. Shading (from white to black) is correlated with the level of phenotype improvement. White, no improvement; light gray, minor improvement; dark gray, significant improvement; black, normal phenotype (NR) or complete rescue of the phenotype (AAV-IS) (From G. Cotugno *et al.* [7]).

Independently of age at vector administration, low levels (6% of normal) of circulating enzyme were sufficient to reduce storage and inflammation in the visceral organs and to ameliorate skull abnormalities; intermediate levels (11% of normal) were required to reduce urinary GAG excretion; high levels (≥50% of normal) were required to rescue the abnormalities of long bones and motor activity (*Figure 1*) [6,7].

AAV2/8-MEDIATED ARSB GENE TRANSFER IN MPS VI CATS

Newborn MPS VI cats, bearing missense ARSB mutations resulting in the expression of inactive enzyme, were injected systemically with AAV2/8-TBG-ARSB (6.6×10^{13} gc/kg). AAV-treated MPS VI cats showed stable and normal levels of circulating ARSB in the absence of immune responses. This was associated with significant reduction of urinary and tissue GAGs levels [6].

More recently, we studied the dose effect of intravascular administrations of AAV2/8-TBG-ARSB in MPS VI cats [6, 8]. In newborn animals, normal circulating ARSB activity was achieved following delivery of high vector doses (6×10^{13} gc/kg, *Table I*) while doses lower than 6×10^{13} gc/kg resulted in below normal levels of circulating ARSB [8]. In addition, levels of circulating ARSB had a characteristic peak-and-drop kinetic suggesting loss of AAV vector genomes in the newborn liver due to hepatocyte proliferation occurring at this age. Consistent with this hypothesis, the delivery at postnatal day 50, an age at which feline liver proliferation is predicted to be less pronounced than in newborns, of AAV2/8 vector doses as low as $0.6-2 \times 10^{12}$ gc/kg resulted in similar to or higher than normal serum ARSB levels in juvenile cats (*Table I*). This was associated with reduction of urinary GAGs and mitral valve thickness, improvement of bone size and improved motor activity [8]. To confirm long-term transgene expression, we measured serum ARSB enzyme activity, urinary GAG levels, and AAV vector genome copies in livers from 12-month-old injected and control (NR and AF cats uninjected or receiving the AAV-*eGFP* vector) animals (*Table I*) [8]. As expected, we observed higher than NR liver ARSB activity in several AAV-injected cats (*Table I*) [8].

Table I. ARSB activity, GAGs, and liver vector genome copies in MPS VI cats treated with AAV vectors.

Animal groups	Serum ARSB	Liver gc/mdg	Liver ARSB	Liver GAGs	Spleen ARSB	Spleen GAGs
NR	9.6 ± 0.5	—	5 ± 0.7	4.4 ± 0.3	14.4 ± 5	8 ± 0,4
AF	1.4 ± 0.1	—	0.02 ± 0.02	14 ± 7.5	0.02 ± 0.02	23 ± 4
p5 ($n = 4$) 6×10^{13} gc/kg	19.1 ± 6*	0.3 ± 0.1	53 ± 15*	4.1 ± 0.1*	1.05 ± 0.6*	5.9 ± 0.6*
p50 ($n = 1$) 6×10^{13} gc/kg	41.5	1.73	630	3.4	2.6*	7.1
p50 ($n = 3$) 6×10^{12} gc/kg	22.5 ± 10*	0.16 ± 0.06	138 ± 63*	4.4 ± 0.3*	4.2 ± 0.4*	5.1 ± 0.4*
p50 ($n=5$) 2×10^{12} gc/kg	19.5 ± 13*	0.02 ± 0.005	82 ± 65	6.7 ± 2.5	2.25 ± 2	9.3 ± 1.5*
p50 ($n=3$) 6×10^{11} gc/kg	4.3 ± 3*	0.09 ± 0.09	3.8 ± 0.1	10.8 ± 3.6	0.05 ± 0.05	14.6 ± 6
p50 ($n=2$) 2×10^{11} gc/kg	3.4 ± 3*	0.005 ± 0.005	16 ± 16*	9 ± 5	0.1 ± 0.1	16 ± 9

Measurements in tissues were done at the time of sacrifice (12 months). Serum ARSB is reported as the average activity measured over time. ARSB activity is expressed as nmol/ml/h for sera and nmol/mg protein/h for tissues. GAG levels are expressed as ug GAG/ug protein. NR: normal untreated cats; p5: cats injected at postnatal day 5; p50: cats injected at postnatal day 50; the AAV vector dose used (genome copies/kilogram, gc/kg) is reported for each group. Gc/mdg: genome copies/molecule of diploid genome. NB. Values are reported as mean ± SE when n ≥ 1. *p-value ≤ 0.05 *versus* AF (From G. Cotugno *et al.* [8]).

This resulted in reduction of liver GAG storage in treated animals, which was more efficient in animals receiving higher vector doses ($6x10^{12}$ - $6x10^{13}$ gc/kg), independent of the age of the cat at treatment (*Table I*). In addition, persistence of liver transduction was confirmed by the presence of detectable AAV vector genome copies at the end of the study. In general, animals receiving higher vector doses and having higher serum enzyme activity have higher liver ARSB activity and AAV vector genome copy numbers (*Table I*) [8].

CONCLUSIONS AND FUTURE PERSPECTIVES

Taken together, the results we have obtained in MPS VI cats and rats treated with AAV2/8 show that production of therapeutic ARSB levels is achieved long term after a single vector administration, resulting in significant amelioration of the MPS VI features. Based on the absence of immune responses to ARSB in MPS VI cats, we propose AAV2/8 liver gene therapy as a therapeutic alternative to ERT to be further tested in MPS VI CRIM+ patients.

ACKNOWLEDGMENTS

This work has been performed with the support of the EC-DG research through the FP6-Network of Excellence, CLINIGENE: LSHB-CT-2006-018933, the FP-7 MEUSIX and a grant from the Italian Telethon Foundation.

REFERENCES

1. Valayannopoulos V, Nicely H, Harmatz P, Turbeville S. Mucopolysaccharidosis VI. *Orphanet J Rare Dis* 2010; 5: 5.

2. Dahms NM, Lobel P, Kornfeld S. Mannose 6-phosphate receptors and lysosomal enzyme targeting. *J Biol Chem* 1989; 264: 12115-8.

3. Harmatz P, Giugliani R, Schwartz IV, Guffon N, Teles EL, Miranda MC, et al. Long-term follow-up of endurance and safety outcomes during enzyme replacement therapy for mucopolysaccharidosis VI: Final results of three clinical studies of recombinant human N-acetylgalactosamine 4-sulfatase. *Mol Genet Metab* 2008; 94: 469-75.

4. Mingozzi F, High KA. Therapeutic *in vivo* gene transfer for genetic disease using AAV: progress and challenges. *Nat Rev Genet* 2011; 12: 341-55.

5. Cotugno G, Aurilio M, Annunziata P, Capalbo A, Faella A, Rinaldi V, et al. Noninvasive repetitive imaging of somatostatin receptor 2 gene transfer with positron emission tomography. *Hum Gene Ther* 2011; 22: 189-96.

6. Tessitore A, Faella A, O'Malley T, Cotugno G, Doria M, Kunieda T, et al. Biochemical, pathological, and skeletal improvement of mucopolysaccharidosis VI after gene transfer to liver but not to muscle. *Mol Ther* 2008; 16: 30-7.

7. Cotugno G, Tessitore A, Capalbo A, Annunziata P, Strisciuglio C, Faella A, et al. Different serum enzyme levels are required for the rescue of the various systemic features in mucopolysaccharidoses. *Hum Gene Ther* 2010; 21: 555-69.

8. Cotugno G, Annunziata P, Tessitore A, O'Malley T, Capalbo A, Faella A, et al. Long-term amelioration of feline mucopolysaccharidosis VI after AAV-mediated liver gene transfer. *Mol Ther* 2011; 19: 461-9.

The CliniBook: Clinical gene transfer
Edited by Odile Cohen-Haguenauer – EDK, Paris © 2012, pp. 46-54

A1-4
Microdystrophin and myostatin gene therapy for Duchenne muscular dystrophy using adeno-associated virus vectors

Helen Foster, Taeyoung Koo, Alberto Malerba, Susan Jarmin,
Takis Athanasopoulos, Keith Foster, George Dickson*

School of Biological Sciences, Royal Holloway, University of London, Egham Hill, Egham, Surrey, TW20 0EX, United Kingdom.
g.dickson@rhul.ac.uk
* Corresponding author

INTRODUCTION – CONCEPTS AND VECTOROLOGY

Duchenne muscular dystrophy (DMD) is a severe muscle wasting disorder caused by a lack of dystrophin protein in skeletal muscle. Loss of dystrophin compromises the integrity of the muscle cell membrane and results in muscle fibres that are highly prone to contraction induced injury. Consequently there are progressive rounds of degeneration and regeneration of the muscle leading to the replacement of muscle fibres with non-contractile fibrotic tissue and fatty infiltrates. Recent reports have suggested that a minimum of 30% of normal dystrophin levels need to be present uniformly in all myofibres to prevent muscular dystrophy in humans [1], which is supported by data from transgenic *mdx* mice. Efficient systemic gene transfer of dystrophin is crucial if restoration of muscle function is to be achieved.

Adeno-associated virus (AAV) mediated gene transfer is widely used for skeletal muscle-directed gene therapy due to the high tropism of AAV vectors for muscle fibres. Transgenes delivered by AAV vectors to the muscle of animal models, including non-human primates have been shown to be stably expressed over several years, demonstrating the potential of AAV vectors to provide "life-long" gene expression. AAV vectors are being investigated for their potential to induce muscle "re-modelling" in dystrophic muscle by the delivery of transgenes to inhibit the myostatin pathway and to also restore dystrophin expression in dystrophic muscle and thereby improve muscle function and stabilise or halt disease progression [2, 3]. However, there is a limitation in the packaging capacity of foreign DNA into AAV vectors. The AAV capsid is able to package a genome of up to 5kb and therefore it is not possible to transfer the 11kb full length dystrophin cDNA into AAV vectors. To overcome this limitation, truncated but functional mini- and micro-dystrophin cDNAs have been engineered by several

research groups and have been tested in both murine and canine models of DMD.
In addition to functionality of the microdystrophin, further considerations need to be made in the treatment of DMD with AAV; these include the ability to efficiently deliver the transgene systemically to all muscles including the heart and diaphragm. Scale up of these processes is required, so that AAV microdystrophin vectors can be assessed in large animal models for efficiency, functionality and immunogenicity before inclusion in clinical trials. Systemic delivery of AAV microdystrophin vectors has previously been demonstrated in mouse models following injection of very high titres of AAV expressing dystrophin under control of a constitutive viral promoter. However, AAV vectors are currently being developed that can achieve efficient gene transfer and expression at lower viral titres with a muscle restrictive promoter driving microdystrophin expression that will be more applicable for use in a clinical setting.

Adeno-associated viral vectors expressing microdystrophin in the *mdx* mouse

A number of groups have conducted extensive studies in the *mdx* mouse following AAV microdystrophin gene transfer. When expressed at a sufficient level, many of these microdystrophin proteins have been demonstrated to improve, but not completely normalise a range of markers of the dystrophic phenotype. Restoration of the dystrophin associated protein complex (DAPC), stabilisation of muscle degeneration and improvements in muscle function have been demonstrated following delivery of microdystrophin at different stages of disease progression [2]. However, the lack of large portions of the dystrophin gene, including some functional domains means that microdystrophin proteins are less able to restore specific force and protect dystrophic muscle from contraction induced injury. Recently the Dickson laboratory has made progress in this area through DNA sequence optimisation and the design of modified microdystrophin genes (*Figure 1*). Sequence optimisation lead to increased levels of dystrophin mRNA and protein and resulted in normalisation of specific force but not resistance to eccentric contractions in *mdx* mice. Further modification of this microdystrophin to include additional functional domains lead to additional improvements in function when administered at sub-optimal doses in *mdx* mice [3, 4] (*Figure 2*).
Another hurdle in the path towards the generalised correction of DMD by AAV microdystrophin gene therapy is that high titres of AAV are required for efficient systemic gene transfer. Such high titres may be toxic and may cause immune responses against the viral proteins. In particular, there is a potential for humoral and cellular immune responses to AAV vectors and transgenes following injection into the *mdx* muscles [5]. To overcome these issues, transient immune suppression to enable re-infusion or use of muscle-specific promoters to avoid expression in antigen presenting cells have been successfully used. We have recently demonstrated that optimisation of codon usage of a eukaryotic gene induces significant increase in levels of mRNA and dystrophin expression in *mdx* mice after intramuscular and systemic AAV gene transfer [3]. The higher expression of an mRNA sequence optimised version of dystrophin may decrease the amount of AAV vectors to be used in systemic administration then reducing the risk of toxicity of the vector. The inclusion of specific domains identified as compulsory for the rescue of the functionality of the dystrophin may allow a reduction of the amount of AAV vectors to be administered for a successful therapy. We demonstrated that the delivery of AAV2/9-microdystrophin incorporating helix 1 of the coiled-coil motif in the CT domain of dystrophin increased the recruitment of some members of the dystrophin associated protein complex including α1-syntrophin and α-dystrobrevin at the sarcolemma of skeletal muscle fibres of *mdx* mice and efficiently

protects *mdx* muscles from muscle damage [4]. An alternate strategy to de-target AAV transduction from non-target tissue can also lower the viral load required for efficient gene transfer to muscle [6].

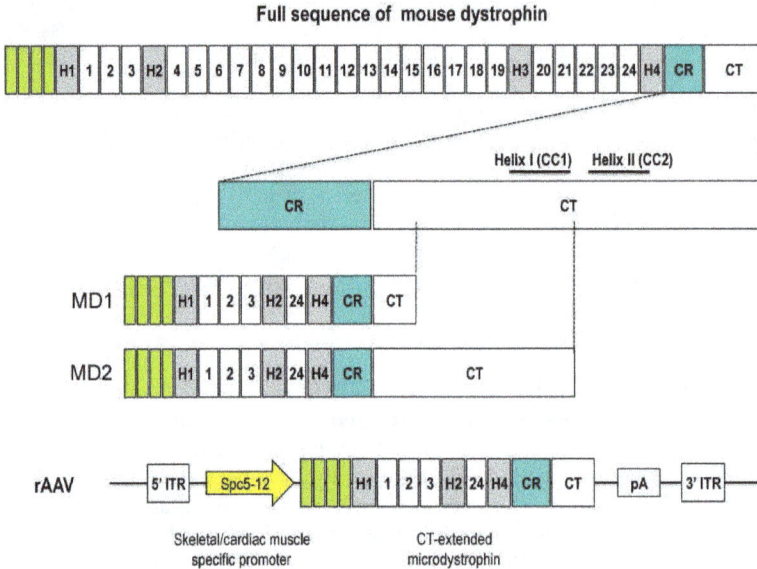

Figure 1. Generation of mouse-specific microdystrophin cDNAs with CT domain extension. The full length dystrophin protein is defined by four structural domains: N-terminus (NT), Rod, Cysteine-rich (CR) and Carboxyl-terminal (CT) domains. The MD1 cDNA incorporates deletions of the Rod domain repeats 4 – 23 and the CT domain. The MD2 cDNAs incorporate additionally coiled coil helix 1 of the CT domain of dystrophin. At the CT end, each microdystrophin contains three amino acids of exon 79 followed by three stop codons. Adapted from Koo *et al.* (2011) [4].

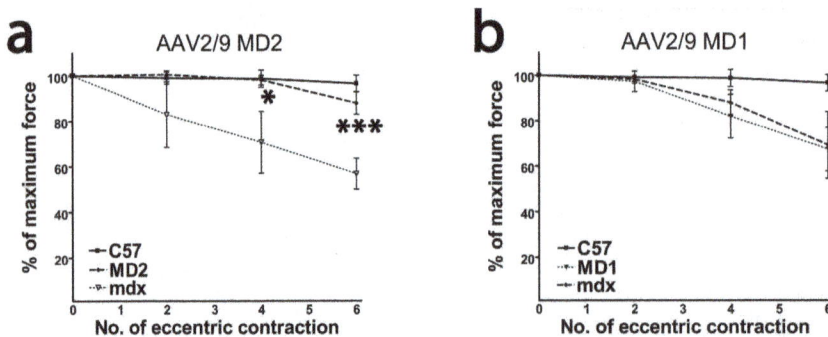

Figure 2. Intramuscular injection of AAV2/9-MD2 leads to muscle protection from lengthening contraction in TA muscles of *mdx* mice. TA muscles of 2 month old *mdx* mice were injected with 2×10^{10} vector genomes of AAV2/9-MD1, or AAV2/9-MD2. 2 months after injection, TA muscles were assessed for force deficit following a series of 6 eccentric contractions. Muscles treated with AAV2/9-MD2 (a) showed a significant improvement in their resistance to contraction-induced injury, while no change was observed in muscle injected with AAV2/9-MD1 (b) compared to saline injected *mdx* muscles. (mean±S.E.M. n = 4-6, one-way ANOVA test, *p < 0.05). Adapted from Koo *et al.* (2011) [4].

ADENO-ASSOCIATED VIRAL VECTORS EXPRESSING MICRODYSTROPHIN IN A DYSTROPHIC DOG MODEL

The golden retriever muscular dystrophy (*GRMD*) dog was the first characterized dog model of DMD. It has been reported that *GRMD* dogs eventually die due to cardiomyopathy. *GRMD* dogs have been identified as having complete dystrophin deficiency with higher phenotypic similarity to human DMD disease than that of *mdx* mouse model. The *GRMD* model has been bred on to a beagle background (*CXMDj*), a smaller dog model which exhibits a similar phenotype to the *GRMD* dog.

To apply AAV mediated gene therapy to DMD patients it is desirable to first test any therapy in large animal models such as the dystrophic dog prior to human clinical trials. It is important to examine both the functionality of the microdystrophin and the immune responses against transgene or AAV vectors in a large animal model such as the canine X-linked muscular dystrophy (*CXMDj*) or golden retriever muscular dystrophy dogs, which are more clinically relevant models for DMD compared to the *mdx* mouse.

A major hurdle facing AAV mediated gene delivery in muscle towards clinical applications is the immune response against the AAV capsid protein or transgene product. Profiling human sera demonstrates worldwide neutralising antibodies to most AAV serotypes [7]. Strong immune responses to capsid have been exhibited following intramuscular injection of AAV2 or AAV6 vectors carrying various transgenes in dogs, in contrast to successful gene delivery in mouse models [8]. Another study demonstrated that a strong cellular and humoral immune response against transgene in the *CXMDj* dog model was activated following delivery of AAV2 (AAV2/2) or 8 (AAV2/8) encoding β-galactosidase [9]. These immune responses have not been encountered in small animal models, but have been observed in juvenile and neonatal muscular dystrophy dogs and random-bred wild-type dogs [8, 10, 11].

These new challenges call on efforts to improve targeted gene delivery, tissue-specific therapeutic gene expression, immune modulation and new vector development and large-scale production technologies. Immune responses can be suppressed with a combination of anti-thymocyte globulin (ATG), cyclosporine (CSP), and mycophenolate mofetil (MMF) and allows long term expression of a canine microdystrophin in the skeletal muscle of *CXMD* dog [10].

It is important to evaluate the serotypes of AAV which renders efficient gene transfer at a low dose of virus in large animals prior to clinical trials. AAV2/8 is one of the promising vector serotypes for preclinical trials in canine models. Several research groups have compared the efficiency of gene transfer between AAV serotype 2 and 8 and found that AAV2/8 vectors showed efficient gene transfer into canine skeletal muscle more widely than AAV2 vectors [9].

Recently we have demonstrated that delivery of AAV2/8 expressing a canine-specific and mRNA sequence-optimized microdystrophin gene controlled by a muscle-specific promoter results in high and stable levels of microdystrophin expression in the (*CXMDj*) dog model of DMD for at least 8 weeks. Following intramuscular injection of AAV2/8 microdystrophin, large areas of dystrophin positive fibres were observed (*Figure 3*); this was associated with stabilisation of the DAPC, a reduction in central nucleation (an important marker of muscle regeneration) and stabilisation of myofibre permeability (*Figure 4*). Importantly, the injections were carried out in the absence of any immunosuppressive regime and unlike other studies in canine models of DMD, no evidence of an immune response was observed [12]. The design of these vectors marks an important step forward to clinical trials.

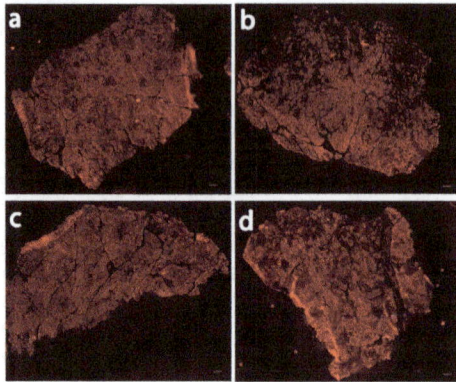

Figure 3. Widespread expression of an mRNA sequence-optimized canine microdystrophin after intramuscular injection of AAV2/8-cMD1 in the *CXMDj* muscles. The (a, b) tibialis cranialis (TA), (c) extensor carpi radialis (ECR) and (d) gastrocnemius (GC) muscles of the CXMDj dog were injected intramuscularly with either 1×10^{13} (a, c), 1×10^{12} (b) or 2×10^{13} vector genome (d) of AAV2/8-cMD1. At 4 weeks (c) or 8weeks (a, b and d) after injection, dystrophin expression was evaluated by immunohistochemistry using NCL-dysB antibody. Dystrophin signal was visualized with Alexafluor 568-conjugated anti-mouse IgG antibody. Scale bar = 300μm. Adapted from Koo *et al.* (2011) [12].

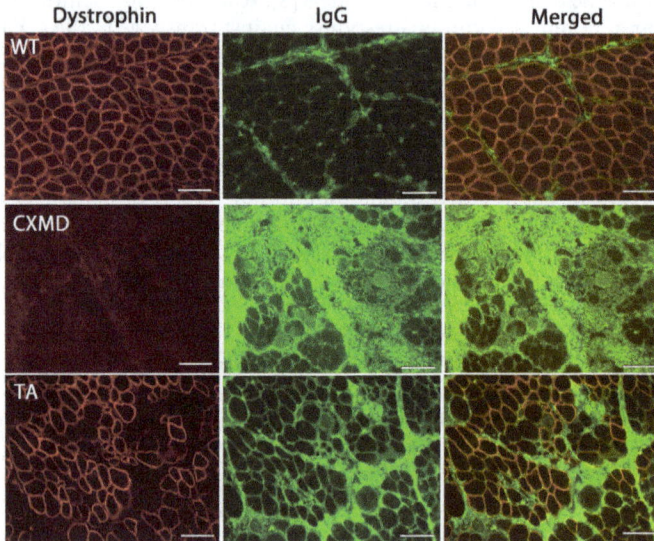

Figure 4. Examination of muscle membrane integrity of muscle of *CXMDj* dog following intramuscular injection of AAV2/8-cMD1. The TA muscle of *CXMDj* dog was injected with 1 x10^{13} vg AAV2/8-cMD1. At 8 weeks post injection, tissues were harvested, cryosectioned and subjected to immuno-histochemistry of serial-sections to examine membrane integrity. Serial-sections were stained using NCL-dysB antibody against microdystrophin or an Alexa 488-anti-canine IgG antibody. The dystrophin signal was visualized with an Alexa 568-conjugated anti-mouse IgG. Right hand panel represents the merged figures between microdystrophin and anti-canine IgG. Age-matched TA muscles of wild-type dog and *CXMDj* dog were assessed in parallel as positive and negative controls, respectively. Magnification bar = 50μm. Adapted from Koo *et al.* (2011) [12].

CLINICAL TRIALS OF AAV MICRODYSTROPHIN IN DMD PATIENTS

To date one AAV, microdystrophin clinical trial has been conducted in DMD patients [13]. Patients received either $2x10^{10}$vg/kg or $1x10^{11}$vg/kg of AAV2.5 CMV microdystrophin *via* intramuscular injection into a biceps muscle. AAV2.5 is a variant of AAV2 which contains five amino acids from AAV1 (1 insertion and 4 substitutions) in the VP1 domain. The AAV2.5 vector expressed a microdystrophin gene under control of the constitutive CMV promoter. Microdystrophin expression was only detected in two of six patients treated and at very low levels (1 and 3 fibres respectively) although vector DNA was detected in all muscle biopsies. A possible explanation is that transduction efficiency of AAV2.5 vectors in human muscle may be low. However, unexpectedly dystrophin specific T cells were detected in four patients. Further analysis revealed that two patients exhibited pre-existing dystrophin specific T cells and that gene transfer may have stimulated a memory T cell response in these patients. In addition, microdystrophin specific T cells were also detected within at least one patient. The detection of both CD4+ and CD8+ dystrophin specific T cells within these patients provides the most likely explanation for the very low levels of dystrophin expression that were observed (no dystrophin specific T cells were detected in highest expressing patient). This unexpected observation, in particular the presence of pre-existing dystrophin specific T-cells, is in contrast to the proposed induction of tolerance to dystrophin by the presence of spontaneous revertant fibres [14]. However, what is unclear is why pre-existing antibodies are detected in some patients and not others. It is speculated that this may be related to disease severity, levels of inflammation within the muscle and timing of the revertant fibre "event". Although this AAV based clinical trial resulted in very few dystrophin positive fibres it has brought to the fore some important considerations for AAV microdystrophin (and other dystrophin replacement strategies) therapies; that the "cellular immune status" of patients with respect to both dystrophin and AAV must be carefully monitored both prior to and post treatment with any vector.

AAV-BASED INHIBITION OF MYOSTATIN IN MODELS OF MUSCULAR DYSTROPHY

Myostatin, a member of the transforming growth factor-beta (TGF-β) super-family of signalling molecules, is a potent inhibitor of muscle growth, expressed mainly by skeletal muscle. Inactivating mutations of myostatin increase muscle mass in species ranging from mice to men [15, 16]. The mature region binds to the Activin receptor type II (ActRIIB), a serine/threonine kinase transmembrane receptor on target cells, leading to an intracellular signalling cascade *via* the Smad2/3/4 complex, activation and translocation to the nucleus and regulated transcription of myogenic genes [17]. Myostatin has also been shown to abolish signalling *via* SMAD3-independent pathways to counter the positive IGF-1/PI3K/AKT mitogenic pathway.

Many strategies have been developed to decrease myostatin expression or its biological activity and are being evaluated in various muscle disorder models currently. These include targeting myostatin binding proteins including myostatin propeptide, follistatin, ActRIIB, GASP-1, and anti-myostatin antibodies as well as RNA interference system based knockdown and strategies that knock down or inhibit the protein's function. Many of these strategies have yielded promising results and increased muscle mass in experimental animals. Within our own lab, an exon skipping regime, to manipulate pre-mRNA levels, has been evaluated *in-vivo* [18]. Preliminary work in the *mdx* mouse demonstrates the feasibility of dual myostatin inhibition and dystrophin restoration by exon skipping strategies [19]. Myostatin inhibition in GRMD dogs leads to muscle hypertrophy and a reduction in muscle fibrosis [20].

CONCLUSIONS AND FUTURE PERSPECTIVES

The design of any future AAV microdystrophin clinical trial must carefully consider not only the functionality of the microdystrophin gene, the AAV serotype used, and the use of tissue restrictive promoters but also the "dystrophin" immune status of the patients. Much progress has recently been made in many of these areas of AAV gene transfer for the treatment of DMD.

Design of the microdystrophin gene is of the upmost importance, with a number of research groups around the world having tested many microdystrophin gene configurations [2]. However, the Dickson laboratory has recently demonstrated a number of improvements to the microdystrophin gene configuration. mRNA sequence optimisation of the microdystrophin gene, such as the inclusion of improved Kozak sequences, codon optimisation and altering GC content had significant results in terms of gene expression and in turn improvement in muscle function [3]. In addition, further modifications have been made to the microdystrophin gene to include additional binding domains, which were demonstrated to further improve functionality [4]. It is possible that the inclusion of other functional domains in the microdystrophin gene may improve function further. Such improvements in microdystrophin gene function and levels of gene expression may also allow a lower effective viral dose to be administered.

In addition to functionality of the microdystrophin, the choice of AAV serotype and route of vector administration are critically important. Many studies have compared the tropism and efficiency of gene transfer of different AAV serotypes in murine and canine muscle, with AAV2/8 and AAV2/9 appearing to have very high tropism for both murine and canine muscle [3, 12, 21]. However, when translating studies to non-human primates (NHP), tropisms identified in other animal models may not be consistent [22] and may be an important factor in the success of clinical trials. Recent data also suggests that route of administration plays an important role in development immune responses to vector and transgene [23]. Therefore, testing of AAV microdystrophin vectors by regional limb perfusion in a dystrophic dog model will be of upmost importance in developing clinically relevant vectors.

Although progress has been made in many areas such as microdystrophin design, use of tissue restrictive promoters to limit immune responses and the development of systemic administration strategies, there are areas where progress and further considerations need to be made. From a safety perspective additional improvements need to be made in efficiency of systemic gene transfer to allow viral doses to be lowered further. If effective gene transfer cannot be achieved *via* a single treatment or gene expression is not as long lived as expected there may also be a need to re-administer AAV vectors. The inclusion of extra levels of gene regulation such as the incorporation of micro RNA target sequences into vectors to prevent off target expression may also be required. Finally, it is increasingly apparent that immune responses to AAV capsid proteins and unexpectedly, the dystrophin protein, need to be considered and managed through the development of immune-suppressive regimes to allow effective clinical trials to be developed.

Whilst dystrophin restoration is the cornerstone for any DMD therapy, attention is being focussed upon the environmental milieu of the muscle to counter the reduced muscle regeneration potential, the loss of muscle and the increase in fibro-fatty lesion. Combined administration strategies to address all the pathological changes within dystrophic muscle will be a natural extension to current phase II/III DMD clinical trials.

ACKNOWLEDGMENTS

This work has been performed with the support of the EC-DG research through the FP6-Network of Excellence, CLINIGENE: LSHB-CT-2006-018933.

REFERENCES

1. Neri M, Torelli S, Brown S, Ugo I, Sabatelli P, Merlini L, *et al*. Dystrophin levels as low as 30% are sufficient to avoid muscular dystrophy in the human. *Neuromuscul Disord* 2007; 17: 913-8.

2. Athanasopoulos T, Graham IR, Foster H, Dickson G. Recombinant adeno-associated viral (rAAV) vectors as therapeutic tools for Duchenne muscular dystrophy (DMD). *Gene Ther* 2004; 11 (suppl 1): S109-21.

3. Foster H, Sharp PS, Athanasopoulos T, Trollet C, Graham IR, Foster K, *et al*. Codon and mRNA sequence optimization of microdystrophin transgenes improves expression and physiological outcome in dystrophic mdx mice following AAV2/8 gene transfer. *Mol Ther* 2008; 16: 1825-32.

4. Koo T, Malerba A, Athanasopoulos T, Trollet C, Boldrin L, Ferry A, *et al*. Delivery of AAV2/9-microdystrophin genes incorporating helix 1 of the coiled-coil motif in the C-terminal domain of dystrophin improves muscle pathology and restores the level of alpha1-syntrophin and alpha-dystrobrevin in skeletal muscles of mdx mice. *Hum Gene Ther* 2011; 22: 1379-88

5. Yuasa K, Sakamoto M, Miyagoe-Suzuki Y, Tanouchi A, Yamamoto H, Li J, *et al*. Adeno-associated virus vector-mediated gene transfer into dystrophin-deficient skeletal muscles evokes enhanced immune response against the transgene product. *Gene Ther* 2002; 9: 1576-88.

6. Asokan A, Conway JC, Phillips JL, Li C, Hegge J, Sinnott R, *et al*. Reengineering a receptor footprint of adeno-associated virus enables selective and systemic gene transfer to muscle. *Nat Biotechnol* 2010; 28: 79-82.

7. Calcedo R, Vandenberghe LH, Gao G, Lin J, Wilson JM. Worldwide epidemiology of neutralizing antibodies to adeno-associated viruses. *J Infect Dis* 2009; 199: 381-90.

8. Wang Z, Allen JM, Riddell SR, Gregorevic P, Storb R, Tapscott SJ, *et al*. Immunity to adeno-associated virus-mediated gene transfer in a random-bred canine model of Duchenne muscular dystrophy. *Hum Gene Ther* 2007; 18: 18-26.

9. Ohshima S, Shin JH, Yuasa K, Nishiyama A, Kira J, Okada T, Takeda S. Transduction efficiency and immune response associated with the administration of AAV8 vector into dog skeletal muscle. *Mol Ther* 2009; 17: 73-80.

10. Wang Z, Kuhr CS, Allen JM, Blankinship M, Gregorevic P, Chamberlain JS, *et al*. Sustained AAV-mediated dystrophin expression in a canine model of Duchenne muscular dystrophy with a brief course of immunosuppression. *Mol Ther* 2007; 15: 1160-6.

11. Kornegay JN, Li J, Bogan JR, Bogan DJ, Chen C, Zheng H, *et al*. Widespread muscle expression of an AAV9 human mini-dystrophin vector after intravenous injection in neonatal dystrophin-deficient dogs. *Mol Ther* 2010; 18: 1501-8.

12. Koo T, Okada T, Athanasopoulos T, Foster H, Takeda S, Dickson G. Long-term functional adeno-associated virusmicrodystrophin expression in the dystrophic CXMDj dog. *J Gene Med* 2011; 13: 497-506.

13. Mendell JR, Campbell K, Rodino-Klapac L, Sahenk Z, Shilling C, Lewis S, *et al*. Dystrophin immunity in Duchenne's muscular dystrophy. *N Engl J Med* 2010; 363: 1429-37.

14. Ferrer A, Wells KE, Wells DJ. Immune responses to dystropin: implications for gene therapy of Duchenne muscular dystrophy. *Gene Ther* 2000; 7: 1439-46.

15. McPherron AC, Lawler AM, Lee SJ. Regulation of skeletal muscle mass in mice by a new TGF-beta superfamily member. *Nature* 1997; 387: 83-90.

16. Schuelke M, Wagner KR, Stolz LE, Hübner C, Riebel T, Kömen W, *et al.* Myostatin mutation associated with gross muscle hypertrophy in a child. *N Engl J Med* 2004; 350: 2682-8.

17. Joulia-Ekaza D, Cabello G. The myostatin gene: physiology and pharmacological relevance. *Curr Opin Pharmacol* 2007; 7: 310-5.

18. Kang JK, Malerba A, Popplewell L, Foster K, Dickson G. Antisense-induced myostatin exon skipping leads to muscle hypertrophy in mice following octa-guanidine morpholino oligomer treatment. *Mol Ther* 2011; 19: 159-64.

19. Kemaladewi DU, Hoogaars WM, van Heiningen SH, Terlouw S, de Gorter DJ, den Dunnen JT, *et al.* Dual exon skipping in myostatin and dystrophin for Duchenne muscular dystrophy. *BMC Med Genomics* 2011; 4: 36.

20. Bish LT, Sleeper MM, Forbes SC, Morine KJ, Reynolds C, Singletary GE, *et al.* Long-term systemic myostatin inhibition via liver-targeted gene transfer in Golden retriever muscular dystrophy. *Hum Gene Ther* 2011, August 30th (*online*).

21. Bish LT, Sleeper MM, Brainard B, Cole S, Russell N, Withnall E, *et al.* Adeno-associated virus (AAV) serotype 9 provides global cardiac gene transfer superior to AAV1, AAV6, AAV7, and AAV8 in the mouse and rat. *Hum Gene Ther* 2008; 19: 1359-68.

22. Gao G, Bish LT, Sleeper MM, Mu X, Sun L, Lou Y, *et al.* Transendocardial delivery of AAV6 results in highly efficient and global cardiac gene transfer in Rhesus macaques. *Hum Gene Ther* 2011; 22: 979-84.

23. Toromanoff A, Adjali O, Larcher T, Hill M, Guigand L, Chenuaud P, *et al.* Lack of immunotoxicity after regional intravenous (RI) delivery of rAAV to nonhuman primate skeletal muscle. *Mol Ther* 2010; 18: 151-60.

The CliniBook: Clinical gene transfer
Edited by Odile Cohen-Haguenauer – EDK, Paris © 2012, pp. 55-61

A1-5
AAV gene therapy for cardiovascular disorders

Serena Zacchigna, Mauro Giacca*

Molecular Medicine Laboratory, International Centre for Genetic Engineering and Biotechnology (ICGEB), Padriciano, 99, 34149 Trieste, Italy.
giacca@icgeb.org
* Corresponding author

Over the past few years, AAV vectors have engendered great interest as safe and effective tools for cardiovascular gene therapy. Indeed, AAV transduces both cardiac and skeletal myocytes at high efficiency with no apparent adverse effects and directs expression of its transgenes for very prolonged periods of time. In addition, novel serotypes are now available (AAV8, AAV9) with improved myocyte tropism. In light of these properties, AAV appears to be the vector of choice to both induce therapeutic angiogenesis and deliver genes of therapeutic value in patients with heart failure, including protein-coding genes and small regulatory RNAs.

This chapter describes the peculiar features of AAV and discusses the pre-clinical and clinical applications of AAV vectors in the cardiovascular field.

Despite remarkable progress made over recent decades in early diagnosis and prevention, cardiovascular disorders (CVD) still represent the leading cause of morbidity and mortality in the Western world and an emerging social problem in developing countries, accounting for roughly 30% of deaths worldwide (http://www.who.int/cardiovascular_diseases/en/). The absolute majority of these deaths are due to chronic diseases, such as ischemic heart disease (IHD) and stroke, which require safe and long lasting therapies, thereby determining a heavy sanitary, social and economic burden. Thus, the development of novel therapeutic strategies able to interfere with the mechanisms of the onset and progression of disease is absolutely warranted. The potential use of gene therapy appears particularly promising for a number of interventional applications in the CVD arena, which include therapy of non-graftable, non-dilatable, multivessel disease, heart failure, hyperlypidemia, genetic cardiomyopathies, and genetically-determined arrhythmias.

Unlike other viruses used as vectors for gene delivery, AAV represents an outstanding tool for cardiovascular gene therapy for the following reasons: (i) AAV vectors efficiently transduce post-mitotic tissues, including all kinds of muscle cells (skeletal muscle, smooth muscle cells and cardiomyocytes), where it drives transgene expression for prolonged periods of time [1]; (ii) AAV vectors do not express any viral protein and are, therefore, poorly immunogenic and inflammatory; it is currently unclear whether, in humans, pre-existing immunity against the virus might nonetheless determine the elimination of the transduced cells over the first weeks post-inoculation, as observed in the liver [2, 3]); (iii) AAV vectors do not integrate into the host cell genome but persist in an episomal form [4], thereby minimizing the problems of both insertional mutagenesis and gene silencing; (iv) AAV vectors can be generated at high titers and transduce cells at a high multiplicity, thus allowing the simultaneous expression of multiple genes from the same cells or tissues [5].

Taken together, these properties have encouraged the pre-clinical and clinical use of AAV vectors for several cardiovascular applications. *Figure 1* reports a schematic representation of the available histological, functional and molecular tools to study the effect of cardiac AAV transduction in rodents.

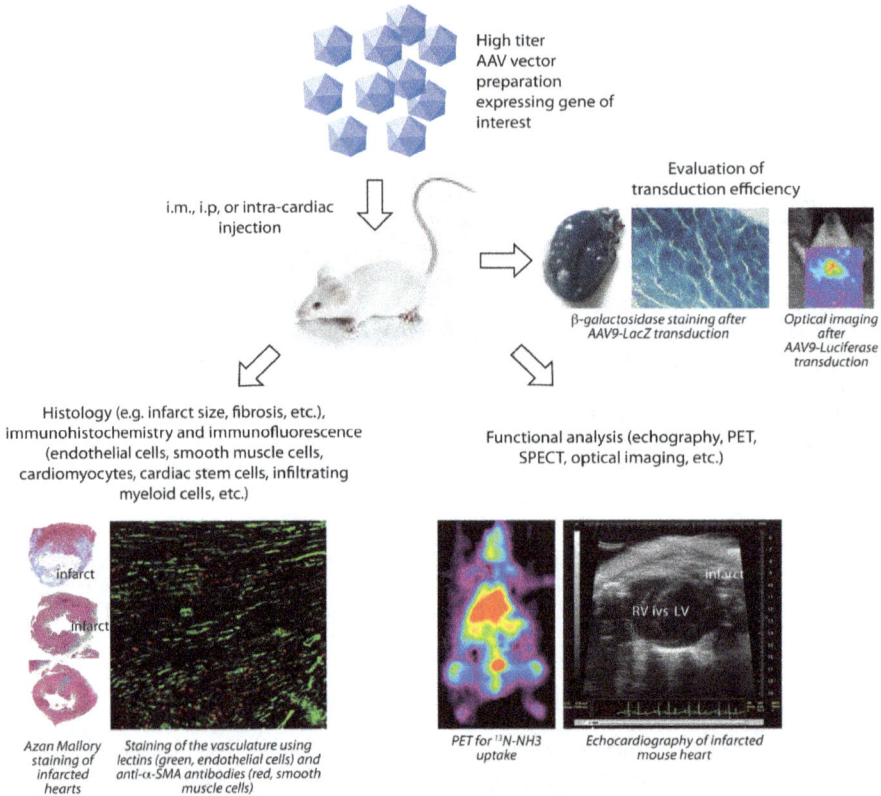

Figure 1. Cardiovascular applications of AAV vectors. The picture shows the available histological, functional and molecular tools to study the effect of cardiac AAV transduction.

AAV FOR THE INDUCTION OF THERAPEUTIC ANGIOGENESIS

One of the most promising strategies in the gene therapy field, which can find application in the treatment of patients with either coronary artery disease (CAD) or peripheral artery disease (PAD), is the delivery of factors able to stimulate new blood vessel formation [6]. Traditionally, the generation of a new vascular network in adult life is believed to occur essentially through capillary sprouting from pre-existing vessels in a process known as angiogenesis. After the identification of several powerful inducers of angiogenesis, such as VEGF (Vascular Endothelial Growth Factor [7]) and FGF (Fibroblast Growth Factor [8]) and the proof of concept of their efficacy in small and large animal models [9], various clinical trials have been undertaken to evaluate the effects of these factors when delivered to CAD and PAD patients as recombinant proteins, naked plasmid DNA or adenoviral vectors. Quite unexpectedly, and in contrast to the brilliant results obtained in the preclinical setting, these trials showed only modest efficacy in the treated patients. Irrespective of the therapeutic gene involved, it appears that the efficiency of gene transfer and the persistence of therapeutic gene expression represent the two major limitations that still hamper clinical success. On one hand, ischemic tissues are often desensitized to growth factor treatment and are thus refractory to short term treatment with recombinant proteins [10]; on the other hand, plasmid DNA delivery is simple and safe but its uptake by cardiac and muscle cells, although much higher than with most other cell types, is still poor and probably not sufficient to sustain the generation of a stable vasculature [10]; finally, adenoviral vectors are burdened with several problems, mainly due to their strong immunogenicity and induction of a strong inflammatory response [11]. Based on these considerations, the viral vector system that appears most suitable for the successful induction of therapeutic angiogenesis is AAV. Over the last few years, more than 100 AAV variants have been isolated from human and non-human primates, some of which show even higher transduction of skeletal muscle (AAV1 and AAV6) and heart (AAV8 and AAV9) than the prototype AAV2 [12]. The AAV-mediated expression of various pro-angiogenic proteins, including different VEGF isoforms and/or other cytokines involved in angiogenesis, on one hand has significantly contributed to a deeper understanding of the molecular mechanisms controlling vessel growth [13, 14], while on the other has resulted in the successful generation of a novel vascular network in different animal models of tissue ischemia [5, 15, 16]. Based on these considerations, although no clinical trials have been initiated as yet, it might be reasonably expected that AAVs will play a central role in clinical experimentation for the induction of therapeutic angiogenesis in the near future.

AAV FOR HEART FAILURE

The term heart failure (HF) refers to a clinical syndrome, occurring when the heart is unable to pump sufficient blood to meet the metabolic requirement of the organism. Despite recent progress in the evaluation and management of HF, prognosis is still poor and more than 60% of affected patients die within 5 years from diagnosis [17]. Recent advances in understanding the molecular correlates of cardiac contraction in given physiological and pathological conditions has paved the way to novel intervention strategies based on gene therapy. Essentially, most approaches attempted so far have aimed at normalizing either the Ca^{2+} cycle or the levels of β-adrenergic stimulation of cardiomyocytes. More specifically, altering the levels or activity of the Ca^{2+} pump SERCA2a and/or of its inhibitor, phospholamban, to restore disturbed Ca^{2+} uptake into the sarcoplasmic reticulum, currently appears as a promising therapeutic strategy for HF [18]. Experimental evidence in hypertensive rats and failing hearts in larger animals have shown that SERCA2a overexpression using AAV vectors significantly improves cardiac function [19]. Based on these results, clinical trials have recently been started using either AAV6 or AAV1 [20]. These represent the first gene therapy trials for HF and their preliminary results indicate safety in the transduction procedure and marginal improvement of heart function, resulting in clinical benefit for approximately half of all patients with HF [21, 22].

AAV FOR THE PREVENTION OF ARTERIAL RESTENOSIS

One of the major achievements in the treatment of CAD patients is percutaneous coronary intervention (PCI), consisting in the introduction of a catheter with a deflated balloon at its extremity, into a stenotic coronary artery, followed by balloon inflation to mechanically dilate the vessel and restore blood perfusion. Despite the great success of this procedure, a significant percentage of cases, up to 40% in some anatomical districts, develop stenosis during the first 6 months following intervention, due to a hyperplastic response of the smooth muscle cells (SMC) of the tunica media [23]. Efficiency of gene therapy to prevent restenosis has been extensively proven in several animal models, in which SMC hyperplasia can be experimentally induced [24]. In these models, the AAV-mediated delivery of genes able to control SMC proliferation and migration, either alone or in combination, has resulted in a significant reduction of the arterial wall thickening, thus preserving vessel function [25, 26]. Progression of this clinical experimentation towards clinical application, however, is compared with the relative efficacy of drug eluting stents, which offer obvious advantages over gene therapy in terms of production, storage and utilization.

AAV FOR CARDIAC ARRHYTHMIA

Cardiac disease is frequently associated with abnormalities in electrical function that can severely impair cardiac performance with potentially fatal consequences. To date, gene therapy research strategies at the preclinical level have targeted three major classes of cardiac arrhythmias: ventricular arrhythmias, atrial fibrillation and bradyarrhythmias, using various vehicles for gene transfer [27]. In this context, AAV-mediated gene delivery has emerged as the preferred choice to achieve long-term gene expression. For instance, the delivery of an AAV vector encoding the voltage-gated potassium channel Kv1.5 has led to the significant restitution of repolarizing currents, and to the partial normalization of the main electrical abnormalities of the long QT syndrome (such as prolongation of the action potential duration and early after-depolarization) in a murine model of the disease [28]. Progression to clinical application will depend on the eventual success of further experimentation in larger models of human disease.

AAV FOR HYPERLIPIDEMIA

The intramuscular injection of AAV vectors has recently been proposed as a potentially safe, minimally invasive procedure for the long-term gene expression of circulating antiatherogenic proteins. For instance, the human apolipoprotein E3 (apoE3) has multiple atheroprotective properties, including receptor-mediated clearance of remnant lipoproteins and diverse lipid-independent antiatherogenic actions at the vessel wall [29]; apoE-deficient ($apoE^{-/-}$) mice develop severe hypercholesterolemia and atherosclerosis. Initial reports of gene transfer using apoE3-expressing adenoviral vectors have shown significant but transient correction of hyperlipidemia, due to the immune clearance of transduced hepatocytes [30], and have prompted studies using alternative recombinant vectors. Also in this case, AAVs, which are nonpathogenic and elicit a relatively muted host response, appear to offer the best potential for lasting transgene expression. Recent experimental evidence indicates that AAV7 and AAV8 efficiently transduce mouse skeletal muscle to deliver microgram quantities of antiatherogenic human apoE3 protein into the circulation [31].

AAV FOR GENETIC CARDIOMYOPATHIES

Cardiomyopathies represent a major cause of morbidity and mortality in both children and adults, currently offering poor therapeutic options. The availability of small and large animal models for the major forms of inherited cardiomyopathy (hypertrophic cardiomyopathy, arrhythmogenic right ventricular cardiomyopathy and dilated cardiomyopathy), as well as for various forms associated to muscular dystrophies, clearly indicates that AAV may be the ideal vector for the treatment of these diseases. Experimental evidence in large animals has shown that the AAV-mediated correction of the abnormal metabolic processes that occur in heart failure (*e.g.* altered calcium metabolism, apoptosis) could normalize the failing myocardial function also in these conditions [27].

In closing, it is worth mentioning that, despite the high efficacy of AAV to transduce cardiomyocytes and skeletal muscle fibers *in vivo*, several unknown factors still limit its even more effective and broader application. In particular, the exquisite tropism of this virus for post-mitotic cells is not yet completely understood [32]. The elucidation of the molecular pathways regulating virus internalization, processing and persistence in the target cells will undoubtedly permit the future development of vectors with improved targeting, tropism and intracellular processing.

ACKNOWLEDGMENTS

This work has been performed with the support of the EC-DG research through the FP6-Network of Excellence, CLINIGENE: LSHB-CT-2006-018933.

REFERENCES

1. Favre D, Provost N, Blouin V, Blancho G, Cherel Y, Salvetti A, Moullier P. Immediate and long-term safety of recombinant adeno-associated virus injection into the nonhuman primate muscle. *Mol Ther* 2001; 4: 559-66.

2. Mingozzi F, High KA. Immune responses to AAV in clinical trials. *Curr Gene Ther* 2011; 11: 321-30.

3. Mingozzi F, High KA. Therapeutic *in vivo* gene transfer for genetic disease using AAV: progress and challenges. *Nat Rev Genet* 2011; 12: 341-55.

4. Schnepp BC, Jensen RL, Chen CL, Johnson PR, Clark KR. Characterization of adeno-associated virus genomes isolated from human tissues. *J Virol* 2005; 79: 14793-803.

5. Arsic N, Zentilin L, Zacchigna S, Santoro D, Stanta G, Salvi S, *et al*. Induction of functional neovascularization by combined VEGF and angiopoietin-1 gene transfer using AAV vectors. *Mol Ther* 2003; 7: 450-9.

6. Carmeliet P, Jain RK. Molecular mechanisms and clinical applications of angiogenesis. *Nature* 2011; 473: 298-307.

7. Carmeliet P, Ng YS, Nuyens D, Theilmeier G, Brusselmans K, Cornelissen I, *et al*. Impaired myocardial angiogenesis and ischemic cardiomyopathy in mice lacking the vascular endothelial growth factor isoforms VEGF164 and VEGF188. *Nat Med* 1999; 5: 495-502.

8. Yanagisawa-Miwa A, Uchida Y, Nakamura F, Tomaru T, Kido H, Kamijo T, *et al*. Salvage of infarcted myocardium by angiogenic action of basic fibroblast growth factor. *Science* 1992; 257: 1401-3.

9. Ylä-Herttuala S, Martin JF. Cardiovascular gene therapy. *Lancet* 2000; 355: 213-22.

10. Rissanen TT, Yla-Herttuala S. Current status of cardiovascular gene therapy. *Mol Ther* 2007; 15: 1233-47.

11. Yang Y, Haecker SE, Su Q, Wilson JM. Immunology of gene therapy with adenoviral vectors in mouse skeletal muscle. *Hum Mol Genet* 1996; 5: 1703-12.

12. Wu Z, Asokan A, Samulski RJ. Adeno-associated virus serotypes: vector toolkit for human gene therapy. *Mol Ther* 2006; 14: 316-27.

13. Tafuro S, Ayuso E, Zacchigna S, Zentilin L, Moimas S, Dore F, Giacca M. Inducible adeno-associated virus vectors promote functional angiogenesis in adult organisms via regulated vascular endothelial growth factor expression. *Cardiovasc Res* 2009; 83: 663-71.

14. Zacchigna S, Pattarini L, Zentilin L, Moimas S, Carrer A, Sinigaglia M, *et al.* Bone marrow cells recruited through the Neuropilin-1 receptor promote arterial formation at the sites of adult neoangiogenesis. *J Clin Invest* 2008; 118: 2062-75.

15. Deodato B, Arsic N, Zentilin L, Galeano M, Santoro D, Torre V, *et al.* Recombinant AAV vector encoding human VEGF165 enhances wound healing. *Gene Ther* 2002; 9: 777-85.

16. Ferrarini M, Arsic N, Recchia FA, Zentilin L, Zacchigna S, Xu X, *et al.* Adeno-associated virus-mediated transduction of VEGF165 improves cardiac tissue viability and functional recovery after permanent coronary occlusion in conscious dogs. *Circ Res* 2006; 98: 954-61.

17. Krum H, Teerlink JR. Medical therapy for chronic heart failure. *Lancet* 2011; 378: 713-21.

18. Hajjar RJ, Schmidt U, Matsui T, Guerrero JL, Lee KH, Gwathmey JK, *et al.* Modulation of ventricular function through gene transfer *in vivo*. *Proc Natl Acad Sci USA* 1998; 95: 5251-6.

19. Miyamoto MI, del Monte F, Schmidt U, DiSalvo TS, Kang ZB, Matsui T, *et al.* Adenoviral gene transfer of SERCA2a improves left-ventricular function in aortic-banded rats in transition to heart failure. *Proc Natl Acad Sci USA* 2000; 97: 793-8.

20. Jessup M, Greenberg B, Mancini D, Cappola T, Pauly DF, Jaski B, *et al.* Calcium upregulation by percutaneous administration of gene therapy in cardiac disease (CUPID): a phase 2 trial of intracoronary gene therapy of sarcoplasmic reticulum Ca^{2+}-ATPase in patients with advanced heart failure. *Circulation* 2011; 124: 304-13.

21. Mearns BM. Gene therapy: can CUPID rescue the broken hearted? *Nat Rev Cardiol* 2011; 8: 481.

22. Giacca M, Baker AH. Heartening results: the CUPID gene therapy trial for heart failure. *Mol Ther* 2011; 19: 1181-2.

23. Chang MW, Barr E, Seltzer J, Jiang YQ, Nabel GJ, Nabel EG, *et al.* Cytostatic gene therapy for vascular proliferative disorders with a constitutively active form of the retinoblastoma gene product. *Science* 1995; 267: 518-22.

24. Isner JM, Walsh K, Rosenfield K, Schainfeld R, Asahara T, Hogan K, Pieczek A. Arterial gene therapy for restenosis. *Hum Gene Ther* 1996; 7: 989-1011.

25. Ramirez-Correa GA, Zacchigna S, Arsic N, Zentilin L, Salvi A, Sinagra G, Giacca M. Potent inhibition of arterial intimal hyperplasia by Timp-1 gene transfer using AAV vectors. *Mol Ther* 2004; 9: 876-84.

26. Camozzi M, Zacchigna S, Rusnati M, Coltrini D, Ramirez-Correa G, Bottazzi B, *et al.* Pentraxin 3 inhibits fibroblast growth factor 2-dependent activation of smooth muscle cells *in vitro* and neointima formation *in vivo*. *Arterioscler Thromb Vasc Biol* 2005; 25: 1837-42.

27. Greener I, Donahue JK. Gene therapy strategies for cardiac electrical dysfunction. *J Mol Cell Cardiol* 2011; 50: 759-65.

28. Kodirov SA, Brunner M, Busconi L, Koren G. Long-term restitution of 4-aminopyridine-sensitive currents in Kv1DN ventricular myocytes using adeno-associated virus-mediated delivery of Kv1.5. *FEBS Lett* 2003; 550: 74-8.

29. Harris JD, Evans V, Owen JS. ApoE gene therapy to treat hyperlipidemia and atherosclerosis. *Curr Opin Mol Ther* 2006; 8: 275-87.

30. Stevenson SC, Marshall-Neff J, Teng B, Lee CB, Roy S, McClelland A. Phenotypic correction of hypercholesterolemia in apoE-deficient mice by adenovirus-mediated *in vivo* gene transfer. *Arterioscler Thromb Vasc Biol* 1995; 15: 479-84.

31. Evans VC, Graham IR, Athanasopoulos T, Galley DJ, Jackson CL, Simons JP, *et al*. Adeno-associated virus serotypes 7 and 8 outperform serotype 9 in expressing atheroprotective human apoE3 from mouse skeletal muscle. *Metabolism* 2010; 60: 491-8.

32. Zentilin L, Giacca M. Adeno-associated virus vectors: versatile tools for *in vivo* gene transfer. *Contrib Nephrol* 2008; 159: 63-77.

The CliniBook: Clinical gene transfer
Edited by Odile Cohen-Haguenauer – EDK, Paris © 2012, pp. 62-70

A1-6
AAV gene therapy for diabetes mellitus

Eduard Ayuso, Veronica Jimenez, David Callejas, Christopher Mann,
Fatima Bosch*

Center of Animal Biotechnology and Gene Therapy and Department of Biochemistry and Molecular Biology, School of Veterinary Medicine, Universitat Autònoma de Barcelona, 08193-Bellaterra, and CIBER de Diabetes y Enfermedades Metabólicas Asociadas (CIBERDEM), Spain.
*Corresponding author:
Center of Animal Biotechnology and Gene Therapy, Edifici H, Universitat Autònoma de Barcelona, 08193 Bellaterra, Spain.
fatima.bosch@uab.es

INTRODUCTION

Diabetes has reached epidemic proportions, with an estimated 55 million people affected in Europe and over 30 million in the 27 EU states. The health costs of diabetes are unsustainable. The two main forms of diabetes mellitus are type 1 (T1D) and type 2 (T2D) [1]. T1D is characterized by a severe lack of insulin production due to the specific destruction of pancreatic β-cells. β-cell loss in T1D is the result of an autoimmune mediated process, where a chronic inflammation called insulitis causes β-cell destruction [2, 3]. T2D results from the reduced ability of the pancreatic β-cells to secrete enough insulin to stimulate glucose utilization by peripheral tissues. As β-cell secretory capacity deteriorates, glucose tolerance worsens and fasting glucose levels progressively increase, eventually culminating in overt hyperglycemia [4]. Defects in both insulin secretion and action contribute to the pathogenesis of T2D, but it is now recognized that insulin deficiency is the crucial constituent, without which T2D does not develop. T1D and T2D are a major cause of morbidity and mortality, decreasing both life quality and life expectancy of millions of affected individuals. Diabetes is a considerable cause of premature mortality, a situation that is likely to worsen, particularly in low- and middle-income countries as diabetes prevalence increases [5]. Investments in developing new and more effective therapies are urgently required to reduce this burden.

T1D is diagnosed when the autoimmune-mediated β-cell destruction is almost complete and patients need insulin-replacement therapy to survive. However, even with insulin-replacement therapy, glycemia is not always properly regulated, and chronic hyperglycemia leads to severe microvascular (retinopathy and nephropathy), macrovascular (stroke, myocardial infarction), and neurological complications. These devastating complications might be prevented by normalization of blood glucose levels. T2D is now becoming manifested in increasingly younger individuals and is caused by the combination of insulin resistance and inadequate insulin secretion. Initially, T2D is treated with oral hypoglycemic agents, typically with adjunct insulin therapy at a later stage of the disease. The distinction between T1D and T2D becomes more difficult in older age groups since patients with T2D may receive insulin therapy [6].

T1D is one of the most common endocrine and metabolic conditions in childhood; its incidence is rapidly increasing, especially among young children. Lifelong insulin treatment is the therapy of choice for T1D. While lifelong treatment with exogenous insulin successfully manages diabetes, correct maintenance of a normoglycemic state can be challenging, exposing diabetic patients to life threatening hypoglycemia and long-term complications of hyperglycemia.

TREATMENTS FOR T1D

The reduction of hyperglycemia and maintenance of normoglycemia is a goal of any therapeutic approach to T1D. The current therapy for most diabetic patients is based on regular subcutaneous injections of mixtures of soluble (short-acting) insulin and lente (long-acting) insulin preparations. Suspensions of soluble insulin particles of different size that give intermediate acting and long-acting components with more sustained action profiles are administered to achieve a constant basal level of the hormone [7]. However, one of the major deficiencies of delayed-action insulin is the variable absorption from subcutaneous tissue [8], mainly because the formulation is a suspension. Moreover, the delayed-action preparations do not generally produce smooth background levels of insulin, resulting in either hyperglycemia or hypoglycemia. Intensive insulin therapy (three or more daily injections) can delay the onset and slow the progression of retinopathy, nephropathy, and neuropathy in T1D patients [9]. However, this kind of treatment is not suitable for all diabetic patients, especially the very young or the old. In addition, patients under intensive insulin treatment present a high risk for hypoglycemia; which is a serious complication that could be lethal. Hypoglycemia is caused by inappropriately raised insulin concentrations or enhanced insulin effect, because of excessive insulin dosage, increased bioavailability, increased sensitivity, and/or inadequate carbohydrate intake [10, 11]. To optimize this dosage, there are insulin pumps which in advanced forms may be controlled directly by a continuous glucose monitor to avoid hypoglycaemia [12].

Alternative approaches to maintain normoglycemia are cell-based therapies that involves transplantation of pancreatic islets or β-cells mainly from cadaveric donors. While some clinical success has been achieved with this approach, particularly with the Edmonton protocol [13, 14], there are still considerable obstacles to be overcome before these strategies will achieve widespread clinical acceptance and improved long-lasting efficacy. In particular, transplanted patients must receive life-long immunosuppression to avoid graft rejection, while the existing autoimmunity may contribute to diminished graft survival or limit the effectiveness of this treatment approach to only a few years at most [15]. As a possible solution to the limited availability of human islets, pig islets may offer an abundant source of tissue and encapsulated islets have been xenotransplanted to non-human primates and, recently, to humans [16, 17]. However, in addition to the lack of long-term efficacy in terms of insulin production and the obvious safety concerns related to the use of non-human tissues that may carry unknown infectious diseases, the use of pig islets actually faces both difficulties with regulatory approval and general public aversion. Stem cell-based technologies have emerged in recent years as a possible approach to treat diabetes; besides issues related to the underlying autoimmune disease, which may require lifelong immunosuppression, the safety and efficacy of these novel technologies needs further assessment (reviewed in [18-21]). To maintain normoglycemia, studies have also focused on the use of surrogate non-β-cells to deliver insulin [22, 23]. These approaches are aimed at lowering blood glucose by delivering insulin under the control of glucose-responsive promoters [24, 25]. However, the slow transcriptional control by glucose delays the insulin secretory response, which may lead to hyperglycemia immediately after meals and to hypoglycemia several hours later. To some extent, this can be circumvented by the use of cells that process and store insulin, such as gut K cells [26], or by inducing β-cell neogenesis in the liver by the expression of key transcription factors involved in the differentiation of pancreatic β cells, such as Pancreatic duodenal homeobox-1 (Pdx-1), NeuroD and Neurogenin-3 (Ngn3) [27-29]. Feasibility, safety, and long-term efficacy of these strategies warrants more studies. While research and clinical efforts are needed to improve existing therapeutic strategies, it is clear that there is a considerable need for new alternative approaches for the treatment of T1D. Notably, gene therapy would offer the potential advantage of a single viral vector administration, which could ideally provide the necessary treatment through the lifetime of the diabetic subject.

ENGINEERING SKELETAL MUSCLE TO INCREASE GLUCOSE UPTAKE

Skeletal muscle is the most important site of glucose removal from blood, accounting for about 70% of glucose disposal after a meal. In addition, skeletal muscle is an excellent target tissue for gene transfer because of its accessibility and its capacity to secrete proteins. Glucose utilization by skeletal muscle is controlled by insulin-stimulated glucose transport through GLUT4 [30] and its phosphorylation by hexokinase II (HK-II) [31]. HK-II has a low K_m for glucose and is inhibited by glucose-6-phosphate, which limits glucose uptake. During diabetes, because of the lack of insulin, GLUT4 translocation to the plasma membrane and HKII mRNA levels and activity decrease [32, 33]. Expression of basal levels of insulin in skeletal muscle of transgenic mice increases glucose uptake [34]. When diabetic, these mice are normoglycemic during fasting but remain hyperglycemic in fed conditions [34]. To reduce diabetic hyperglycemia, the hepatic glucose phosphorylating enzyme glucokinase (Gck) has also been expressed in skeletal muscle [35]. In contrast to HK-II, Gck has a high K_m for glucose (about 8mM), it is not inhibited by glucose 6-phosphate, and it shows kinetic cooperativity with glucose [31]. These features allow glucose to be taken up only when it is at high concentrations, as already reported in pancreatic β-cells [36]. Expression of Gck in skeletal muscle increases glucose disposal and reduces diabetic hyperglycemia [35, 37, 38]. However, expression of Gck alone cannot normalize glycemia in type 1 diabetes because of the lack of insulin-mediated glucose transport. To this end, we have found that the expression of Gck in skeletal muscle of fed diabetic transgenic mice in conjunction with the administration of low doses of soluble, short acting, insulin leads to the normalization of glycemia [35]. Altogether these results suggest that basal production of insulin by genetically engineered skeletal muscle allow to maintain normoglycemia between meals. After feeding, blood glucose levels rise and the expression of Gck might be used to increase glucose utilization and normalization of glycemia. Thus, we have shown that co-expression of Gck and insulin in skeletal muscle of double transgenic mice reverts diabetic alterations [39], indicating that an approach of this kind might be useful to treat T1D.

To develop a gene therapy approach based on this strategy an efficient and safe method for gene transfer to skeletal muscle is required. Adeno-associated virus (AAV)-based vectors are one of the preferred tools for gene transfer. The high transduction efficiency *in vivo* in a variety of post-mitotic tissues and the relatively low immunogenicity contributed to the AAV vectors use in a variety of preclinical studies [40]. Translation of preclinical results into the clinical arena resulted in promising results, confirming the ability of AAV vectors to safely transduce liver, muscle, and neurological tissue in humans [41-43]. Importantly, several groups showed that a single administration of AAV vectors leads to long-term expression of the transgene product [44, 45]. Among the repertoire of AAV serotypes, AAV1 is probably the most efficient vector for transduction of skeletal muscle by direct injection and human clinical trials have shown that this vector is safe and transgene expression could persist a long time after the administration [43].

We used AAV1 vectors to co-express Gck and insulin genes into skeletal muscle of diabetic mice. These mice restored and maintained normoglycemia in fed and fasted conditions for >4 months after STZ administration [39]. Insulin and Gck treated mice also showed increased skeletal muscle glucose uptake, normalization of liver glucose metabolism (increased glucose uptake and glycogen synthesis and reduced hepatic glucose production) and improved glucose tolerance. Moreover, these mice presented with normal food and fluid intake and normalisation of abdominal fat pad and skeletal muscle weights [39]. These results suggest that secretion of basal levels of insulin, in conjunction with increased glucose uptake by the skeletal muscle, permit a tight regulation of glycemia [39]. As a step towards the development of clinical trials in patients, a pre-clinical study in diabetic dogs is undergoing. Feasibility, efficacy, duration of effects as well as biochemical and safety issues are under investigation. Circulating levels of human C-peptide were detected for several years after a single intramuscular injection of AAV1 vectors expressing human insulin. Moreover, dogs treated with the combination of insulin and Gck vastly improved ability to dispose of glucose suggesting the concerted action of both genes. Although further studies are required, these preliminary results suggest that engineering skeletal muscle to produce insulin and glucokinase may be a potential therapy for the treatment of T1D.

ENGINEERING THE PANCREAS FOR THE TREATMENT AND PREVENTION OF DIABETES MELLITUS

Genetic engineering of skeletal muscle to produce insulin and increase glucose uptake could be considered as a treatment but not as a cure for T1D. To develop a curative therapy it will be necessary to target the primary affected organ in T1D, that is the pancreas. Despite the progress in *in vivo* tissue engineering, effective gene transfer to the pancreas has remained challenging due to its anatomic location and complex structure, with the risk of pancreatitis being of serious concern. In the past years, viral and non-viral mediated approaches have been tested for targeting the pancreas with different outcomes. Systemic administration of DNA-phospholipid gas-filled microbubbles in combination with ultrasound technology achieved short-term transduction of rat beta cells [46]. However, this technology is not broadly available and difficult to manage. Systemic delivery of adenoviral (Ad) vectors fail to transduce the pancreas, however, when these vectors are delivered either by direct pancreatic injection or through the pancreatic duct transduction of exocrine and few endocrine cells was observed [47, 48]. In contrast, the systemic delivery of Ad vectors under clamped hepatic circulation described by our laboratory resulted in preferential transduction of beta cells in mice [49]. Similarly, transduction of endocrine, but also exocrine, pancreas was observed after injection of Ad vectors into pancreatic vessels of healthy and diabetic dogs [50]. Nevertheless, transgene expression was transient due to the inherent immunogenicity of first-generation Ad vectors. Lentiviral vectors (LV) mediate long-term transgene expression because of their ability to integrate into the host genome. LV delivered intraductally were shown to be able to transduce ductal and acinar cells, but only a minimal percentage of endocrine cells [51, 52]. Conversely, AAV vectors have been described to be more efficient than adenoviral and lentiviral vector in transducing the pancreas [47, 53]. Single stranded AAV (ssAAV) vectors of serotype 8 and 9 (AAV8 and AAV9) have shown modest transduction of exocrine and endocrine pancreas when delivered systemically [54, 55], intrapancreatically [47, 53], intraductally [56] or through the intrapancreatic vessels [57]. Interestingly, double stranded AAV (dsAAV) of serotypes 6 and 8 resulted in higher beta cell transduction compared to ssAAV [58]. However, a major restriction to the use of dsAAV is their very low cloning capacity of no more than 2.2kb and difficulties in vector generation, which preclude transfer of many genes of interest to the pancreas. We performed a detailed comparative study of several serotypes of ssAAV to transfer genes to the pancreas *in vivo*. Our results demonstrated that intraductal delivery of ssAAV vectors of serotypes 6, 8 and 9 led to highly efficient and long-term transduction of beta cells (*Figure 1*), with AAV6 and AAV8 showing the highest efficiency [59]. However, alpha cells were poorly transduced. Acinar cells were transduced by the three serotypes tested and ductal cells only by AAV6. In addition, intraductal delivery resulted in higher AAV-mediated transduction of the pancreas than did systemic administration. We also assayed a gene therapy approach to prevent T1D in an autoimmune murine model of the disease based on this technology. Intraductal delivery of AAV9 vectors encoding for the beta cell anti-apoptotic and mitogenic hepatocyte growth factor (HGF) preserved beta cell mass, diminished lymphocytic infiltration of the islets and protected mice from autoimmune diabetes [59]. Similarly, others have shown that delivery of GLP-1, IL-4 and CCL-22 to murine beta-cells by using dsAAV8 protects against the development of diabetes [60, 61].

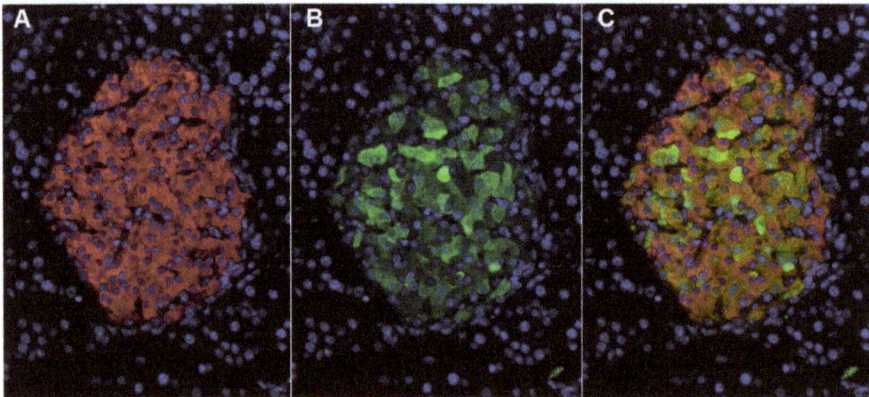

Figure 1. Transduction of beta cells by AAV vectors delivered intraductally. Immunohistochemical analysis of insulin (A), GFP (B) and merged (C) in islets of mice injected intraductally with 3×10^{12}vg of AAV8 encoding the GFP reporter gene driven by the CAG ubiquitous promoter. Animals were analysed 1 month after injection. Original magnification 400x.

Altogether these data demonstrate the value of AAV vectors as a tool for genetic engineering of the pancreas for both the study of islet physiopathology and the assessment of new gene therapy approaches for diabetes.

CONCLUSIONS AND PERSPECTIVES

AAV-mediated genetic engineering of tissues constitute a novel approach to treat T1D. In mice and dogs we demonstrated that co-expression of insulin together with glucokinase in skeletal muscle resulted in normalization of glycemia in diabetic animals. Although further studies are required to assess the safety of the approach, our data open novel possibilities for developing a long-term therapy based on a single administration of the vectors.

On the other hand, preliminary results in mice demonstrated that direct intervention into the pancreas might be useful to prevent and, eventually, treat the disease. Although these strategies are still far from the bedside, the retrograde pancreatic intraductal injection could potentially be adapted to humans through a minimally invasive clinical procedure called endoscopic retrograde cholangiopancreatography [62]. The conjunction of both increasing number of encouraging preclinical studies in animals, together with the positive results obtained with AAV in the clinic, indicate that gene therapy for diabetes is likely to reach the clinical phase in the coming years.

ACKNOWLEDGEMENTS

Work in our laboratory relevant to this review was supported by grants from Ministerio de Ciencia e Innovación, Plan Nacional I+D+I (SAF2008-00962) and Generalitat de Catalunya (2009 SGR-224), Spain, and from European Commission DG Research FP6-Network of Excellence, CLINIGENE, LSHB-CT-2006-018933.

REFERENCES

1. Report of the expert committee on the diagnosis and classification of diabetes mellitus. *Diabetes Care* 1997; 20: 1183-97.

2. Eizirik DL, Mandrup-Poulsen T. A choice of death: the signal-transduction of immune-mediated beta-cell apoptosis. *Diabetologia* 2001; 44: 2115-33.

3. Mathis D, Vence L, Benoist C. Beta-cell death during progression to diabetes. *Nature* 2001; 414: 792-8.

4. Kahn SE, Hull RL, Utzschneider KM. Mechanisms linking obesity to insulin resistance and type 2 diabetes. *Nature* 2006; 444: 840-6.

5. Roglic G, Unwin N. Mortality attributable to diabetes: estimates for the year 2010. *Diabetes Res Clin Pract* 2009; 87: 15-9.

6. Diabetes Atlas, 4th edition. International Diabetes Federation, 2009.

7. Heine RJ, Bilo HJ, Sikkenk AC, van der Veen EA. Mixing short and intermediate acting insulins in the syringe: effect on postprandial blood glucose concentrations in type I diabetics. *Br Med J (Clin Res Ed)* 1985; 290: 204-5.

8. Binder C, Lauritzen T, Faber O, Pramming S. Insulin pharmacokinetics. *Diabetes Care* 1984; 7: 188-99.

9. The Diabetes Control and Complications Trial Research Group. The effect of intensive treatment of diabetes on the development and progression of long-term complications in insulin-dependent diabetes mellitus. *N Engl J Med* 1993; 329: 977-86.

10. Cryer PE. Hypoglycemia risk reduction in type 1 diabetes. *Exp Clin Endocrinol Diabetes* 2001; 109 (suppl 2): S412-23.

11. Cryer PE. Hypoglycaemia: the limiting factor in the glycaemic management of Type I and Type II diabetes. *Diabetologia* 2002; 45: 937-48.

12. Choudhary P, Amiel SA. The use of technology to reduce hypoglycemia. *Pediatr Endocrinol Rev* 2010; 7 (suppl 3): 384-95.

13. Correa-Giannella ML, Raposo do Amaral AS. Pancreatic islet transplantation. *Diabetol Metab Syndr* 2009; 1: 9.

14. Shapiro AM, Lakey JR, Ryan EA, Korbutt GS, Toth E, Warnock GL, *et al*. Islet transplantation in seven patients with type 1 diabetes mellitus using a glucocorticoid-free immunosuppressive regimen. *N Engl J Med* 2000; 343: 230-8.

15. Ryan EA, Paty BW, Senior PA, Bigam D, Alfadhli E, Kneteman NM, *et al*. Five-year follow-up after clinical islet transplantation. *Diabetes* 2005; 54: 2060-9.

16. Elliott RB, Escobar L, Tan PL, Muzina M, Zwain S, Buchanan C. Live encapsulated porcine islets from a type 1 diabetic patient 9.5 yr after xenotransplantation. *Xenotransplantation* 2007; 14: 157-61.

17. Hering BJ, Walawalkar N. Pig-to-nonhuman primate islet xenotransplantation. *Transpl Immunol* 2009; 21: 81-6.

18. Aguayo-Mazzucato C, Bonner-Weir S. Stem cell therapy for type 1 diabetes mellitus. *Nat Rev Endocrinol* 2010; 6: 139-48.

19. Champeris Tsaniras S, Jones PM. Generating pancreatic beta-cells from embryonic stem cells by manipulating signaling pathways. *J Endocrinol* 2010; 206: 13-26.

20. Tateishi K, He J, Taranova O, Liang G, D'Alessio AC, Zhang Y. Generation of insulin-secreting islet-like clusters from human skin fibroblasts. *J Biol Chem* 2008; 283: 31601-7.

21. Maehr R, Chen S, Snitow M, Ludwig T, Yagasaki L, Goland R, *et al*. Generation of pluripotent stem cells from patients with type 1 diabetes. *Proc Natl Acad Sci USA* 2009; 106: 15768-73.

22. Trucco M. Regeneration of the pancreatic beta cell. *J Clin Invest* 2005; 115: 5-12.

23. Dong H, Woo SL. Hepatic insulin production for type 1 diabetes. *Trends Endocrinol Metab* 2001; 12: 441-6.

24. Won JC, Rhee BD, Ko KS. Glucose-responsive gene expression system for gene therapy. *Adv Drug Deliv Rev* 2009; 61: 633-40.

25. Han J, McLane B, Kim EH, Yoon JW, Jun HS. Remission of diabetes by insulin gene therapy using a hepatocyte-specific and glucose-responsive synthetic promoter. *Mol Ther* 2011; 19: 470-8.

26. Cheung AT, Dayanandan B, Lewis JT, Korbutt GS, Rajotte RV, Bryer-Ash M, *et al*. Glucose-dependent insulin release from genetically engineered K cells. *Science* 2000; 290: 1959-62.

27. Ferber S, Halkin A, Cohen H, Ber I, Einav Y, Goldberg I, *et al*. Pancreatic and duodenal homeobox gene 1 induces expression of insulin genes in liver and ameliorates streptozotocin-induced hyperglycemia. *Nat Med* 2000; 6: 568-72.

28. Kojima H, Fujimiya M, Matsumura K, Younan P, Imaeda H, Maeda M, Chan L. NeuroD-beta-cellulin gene therapy induces islet neogenesis in the liver and reverses diabetes in mice. *Nat Med* 2003; 9: 596-603.

29. Yechoor V, Liu V, Espiritu C, Paul A, Oka K, Kojima H, Chan, L. Neurogenin3 is sufficient for transdetermination of hepatic progenitor cells into neo-islets *in vivo* but not transdifferentiation of hepatocytes. *Dev Cell* 2009; 16: 358-73.

30. Kahn BB. Lilly lecture 1995. Glucose transport: pivotal step in insulin action. *Diabetes* 1996; 45: 1644-54.

31. Printz RL, Magnuson MA, Granner DK. Mammalian glucokinase. *Annu Rev Nutr* 1993; 13: 463-96.

32. Postic C, Leturque A, Printz RL, Maulard P, Loizeau M, Granner DK, Girard J. Development and regulation of glucose transporter and hexokinase expression in rat. *Am J Physiol* 1994; 266: E548-59.

33. Printz RL, Koch S, Potter LR, O'Doherty RM, Tiesinga JJ, Moritz S, Granner DK. Hexokinase II mRNA and gene structure, regulation by insulin, and evolution. *J Biol Chem* 1993; 268: 5209-19.

34. Riu E, Mas A, Ferre T, Pujol A, Gros L, Otaegui P, *et al*. Counteraction of type 1 diabetic alterations by engineering skeletal muscle to produce insulin: insights from transgenic mice. *Diabetes* 2002; 51: 704-11.

35. Otaegui PJ, Ferre T, Pujol A, Riu E, Jimenez R, Bosch F. Expression of glucokinase in skeletal muscle: a new approach to counteract diabetic hyperglycemia. *Hum Gene Ther* 2000; 11: 1543-52.

36. Matschinsky FM. Banting lecture 1995. A lesson in metabolic regulation inspired by the glucokinase glucose sensor paradigm. *Diabetes* 1996; 45: 223-41.

37. Jimenez-Chillaron JC, Newgard CB, Gomez-Foix AM. Increased glucose disposal induced by adenovirus-mediated transfer of glucokinase to skeletal muscle *in vivo*. *Faseb J* 1999; 13: 2153-60.

38. Otaegui PJ, Ontiveros M, Ferre T, Riu E, Jimenez R, Bosch F. Glucose-regulated glucose uptake by transplanted muscle cells expressing glucokinase counteracts diabetic hyperglycemia. *Hum Gene Ther* 2002; 13: 2125-33.

39. Mas A, Montane J, Anguela XM, Munoz S, Douar AM, Riu E, *et al*. Reversal of type 1 diabetes by engineering a glucose sensor in skeletal muscle. *Diabetes* 2006; 55: 1546-53.

40. Daya S, Berns KI. Gene therapy using adeno-associated virus vectors. *Clin Microbiol Rev* 2008; 21: 583-93.

41. Nathwani AC, Tuddenham EG, Rangarajan S, Rosales C, McIntosh J, Linch DC, *et al*. Adenovirus-associated virus vector-mediated gene transfer in hemophilia B. *N Engl J Med* 2012 (in press).

42. LeWitt PA, Rezai AR, Leehey MA, Ojemann SG, Flaherty AW, Eskandar EN, *et al*. AAV2-GAD gene therapy for advanced Parkinson's disease: a double-blind, sham-surgery controlled, randomised trial. *Lancet Neurol* 2011; 10: 309-19.

43. Flotte TR, Trapnell BC, Humphries M, Carey B, Calcedo R, Rouhani F, *et al*. Phase 2 clinical trial of a recombinant adeno-associated viral vector expressing alpha(1)-antitrypsin: interim results. *Hum Gene Ther* 2011; 22: 1239-47.

44. Simonelli F, Maguire AM, Testa F, Pierce EA, Mingozzi F, Bennicelli JL, *et al*. Gene therapy for Leber's congenital amaurosis is safe and effective through 1.5 years after vector administration. *Mol Ther* 2010; 18: 643-65.

45. Niemeyer GP, Herzog RW, Mount J, Arruda VR, Tillson DM, Hathcock J, *et al*. Long-term correction of inhibitor-prone hemophilia B dogs treated with liver-directed AAV2-mediated factor IX gene therapy. *Blood* 2009; 113: 797-806.

46. Chen S, Ding JH, Bekeredjian R, Yang BZ, Shohet RV, Johnston SA, *et al*. Efficient gene delivery to pancreatic islets with ultrasonic microbubble destruction technology. *Proc Natl Acad Sci USA* 2006; 103: 8469-74.

47. Wang AY, Peng PD, Ehrhardt A, Storm TA, Kay MA. Comparison of adenoviral and adeno-associated viral vectors for pancreatic gene delivery *in vivo*. *Hum Gene Ther* 2004; 15: 405-13.

48. Taniguchi H, Yamato E, Tashiro F, Ikegami H, Ogihara T, Miyazaki J. Beta-cell neogenesis induced by adenovirus-mediated gene delivery of transcription factor pdx-1 into mouse pancreas. *Gene Ther* 2003; 10: 15-23.

49. Ayuso E, Chillon M, Agudo J, Haurigot V, Bosch A, Carretero A, *et al*. *In vivo* gene transfer to pancreatic beta cells by systemic delivery of adenoviral vectors. *Hum Gene Ther* 2004; 15: 805-12.

50. Ayuso E, Chillon M, Garcia F, Agudo J, Andaluz A, Carretero A, *et al. In vivo* gene transfer to healthy and diabetic canine pancreas. *Mol Ther* 2006; 13: 747-55.

51. Xu X, D'Hoker J, Stange G, Bonne S, De Leu N, Xiao X, *et al.* Beta cells can be generated from endogenous progenitors in injured adult mouse pancreas. *Cell* 2008; 132: 197-207.

52. Collombat P, Xu X, Ravassard P, Sosa-Pineda B, Dussaud S, Billestrup N, *et al.* The ectopic expression of Pax4 in the mouse pancreas converts progenitor cells into alpha and subsequently beta cells. *Cell* 2009; 138: 449-62.

53. Cheng H, Wolfe SH, Valencia V, Qian K, Shen L, Phillips MI, *et al.* Efficient and persistent transduction of exocrine and endocrine pancreas by adeno-associated virus type 8. *J Biomed Sci* 2007; 14: 585-94.

54. Nakai H, Fuess S, Storm TA, Muramatsu S, Nara Y, Kay MA. Unrestricted hepatocyte transduction with adeno-associated virus serotype 8 vectors in mice. *J Virol* 2005; 79: 214-24.

55. Inagaki K, Fuess S, Storm TA, Gibson GA, McTiernan CF, Kay MA, Nakai H. Robust systemic transduction with AAV9 vectors in mice: efficient global cardiac gene transfer superior to that of AAV8. *Mol Ther* 2006; 14: 45-53.

56. Loiler SA, Tang Q, Clarke T, Campbell-Thompson ML, Chiodo V, Hauswirth W, *et al.* Localized gene expression following administration of adeno-associated viral vectors via pancreatic ducts. *Mol Ther* 2005; 12: 519-27.

57. Maione F, Molla F, Meda C, Latini R, Zentilin L, Giacca M, *et al.* Semaphorin 3A is an endogenous angiogenesis inhibitor that blocks tumor growth and normalizes tumor vasculature in transgenic mouse models. *J Clin Invest* 2009; 119: 3356-72.

58. Wang Z, Zhu T, Rehman KK, Bertera S, Zhang J, Chen C, *et al.* Widespread and stable pancreatic gene transfer by adeno-associated virus vectors via different routes. *Diabetes* 2006; 55: 875-84.

59. Jimenez V, Ayuso E, Mallol C, Agudo J, Casellas A, Obach M, *et al. In vivo* genetic engineering of murine pancreatic beta cells mediated by single-stranded adeno-associated viral vectors of serotypes 6, 8 and 9. *Diabetologia* 2011; 54: 1075-86.

60. Riedel MJ, Gaddy DF, Asadi A, Robbins PD, Kieffer TJ. DsAAV8-mediated expression of glucagon-like peptide-1 in pancreatic beta-cells ameliorates streptozotocin-induced diabetes. *Gene Ther* 2010; 17: 171-80.

61. Montane J, Bischoff L, Soukhatcheva G, Dai DL, Hardenberg G, Levings MK, *et al.* Prevention of murine autoimmune diabetes by CCL22-mediated Treg recruitment to the pancreatic islets. *J Clin Invest* 2011; 121: 3024-8.

62. Hendrick LM, Harewood GC, Patchett SE, Murray FE. Utilization of resource leveling to optimize ERCP efficiency. *Ir J Med Sci* 2011; 180: 143-8.

The CliniBook: Clinical gene transfer
Edited by Odile Cohen-Haguenauer – EDK, Paris © 2012, pp. 71-82

A1-7
Approaches to large scale production of AAV-vectors

Otto-Wilhelm Merten[1], Philippe Moullier[2]*

[1]*Généthon, 1 rue de l'Internationale, BP60, F-91000 Évry, France.*
[2]*CHU de Nantes, Laboratoire de Thérapie génique, Inserm UMR649, 30 boulevard Jean-Monnet, F-44035 Nantes Cedex 1, France.*
moullier@ufl.edu
*Corresponding author

Introduction

Adeno-associated virus based vectors are efficient vehicles for gene therapy in humans. An important set of data has been accumulated from various pre-clinical models (rodents, dogs, monkeys), providing evidences of the quasi-absence of pathogenicity or toxicity, an excellent safety profile and the ability to confer long-term gene expression in a wide range of tissues [1]. In addition, in recent years, an increasing number of clinical trials with AAV vectors has been conducted for the treatment of various rare diseases, including those affecting retina [2-4], the central nervous system [5], liver [6, 7] and muscle tissues [8]. In dependence of the target tissue (disease to be treated) the AAV amounts needed for performing clinical trials can vary considerably. Whereas for ocular treatment, vector amounts of $5x10^{10}$ to 10^{12} vg/eye are used/proposed, the estimated efficient dose for the systemic delivery of AAV for the treatment of neuro-muscular diseases ranges between 1 and $2x10^{13}$ vg/kg patient tissue. This signifies for instance that for a phase 1 clinical trial with loco-regional delivery at least $5x10^{16}$ vg of AAV have to be manufactured (this number includes the amount needed for the QC analytics). However, this signifies also that a highly efficient large scale manufacturing process is needed for producing these and in the future much higher vector quantities for further advanced clinical trials.

Scalable AAV vector production systems

Transfection based production systems

Although the traditional laboratory scale vector production method based on the transfection of adherently growing cells, such as HEK293 using initially three [9-11] and after optimisation two plasmids [12, 13] providing the recombinant AAV vector, the adenoviral helper functions (E2A, E4, VA RNA) as well as the AAV *rep-cap* genes, is very versatile. It allows the easy switch from one serotype to another one and/or from one transgene to be transferred to another one by essentially keeping the AAV2 derived ITRs and *rep* functions [14]. However on another side, it is hampered by a limited scalability. Traditional scale-up consisted in the use of CellFactories [15] or similar multitray culture devices, roller bottles [16] and CellCubes (Brown *et al*. pers. commun.), essentially for increasing the transfectable cell number by increasing the available cell culture surface. However, *in fine* no real scale-up is feasible with such culture systems and other scalable manufacturing systems have to be envisaged.

The most obvious approach is a suspension culture approach in which after adaptation to suspension growth HEK293 or HEK293T cells are transfected in serum-free media using either calcium phosphate or polyethyleneimine (PEI) as transfection agent. In addition to induction of cell aggregation, the calcium phosphate precipitation method usually requires exchanging the medium before and after transfection and its transfection efficiency is heavily impacted by several medium parameters, such as pH, Ca-concentration, phosphate-concentration, impurities, etc. – all drawbacks which are not encountered when using the PEI method. The use of PEI appears to be more advanced, due to its reproducibility, reliability and its independence of variations in transfection conditions. Several groups have established it in spinner flasks and evaluated its scalability [17, 18]. Thus the PEI-method is more adapted for large scale production of AAV vectors than the calcium phosphate transfection method.

Based on the data published by Durocher *et al*. [17] generation of 9.3×10^{13} vg of AAV is feasible using a 3L reactor culture, for producing 5×10^{16} vg of AAV for a phase 1 clinical trial (see above) a reactor culture of about 1600L would be required. Although the PEI based transfection method for the production of AAV was shown to be feasible, scale-up to scales beyond a 100L scale seems to be impractical due to the high costs associated with the elevated quantities of plasmids. In addition, even when using a transfection method characterized by a high reliability and reproducibility as the PEI based transfection method, all transfections are characterized by a certain inherent variability which might be unacceptable for large scale productions.

Advanced scalable AAV production systems

To overcome the limited scalability of the above mentioned method, three different (scalable) AAV vector production systems have been developed.

1. The first one is based on the use of stable HeLa- or A549 cell clones containing either only the AAV *rep-cap* genes [19-22] (packaging cells) or the AAV *rep-cap* genes and the rAAV-vector DNA [23-27] (producer cells). Often the establishment of the producer cell lines is based on the packaging cell lines.

In the case of the packaging cells, for AAV production they are infected with a conditionally replication-defective helper ts-E2b adenovirus and 24h later with a ΔE1-adenovirus – AAV hybridvirus (both adenoviruses are modified for avoiding their production during AAV production) [28]. Although scale-up in suspension reactors is theoretically possible, data are only available for adherently grown cultures [28]. Productivities ranging from 3×10^4 to 6×10^5 vg/c have been reported using 15 cm^2 plates [29] (*Table I*).

In the case of producer cells, for AAV generation, they have to be infected with wt-adenovirus [30, 31] or conditionally replication defective adenovirus [25, 30]. The productivities are rather similar to those observed for that of packaging cell lines (>10^4 vg/c) (*Table I*). Farson *et al*. [25] has evaluated the production of AAV in serum-free medium at a 15L reactor scale, leading to the production 4.2×10^{13} vg in total which is, however, rather low, probably due to insufficient cell growth in the reactor. Thorne (pers. commun.) reported on scale-up to 100L.

Table I. Comparison of different AAV production methods in view of the large scale production of AAV vectors.

Production method	Yield (vg/c)	Scale-up	Yield per production unit (vg)	Number of production units for producing 5×10^{16} purified AAV particles*	Generation of rcAAV	Ref.
293, triple transfection ****	$10 – 10^3/10^4$	15 cm² plates or CellFactory	Per 100 15cm² plates: 6-9x10¹² vg/10⁹ c 1-2x10¹² vg/CellFactory	25000	1/10³ – 1/10⁶ vg	[29] unpubl. results
HeLa (B50) or A549 (K209) based **packaging cell**, rAAV production induced by infection with wtAd5 or Ad sub100r + Ad-AAV hybrid virus	$3 \times 10^4 – 5 \times 10^5$	Adherent growth, in principle, adaptable to suspension growth in suspension	Per 100 15cm² plates: 3.4x10¹³ vg/10⁹ c – 60x10¹³ vg/10⁹ c	15cm² plates 735300- 41700	<1/10¹¹ vg	[22, 29]
A549 based **producer cell**, rAAV production induced by infection with a wtAd or tsAd	$>10^4$	**Suspension culture – reactor scale: 15 L, scale-up possible**	Per 15L STR**: 4.2x10¹³	Reactor volume: L 89300	<1/10⁹ vg	[25]
HeLa based + wtAd	Up to 10^5		Calculated (base: 10⁵ vg/c, 10⁹ c/L)	2500		[24]
rHSV-1 expression system: sBHK cells are infected with 2 different rHSV-1 vectors	sBHK: 5.5x10⁴ – 1.2x10⁵	**sBHK: suspension culture – WAVE reactor: 10 L, scale-up possible**	For 10L WAVE reactor: 2.4x10¹⁴ DRP/L (AAV1)	Reactor volume: L 1000	Absence (limit of detection?)	[37, 53]
Baculovirus system: Sf9 infected with 2 different rec. baculoviruses	$10^4 – 10^5$	**Suspension culture: 200L STR, larger scale possible**	For 200L SUB***: 8.3x10¹³ vg/L (AAV6) (4x10⁶ c/ml)	Reactor volume: L 300	<1/10¹¹ vg	[38]
Original system – use of 3 different rec. baculoviruses		**50L STR**	For 50L STR: 9.4x10¹³ vg/L (AAV1) (1x10⁶ c/ml)	2600		[52] Merten, ESGCT 2009, Clinigene Industrial Symposium

Note: *assumption: purification yield = 20%, thus 5 times more bulk product has to be manufactured, the number of production units takes this fact into account; **STR = stirred tank reactor; ***SUB = single use bioreactor (Hyclone); ****the yield per production unit and the number of production units needed for the production of 5×10^{16} vg is estimated for the underlined items.

In general, the generation of stable cell lines as cell factories for rAAVs is better suited for large-scale production than transient transfection. Nevertheless, generation of such cells is generally tedious and time consuming with a low frequency of clone output. Recently, Yuan *et al.* [32] reported the development of a new versatile 293-based packaging/producer cell line which can be established *via* a one step cloning and a single plasmid transfection with a plasmid containing the AAV helper functions and the recombinant AAV vector. The *rep/cap* functions are inducible *via* infection by using a recombinant adenovirus harbouring the Cre recombinase gene (Ad-CRE) leading to the removal of an intron with three polyadenylation elements framed by lox-sites, which disrupt all *rep* transcripts. These cells produce vector levels ranging from 0.9×10^5 to 1.3×10^5 vg/cell using a 10 stack CellFactory system. The vector amount produced with such a system was $5-8 \times 10^{13}$ vg. When adapted to suspension culture, production in reactor systems can be envisaged and will probably lead to high amounts of vector particles.

2. The second scalable system is based on the use of HSV-1. It could be demonstrated that replication defective HSV vectors that lacked the ICP-27 gene are the most interesting ones with respect to specific AAV yields in mammalian cells [33-35]. A highly efficient rHSV-based rAAV complementation system has been reported [36], that uses two rHSV vectors, one harboring the ITR-flanked gene of interest (= rAAV-vector) and the second one bearing the *rep* and *cap* genes. Both vectors have proven to be stable during serial expansion. Using this production system, practically similar AAV yields were reported [37], when using HEK 293 cells grown in 10 stack CellFactories and BHK cells grown in suspension in WAVE reactors, reaching 74600 and 85400 DNase-resistant AAV particles (DRP)/cell (= comparable to vg/cell), respectively. The BHK-based production system has the advantage of a lower required MOI for both complementation vectors as well as a more simple scalability. Thomas *et al.* [37] reported average volumetric productivities of 2.4×10^{14} DRP/L when using disposable 10L reactors.

3. The third and more recent production system is based on the use of insect cells (Sf9 cells), which are infected with three recombinant baculoviruses providing the AAV *rep* and *cap* genes on two separate baculoviruses and the rAAV vector on a third baculovirus [38]. The most important improvement concerns the genetic stabilization of the rep construct and in parallel the reduction of the number of the required baculoviruses to two, providing the AAV *rep* and *cap* functions on one and the rAAV vector on the second baculovirus [39]. The volumetric production yields are in the range of about 1×10^{14} vg/L (AAV1) when using 10L/50L stirred tank reactors thus achieving productivities comparable to the HSV-1 based production system (see below).

• *Comparison of different production systems: Table I* compares the different production systems as well as the presently established production scales. Concerning the specific vector yield per cell, all expression systems except the transfection system based on HEK293 cells are comparable and the specific yield ranges between 10^4 and 6×10^5 vg/c. However, as already mentioned, a really scalability of an expression system is based on the use of a suspension process. In this context, the transfection system is limited in scalability even if put into a suspension process (*vide supra*) and a packaging cells based process (using rHeLa or rA549 cells) could be adapted to suspension, however, up to now no open scientific literature has really reported on this possibility. Thus when keeping both expression systems, the production of 5×10^{16} vg for a phase 1 clinical study would demand either 25000 CF-10 CellFactories (in the case of the transfection system) or $41700 - 735300$ 15 cm^2 plates (numbers are depending on production levels) in the case of the use of packaging cells.

All other AAV production systems have been adapted to a suspension process. The comparison of the processes based on producer cells (*e.g.* rHeLa – here, only calculated assuming that the cells produce about 10^5 vg/c and that a normal producer culture achieves cell densities of 10^9 c/L), on the recombinant HSV-1/sBHK and the Sf9/Baculovirus system indicates that relatively comparable vector amounts at a liter scale can be obtained. In view of our example, this would mean that reactor scales ranging from 1000 to 3000L have to be set-up in order to produce the required quantities. The differences between the three expression systems are negligible and can probably be explained by differences in the titration methods – in any case, the magnitude of reactor scale is identical for the three production systems.

With respect to potential contaminations by rcAAV, for all expression systems except for the transfection based production system, the absence of the generation of rcAAV/rep positive AAV could be shown (= always below detection limit of the analytical method used). However, concerning the transfection based production systems often contaminations by rcAAV/rep-positive AAV due to homologous or non-homologous recombination events have been reported [10, 40].

Our choice of the large-scale AAV vector production system (Sf9/baculovirus system) and scale-up

The choice for the Sf9/baculovirus system was based on the following facts and considerations: recombinant baculovirus derived from the *Autographa californica* multiple nucleopolyhedrosis virus (AcMNPV) is widely employed for large-scale production of heterologous proteins in cultured insect cells [41-43] for the following reasons: (1) the strong *polyhedrin* or *p10* promoters enable high-level expressions of foreign proteins; (2) insect cells are able to grow in suspension culture in serum-free media and thus are easy to scale up; and (3) the proteins synthesized in insect cells are processed and modified posttranslationally, to some extent, as in mammalian cells and often retain biological activity, and it could be shown that virus-like particles [44, 45], including AAV [46] can be produced with this expression system. Moreover, the establishment of new baculoviruses is much more straight forward than the development of new packaging or producer cell lines which represents a rather time intensive process. In addition to these advantages, the Sf9/baculovirus system is characterized by a high safety profile (baculovirus is non-pathogenic for vertebrates [47], Sf9 cells are non-tumorigenic [48, 49], animal-free culture media are available, making it to date superior to all other scalable AAV production systems.

The basic technology (bacmids necessary for the AAV production) as published by Urabe *et al.* [38] and subsequent improvements (reduction from the triple to the dual baculovirus system by Smith *et al.* [39] were transferred from the NIH (R. Kotin) to Généthon and established at a spinner (100 – 400mL) and later at a bioreactor (2 – 10L) scale using classical glass vessel stirred tank reactors designed for animal cell culture, for the production of AAV1 and AAV8 vectors.

These culture scales are insufficient for the production of clinical vector lots for the treatment of neuro-muscular diseases because for instance a 10L reactor can produce about 10^{15} vg (AAV1) which gives about 4.6×10^{14} vg after purification. Thus, large-scale reactor systems for the GMP production are indispensable. In this context, a choice of high importance has to be done: use of a stain-less steel production line versus disposable manufacturing systems.

Since we are dealing with a GMP manufacturing plant of viral vector lots for clinical trials, its conception is based on the idea that a highly flexible production unit is necessary in order to be able to easily switch from one manufacturing process to another one when other vectors have to be produced or when new manufacturing technologies have to be implemented. In addition, the reduction of costs related to rinsing, cleaning, sanitization, and sterilization as well as their validation is of certain interest (money-wise as well as time-wise). Based on these considerations, the decision was taken to invest into disposable manufacturing system. In addition, to the above-mentioned considerations, further advantages are the fast switch from a finished production run to the next production with only minimal down-time representing essentially a plug and play concept.

In the recent years, several disposable reactor systems have been commercialized, thus it was necessary to evaluate the most interesting ones. For large scale AAV production the WAVE bag reactor systems have been excluded because their scalability as well as oxygen transfer is limited, however, they have been tested and were retained for the production of baculoviral seed lots as well as for intermediate biomass amplification for the seeding the production reactor. Thus, the following disposable reactor systems have been evaluated: SUB from Hyclone (50L), Nucleo from ATMI (20L), Cultibag STR from Sartorius (50L).

In addition to culture performance and vector production, the criteria for the choice of the disposable reactor system were the following: availability of the whole package (reactor system), investment/consumable costs, simple handling, user-friendly software, rapidity of maintenance, availability of plastic bags, and financial health of the producer/vendor company.

The comparisons were done using the following standard conditions: the cultures were started with an inoculation cell number of about $3x10^5$ c/ml using SFM900II medium and infected with 3 different baculoviruses at an MOI of 5 in total after having attained $0.8-1.5x10^6$ c/ml in view of the production of AAV1-GFP vectors. Since standard culture conditions (pH 6.2, $pO_2=50\%$, temperature: 27°C, agitation conditions as proposed by the vendors) were used cell growth was only negligibly influenced by the different reactor scales and specific growth rates ranging from 0.0194±0.0035/h (2L standard stirred tank reactor from Sartorius, n=6) to 0.0258±0.0065/h (20L 'Nucleo' reactor from ATMI, n=6). The specific growth rates observed in the 10L stirred tank reactor from Sartorius, the 50L 'SUB' from Hyclone and the 50L 'Cultibag STR' from Sartorius were rather similar (0.024/h) (*Table II*) and the differences were non-significant. These values indicate that cell growth was essentially identical for the different systems tested.

Table II. Comparison of different reactor systems for specific cell growth of Sf9 cells.

	Traditional stirred tank glass reactor (STR – Sartorius)		Disposable bioreactors		
	2L (n=6)	10L (n=4)	SUB 50L (Hyclone) (n=3)	Nucleo 20L (ATMI) (n=6)	Cultibag STR 50L (Sartorius) (n=4)
μ (1/h)	0.0194±0.0035	0.0248±0.0011	0.0240±0.0026	0.0258±0.0065	0.0246±0.0023

However, biomass is only an intermediate objective because *in fine* it is the final vector amount, which mainly counts and which can be produced per reactor unit.

Since different maximal reactor volumes were used, the comparison of the reactors was done based on the specific vector production rates (*Table III*). The 2L and 10L cultures showed specific productivities (TU/c - transducing units/c, which is possible because the model vector produced was an AAV1-GFP) of 1±0.6 whereas those observed for the disposable reactors ranged between 3.69±1.5 (for the SUB reactor from

Hyclone) and 10.21±6.87 (for the Nucleo reactor from ATMI). With respect to the specific productivities expressed as number of total vector particles produced per cell (vp/c) the values ranged between $0.51x10^6±0.29x10^6$ vp/c (for the cultures performed in the SUB from Hyclone) and $3.73x10^6±1.01x10^6$ vp/c (for the cultures performed in the Cultibag STR from Sartorius). Despite the apparent variabilities in particular, between the different small scale and large scale reactor systems, they were not statistically significant (use of t-test). The differences (for TU/c as well as for vp/c) can essentially be explained by variability in the baculovirus seed material (probably due to inactivation because of the storage duration of the different baculoviruses when stored at 4°C in the dark over several months [50]. It has to be kept in mind that the different cultures were performed over a period of more than one year. In addition, the assessment was performed with the original triple baculovirus system (as developed by Urabe *et al.* [38]) meaning also that a supplementary variability was introduced when compared to the more recent two baculovirus system [39].

Table III. Comparison of different reactor systems for specific vector productivities (vp/c [number of viral particles/c], TU/c [number of transducing units/c]).

	Traditional stirred tank glass reactor (STR – Sartorius)		Disposable bioreactors		
	2L (n=6)	10L (n=4)	SUB 50L (Hyclone) (n=3)	Nucleo 20L (ATMI) (n=6)	Cultibag STR 50L (Sartorius) (n=4)
vp/c	$1.2x10^6 ± 1.1x10^6$	$0.72x10^6 ± 0.22x10^6$	$0.51x10^6 ± 0.29x10^6$	$2.5x10^6 ± 2.37x10^6$	$3.73x10^6 ± 1.01x10^6$
TU/c	$1.0 ± 0.6$	$1.1 ± 0.6$	$3.69 ± 1.5$	$10.21 ± 6.87$	$5.42 ± 8.00$

Note: no indications on the specific productivities expressed in vector genome per cell can be given because during the time of the assessment of the different reactor systems no vg-based vector titrations were performed.

Since neither the culture data nor the vector production data indicated significant differences between the three assessed disposable reactor systems, the choice was based on other criteria which were essentially in favour for the Cultibag STR system (Sartorius). These criteria included the availability of a whole package (reactor system and control system, for instance, at that time not available for the SUB system (Hyclone)), simplicity of handling (*e.g.* installation of a new culture bag), user-friendly software (we were already familiar with the software because of the equipment with small scale laboratory reactors from Sartorius), rapidity of maintenance, etc.

IMPLEMENTATION OF THE DISPOSABLE LARGE-SCALE CULTURE SYSTEM

The implementation of the Cultibag STR system from Sartorius allows the reproducible production of AAV vectors at a 50L scale. Since the final aim is the availability of a completely disposable manufacturing facility, all culture units necessary for the amplification of the biomass for starting the production reactor as well as the production of the viral seed stock make use of disposables (disposable spinner flasks, WAVE reactor). The cell culture process at the production scale takes only 7 days (from seeding up to harvesting). After production, the bulk is harvested, treated with detergent for lysing producer cells and baculoviruses, and further treated *via* clarification, AVB-chromatography, diafiltration/concentration and final sterile filtration (thus, corresponding essentially to the process described by Smith *et al.* [39]). This process was used for the production of AAV1 vectors with 3 different transgenes (GFP (as model), human γ-sarcoglycan, U7-exon-skipping). In average, 10L glass and 50L disposable reactor cultures produce $1.1x10^{15}$ vg and $4.7x10^{15}$ vg in total, respectively, leading to total vector quantities of $4.6x10^{14}$ vg and $1.8x10^{15}$ vg, respectively, after purification. Thus, the purification yields range from 40 to 50%. The final production concentration is ranging between $8.5x10^{12}$ and $5.0x10^{13}$ vg/ml. For clinical purposes, the whole manufacturing has to be performed under GMP conditions, and the final product has to be rigorously analysed (*e.g.,* see Wright and Zelenaia [51]) including assays specific for the Sf9/baculovirus system (including tests for the detection of residual baculovirus protein, residual host cell protein, residual baculovirus DNA/DNA sequences, residual host cell DNA/DNA sequences, etc.). The present production system can efficiently be scaled up to 200L (*Figure 1*) or even 1000L, by simply using a larger culture bag. The culture and production parameters as well as reactor productivities are comparable for the different scales; this was evaluated and confirmed in our hands at the 200L scale (not shown).

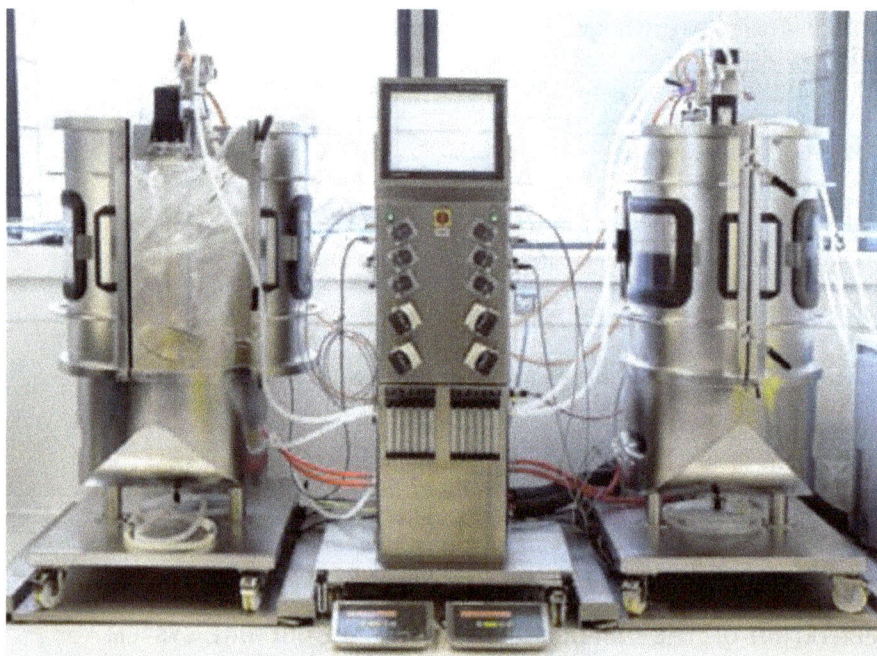

Figure 1. Presentation of the disposable Cultibag STR 200L stirred tank reactor used for the production of AAV using the Sf9/baculovirus system.

Finally with respect to the above mentioned example, the production of about $5x10^{16}$ vg for a phase I clinical study would either demand 3x1000L reactor runs or 13x200L reactor runs without modification of the production conditions or optimisation. However, optimisation of the process will certainly lead to higher reactor yields and thus to a reduction in the required production volume – issues, which are treated by us as well as by others active in this field (*e.g.* Cecchini *et al.* [52]).

CONCLUSIONS

The use of one of the scalable production systems of AAV vectors will permit the large scale production of AAV vector amounts required for the execution of clinical studies in the frame of the development of therapeutic strategies for the treatment of neuro-muscular diseases. We have chosen the SF9/baculovirus expression system mainly due to safety considerations but also to production features and could show that scalable production is possible by using one or the other disposable large scale reactor system without major differences in with respect to growth and vector production. Based on these and further criteria the disposable Cultibag STR reactor system was chosen allowing the production of high quantities of AAV vectors. Further scale-up will lead us to the production scale necessary for producing the vector quantities required for performing a loco-regional phase 1 study for the treatment of neuro-muscular diseases.

ACKNOWLEDGMENTS

This work has been performed with the support of the EC-DG research through the FP6-Network of Excellence, CLINIGENE: LSHB-CT-2006-018933.

REFERENCES

1. Warrington KH Jr, Herzog RW. Treatment of human disease by adeno-associated viral gene transfer. *Hum Genet* 2006; 119: 571-603.

2. Bainbridge JW, Smith AJ, Barker SS, *et al*. Effect of gene therapy on visual function in Leber's congenital amaurosis. *N Engl J Med* 2008; 358: 2231-9.

3. Maguire AM, High K, Auricchio A, *et al*. Age-dependent effects of RPE65 gene therapy for Leber's congenital amaurosis: a phase 1 dose-escalation trial. *Lancet* 2009; 374: 1597-605.

4. Simonelli F, Maguire AM, Testa F, *et al*. Gene therapy for Leber's congenital amaurosis is safe and effective through 1.5 years after vector administration. *Mol Ther* 2010; 18: 643-50.

5. Palfi S. Towards gene therapy for Parkinson's disease. *Lancet Neurol* 2008; 7: 375-6.

6. High KA. Clinical gene transfer studies for hemophilia B. *Semin Thromb Hemost* 2004; 30: 257-67.

7. Manno CS, Pierce GF, Arruda VR, *et al*. Successful transduction of liver in hemophilia by AAV-Factor IX and limitations imposed by the host immune response. *Nat Med* 2006; 12: 342-7.

8. Rodino-Klapac LR, Janssen PM, Montgomery CL, Coley BD, Chicoine LG, Clark KR, Mendell JR. A translational approach for limb vascular delivery of the micro-dystrophin gene without high volume or high pressure for treatment of Duchenne muscular dystrophy. *J Transl Med* 2007; 5: 45.

9. Matsushita T, Elliger S, Elliger C, Podsakoff G, Villarreal L, Kurtzman GJ, Iwaki Y, Colosi P. Adeno-associated virus vectors can be efficiently produced without helper virus. *Gene Ther* 1998; 5: 938-45.

10. Salvetti A, Orève S, Chadeuf G, Favre D, Cherel Y, Champion-Arnaud P, David-Ameline J, Moullier P. Factors influencing recombinant adeno-associated virus production. *Hum Gene Ther* 1998; 9: 695-706.

11. Xiao X, Li J, Samulski RJ. Production of high-titer recombinant adeno-associated virus vectors in the absence of helper adenovirus. *J Virol* 1998; 72: 2224-323.

12. Collaco RF, Cao X, Trempe JP. A helper virus-free packaging system for recombinant adeno-associated virus vectors. *Gene* 1999; 238: 397-405.

13. Grimm D, Kern A, Pawlita M, Ferrari F, Samulski R, Kleinschmidt J. Titration of AAV-2 particles via a novel capsid ELISA: packaging of genomes can limit production of recombinant AAV-2. *Gene Ther* 1999; 6: 1322-30.

14. Rabinowitz JE, Rolling F, Li C, Conrath H, Xiao W, Xiao X, Samulski RJ. Cross-packaging of a single adeno-associated virus (AAV) type 2 vector genome into multiple AAV serotypes enables transduction with broad specificity. *J Virol* 2002; 76: 791-801.

15. Drittanti L, Jenny C, Poulard K, *et al*. Optimized helper virus-free production of high-quality adeno-associated virus vectors. *J Gene Med* 2001; 3: 59-71.

16. Liu YL, Wagner K, Robinson N, Sabatino D, Margaritis P, XiaoW, Herzog RW. Optimized production of high-titer recombinant adenoassociated virus in roller bottles. *BioTechniques* 2003; 34: 184-9.

17. Durocher Y, Pham PL, St-Laurent G, *et al*. Scalable serum-free production of recombinant adeno-associated virus type 2 by transfection of 293 suspension cells. *J Virol Methods* 2007; 144: 32-40.

18. Feng L, Guo M, Zhang S, Chu J, Zhuang Y, Zhang S. Improvement in the suspension-culture production of recombinant adeno-associated virus-LacZ in HEK-293 cells using polyethyleneimine-DNA complexes in combination with hypothermic treatment. *Biotechnol Appl Biochem* 2008; 50: 121-32.

19. Clark KR, Voulgaropoulou F, Johnson PR. A stable cell line carrying adenovirus-inducible rep and cap genes allows for infectivity titration of adeno-associated virus vectors. *Gene Ther* 1996; 3: 1124-32.

20. Fan PD, Dong JY. Replication of rep-cap genes is essential for the high-efficiency production of recombinant AAV. *Hum Gene Ther* 1997; 8: 87-98.

21. Gao GP, Alvira MR, Wang L, Calcedo R, Johnston J, Wilson JM. Novel adeno-associated viruses from rhesus monkeys as vectors for human gene therapy. *Proc Natl Acad Sci USA* 2002; 99: 11854-9.

22. Gao GP, Lu F, Sanmiguel JC, *et al*. Rep/Cap gene amplification and high-yield production of AAV in an A549 cell line expressing Rep/Cap. *Mol Ther* 2002; 5: 644-649.

23. Blouin V, Brument N, Toublanc E, Raimbaud I, Moullier P, Salvetti A. Improving rAAV production and purification: towards the definition of a scaleable process. *J Gene Med* 2004; 6 (suppl 1): 223-8.

24. Chadeuf G, Favre D, Tessier J, Provost N, Nony P, Kleinschmidt J, Moullier P, Salvetti A. Efficient recombinant adeno-associated virus production by a stable rep-cap HeLa cell line correlates with adenovirus-induced amplification of the integrated rep-cap genome. *J Gene Med* 2000; 2: 260-8.

25. Farson D, Harding TC, Tao L, *et al*. Development and characterization of a cell line for large-scale, serum-free production of recombinant adeno-associated viral vectors. *J Gene Med* 2004; 6: 1369-81.

26. Liu X, Voulgaropoulou F, Chen R. Johnson PR, Clark KR. Selective rep-cap gene amplification as a mechanism for high-titer recombinant AAV production from stable cell lines. *Mol Ther* 2000; 2: 394-403.

27. Mathews LC, Gray JT, Gallagher MR, Snyder RO. Recombinant adeno-associated viral vector production using stable packaging and producer cell lines. *Methods Enzymol* 2002; 346: 393-413.

28. Zhang H, Xie J, Xie Q, Wilson JM, Gao G. Adenovirus-adeno-associated virus hybrid for large-scale recombinant adeno-associated virus production. *Hum Gene Ther* 2009; 20: 922-9.

29. Gao GP, Qu G, Faust LZ, Engdahl RK, Xiao W, Hughes JV, Zoltick PW, Wilson JM. High-titer adeno-associated viral vectors from a Rep/Cap cell line and hybrid shuttle virus. *Hum Gene Ther* 1998; 9: 2353-62.

30. Jenny C, Toublanc E., Danos O, Merten OW. Serum-free production of rAAV-2 using HeLa derived producer cells. *Cytotechnology* 2005; 49: 11-23.

31. Tatalick LM, Gerard CJ, Takeya R, Price DN, Thorne BA, Wyatt LM, Anklesaria P. Safety characterization of HeLa-based cell substrates used in the manufacture of a recombinant adeno-associated virus-HIV vaccine. *Vaccine* 2005; 23: 2628-38.

32. Yuan Z, Qiao C, Hu P, Li J, Xiao X. A versatile AAV producer cell line method for scalable vector production of different serotypes. *Hum Gene Ther* 2011; 22: 613-24.

33. Booth MJ, Mistry A, Li X, Thrasher A, Coffin RS. Transfection-free and scalable recombinant AAV vector production using HSV/AAV hybrids. *Gene Ther* 2004; 11: 829-37.

34. Conway J, Rhys CM, Zolotukhin I, Zolotukhin S, Muzyczka N, Hayward GS, Byrne BJ. High-titer recombinant adeno-associated virus production utilizing a recombinant herpes simplex virus type I vector expressing AAV-2 Rep and Cap. *Gene Ther* 1999; 6: 986-93.

35. Conway JE, Zolotukhin S, Muzyczka N, Hayward GS, Byrne BJ. Recombinant adeno-associated virus type 2 replication and packaging is entirely supported by a herpes simplex virus type 1 amplicon expressing Rep and Cap. *J Virol* 1997; 71: 8780-9.

36. Kang W, Wang L, Harrell H, *et al.* An efficient rHSV-based complementation system for the production of multiple rAAV vector serotypes. *Gene Ther* 2009; 16: 229-39.

37. Thomas DL, Wang L, Niamke J, *et al.* Scalable recombinant adeno-associated virus production using recombinant herpes simplex virus type 1 coinfection of suspension-adapted mammalian cells. *Hum Gene Ther* 2009; 20: 861-70.

38. Urabe M, Ding C, Kotin RM. Insect cells as a factory to produce adeno-associated virus type 2 vectors. *Hum Gene Ther* 2002; 13: 1935-43.

39. Smith RH, Levy JR, Kotin RM. A simplified baculovirus-AAV expression vector system coupled with one-step affinity purification yields high-titer rAAV stocks from insect cells. *Mol Ther* 2009; 17: 1888-96.

40. Park JY, Lim BP, Lee K, Kim YG, Jo EC. Scalable production of adeno-associated virus type 2 vectors via suspension transfection. *Biotechnol Bioeng* 2006; 94: 416-30.

41. Condreay JP, Kost TA. Baculovirus expression vectors for insect and mammalian cells. *Curr Drug Targets* 2007; 8: 1126-31.

42. Hitchman RB, Possee RD, King LA. Baculovirus expression systems for recombinant protein production in insect cells. *Recent Pat Biotechnol* 2009; 3: 46-54.

43. Jarvis DL. Baculovirus-insect cell expression systems. *Methods Enzymol* 2009; 463: 191-222.

44. Casal JI. Use of the baculovirus expression system for the generation of virus-like particles. *Biotechnol Genet Eng Rev* 2001; 18: 73-87.

45. van Oers MM. Vaccines for viral and parasitic diseases produced with baculovirus vectors. *Adv Virus Res* 2006; 68: 193-253.

46. Ruffing M, Zentgraf H, Kleinschmidt JA. Assembly of virus like particles by recombinant structural proteins of adeno-associated virus type 2 in insect cells. *J Virol* 1992; 66: 6922-30.

47. Tiga ST, zu Altenschildesche GM, Doerfler W. Autographa Californica nuclear polyhedrosis virus (AcNPV) FNA does not pesist in mass cultures of mammalian cells. *Virology* 1983; 125: 107-17.

48. Cox MMJ, Anderson DK. Production of a novel influenza vaccine using insect cells: protection against drifted strains. *Influenza Other Respi Viruses* 2007; 1: 35-40.

49. McPherson CE. Development of a novel recombinant influenza vaccine in insect cells. *Biologicals* 2008; 36: 350-3.

50. Jorio H, Tran R, Kamen A. Stability of serum-free and purified baculovirus stocks under various storage conditions. *Biotechnol Prog* 2006; 22: 319-25.

51. Wright JF, Zelenaia O. Vector characterization methods for quality control testing of recombinant adeno-associated viruses. *Methods Mol Biol* 2011; 737: 247-278.

52. Cecchini S, Virag T, Kotin RM. Reproducible high yields of recombinant adeno-associated virus produced using invertebrate cells in 0.02- to 200-liter cultures. *Hum Gene Ther* 2011; 22: 1021-1030.

53. Clément N, Knop DR, Byrne BJ. Large-scale adeno-associated viral vector production using a herpesvirus-based system enables manufacturing for clinical studies. *Hum Gene Ther* 2009; 20: 796-806.

The CliniBook: Clinical gene transfer
Edited by Odile Cohen-Haguenauer – EDK, Paris © 2012, pp. 83-90

A1-8
Reference materials for the characterization of adeno-associated viral vectors

EDUARD AYUSO[1]*, VÉRONIQUE BLOUIN[2], CHRISTOPHE DARMON[2,3], FATIMA BOSCH[1], MARTIN LOCK[4], RICHARD O. SNYDER[2,5], PHILIPPE MOULLIER[2,3,5]

[1]*Center of Animal Biotechnology and Gene Therapy and Department of Biochemistry and Molecular Biology, Universitat Autònoma de Barcelona, Bellaterra, Spain.*
[2]*Inserm UMR 1089, Nantes, France.*
[3]*EFS-Atlantic Bio GMP, Saint-Herblain, France.*
[4]*Gene Therapy Program, Department of Pathology and Laboratory Medicine, University of Pennsylvania, Philadelphia, USA.*
[5]*Department of Molecular Genetics and Microbiology, University of Florida, Gainesville, USA.*
E. Ayuso and V. Blouin contributed equally
eduard.ayuso@uab.es
* *Corresponding author*

INTRODUCTION

Recombinant adeno-associated viral (rAAV) vectors are increasingly being used in gene therapy applications because of their many desirable properties. rAAV vectors have an excellent safety profile, as they are non-replicating, poorly immunogenic and have not been associated with any disease in humans. rAAV vectors efficiently transduce post-mitotic cells and several pre-clinical studies demonstrate that rAAV vector-mediated gene transfer results in long-term gene expression, up to several years, in small and large animal models of various diseases [1-7]. In addition, they do not integrate efficiently into the host genome, thereby considerably reducing the risk of insertional mutagenesis [8, 9]. Over the last few years, translation of preclinical data into the clinical arena in the form of over 80 different AAV-based clinical trials has resulted in promising results, confirming the ability of AAV vectors to safely transduce liver, muscle, and neurons in humans [10-13]. Furthermore, therapeutic benefit has been observed [12, 14-19].

In addition to the excellent safety profile and the prolonged expression of transgenes, nowadays it is possibile to obtain high titer and high pure AAV vector preparations using different production methods [20].

Despite the progress in the field, there is a lack of standardization and inability to compare titer values between preclinical and clinical studies for vectors made in different laboratories. To share and compare pharmacodynamic, pharmacokinetic, toxicologic, and efficacy data from these studies, it would be necessary to determine equivalent titer units to obtain a common dosage unit. Therefore, highly characterized reference standard stock materials (RSM) of rAAV are required to facilitate these comparisons. A RSM allows researchers to normalize their titer values to the common standard, thus allowing each group to state its titers in units that could be compared to those used in other studies; this comparison could also happen retrospectively. This need is not new to the field of gene therapy and has previously been addressed for adenoviral vectors. The Adenovirus Reference Material Working Group (ARMWG) developed and characterized the adenovirus reference material (ARM) for the purpose of normalizing titers and doses of gene therapy vectors based on adenovirus type 5 [21].

Today, an AAV serotype 2 (AAV2) RSM has been produced and characterized and is available to all members of the research community while an AAV serotype 8 (AAV8) RSM has been produced and is currently being characterized prior to release for use by the community [22, 23]. The RSMs will be used primarily to calibrate the internal standards and analytical methods used by individual laboratories in order to interrelate the doses used in different nonclinical and clinical studies. When reporting titers in the literature or to regulatory authorities, the relationship to an RSM could be included. The RSMs have been designed in a form suitable for nonclinical and clinical data support, together with the profile and information regarding the development of each RSM (*Figure 1*).

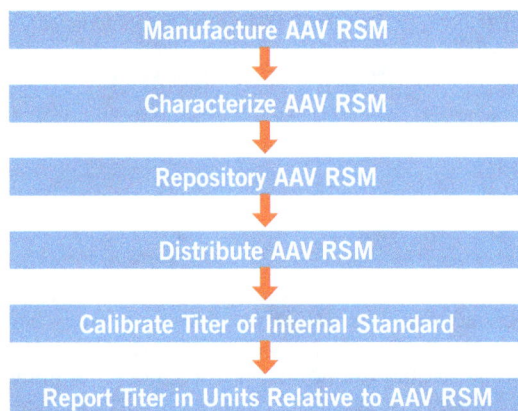

Figure 1. The AAV RSMs were manufactured and characterized to meet the amount and specifications designated by each Working Group. Once characterized and statistically analyzed, the RSMs were transferred to a repository where researchers can request vials of the RSMs. Each laboratory uses an RSM to calibrate their own internal product-specific standards and can report their vector product titers in units relative to the RSM.

AAV2 REFERENCE MATERIAL

As the first serotype used to generate vectors, AAV2 is so far the best characterized serotype for gene transfer studies in experimental animals and human subjects [10, 12, 16, 24-29].

The AAV2 Reference Standard Working Group (AAV2RSWG) was formed to produce and characterize an AAV2-green fluorescent protein (AAV2-GFP) viral vector RSM derived from the vector plasmid pTR-UF-11(ATCC # MBA-331) [30]. The AAV2RSWG is a volunteer organization and comprises members from both industry and universities in nine different countries, and the International Society for BioProcess Technology (www.ISBioTech.org), under the guidance of the FDA and NIH [22, 31].

The production and purification of the rAAV2 RSM were carried out at the Vector Core of the University of Florida's Powell Gene Therapy Center (Gainesville, FL), using helper virus-free transient transfection and chromatographic purification [31]. The production process involved cotransfection of batches of ten 10-layer Cell Factories containing HEK293 cells with an AAV2 genome/eGFP trans-gene plasmid and a second plasmid encoding the AAV2 capsid proteins and necessary helper functions. The transfected cells were harvested and the vector was purified by sequential rounds of column chromatography. The purified bulk material was vialed, confirmed negative for microbial contamination, and then distributed for characterization along with standard assay protocols and assay reagents to 16 laboratories worldwide.

A Quality Control subcommittee of the AAV2RSWG was formed for the purpose of characterizing the rAAV2 RSM. In consultation with members of the AAV2RSWG, the committee selected the following characterization assays: (1) capsid titer by A20 enzyme-linked immunosorbent assay (ELISA; Progen Biotechnik, Heidelberg, Germany); (2) vector genome titer by quantitative polymerase chain reaction (qPCR); (3) infectious titer by median tissue culture infective dose (TCID50) with qPCR readout and by transduction (green fluorescent protein [GFP] readout); and (4) purity and capsid identification by sodium dodecyl sulfate-polyacrylamide gel electrophoresis (SDS-PAGE).

Testing proceeded from July 2008 to March 2009, at which point the quantitative data were collated and statistically analyzed. Preliminary analysis showed significant variance and non-normal data distribution with all of the assays except for particle titer determination. Using statistical transformation and modeling of the raw data, mean titers and confidence intervals were determined for capsid particles, vector genomes, transducing units, and infectious units (*Table I*) [23]. Further analysis confirmed the identity of the reference material as AAV2 and the purity relative to nonvector proteins as greater than 94%. Importantly, high variance in the titers was observed despite providing a standardized protocol and reagents to the testing group and highlights the need within the AAV community for a reference standard with which assay titers can be normalized.

The rAAV2 RSM has been deposited at the American Type Culture Collection (ATCC # VR-1616) and is available to the scientific community to calibrate laboratory-specific internal titer standards.

Table I. rAAV2 reference standard material titers estimates (adapted from [23]).

Titer Units (method)	Mean	Lower 95% confidence limit for the mean	Lower 95% confidence limit for the mean	± 2 SD	± 3 SD
Particles/ml (ELISA)	9.18×10^{11}	7.89×10^{11}	1.05×10^{12}	3.73×10^{11}–1.45×10^{12}	1.04×10^{11}–1.78×10^{12}
Vector Genomes/ml (qPCR)	3.28×10^{10}	2.70×10^{10}	4.75×10^{10}	9.00×10^{8}–1.04×10^{11}	0–1.66×10^{11}
Transducing units/ml (green cells)	5.09×10^{8}	2.00×10^{8}	9.60×10^{8}	0–2.47×10^{9}	0–4.00×10^{9}
Infectious units/ml (TCID$_{50}$)	4.37×10^{9}	2.06×10^{9}	9.26×10^{9}	5.15×10^{8}–3.71×10^{10}	1.77×10^{8}–1.08×10^{11}

AAV8 REFERENCE MATERIAL

Most of the 54 clinical trials to date have involved AAV2 vectors (www.wiley.co.uk/genmed/clinical), but vector systems based on other AAV serotypes are being rapidly developed. AAV8 is becoming widely utilized for gene transfer [32]. Because the tropism of AAV8 is distinct from that of AAV2, different cells and organs can be targeted for transduction. In Europe the effort has begun to generate an AAV8 RSM. Members of the AAV8RSWG have been assembled, including 3 from industry and 17 from academia, from 10 countries [22].

The AAV8 Reference Standard Material (AAV8 RSM) has been produced in the frame of the CLINIGENE Network of Excellence. The project entitled "*A European AAV8 Reference Standard Material (AAV8 RSM): a Clinigene initiative*" was carried out by two laboratories who harmonized their production protocols, *i.e.* The Laboratoire de Thérapie Génique - UMR 649 in Nantes, France (P. Moullier) and the Center of Animal Biotechnology and Gene Therapy at Universitat Autonoma de Barcelona, Spain (F. Bosch). The final filling operation was carried out at EFS-Atlantic Bio GMP (ABG), a GMP facility, Nantes, France in an ISO5 cleanroom environment.

The AAV8-RSM is a pseudotyped AAV2 genome vector with capsid serotype 8 [32] expressing the GFP protein. To harmonize the two reference standards, the AAV8 RSS contain the same vector genome derived from pTR-UF-11 that was used for the AAV2 RSM.

The bulk of AAV8-RSM was produced using a HEK293 transfection-based protocol ie: HEK293 cells were amplified and transfected by the vector plasmid pTR-UF11 and the helper plasmid pDP8 harboring the *rep* gene from AAV2, the *cap* gene from AAV8, the adenovirus helper genes E2A, E4, VA-RNA and the ampicillin resistance gene. The protocol followed was recently described [33]. Briefly, two to three days post-transfection, the cells and the supernatant were harvested and pelleted. The cell pellet was then discarded and the supernatant was PEG-precipitated, treated with benzonase and purified by double Cesium-Chloride gradients ultracentrifugations followed by a dialysis step against Phosphate Buffer Saline with Calcium and Magnesium (DPBS) .

The purified bulk was then tested for vector genome titer, bioburden, mycoplasma and endotoxin prior to fill and finish. Final formulation and sterile filtration steps were then carried out in a ISO5 cleanroom where purified bulk was then diluted with DPBS (final volume 525mL), sterile filtered by 0,22m filtration, to generate the filtered formulated bulk. A total of 4088 vials containing 0,125mL were subsequently filled into 1.2 mL polypropylene low-binding cryovials. The AAV8 RSM has already been transferred to ATCC who will store and distribute the vials to users (ATCC # VR-1816), once the final Quality Controls assays will have been performed and the lot released. The final QC plan has been finalized by the AAV8 RSM Working Group, the assays are being beta tested, and the characterization of the AAV8 RSM will be performed in the coming months. However, the QC tests are similar to those used for the AAV2-RSM, towards harmonization between the two standards. The same testing laboratories have been solicited and ATCC will provide them with vials of the AAV8-RSM as needed. The University of Pennsylvania beta-tested the SOPs for AAV2-RSM and will coordinate both the characterization of the AAV8-RSM and beta-testing of the related protocols. Beyond the safety assays the QC plan includes assays for infectious titer, vector genome titer, and purity/identity assay (SDS-PAGE, silver stain, Western blot). Furthermore, the University of Pennsylvania is collaborating on the development of an AAV8 specific Capsid ELISA titer assay with PROGEN Gmbh, Germany. Statistical analysis of the data obtained from the different testing labs will be conducted at the University of Florida, as was previously performed for the AAV2-RSM. A stability study will also be conducted on an annual basis, including, at least the following assays: (i) infectious titer, (ii) vector genome titer and (iii) capsid integrity.

CONCLUSIONS

Following the example set by the Adenoviral Reference Material Working Group for developing the adenovirus reference material (ATCC # VR-1516) [21], the members of the AAV community are developing two high-quality AAV RSMs. The AAV2 RSM has been completely characterized and is available for the scientific community [23], and in the coming months, the AAV8 RSM will be characterized and made available through the ATCC.

Nevertheless, with more than 100 serotypes isolated so far from humans and non-human primates [32, 34]; together with an increasing number of engineered capsids [35-39] the repertoire of recombinant AAV vectors entering preclinical and clinical development is expected to increase in the near future. While having a large array of serotypes to choose from, with different tropism and seroprevalence, constitutes a great asset for the advancement of the field, each new serotype and capsid variant poses a new challenge from production, purification to characterization.

It is possible that for nonbiological assays such as vector genome titration, the AAV2/AAV8 RSM could be used for the calibration of other AAV serotypes. Because the vector capsid is not directly involved in these types of assays, it might be argued that there is no capsid specificity and that the capsid serotype would not have an impact. Regarding biological assays such as infectious titer, the paramount roles of the capsid, the required target cell line, and the helper virus preclude the use of a single RSM to calibrate other serotypes. Nevertheless, a side-by-side comparison of AAV2 *vs* AAV8 RSM will help determine whether other RSMs shall be required, or conversely if, referring to AAV2/AAV8 data would be sufficient for standardization .

In summary, the use of AAV RSMs will facilitate comparisons among nonclinical or clinical studies, the manufacture of more consistent and higher-quality vectors, and ultimately help establish accurate or appropriate regulatory policy.

ACKNOWLEDGMENTS

The AAV8 RSM has been performed with the support of the EC-DG research through the FP6-Network of Excellence, CLINIGENE: LSHB-CT-2006-018933. The AAV2 RSM work was supported by NIH grant U42RR11148. We acknowledge the generosity of members of the AAV RSM Working Groups, the laboratories who participated in the production of the AAV2 RSM and AAV8 RSM and characterization of the AAV2 RSM, along with ATCC, Nunc, Aldevron, Corning, Fisher Thermo Scientific, Indiana University Vector Production Facility, HyClone, PAA laboratories GmbH, LabClinics SA, Mediatech, Plasmid Factory, Progen, and ISBioTech. ROS may be entitled to royalties on technology discussed in this article. ROS owns equity in a gene therapy company that is commercializing AAV for gene therapy applications.

This work has been performed with the support of the EC-DG research through the FP6-Network of Excellence, CLINIGENE: LSHB-CT-2006-018933.

REFERENCES

1. Goyenvalle A, Vulin A, Fougerousse F, Leturcq F, Kaplan JC, Garcia L, Danos O. Rescue of dystrophic muscle through U7 snRNA-mediated exon skipping. *Science* 2004; 306: 1796-19.

2. Herzog RW, Hagstrom JN, Kung SH, Tai SJ, Wilson JM, Fisher KJ, High KA. Stable gene transfer and expression of human blood coagulation factor IX after intramuscular injection of recombinant adeno-associated virus. *Proc Natl Acad Sci USA* 1997; 94: 5804-9.

3. Jiang H, Pierce GF, Ozelo MC, de Paula EV, Vargas JA, Smith P, *et al*. Evidence of multiyear factor IX expression by AAV-mediated gene transfer to skeletal muscle in an individual with severe hemophilia B. *Mol Ther* 2006; 14: 452-5.

4. Jiang H, Lillicrap D, Patarroyo-White S, Liu T, Qian X, Scallan CD, *et al*. Multiyear therapeutic benefit of AAV serotypes 2, 6, and 8 delivering factor VIII to hemophilia A mice and dogs. *Blood* 2006; 108: 107-15.

5. Mas A, Montane J, Anguela XM, Munoz S, Douar AM, Riu E, *et al*. Reversal of type 1 diabetes by engineering a glucose sensor in skeletal muscle. *Diabetes* 2006; 55: 1546-53.

6. Song S, Morgan M, Ellis T, Poirier A, Chesnut K, Wang J, *et al*. Sustained secretion of human alpha-1-antitrypsin from murine muscle transduced with adeno-associated virus vectors. *Proc Natl Acad Sci USA* 1998; 95: 14384-8.

7. Mingozzi F, Hasbrouck NC, Basner-Tschakarjan E, Edmonson SA, Hui DJ, Sabatino DE, *et al*. Modulation of tolerance to the transgene product in a nonhuman primate model of AAV-mediated gene transfer to liver. *Blood* 2007; 110: 2334-41.

8. Li H, Malani N, Hamilton SR, Schlachterman A, Bussadori G, Edmonson SE, *et al*. Assessing the potential for AAV vector genotoxicity in a murine model. *Blood* 2011; 117: 3311-9.

9. Nakai H, Montini E, Fuess S, Storm TA, Grompe M, Kay MA. AAV serotype 2 vectors preferentially integrate into active genes in mice. *Nat Genet* 2003; 34: 297-302.

10. Kaplitt MG, Feigin A, Tang C, Fitzsimons HL, Mattis P, Lawlor PA, *et al*. Safety and tolerability of gene therapy with an adeno-associated virus (AAV) borne GAD gene for Parkinson's disease: an open label, phase I trial. *Lancet* 2007; 369: 2097-105.

11. Stroes ES, Nierman MC, Meulenberg JJ, Franssen R, Twisk J, Henny CP, *et al*. Intramuscular administration of AAV1-lipoprotein lipase S447X lowers triglycerides in lipoprotein lipase-deficient patients. *Arterioscler Thromb Vasc Biol* 2008; 28: 2303-4.

12. Manno CS, Pierce GF, Arruda VR, Glader B, Ragni M, Rasko JJ, *et al*. Successful transduction of liver in hemophilia by AAV-Factor IX and limitations imposed by the host immune response. *Nat Med* 2006; 12: 342-7.

13. Flotte TR, Trapnell BC, Humphries M, Carey B, Calcedo R, Rouhani F, *et al*. Phase 2 clinical trial of a recombinant adeno-associated viral vector expressing alpha1-antitrypsin: interim results. *Hum Gene Ther* 2011; 10: 1239-47.

14. Raj D, Davidoff AM, Nathwani AC. Self-complementary adeno-associated viral vectors for gene therapy of hemophilia B: progress and challenges. *Exp Rev Hematol* 2011; 4: 539-49.

15. LeWitt PA, Rezai AR, Leehey MA, Ojemann SG, Flaherty AW, Eskandar EN, *et al*. AAV2-GAD gene therapy for advanced Parkinson's disease: a double-blind, sham-surgery controlled, randomised trial. *Lancet Neurol* 2011; 10: 309-19.

16. Hauswirth WW, Aleman TS, Kaushal S, Cideciyan AV, Schwartz SB, Wang L, *et al*. Treatment of leber congenital amaurosis due to RPE65 mutations by ocular subretinal injection of adeno-associated virus gene vector: short-term results of a phase I trial. *Hum Gene Ther* 2008; 19: 979-90.

17. Bainbridge JW, Smith AJ, Barker SS, Robbie S, Henderson R, Balaggan K, *et al*. Effect of gene therapy on visual function in Leber's congenital amaurosis. *N Engl J Med* 2008; 358: 2231-9.

18. Maguire AM, Simonelli F, Pierce EA, Pugh EN Jr, Mingozzi F, Bennicelli J, *et al.* Safety and efficacy of gene transfer for Leber's congenital amaurosis. *N Engl J Med* 2008; 358: 2240-8.

19. Maguire AM, High KA, Auricchio A, Wright JF, Pierce EA, Testa F, *et al.* Age-dependent effects of RPE65 gene therapy for Leber's congenital amaurosis: a phase 1 dose-escalation trial. *Lancet* 2009; 374: 1597-605.

20. Ayuso E, Mingozzi F, Bosch F. Production, purification and characterization of adeno-associated vectors. *Curr Gene Ther* 2010; 10: 423-36.

21. Hutchins B. Development of a reference material for characterizing adenovirus vectors. *Bioprocessing Journal* 2002; 1: 25-8.

22. Moullier P, Snyder RO. International efforts for recombinant adeno-associated viral vector reference standards. *Mol Ther* 2008; 16: 1185-8.

23. Lock M, McGorray S, Auricchio A, Ayuso E, Beecham EJ, Blouin-Tavel V, *et al.* Characterization of a recombinant adeno-associated virus type 2 reference standard material. *Hum Gene Ther* 2010; 21: 1273-85.

24. Mount JD, Herzog RW, Tillson DM, Goodman SA, Robinson N, McCleland ML, *et al.* Sustained phenotypic correction of hemophilia B dogs with a factor IX null mutation by liver-directed gene therapy. *Blood* 2002; 99: 2670-6.

25. Mueller C, Flotte TR. Clinical gene therapy using recombinant adeno-associated virus vectors. *Gene Ther* 2008; 15: 858-63.

26. Flotte TR. Recent developments in recombinant AAV-mediated gene therapy for lung diseases. *Curr Gene Ther* 2005; 5: 361-6.

27. Adriaansen J, Tas SW, Klarenbeek PL, Bakker AC, Apparailly F, Firestein GS, *et al.* Enhanced gene transfer to arthritic joints using adeno-associated virus type 5: implications for intra-articular gene therapy. *Ann Rheum Dis* 2005; 64: 1677-84.

28. Acland GM, Aguirre GD, Ray J, Zhang Q, Aleman TS, Cideciyan AV, *et al.* Gene therapy restores vision in a canine model of childhood blindness. *Nat Genet* 2001; 28: 92-5.

29. Niemeyer GP, Herzog RW, Mount J, Arruda VR, Tillson DM, Hathcock J, *et al.* Long-term correction of inhibitor-prone hemophilia B dogs treated with liver-directed AAV2-mediated factor IX gene therapy. *Blood* 2009; 113: 797-806.

30. Burger C, Gorbatyuk OS, Velardo MJ, Peden CS, Williams P, Zolotukhin S, *et al.* Recombinant AAV viral vectors pseudotyped with viral capsids from serotypes 1, 2, and 5 display differential efficiency and cell tropism after delivery to different regions of the central nervous system. *Mol Ther* 2004; 10: 302-17.

31. Potter M, Phillipsber G, Phillipsberg T, Petersen M, Sanders D, Fife J, *et al.* Manufacture and stability study of the recombinant adeno-associated virus serotype 2 reference standard. *Bioprocessing Journal* 2008; 7: 8-14.

32. Gao GP, Alvira MR, Wang L, Calcedo R, Johnston J, Wilson JM. Novel adeno-associated viruses from rhesus monkeys as vectors for human gene therapy. *Proc Natl Acad Sci USA* 2002; 99: 11854-9.

33. Ayuso E, Mingozzi F, Montane J, Leon X, Anguela XM, Haurigot V, *et al.* High AAV vector purity results in serotype- and tissue-independent enhancement of transduction efficiency. *Gene Ther* 2010; 17: 503-10.

34. Gao G, Vandenberghe LH, Alvira MR, Lu Y, Calcedo R, Zhou X, Wilson JM. Clades of adeno-associated viruses are widely disseminated in human tissues. *J Virol* 2004; 78: 6381-6388.

35. Zhong L, Li B, Mah CS, Govindasamy L, Agbandje-McKenna M, Cooper M, *et al.* Next generation of adeno-associated virus 2 vectors: point mutations in tyrosines lead to high-efficiency transduction at lower doses. *Proc Natl Acad Sci USA* 2008; 105: 7827-32.

36. Chen YH, Chang M, Davidson BL. Molecular signatures of disease brain endothelia provide new sites for CNS-directed enzyme therapy. *Nat Med* 2009; 15: 1215-8.

37. Perabo L, Endell J, King S, Lux K, Goldnau D, Hallek M, Buning H. Combinatorial engineering of a gene therapy vector: directed evolution of adeno-associated virus. *J Gene Med* 2006; 8: 155-62.

38. Koerber JT, Klimczak R, Jang JH, Dalkara D, Flannery G, Schaffer DV. Molecular evolution of adeno-associated virus for enhanced glial gene delivery. *Mol Ther* 2009; 17: 2088-95.

39. Choi VW, McCarty DM, Samulski RJ. AAV hybrid serotypes: improved vectors for gene delivery. *Curr Gene Ther* 2005; 5: 299-310.

TECHNOLOGIES

Retrovirus mediated gene transfer state-of-the-art

COORDINATED BY
PEDRO E. CRUZ
AND
MANUEL J.T. CARRONDO

The CliniBook: Clinical gene transfer
Edited by Odile Cohen-Haguenauer – EDK, Paris © 2012, pp.93-99

A2-1
Highlights on retrovirus mediated gene transfer

PEDRO E. CRUZ[1,2]*, MANUEL J.T. CARRONDO[1]

[1]*IBET, Apartado 12, 2781-901 Oeiras, Portugal.*
[2]*ECBio, S.A., R. Henrique Paiva Couceiro, 27, 2700-451 Amadora, Portugal.*
pcruz@itqb.unl.pt
* Corresponding author

OVERVIEW

During the five years of Clinigene the Retrovirus platform has focused on solving a number of bottlenecks that hampered the use of these vectors in the clinic. Specifically, safety issues related to the integration in the host cell genome and manufacturing limitations related to vector titre and stability were addressed. Several partners focused on improving vector design for example by using genetic insulators or on the optimisation of self-inactivating vectors. Others concentrated their efforts on developing new and safer producer cells and improved production and purification processes.

After the creation of the Biosafety platform most of the safety issues span-off but vector design and production bridged these two platforms with clear positive results.

Regarding the translation to the clinic, the trials on ADA-SCID conducted in Milan resulted in the hallmark not only for this platform but also for the gene therapy field itself. Other trials resulting from the work performed in the Retrovirus platform, namely for Cancer, X-SCID and Fanconi's anemia, using new improved and safer vectors will continue to show the potential of this technology and demonstrate its impact in the society human health improvement.

INTRODUCTION

Retroviral vectors were used in the first gene therapy clinical trial starting in 1990 for the treatment of adenosine deaminase deficiency (ADA) [1].

Today, retroviral vectors are still amongst the most widely used vectors in gene therapy clinical trials, mainly on the treatment of genetic diseases but also to target pathologies of other origins, such as cancers or neurological disorders.

One of the most relevant characteristics of retroviral vectors in what gene therapy is concerned is the integration of the genetic material into the host-cell genome, resulting in long-term transgene expression. This makes them particularly competent for the treatment of monogenic diseases. Indeed, retroviruses have been used in the treatment of X-linked severe combined immunodeficiency, one of the most relevant successes of gene therapy [2]. This recent demonstration of life-saving immune reconstitution in trials for X-SCID fully confirms the efficacy of both gene transfer approach and retroviral vectors.

BOTTLENECKS AND CHALLENGES

In the last five years significant research has been made at different levels. Due to the foreseen increase in the demand of retroviral vectors for phase III clinical trials, in Clinigene NoE several bottlenecks and limitations were specifically targeted to allow large-scale production and widespread application of these vectors while maintaining good safety profile (*Table I*). The areas of focus included efficacy and safety, quality and manufacture, biosafety studies and clinical trials.

Table I. Bottlenecks and technical limitations in the development of retrovirus-based gene therapy vectors and solutions found in Clinigene NoE.

Bottlenecks	Technical limitations	Solutions found
• Integration - insertional mutagenesis • Safe vectors • Vector targeting • Producer cell characterisation	• Production - vector titers • Purification - yields • Vector stability	• New vectors designs including new SIN and insulated vectors • Development of characterised packaging cells with specific integration sites • Novel purification, formulation and storage protocols

EFFICACY AND SAFETY

MLV LTR driven retroviral vectors have been shown to activate proto-oncogenes. This risk is a major concern that hampers potential therapeutic applications of retroviral vectors.

The development of SIN retroviral vectors, lacking enhancer/promoter elements at viral LTR's has significantly reduced the oncogenic potential, confirming the importance of retroviral vector design in vector safety [3]. Further improvements on SIN vectors included the use of physiological promoters and led to significant decrease in the ability to induce clonal dominance in hematopoietic stem cells [4].

• One of these new vectors, a gammaretroviral SIN vector expressing IL2RG from the internal EF1a promoter has been used in an international clinical trial that started in December 2010 (ICH London, Necker Hospital Paris, Cincinnati Children's Hospital, UCLA). This vector has a significantly lower genotoxicity in comparison with MFG-gc shown in cell-based assay and C57BL6 model (collaboration with Cincinnati Children's Hospital and Harvard Medical School).

• A different approach followed to devise safer vectors was the development of new genetic insulator elements. Genetic insulators are *cis*-elements that act as boundary, inhibiting enhancer or silencer interactions between the integrated transgene and the surrounding chromatin. Due to the deletions of enhancer-promoter sequences from the 3'U3 region in SIN viral vectors mentioned above, these elements could be introduced to further improve vector performance. The implementation of genetic insulator elements in SIN retroviral vectors contributed to the reduction of genotoxicity potential, as shown in cell culture-based immortalization assays [4-6].

The development of more powerful insulators and research on their efficacy is still ongoing as described by Cohen-Haguenauer *et al.* ([7] and *ibid.*, see chapter A3-4).

• Along with the research on improving gammaretroviral vectors, a novel alpharetroviral SIN vector platform based on Rous sarcoma virus (RSV) was also developed. These vectors can be an alternative as they show a more neutral integration spectrum, with advantages on safety. Furthermore, the low titers commonly observed in SIN vectors were circumvented by codon optimization of the Gag/Pol expression construct and further optimization steps leading to titers over 10^7 infectious particle per ml in human cells [8].

• Improved SIN vectors and the alpharetroviral vector platform are described below by Baum *et al* (See chapter A2-2).

• In parallel with the development of non-replicative vectors, important developments were achieved by using replicant competent retroviruses to deliver RNAi to tumour cells *in vitro* and *in vivo*. Although the major goal was to study gene function of tumour biology, efficacy was also evaluated. *In vitro* studies were done to determine the delivery and knockdown efficiencies of a miRNA-adapted shRNA expression cassette inserted between env and 3' LTR by silencing Luciferase and eGFP *in vitro*. Proof of concept *in vivo* was performed by silencing PLK1, in a HT1080 tumor by intratumoural application. Significant reduction in the increase of tumor volume after 25 days was observed [9]. Tumour specificity and long-term down regulation of the desired target gene were confirmed. This approach is further described in a sub-chapter (See chapter A2-3) below by Schaser and collaborators.

QUALITY/MANUFACTURE

The work on the production of retroviral vectors was done at different levels: producer cell creation, culture medium optimization and production process development - bioreaction, downstream processing and storage.

One of the main strategies in cell line creation used targeted genome integration to derive well-defined high-titer retroviral modular producer cells. Two cell lines were created; Flp293A and 293 FLEX, both derived from 293 cells, which produce retroviral vectors pseudotyped with amphotropic and GaLV envelopes, respectively [10, 11]. In this new approach, a favorable chromosomal site for stable and high retroviral vector production is first identified and tagged. Due to the presence of two heterologous non-compatible FRT sites flanking the tagged retroviral genome, this defined chromosomal site can be re-used of by means of recombinase mediated cassette exchange. Details on the cell line creation process can be found below in the sub-chapter (See chapter A2-4) by Coroadinha and co-workers.

The resulting producer cell clones are genetically identical and yield reproducibly high levels of viruses (up to 2.5×10^7 infectious particles per 10^6 cells in 24h were obtained within three weeks) even for different transgenes. Furthermore, the single, defined integration site in modular producer cell lines provides the high level of safety needed for the implementation of these vectors into the clinic.

The amount of retroviral vectors required, per patient ranges between 10^9-10^{10} [12]. This corresponds to 1-10L volume of culture per patient for the titers usually obtained in the order of 10^6-10^7 infectious particles per mL. Along with the low titers, the stability of retroviral vectors (with half lives of 2-9 h at the normal production temperature of 37°C), also make difficult the establishment of efficient production processes [13]. Within Clinigene, several production steps were optimized including the culture conditions, the times of harvesting and, at the end, the purification process and storage conditions.

Culture conditions and medium composition have a significant impact on viral titres due to their effect upon producer cell metabolism. This has been studied in order to better understand how medium constituents, such as sugars, influence vector productivity and stability. Specifically, it was shown that elevated medium osmolality, created by addition of osmolytes or elevated sugar concentrations to the culture medium, increases specific retrovirus productivity and stability, which has also been related with alterations in producer cell lipid metabolism [14].

Regulatory agencies quality requirements strongly suggest that serum be eliminated from culture. The use of serum-free media is an important step regarding prevention of immunological response to viral preparation and also helps development of purification strategies. Several human derived producer cell lines have been adapted to reduced-serum or serum-free medium while maintaining high titres [15].

Currently, the purification of retroviral vectors for clinical applications involves the use of different separation technologies, usually based on chromatography and membrane processes [16]. The main goal under Clinigene in this line of work was the development of fast and efficient purification strategies.

Membrane separation techniques were applied for clarification, concentration and partial purification of retroviral supernatants. Ultrafiltration was optimized to concentrate and wash feed streams prior to chromatography. Indeed, chromatography is the heart of the purification strategies tested but due to the low stability of retroviral vectors, the definition of the conditions for chromatographic purification, including the chromatographic medium and buffers used, is of extreme relevance. Anion exchange chromatography (AEXc) offers milder conditions and elevated purification factors. AEXc is based on the adsorption of negatively charged retroviral vectors to positively charged resins. Using AEXc it was possible to obtain in this step up to 70% recovery of infectious particles [14]. Size exclusion chromatography (SEC) has also been efficiently applied to the separation of retroviruses from cellular and medium contaminants but it is difficult to scale up and has a very low throughput. A scaleable purification process involving microfiltration, ultrafiltration and AEXc was developed providing a global yield of 26% in infectious retroviral particles with a final vector titer of 3.2×10^8 infectious particles per mL [16].

Finally, it was demonstrated that AEXc enables the separation of gp70 proteins as well as envelope protein-free vectors constituting a significant improvement to the quality of retroviral preparations for gene therapy applications [17].

The use of purified vectors created the need for new stabilizing formulations as pure vectors are more sensitive than those from clarified supernatants. For this purpose, the identification of the inactivation mechanisms, mainly related to the inactivation of reverse transcriptase was extremely important [18]. Vector stabilization at 4°C after purification could be achieved by adding recombinant human albumin (rHSA) to the storage buffer [19]. For freezing, the addition of cryoprotectants (*e.g.*, sucrose and trehalose) is necessary to decrease the loss of infectivity of viral vectors and thus enhances their stability during long term storage [20].

The advances made in the quality and manufacture of retroviral vectors mentioned above had a proof of concept on the production a 8.9kb collagen VII therapeutic vector for the treatment of epidermolysis bullosa. The modular cells were used to produce vectors under optimized conditions. Vectors were subsequently purified and shown to infect target cells - keratynocyte cell lines and primary cells [21]. Overall, it was shown that therapeutic virus production from bench to bedside could be done safer, faster, and cheaper.

BIOSAFETY STUDIES

The need for safer vectors promoted the development of assays for their assessment. *In vivo* assays and cell based assays such as *in vitro* immortalization (IVIM) assay developed by Modlich and co-workers [3] have been used to systematically evaluate and compare the performance of different retroviral vectors in respect to their cell transforming potential. IVIM assay has been shown to be particularly robust method to measure the impact of vector content and insertion pattern on insertional genotoxicity. The insertional preferences and cell transforming potential of different viral vectors upon transduction of hematopoietic cells can be determined in a fast and expedite way. Moreover, it is envisioned that further developments of this method will allow its broader application in different cell lineages. As for *in vivo* tests, insertional genotoxicity assays were performed in C57BL6 serial BMT model [22] and *cdkn2a$^{-/-}$* cancer prone mice ([23] and *ibid.*). The use of highthroughput integration sites analysis is detailed by Schmidt and von Kalle (See B2-3) in a dedicated chapter (*ibid.*), based on improved techniques [24].

CLINICAL TRIALS

To date, retroviral vector gene delivery has been applied in many diseases in phase I clinical trials. Presently, clinical trials involving retroviral vectors cover a broad range of pathologies from genetic to cardiovascular and infectious diseases, neurodegenerative disorders and also ocular pathologies, besides an extensive variety of cancers, which still constitute the major target. An updated overview on the current applications of retroviral vectors in gene therapy clinical trials can be found in www.clinigene.eu.

The cure of ADA-SCID by introducing a function adenosine deaminase enzyme in patients haematopoietic stem cells [2] has become a hallmark for gene therapy and an encouraging result for all groups working in the development of retroviral vectors. The ADA-SCID clinical trials are described in a dedicated chapter below by Aiuti and co-workers (See chapter C1-3).

FUTURE DIRECTIONS

Retroviral vectors are one of the preferentially used tools for gene therapy applications due to their advantages relatively to other vectors. Indeed, the success of their application in both phase I and II clinical trials is now opening prospects to phase III trials. The research undertaken in Clinigene in the last five years was key to support large-scale production of these vectors. Despite the advances in packaging cells and the vectors themselves, several steps of the vector production process can still be improved. Reduction of costs for large-scale GMP production and certification of clinical grade vectors are important issues. Herein, the most recent strategies together with future innovations will certainly be valuable to increase productivity, stability, quality and safety of retroviral vectors for clinical applications.

As the number and scale of clinical trials increase international harmonisation of requirements for clinical grade vector production (specially between EU and USA) would significantly contribute for the clinical development and application of these vectors.

ACKNOWLEDGMENTS

This work has been performed with the support of the EC-DG research through the FP6-Network of Excellence, CLINIGENE: LSHB-CT-2006-018933.

REFERENCES

1. Blaese RM, Culver KW, Miller AD, Carter CS, Fleisher T, Clerici M, *et al*. T lymphocyte-directed gene therapy for ADA- SCID: initial trial results after 4 years. *Science* 1995; 270: 475-80.

2. Aiuti A, Cattaneo F, Galimberti S, Benninghoff U, Cassani B, Callegaro L, *et al*. Gene therapy for immunodeficiency due to adenosine deaminase deficiency. *N Engl J Med* 2009; 360: 447-58.

3. Modlich U, Bohne J, Schmidt M, von Kalle C, Knoss S, Schambach A, Baum C. Cell-culture assays reveal the importance of retroviral vector design for insertional genotoxicity. *Blood* 2006; 108: 2545-53.

4. Zychlinski D, Schambach A, Modlich U, Maetzig T, Meyer J, Grassman E, *et al*. Physiological promoters reduce the genotoxic risk of integrating gene vectors. *Mol Ther* 2008; 16: 718-25.

5. Modlich U, Navarro S, Zychlinski D, Maetzig T, Knoess S, Brugman MH, *et al*. Insertional transformation of hematopoietic cells by self-inactivating lentiviral and gammaretroviral vectors. *Mol Ther* 2009; 17: 1919-28.

6. Gaussin A, Modlich U, Bauche C, Niederlander NJ, Schambach A, Duros C, *et al*. CTF/NF1 transcription factors act as potent genetic insulators for integrating gene transfer vectors. *Gene Ther* 2011; May 12 (*online*).

7. Duros C, Artus A, Gaussin A, Scholtz S, Cesana D, Montini E, *et al*. Insulated lentiviral vectors towards safer gene transfer to stem cells. In: *2011 Annual meeting of the Society of gene and cell therapy*. Seattle-Washington, 2011.

8. Suerth JD, Maetzig T, Galla M, Baum C, Schambach A. Self-inactivating alpharetroviral vectors with a split-packaging design. *J Virol* 2010; 84: 6626-35.

9. Schaser T, Wrede C, Duerner L, Sliva K, Cichutek K, Schnierle B, Buchholz CJ. RNAi-mediated gene silencing in tumour tissue using replication-competent retroviral vectors. *Gene Ther* 2011; 18: 953-60.

10. Schucht R, Coroadinha AS, Zanta-Boussif MA, Verhoeyen E, Carrondo MJ, Hauser H, Wirth D. A new generation of retroviral producer cells: predictable and stable virus production by Flp-mediated site-specific integration of retroviral vectors. *Mol Ther* 2006; 14: 285-92.

11. Coroadinha AS, Schucht R, Gama-Norton L, Wirth D, Hauser H, Carrondo MJ. The use of recombinase mediated cassette exchange in retroviral vector producer cell lines: predictability and efficiency by transgene exchange. *J Biotechnol* 2006; 124: 457-68.

12. Cruz PE, Rodrigues T, Carmo M, Wirth D, Amaral AI, Alves PM, Coroadinha AS. Manufacturing of retroviruses. *Methods Mol Biol* 2011; 737: 157-82.

13. Merten OW. State-of-the-art of the production of retroviral vectors. *J Gene Med* 2004; 6 (suppl 1): S105-24.

14 Coroadinha AS, Silva AC, Pires E, Coelho A, Alves PM, Carrondo MJ. Effect of osmotic pressure on the production of retroviral vectors: enhancement in vector stability. *Biotechnol Bioeng* 2006; 94: 322-9.

15. Rodrigues AF, Carmo M, Alves PM, Coroadinha AS. Retroviral vector production under serum deprivation: the role of lipids. *Biotechnol Bioeng* 2009; 104: 1171-81.

16. Rodrigues T, Carvalho A, Carmo M, Carrondo MJ, Alves PM, Cruz PE. Scaleable purification process for gene therapy retroviral vectors. *J Gene Med* 2007; 9: 233-43.

17. Rodrigues T, Alves A, Lopes A, Carrondo MJ, Alves PM, Cruz PE. Removal of envelope protein-free retroviral vectors by anion-exchange chromatography to improve product quality. *J Sep Sci* 2008; 31: 3509-18.

18. Carmo M, Panet A, Carrondo MJ, Alves PM, Cruz PE. From retroviral vector production to gene transfer: spontaneous inactivation is caused by loss of reverse transcription capacity. *J Gene Med* 2008; 10: 383-91.

19. Carmo M, Alves A, Rodrigues AF, Coroadinha AS, Carrondo MJ, Alves PM, Cruz PE. Stabilization of gammaretroviral and lentiviral vectors: from production to gene transfer. *J Gene Med* 2009; 11: 670-8.

20. Cruz PE, Silva AC, Roldao A, Carmo M, Carrondo MJ, Alves PM. Screening of novel excipients for improving the stability of retroviral and adenoviral vectors. *Biotechnol Prog* 2006; 22: 568-76.

21. Carrondo M, Panet A, Wirth D, Coroadinha AS, Cruz P, Falk H, *et al.* Integrated strategy for the production of therapeutic retroviral vectors. *Hum Gene Ther* 2011; 22: 370-9.

22. Kustikova OS, Schiedlmeier B, Brugman MH, Stahlhut M, Bartels S, Li Z, Baum C. Cell-intrinsic and vector-related properties cooperate to determine the incidence and consequences of insertional mutagenesis. *Mol Ther* 2009; 17: 1537-47.

23. Montini E, Cesana D, Schmidt M, Sanvito F, Bartholomae CC, Ranzani M, *et al.* The genotoxic potential of retroviral vectors is strongly modulated by vector design and integration site selection in a mouse model of HSC gene therapy. *J Clin Invest* 2009; 119: 964-75.

24. Gabriel R, Eckenberg R, Paruzynski A, Bartholomae CC, Nowrouzi A, Arens A, *et al.* Comprehensive genomic access to vector integration in clinical gene therapy. *Nat Med* 2009; 15: 14316.

The CliniBook: Clinical gene transfer
Edited by Odile Cohen-Haguenauer – EDK, Paris © 2012, pp. 100-111

A2-2
Retroviral vector development: reducing genotoxicity of integrated DNA and creating virus-like particles for transient cell modification

MELANIE GALLA, TOBIAS MAETZIG, JULIA D. SUERTH, UTE MODLICH, AXEL SCHAMBACH, CHRISTOPHER BAUM*

Hannover Medical School (MHH) Institute of Experimental Haematology,
Carl-Neuberg-Str. 1, D-30625 Hannover, Germany.
baum.christopher@mh-hannover.de
* Corresponding author

Since the early 1980s, retrovirus-based vectors are increasingly used to stably integrate recombinant DNA into target cells [1-3]. Typical applications include the transfer of genes into hematopoietic stem cells (HSCs) or other cells with high proliferative capacity, such as T lymphocytes. The first retroviral vectors were based on Moloney murine leukemia virus (MoMLV), a simple gamma-retrovirus [1]. Modifications introduced two decades ago typically affected the enhancer-promoter region, and the replacement of a potential repressor element that overlapped with the MoMLV primer binding site by an epigenetically neutral sequence, with the aim to increase transcription levels in hematopoietic cells [4-7]. These modifications maintained the original design of intact long terminal repeats (LTRs), and thus, efforts were also made to improve the post-transcriptional processing of the rather large untranslated regions in the LTR-driven transcript, by removing aberrant reading frames and introducing alternative splice sites [8, 9].

Gamma-retroviral vectors are paradigmatic for the establishment of stable packaging cells, which use a split-genome design to reduce the risk of recombination events that may form replication-competent retroviruses (RCR) [1, 2]. Progress made with the development of suitable pseudotypes and improvements of gene expression cassettes have led to a series of clinical trials, primarily targeting HSCs or T-lymphocytes, with long-term success achieved in some applications [10]. The advent of lentiviral vectors, capable of transducing resting cells, has illustrated the great potential of the extended world of retroviruses for vector development [11]. We thus aimed for a holistic approach, exploring and combining principles of different members of the *Retroviridae* family, as a basis to develop new and translationally useful principles for therapeutic cell modification [12].

SIN VECTOR DEVELOPMENT

Limitations of the first generation of clinically used gamma-retroviral vectors were largely caused by the maintenance of the original genome architecture. The presence of potent, unspecific enhancer-promoter sequences in the U3 region of the LTRs not only promotes the potential formation of RCRs, it also increases the risk of insertional host gene activation by various mechanisms. While RCRs were only observed in one clinically relevant application (a non-human primate model) [13], insertional mutagenesis was identified as a major dose limiting adverse event in pre-clinical models [14, 15] and unfortunately also in clinical trials (targeting X-linked severe combined immunodeficiency, Wiskott-Aldrich Syndrome and Chronic Granulomatous Disease) [16-19].

The "self-inactivating" (SIN) design, which avoids enhancer-promoter sequences in the U3 region, addresses both risks, RCR formation and insertional mutagenesis. The development of SIN retroviral vectors was already proposed in 1986 [20], but at that time the vector production technology was not sufficiently advanced to allow SIN vector production at a scale and with a titer required for clinical application. With the aim to increase vector potency and safety, we made several contributions to SIN vectorology over the past years:

A substantial deletion was engineered in the gamma-retroviral U3 region, extending the region deleted in the first generation SIN vectors and thus encompassing all known enhancer and promoter sequences [21]. The resulting vectors could be produced at high titers by transient transfection, similar to LTR-driven constructs, after we modified the "genomic" promoter (the promoter driving full-length mRNA in the packaging cells) [22]. With collaborators, stable packaging cells were generated to support gamma-retroviral SIN vector production in a system that relies on recombinase-mediated cassette-exchange in a master packaging clone [23] (also see Coroadinha *et al., ibid.*).

We also developed variants of the widely used woodchuck hepatitis virus post-transcriptional regulatory element (WPRE) [24], originally introduced by Hope *et al.* to increase lentiviral vector titers and expression [25]. We described several versions of the WPRE that have residual reading frames destroyed and a cryptic promoter for the hepadnaviral X-protein deleted [24], now used for clinical grade vector development by several investigators, in lentiviral or gamma-retroviral vectors and also in transposons and adeno-associated viral vectors.

Following a systematic comparison of SIN vector potency in the gamma-retroviral and lentiviral context [26], a gamma-retroviral SIN vector was created for a second-generation clinical trial to treat children suffering from X-linked severe combined immunodeficiency (SCID-X1) by gene therapy [27]. This allowed the clinical investigators to change only one variable in their otherwise successful clinical trial design [28]. This variable is the most likely cause of the insertional leukemias occurring as adverse events in two first generation clinical trials, *i.e.* proto-oncogene upregulation induced by the insertion of an LTR-driven expression cassette [29, 30]. The new gamma-retroviral SIN vector was shown to be sufficiently potent to restore the development of lymphocytes in preclinical models [27], and its backbone had a significantly lower risk of insertional mutagenesis according to the results of transformation assays [31]. The new gamma-retroviral SIN vector to correct SCID-X1 was produced in large scale through a collaboration with Cincinnati Children's Hospital Medical Center [32] and shared with several clinical investigators in the USA, France and UK to commence the first transatlantic multicenter clinical trial in gene therapy. Other gamma-retroviral SIN vectors developed on the same platform showed promising performance in a preclinical model of mucopolysaccharidosis I [33].

Furthermore, in collaboration with other investigators we tested the effects of codon-optimization of expression units delivered by various forms of gamma-retroviral and lentiviral vectors, including vectors used for cellular reprogramming. Using an own algorithm in combination with the suggestions made from commercial suppliers, we designed codon-optimized vectors to express various cDNAs (*IL2RG*, *WASP*, *RAG1*, *BTK*, *OCT4*, *KLF4*, *SOX2*, and others) [34-38]. A codon-optimized multicistronic lentiviral construct that we designed to express the canonical "Yamanaka" transcription factors for reprogramming of somatic cells to induced pluripotent cells (OCT4, KLF4, SOX2, c-MYC) [39] has been shown to work very efficiently, allowing live-cell monitoring of the reprogramming process [34], with potential excision of the reprogramming cassette by transient delivery of Flp recombinase protein in established pluripotent cell clones. This vector is now used by various distinguished laboratories contributing to the emerging discipline of cell reprogramming with the aim of generating novel cell sources for biological studies and therapeutic applications.

QUANTITATIVE GENOTOXICITY ASSAYS

Determining the impact of vector modifications on the risk of insertional mutagenesis required the development of robust, sensitive and quantitative assays. Triggered by an observation of N. Copeland's laboratory [40], we introduced an *in vitro* immortalization assay that scores insertional mutants with insertional upregulation of either *Evi-1* or *Prdm16*, two proto-oncogenes that have been associated with clonal outgrowth in clinical trials [31, 41-44]. This assay allows a precise determination of the incidence and proliferative fitness of insertional mutants as a function of any of the following variables: target cell type, culture conditions, vector copy number, vector enhancer or promoter, vector architecture (LTR vs. SIN), presence of additional regulatory elements such as WPRE or insulators, and vector integration pattern [31, 41-45].
Our results indicate that the modification of the integration pattern is most important for vectors containing strong enhancers, and can reduce the risk of insertion events by up to 10-fold in this setting [31, 42]. Furthermore, by redesigning the transgene expression cassette, even when maintaining the rather disadvantageous insertion pattern of gamma-retroviral vectors, the risk of insertion events can be attenuated below the detection limit of the assay (more than 10-fold increased safety compared to conventional LTR vectors) [31]. Insulators can reduce the fitness of mutants induced by vectors that contain strong internal enhancers [31, 43, 45], and we hypothesized that the resulting reduced proliferation rate may lower the risk to acquire secondary mutations. However, an insulator that is sufficiently potent to fully shield strong enhancers, such as those derived from murine leukemia viruses, still needs to be defined. A remaining limitation of this *in vitro* immortalization assay is that it does not reflect the risk of gene disruption events, which are potentially more likely for lentiviral than for gamma-retroviral vectors, owing to the canonical features of the integrase, its cellular interaction partners and the epigenetic landscape of the cellular genome [46-48]. Nevertheless, the assay was successfully used to test the insertional risk of several vectors proposed for new clinical trials, typically in academic collaborations supported by network grants. So far, the results obtained in this assay were largely consistent with, and sometimes even more sensitive than data obtained in more cumbersome transplantation models [15, 49-52].

ALPHA-RETROVIRAL VECTOR DEVELOPMENT

The propensity to target genomic transcriptional start sites and CpG-rich regulatory elements for integration of the transgene can be considered as a potential disadvantage of SIN gamma-retroviral vectors. Lentiviral vectors do not seem to offer a perfect solution since they have a clear preference for integration within transcribed gene regions, thus potentially causing problems by gene truncation or fusion transcripts [46, 47]. In contrast, the alpha-retroviruses are known to have a relatively neutral integration pattern [53, 54]. This was a first and most obvious reason to explore the development of alpha-retroviral SIN vectors for clinical applications.

Secondly, the removal of residual splice sites can be important to reduce the risk of RNA-processing mediated insertional mutagenesis. Like lentiviral vectors, SIN gamma-retroviral vectors can only be produced at optimal titers when the major splice donor remains in the vector backbone. Interestingly, in the Rous sarcoma virus (RSV), the prototypical alpha-retrovirus, the major splice donor is located in Gag, and not in the 5' untranslated leader region shortly downstream of the primer binding site, as in MoMLV or HIV-1. Therefore, in the case of alpha-retroviruses, the removal of Gag from vector constructs also deletes the major splice donor, yet without compromising the titer [55].

A third potential advantage of an alpha-retroviral SIN vector system would be the failure of the original Rous sarcoma virus (RSV) to replicate in human cells. Thus, even if RCR genomes may be formed, they are unlikely to spread in human cells, in contrast to gamma-retroviral or lentiviral RCR for which no such limitation is known.

A fourth interesting feature of RSV is its large proviral genome, which not only comprises the canonical *gag-pol* and *env* genes but also the *src* oncogene. If replaceable, this may offer space for relatively large transgene cassettes.

The final argument in favor of an alpha-retroviral vector system is the absence of an overt toxicity in cells stably expressing the proteins encoded by *gag* and *pol*. This may promote the establishment of stable packaging cells, following the principles known for gamma-retroviral vectors.

Based on these considerations, we were able to develop a novel alpha-retroviral SIN vector platform in which all viral coding sequences and the major splice sites were removed from the gene vector. Furthermore, the enhancer-promoter of the U3 region was deleted. In total, we thus removed >8kb of retroviral sequences from the vector backbone. This created space for the insertion of new gene cassettes [55]. The exact packaging limit remains to be defined.

Removing the enhancer-promoter sequences allowed the transcriptional control of the gene(s) of interest to originate from the internal promoter. Typically used cellular promoters such as PGK or EF1α functioned well in the alpha-retroviral context, although the expression levels were slightly lower than those obtained with lentiviral or gamma-retroviral vectors. Other promoters are under investigation.

Vector production in human cells was accomplished with codon-optimization of the gag-pol message [55]. Preliminary data suggest that this modification still does not support replication in human cells. Titers achieved with three-plasmid split packaging systems are in the same range as known for gamma-retroviral and lentiviral production systems. Pseudotyping was shown to be possible with a variety of clinically used envelope proteins, including vesicular stomatitis virus glycoprotein [56], the RD114/TR variant based on a feline endogenous retrovirus [57], and the ecotropic and amphotropic envelopes of MoMLV [55].

The host range of the alpha-retroviral vector particles depended on the pseudotype. Similar as gamma-retroviruses but different from lentiviruses, the alpha-retroviral vectors require mitosis to integrate the transgene into cellular chromosomes. However, there is some evidence that certain terminally differentiated cells are also susceptible to alpha-retroviral transduction [58, 59]. For the newly developed, pseudotyped alpha-retroviral SIN vectors, the range of cell types that can be transduced by *in vivo* application remains to be established. A restricted *in vivo* host range is a potential safety advantage in case of inadvertent contamination of *ex vivo* treated cells with residual infectious vector particles. Indeed, careful studies performed with cells exposed to lentiviral vectors have indicated that transmission of replication-deficient vectors is a relevant concern [60].

Taken together, our data suggest that alpha-retroviral SIN vectors are an interesting alternative, especially for those applications for which gamma-retroviral protocols have already led to a clinical benefit (such as immunodeficiency syndromes, modification of T-lymphocytes with new antigen receptors or genetic correction of keratinocytes).

RETROVIRAL DELIVERY OF EPISOMAL DNA

In the context of lentiviral vectors, a prominent study established the potential utility of episomal circular intermediates of the retroviral life cycle to confer a therapeutic activity in terminally differentiated retinal cells [61]. Targeted mutations in catalytic core of the Integrase enzyme, encoded in the retroviral *pol* reading frame, efficiently block chromosomal integration of proviral DNA [62-65]. We generated a similar principle by deleting attachment sites of the viral Integrase from the LTR [66]. However, whatever mechanism is used to inhibit the Integrase, residual integration events also occur for retroviral/lentiviral episomes. As these events follow a non-Integrase mediated mechanism and are rare, especially in postmitotic cells, episomal retroviral/lentiviral vectors hold promise for a large number of applications. We derived a series of such integration-deficient vectors based on both, lentiviral and gamma-retroviral vectors, and equipped these vectors with bicistronic promoters [67], previously shown to work well in integration-proficient lentiviral vectors to co-express fluorescent proteins along with another gene of interest [68]. Having obtained evidence that RNA double strand formation reduces the titer of retrovirus-based vectors containing bidirectional promoters, we developed a strategy to increase titers by the co-expression of an accessory viral protein in the packaging cells [67].

The increasing repertoire of episomal retrovirus-based vectors offers a broadly applicable platform for the transient modification of proliferating cells, and the quasi permanent modification of resting cells. As for integrating vectors, gene dosage effects can be addressed with the choice of the promoter and the copy number of the transgene cassette.

RETROVIRAL TRANSDUCTION OF mRNA AND PROTEIN

In the course of our studies investigating the mechanisms of splice regulation in gamma-retroviruses [69], we observed that gamma-retroviral vectors which were deficient to initiate reverse transcription still delivered the biological activity encoded by the proviral genome into target cells, given that the cDNA was placed in the position of the gag-pol transcription unit. Since our gamma-retroviral vectors were designed to have all aberrant translational start codons upstream of gag deleted, we wondered whether retroviral particles that fail to initiate reverse transcription may allow translation of their genomic mRNA in target cells, following disassembly of the capsid. A series of experiments confirmed this hypothesis [66, 70]. We thus developed vectors that are deficient in reverse transcription [66, 70, 71], utilizing an artificial primer binding site that fails to recognize any naturally occurring cellular tRNA [72]. The comparison of the vector genomes shown in *Figure 1* reveals that gamma-retroviral, and potentially also alpha-retroviral vectors, are especially suitable for this approach, as their genomic messages can be recoded to promote translational initiation behind the packaging signal in the 5' untranslated region, owing to the complete deletion of the gag reading frame. For lentiviral vectors, minimized "leader" sequences have also been described but typically suffer from reduced titers [73]. Anyhow, for the transfer of mRNA into the cellular cytoplasm the canonical advantage of lentiviral vectors to transduce resting cells is no longer of interest.

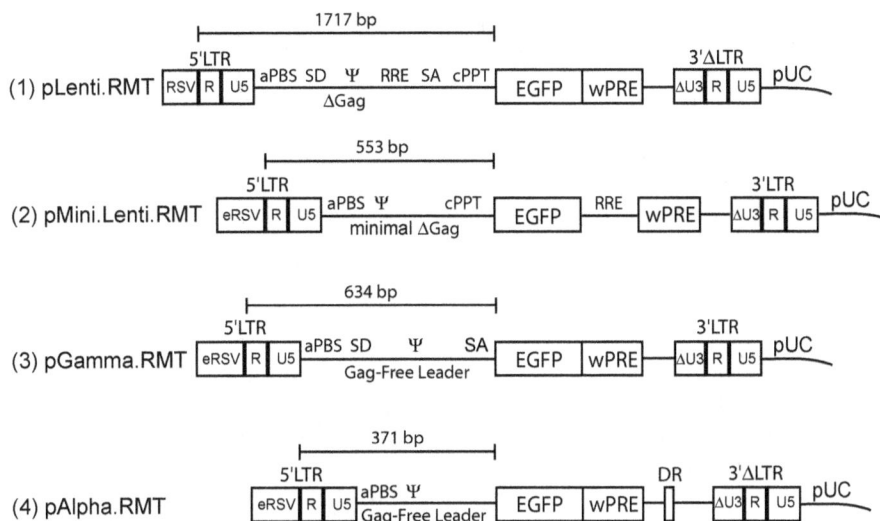

Figure 1. A comparison of the untranslated regions of lentiviral vectors (1), lentiviral vectors with a minimized leader region (2), and the current generations of gamma-retroviral (3) and alpha-retroviral (4) vectors. Shown are the configurations designed for retrovirus particle-mediated transfer of mRNA (RMT), thus incorporating an artificial primer binding site (aPBS). After disassembly of the particle and release of the mRNA, ribosomal scanning starts from the cap-site at the beginning of the R region of the 5'LTR, explaining why RMT vectors need to be devoid of aberrant reading frames in the 5' untranslated region. This is the case for gamma-retroviral vectors (3) and can also be achieved, with minor modifications, for alpha-retroviral vectors (4).

In recent work, we could greatly increase the potency of this new principle of retrovirus-particle-mediated mRNA transduction (RMT) by further improving the codon usage of the transcription unit embedded into the particles [71]. Modifications that increased the biological activity of the encoded protein further augmented the potency of RMT. We could thus deliver the *Sleeping Beauty* transposase, as developed by Z. Ivics and Z. Iszvak [74], at levels that lead to very efficient transposition of transfected transposable elements in target cells, simultaneously avoiding a newly discovered cytotoxicity of the transposase by short-lived, dose-controlled mRNA delivery [71]. Further applications of RMT include the delivery of other DNA-modifying enzymes such as the recombinases Flp or Cre [66, 71]. Whether the approach will be potent enough to induce changes in cell fate by delivery of key transcription factors remains to be determined.

A further new principle that we introduced in the course of our studies of the life cycle of retroviral particles was the delivery of proteins, rather than nucleic acids, embedded into the *gag-pol* reading frame of MoMLV. Having defined several positions that tolerated the incorporation of EGFP, we went on to flank the protein of interest with consensus sequences for the retroviral protease. The hypothesis of this work was that the newly formed gag-pol polyprotein, with the foreign protein unit contained in-frame, would participate in the formation of retrovirus particles, which then start to release the protein of interest only after budding, following the activation of the protease in the nascent particle. Functional and biochemical studies confirmed this hypothesis [75]. We went on to demonstrate that intact functional proteins such as the recombinase Flp can be transferred to target cells using this approach. Following the example of RMT, we name this principle retrovirus particle-mediated protein transfer (RPT). Proof-of-concept has been shown with the excision of a lentiviral reprogramming vector from induced pluripotent stem cells [75].

As opposed to previously described strategies that delivered foreign protein *via* fusion with accessory retroviral proteins [76], incorporation into gag may allow a maximum of ~5000 protein units to be delivered per particle. However, it is possible that the majority of the protein delivered by RPT may still follow the intracellular fate of the retroviral particles, with proteolytic degradation, even though the foreign protein can be efficiently released from the Gag polyprotein. We are thus analyzing intracellular particle fate and mechanisms of particle disassembly to further increase the potential of this approach.

SUMMARY AND OUTLOOK

The therapeutic potential of retroviral vectors is far from being fully explored. Our approach is to take advantage of the large spectrum of evolutionary optimized principles offered in the extended world or retroviruses: we thus analyze various families of retroviruses for potentially useful features to develop new principles for the delivery of integrated DNA, episomal DNA, mRNA or proteins. We focus on gamma-retroviral vectors and the new generation of alpha-retroviral vectors when developing systems that allow robust production in stable packaging conditions; we also prefer gamma-retroviruses and in the future maybe also alpha-retroviruses for the delivery of mRNA or protein, taking advantage of their relatively simple genome configuration; we prefer lentiviral vectors for applications targeting resting cells. Eventually, hybrid vectors may combine the best features of these worlds. Robust quantitative assays are needed to determine potency and safety before clinical application. Rational vector development in combination with a fair risk/benefit evaluation will set the stage for new clinical trials, hopefully resulting in reliable and cost-effective medicinal products.

ABBREVIATIONS

iPS cells, induced pluripotent stem cells;
LTR, long terminal repeat;
MoMLV, Moloney murine leukemia virus;
RSV, Rous sarcoma virus;
SCID, severe combined immunodeficiency;
SIN, self-inactivating.

ACKNOWLEDGEMENTS

The authors are grateful for the support of their work by the German research Council (DFG), the German Ministry of Research and Education (BMBF), the Food and Drug Administration (FDA) and the European Union EC-DG research through the FP6-Network of Excellence, CLINIGENE: LSHB-CT-2006-018933, and the FP7-Integrated Project PERSIST.

REFERENCES

1. Miller AD. Retroviral vectors. *Curr Top Microbiol Immunol* 1992; 158: 1-24.

2. Mann R, Mulligan RC, Baltimore D. Construction of a retrovirus packaging mutant and its use to produce helper-free defective retrovirus. *Cell* 1983; 33: 153-9.

3. Williams DA, Lemischka IR, Nathan DG, Mulligan RC. Introduction of new genetic material into pluripotent haematopoietic stem cells of the mouse. *Nature* 1984; 310: 476-80.

4. Grez M, Akgün E, Hilberg F, Ostertag W. Embryonic stem cell virus, a recombinant murine retrovirus with expression in embryonic stem cells. *Proc Natl Acad Sci USA* 1990; 87: 9202-6.

5. Baum C, Hegewisch-Becker S, Eckert HG, Stocking C, Ostertag W. Novel retroviral vectors for efficient expression of the multidrug-resistance (mdr-1) gene in early hemopoietic cells. *J Virol* 1995; 69: 7541-7.

6. Challita PM, Skelton D, el-Khoueiry A, Yu XJ, Weinberg K, Kohn DB. Multiple modifications in cis elements of the long terminal repeat of retroviral vectors lead to increased expression and decreased DNA methylation in embryonic carcinoma cells. *J Virol* 1995; 69: 748-55.

7. Wolf D, Goff SP. Embryonic stem cells use ZFP809 to silence retroviral DNAs. *Nature* 2009; 458: 1201-4.

8. Schambach A, Wodrich H, Hildinger M, Bohne J, Kräusslich HG, Baum C. Context dependence of different modules for posttranscriptional enhancement of gene expression from retroviral vectors. *Mol Ther* 2000; 2: 435-45.

9. Hildinger M, Abel KL, Ostertag W, Baum C. Design of 5' untranslated sequences in retroviral vectors developed for medical use. *J Virol* 1999; 73: 4083-9.

10. Cavazzana-Calvo M, Thrasher A, Mavilio F. The future of gene therapy. *Nature* 2004; 427: 779-81.

11. Naldini L, Blömer U, Gallay P, Ory D, Mulligan R, Gage FH, *et al*. In vivo gene delivery and stable transduction of nondividing cells by a lentiviral vector. *Science* 1996; 272: 263-7.

12. Baum C, Schambach A, Bohne J, Galla M. Retrovirus vectors: toward the plentivirus? *Mol Ther* 2006; 13: 1050-63.

13. Donahue RE, Kessler SW, Bodine D, McDonagh K, Dunbar C, Goodman S, *et al*. Helper virus induced T cell lymphoma in nonhuman primates after retroviral mediated gene transfer. *J Exp Med* 1992; 176: 1125-35.

14. Li Z, Düllmann J, Schiedlmeier B, Schmidt M, von Kalle C, Meyer J, *et al*. Murine leukemia induced by retroviral gene marking. *Science* 2002, 296: 497.

15. Modlich U, Kustikova OS, Schmidt M, Rudolph C, Meyer J, Li Z, *et al*. Leukemias following retroviral transfer of multidrug resistance 1 (MDR1) are driven by combinatorial insertional mutagenesis. *Blood* 2005. 105: 4235-46.

16. Hacein-Bey-Abina S, Von Kalle C, Schmidt M, McCormack MP, Wulffraat N, Leboulch P, *et al.* LMO2-associated clonal T cell proliferation in two patients after gene therapy for SCID-X1. *Science* 2003; 302: 415-9.

17. Hacein-Bey-Abina S, von Kalle C, Schmidt M, Le Deist F, Wulffraat N, McIntyre E, *et al.* A serious adverse event after successful gene therapy for X-linked severe combined immunodeficiency. *N Engl J Med* 2003; 348: 255-6.

18. Persons DA, Baum C. Solving the problem of gamma-retroviral vectors containing long terminal repeats. *Mol Ther* 2011; 19: 229-31.

19. Stein S, Ott MG, Schultze-Strasser S, Jauch A, Burwinkel B, Kinner A, *et al.* Genomic instability and myelodysplasia with monosomy 7 consequent to EVI1 activation after gene therapy for chronic granulomatous disease. *Nat Med* 2010; 16: 198-204.

20. Yu SF, von Rüden T, Kantoff PW, Garber C, Seiberg M, Rüther U, *et al.* Self-inactivating retroviral vectors designed for transfer of whole genes into mammalian cells. *Proc Natl Acad Sci USA* 1986; 83: 3194-8.

21. Kraunus J, Schaumann DH, Meyer J, Modlich U, Fehse B, Brandenburg G, *et al.* Self-inactivating retroviral vectors with improved RNA processing. *Gene Ther* 2004; 11: 1568-78.

22. Schambach A, Mueller D, Galla M, Verstegen MM, Wagemaker G, Loew R, *et al.* Overcoming promoter competition in packaging cells improves production of self-inactivating retroviral vectors. *Gene Ther* 2006; 13: 1524-33.

23. Loew R, Meyer Y, Kuehlcke K, Gama-Norton L, Wirth D, Hauser H, *et al.* A new PG13-based packaging cell line for stable production of clinical-grade self-inactivating gamma-retroviral vectors using targeted integration. *Gene Ther* 2010; 17: 272-80.

24. Schambach A, Bohne J, Baum C, Hermann FG, Egerer L, von Laer D, Giroglou T. Woodchuck hepatitis virus post-transcriptional regulatory element deleted from X protein and promoter sequences enhances retroviral vector titer and expression. *Gene Ther* 2006; 13: 641-5.

25. Zufferey R, Donello JE, Trono D, Hope TJ. Woodchuck hepatitis virus posttranscriptional regulatory element enhances expression of transgenes delivered by retroviral vectors. *J Virol* 1999; 73: 2886-92.

26. Schambach A, Bohne J, Chandra S, Will E, Margison GP, Williams DA, Baum C. Equal potency of gammaretroviral and lentiviral SIN vectors for expression of O6-methylguanine-DNA methyl-transferase in hematopoietic cells. *Mol Ther* 2006; 13: 391-400.

27. Thornhill SI, Schambach A, Howe SJ, Ulaganathan M, Grassman E, Williams D, *et al.* Self-inactivating gammaretroviral vectors for gene therapy of X-linked severe combined immunodeficiency. *Mol Ther* 2008; 16: 590-8.

28. Alexander BL, Ali RR, Alton EW, Bainbridge JW, Braun S, Cheng SH, *et al.* Progress and prospects: gene therapy clinical trials (part 1). *Gene Ther* 2007; 14: 1439-47.

29. Howe SJ, Mansour MR, Schwarzwaelder K, Bartholomae C, Hubank M, Kempski H, *et al.* Insertional mutagenesis combined with acquired somatic mutations causes leukemogenesis following gene therapy of SCID-X1 patients. *J Clin Invest* 2008; 118: 3143-50.

30. Hacein-Bey-Abina S, Garrigue A, Wang GP, Soulier J, Lim A, Morillon E, et al., Insertional oncogenesis in 4 patients after retrovirus-mediated gene therapy of SCID-X1. *J Clin Invest* 2008; 118: 3132-42.

31. Zychlinski D, Schambach A, Modlich U, Maetzig T, Meyer J, Grassman E, *et al.* Physiological promoters reduce the genotoxic risk of integrating gene vectors. *Mol Ther* 2008; 16: 718-25.

32. Van der Loo JC, Swaney WP, Grassman E, Terwilliger A, Higashimoto T, Schambach A, *et al.* Scale-up and manufacturing of clinical-grade self-inactivating gamma-retroviral vectors by transient transfection. *Gene Ther* 2011; July 14 (*online*).

33. Metcalf JA, Ma X, Linders B, Wu S, Schambach A, Ohlemiller KK, *et al*. A self-inactivating gamma-retroviral vector reduces manifestations of mucopolysaccharidosis I in mice. *Mol Ther* 2010; 18: 334-42.

34. Warlich E, Kuehle J, Cantz T, Brugman MH, Maetzig T, Galla M, *et al*. Lentiviral vector design and imaging approaches to visualize the early stages of cellular reprogramming. *Mol Ther* 2011; 9: 782-9.

35. Pike-Overzet K, Rodijk M, Ng YY, Baert MR, Lagresle-Peyrou C, Schambach A, *et al*. Correction of murine Rag1 deficiency by self-inactivating lentiviral vector-mediated gene transfer. *Leukemia* 2011; 25: 1471-83.

36. Huston MW, van Til NP, Visser TP, Arshad S, Brugman MH, Cattoglio C, *et al*. Correction of murine SCID-X1 by lentiviral gene therapy using a codon-optimized IL2RG gene and minimal pre-transplant conditioning. *Mol Ther* 2011; 19: 1867-77.

37. Avedillo Díez I, Zychlinski D, Coci EG, Galla M, Modlich U, Dewey RA, *et al*. Development of novel efficient SIN vectors with improved safety features for Wiskott-Aldrich syndrome stem sell based gene therapy. *Mol Pharm* 2011; 8 :1525-37.

38. Ng YY, Baert MR, Pike-Overzet K, Rodijk M, Brugman MH, Schambach A, *et al*. Correction of B-cell development in Btk-deficient mice using lentiviral vectors with codon-optimized human BTK. *Leukemia* 2010; 24: 1617-30.

39. Takahashi K, Yamanaka S. Induction of pluripotent stem cells from mouse embryonic and adult fibroblast cultures by defined factors. *Cell* 2006; 126: 663-76.

40. Du Y, Jenkins NA, Copeland NG. Insertional mutagenesis identifies genes that promote the immortalization of primary bone marrow progenitor cells. *Blood* 2005; 106: 3932-9.

41. Maetzig T, Brugman MH, Bartels S, Heinz N, Kustikova OS, Modlich U, *et al*. Polyclonal fluctuation of lentiviral vector-transduced and expanded murine hematopoietic stem cells. *Blood* 2011; 117 :3053-64.

42. Modlich U, Navarro S, Zychlinski D, Maetzig T, Knoess S, Brugman MH, *et al*. Insertional transformation of hematopoietic cells by self-inactivating lentiviral and gammaretroviral vectors. *Mol Ther* 2009; 17: 1919-28.

43. Arumugam PI, Higashimoto T, Urbinati F, Modlich U, Nestheide S, Xia P, *et al*. Genotoxic potential of lineage-specific lentivirus vectors carrying the beta-globin locus control region. *Mol Ther* 2009; 17: 1929-37.

44. Modlich U, Bohne J, Schmidt M, von Kalle C, Knöss S, Schambach A, Baum C. Cell-culture assays reveal the importance of retroviral vector design for insertional genotoxicity. *Blood* 2006; 108: 2545-53.

45. Gaussin A, Modlich U, Bauche C, Niederländer NJ, Schambach A, Duros C, *et al*. CTF/NF1 transcription factors act as potent genetic insulators for integrating gene transfer vectors. *Gene Ther* 2011; May 12 (*online*).

46. Wu X, Li Y, Crise B, Burgess SM. Transcription start regions in the human genome are favored targets for MLV integration. *Science* 2003; 300: 1749-51.

47. Schröder AR, Shinn P, Chen H, Berry C, Ecker JR, Bushman F. HIV-1 integration in the human genome favors active genes and local hotspots. *Cell* 2002; 110: 521-9.

48. Wang GP, Ciuffi A, Leipzig J, Berry CC, Bushman FD. HIV integration site selection: analysis by massively parallel pyrosequencing reveals association with epigenetic modifications. *Genome Res* 2007; 17: 1186-94.

49. Modlich U, Schambach A, Brugman MH, Wicke DC, Knoess S, Li Z, *et al*. Leukemia induction after a single retroviral vector insertion in Evi1 or Prdm16. *Leukemia* 2008; 22: 1519-28.

50. Kustikova OS, Schiedlmeier B, Brugman MH, Stahlhut M, Bartels S, Li Z, Baum C. Cell-intrinsic and vector-related properties cooperate to determine the incidence and consequences of insertional mutagenesis. *Mol Ther* 2009; 17: 1537-47.

51. Montini E, Cesana D, Schmidt M, Sanvito F, Bartholomae CC, Ranzani M, *et al*. The genotoxic potential of retroviral vectors is strongly modulated by vector design and integration site selection in a mouse model of HSC gene therapy. *J Clin Invest* 2009; 119: 964-75.

52. Montini E, Cesana D, Schmidt M, Sanvito F, Ponzoni M, Bartholomae C, *et al*. Hematopoietic stem cell gene transfer in a tumor-prone mouse model uncovers low genotoxicity of lentiviral vector integration. *Nat Biotechnol* 2006; 24: 687-96.

53. Hu J, Ferris A, Larochelle A, Krouse AE, Metzger ME, Donahue RE, *et al*. Transduction of rhesus macaque hematopoietic stem and progenitor cells with avian sarcoma and leukosis virus vectors. *Hum Gene Ther* 2007; 18: 691-700.

54. Mitchell RS, Beitzel BF, Schroder AR, Shinn P, Chen H, Berry CC, *et al*. Retroviral DNA integration: ASLV, HIV, and MLV show distinct target site preferences. *PLoS Biol* 2004; 2: E234.

55. Suerth JD, Maetzig T, Galla M, Baum C, Schambach A. Self-inactivating alpharetroviral vectors with a split-packaging design. *J Virol* 2010; 84: 6626-35.

56. Emi N, Friedmann T, Yee J.K. Pseudotype formation of murine leukemia virus with the G protein of vesicular stomatitis virus. *J Virol* 1991; 65: 1202-7.

57. Sandrin V, Muriaux D, Darlix JL, Cosset FL. Intracellular trafficking of Gag and Env proteins and their interactions modulate pseudotyping of retroviruses. *J Virol* 2004; 78: 7153-64.

58. Greger JG, Katz RA, Taganov K, Rall GF, Skalka AM. Transduction of terminally differentiated neurons by avian sarcoma virus. *J Virol* 2004; 78: 4902-6.

59. Hatziioannou T, Goff SP. Infection of nondividing cells by Rous sarcoma virus. *J Virol* 2001; 75: 9526-31.

60. O'Neill LS, Skinner AM, Woodward JA, Kurre P. Entry kinetics and cell-cell transmission of surface-bound retroviral vector particles. *J Gene Med* 2010; 12: 463-76.

61. Yáñez-Muñoz RJ, Balaggan KS, MacNeil A, Howe SJ, Schmidt M, Smith AJ, *et al*. Effective gene therapy with nonintegrating lentiviral vectors. *Nat Med* 2006; 12: 348-53.

62. Karwacz K, Mukherjee S, Apolonia L, Blundell MP, Bouma G, Escors D, *et al*. Nonintegrating lentivector vaccines stimulate prolonged T-cell and antibody responses and are effective in tumor therapy. *J Virol* 2009; 83: 3094-103.

63. Apolonia L, Waddington SN, Fernandes C, Ward NJ, Bouma G, Blundell MP, *et al*. Stable gene transfer to muscle using non-integrating lentiviral vectors. *Mol Ther* 2007; 15: 1947-54.

64. Philpott NJ, Thrasher AJ. Use of nonintegrating lentiviral vectors for gene therapy. *Hum Gene Ther* 2007; 18: 483-9.

65. Nightingale SJ, Hollis RP, Pepper KA, Petersen D, Yu XJ, Yang C, *et al*. Transient gene expression by nonintegrating lentiviral vectors. *Mol Ther* 2006; 13: 1121-32.

66. Galla M, Will E, Kraunus J, Chen L, Baum C. Retroviral pseudotransduction for targeted cell manipulation. *Mol Cell* 2004; 16: 309-15.

67. Maetzig T, Galla M, Brugman MH, Loew R, Baum C, Schambach A. Mechanisms controlling titer and expression of bidirectional lentiviral and gammaretroviral vectors. *Gene Ther* 2010; 17: 400-11.

68. Amendola M, Venneri MA, Biffi A, Vigna E, Naldini L. Coordinate dual-gene transgenesis by lentiviral vectors carrying synthetic bidirectional promoters. *Nat Biotechnol* 2005; 23: 108-16.

69. Kraunus J, Zychlinski D, Heise T, Galla M, Bohne J, Baum C. Murine leukemia virus regulates alternative splicing through sequences upstream of the 5' splice site. *J Biol Chem* 2006; 281: 37381-90.

70. Galla M, Schambach A, Towers GJ, Baum C. Cellular restriction of retrovirus particle-mediated mRNA transfer. *J Virol* 2008; 82: 3069-77.

71. Galla M, Schambach A, Falk CS, Maetzig T, Kuehle J, Lange K, *et al*. Avoiding cytotoxicity of transposases by dose-controlled mRNA delivery. *Nucleic Acids Res* 2011; 39: 7147-60.

72. Lund AH, Duch M, Lovmand J, Jørgensen P, Pedersen FS. Complementation of a primer binding site-impaired murine leukemia virus-derived retroviral vector by a genetically engineered tRNA-like primer. *J Virol* 1997; 71: 1191-5.

73. Berkowitz RD, Hammarskjöld ML, Helga-Maria C, Rekosh D, Goff SP. 5' regions of HIV-1 RNAs are not sufficient for encapsidation: implications for the HIV-1 packaging signal. *Virology* 1995; 212: 718-23.

74. Mátés L, Chuah MK, Belay E, Jerchow B, Manoj N, Acosta-Sanchez A, *et al*. Molecular evolution of a novel hyperactive Sleeping Beauty transposase enables robust stable gene transfer in vertebrates. *Nat Genet* 2009; 41: 753-61.

75. Voelkel C, Galla M, Maetzig T, Warlich E, Kuehle J, Zychlinski D, *et al*. Protein transduction from retroviral Gag precursors. *Proc Natl Acad Sci USA* 2010; 107: 7805-10.

76. Link N, Aubel C, Kelm JM, Marty RR, Greber D, Djonov V, *et al*. Therapeutic protein transduction of mammalian cells and mice by nucleic acid-free lentiviral nanoparticles. *Nucleic Acids Res* 2006; 34: e16.

The CliniBook: Clinical gene transfer
Edited by Odile Cohen-Haguenauer – EDK, Paris © 2012, pp. 112-117

A2-3
Replication-competent γ-retroviral vectors for tumor therapy

THOMAS SCHASER[1], LYDIA DÜRNER[2], KLAUS CICHUTEK, CHRISTIAN J. BUCHHOLZ*

Division of Medical Biotechnology, Paul-Ehrlich-Institut, Langen, Germany.
Current addresses: [1]Miltenyi Biotec GmbH, Bergisch Gladbach, Germany. [2]Pharma
Research and Early Development, Roche Glycart AG, CH-8952 Schlieren, Switzerland.
christian.buchholz@pei.de
* Corresponding author

INTRODUCTION

Selective infection of tumor cells combined with the transfer of anti-tumoral genes is an attractive strategy for cancer therapy. Especially, as efficient therapy requires wide or complete dispersion of the anti-tumoral gene within the tumor tissue as observed in numerous clinical trials with replication-incompetent vector systems. Besides a number of different oncolytic viruses such as adenovirus, measles virus or herpes virus, γ-retroviruses, especially murine leukemia virus (MLV), are being developed for tumor therapy because of their intrinsic selectivity for mitotically active cells. Moreover, γ-retroviruses can integrate into the host cell genome without causing cytopathic effects, thus offering the unique potential for persistence of the virus and a potentially permanent anti-tumoral effect [1].

To achieve cell killing, a suicide gene is added to the MLV genome, resulting in so called replication-competent retroviral (RCR) vectors. The mode of anti-tumoral activity is defined by the type of therapeutic gene that is inserted into the MLV genome. For example, the gene coding for the yeast cytosine deaminase (CD) was successfully distributed to glioma cells *in vitro* as the virus replicates [2]. Therapeutic efficacy was shown by reduced viability of tumor cells upon administration of the prodrug 5′fluorocytosin (5′-FC) into the chemotherapeutic compound 5′fluorouracil (5′-FU). This system has also been tested in preclinical studies: mice with pre-established primary gliomas showed extended survival rates after single, intra-cerebral MLV inoculation and subsequent intraperitoneal prodrug treatment. In addition, anti-tumoral efficacy was also shown for another suicide gene, the purine nucleoside phosphorylase, in an experimental glioma mouse model and a colorectal tumor mouse model transferring cytosine deaminase [3, 4].

The beneficial outcome of these studies has advanced RCR vectors to a phase I clinical trial (NCT01156584; clinicaltrials.gov), in which patients with recurrent glioblastoma multiforme will be treated with MLV transferring CD by local intra-tumoral injection. For most types of tumors, systemic, rather than local applications will be required to achieve therapeutic benefit. However, intravenously applied MLV does not only infect tumor cells, but also extra-tumoral tissue, especially spleen and bone marrow [5, 6]. Moreover, replication-defective retroviral vectors used for genetic modification of hematopoietic stem cells in clinical trials have induced leukemia in a number of patients [7]. Therefore a targeting strategy for systemically applied RCR vectors is needed to prevent infection of non-tumorous tissue.

During the Clinigene project, we have improved MLV-based RCR vectors in two directions. First, targeting at the stage of cell entry has been achieved to restrict virus spreading solely to tumor cells [6]. Second, we have extended the types of anti-tumoral genes that can be transferred to inhibitory RNA (RNAi) allowing silencing of any target gene of choice by RCR vectors [8].

CELL ENTRY TARGETED RCR VECTORS

Restricting virus infection at the level of cell entry is expected to enhance gene delivery by diminishing the loss of virus to non-target cells and to increase the safety of gene delivery. For γ-retroviruses, an efficient cell entry targeting system is based on protease-activatable envelope (Env) proteins [9]. In this system, viruses remain non-infectious until the Env protein becomes activated by cleavage through a tumor specific protease that recognizes an engineered protease substrate (*Figure 1*). Tumors are known to express specific active proteases to facilitate dissemination of tumor cells and to promote angiogenesis. To engineer viruses conditionally replicating in cancer cells, we coupled infectivity to proteolytic activity of the target cell. A CD40L blocking domain fused to the envelope inhibited cell entry unless it is cleaved off at a protease substrate linker by tumor-associated proteases such as the matrix metalloproteases (MMP) [10].

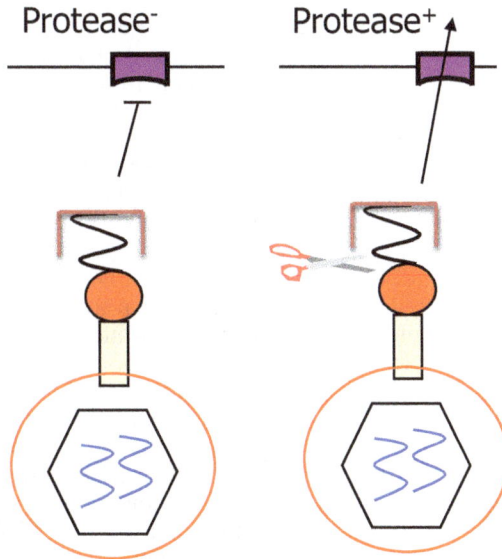

Figure 1. Proteolytic activation of RCR vectors. The RCR vector particle is shown with a single envelope protein, which is modified with a blocking domain that prevents cell entry and gene delivery (left). When the linker between the envelope protein and the blocking domain becomes cleaved by proteases released from the target cell, the envelope protein is activated and mediates cell entry via the natural receptor (right).

From retroviral protease substrate libraries in which the peptide linker was randomly diversified, variants were selected on given tumor cell lines. Selected virus clones showed enhanced dissemination efficiency through MMP-positive tumor cells *in vitro* and spread through the complete tumor tissue in SCID mouse tumor xenografts. In a comparative study, we analysed spreading of non-targeted and of protease activatable, tumor-targeted MLVs to tumor and non-tumoral organs in immunodeficient mice [6]. Both virus types were able to efficiently infect tumor cells after systemic administration. The non-targeted virus, however, also infected non-tumoral organs like bone marrow, spleen and liver efficiently. In contrast, the targeted viruses revealed in a quantitative analysis of virus spreading an up to 500-fold more selective infection of tumor tissue than the non-targeted virus.

In the described study, immunodeficient mice were analyzed for the biodistribution of MLV. It is likely that infection of non-tumoral organs is especially efficient in immuno-deficient mice. Indeed, Hiraoka *et al.* [3] demonstrated the absence of MLV infection in non-tumor tissue of an immunocompetent colorectal cancer metastasis model using a highly sensitive quantitative PCR approach detecting the *env* gene at a similar sensi-tivity as by Duerner *et al.* [6]. Solly *et al.* [5] showed that low infection levels of repli-cation-competent retroviral vectors in immunodeficient mice were reduced to undetectable levels in immunocompetent mice. However, immunodeficient mice may more closely reflect the often immunosuppressed status of end-stage cancer patients that will be the most likely patient population for first in man studies with replication-competent MLV vectors.

RNAi TRANSFER TO TUMOR TISSUE BY RCR VECTORS

RNA interference (RNAi)-mediated downregulation of gene expression represents a powerful technology in functional genomics and biomedical drug research. Currently, two types of RNAi delivery can be distinguished. Small interfering RNA (siRNA) is chemically synthesised and either transfected into cells for *in vitro* studies or injected in large amounts for *in vivo* gene silencing. High dosage administrations of unmodified, saline-formulated siRNAs are able to confer target gene knockdown after intravitreal, intranasal or orthotracheal application [11]. The systemic application of unmodified siRNAs has proven ineffective due to the rapid renal excretion and the high RNase activity in serum. Moreover, as siRNA only induces transient gene silencing, its efficacy is limited. Small hairpin RNA (shRNA) is transcribed from a DNA expression con-struct and delivered with a vector system. It has been shown that shRNAs flanked with microRNA derived sequences are more active than shRNAs without [12]. Depending on the vector type used, shRNA delivery results in long-term or even permanent gene silencing.

Lentiviral and γ-retroviral vectors transferring shRNA expression cassettes confer sta-ble gene-silencing. In contrast to lentiviral vectors, the tropism of γ-retroviral vectors is restricted to dividing cells. This makes γ-retroviral vectors especially suitable to trans-fer shRNA to tumor cells and tissue. The limited transduction rate of replication-de-ficient γ-retroviral vectors, especially *in vivo*, may be overcome by using RCR vectors (*Figure 2*). The initial description of an RCR vector encoding an shRNA expression cassette showed that such vectors are genetically stable, fully replication-competent and allow efficient gene silencing in cultivated cells [13].

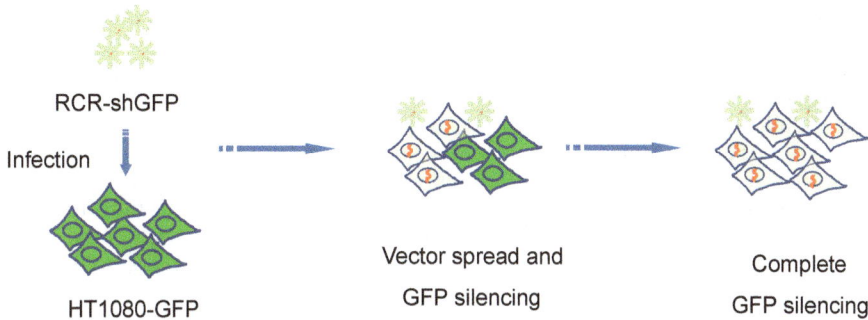

Figure 2. RNAi delivery by RCR vectors. Schematic diagram illustrating the concept of RNAi delivery *via* RCR vectors. HT1080 cells stably expressing GFP are shown in green, the GFP gene targeted shRNA encoded by the RCR vector in red. Over time, RCR vectors spread through the cells thereby propagating the shRNA encoding RCR genome which in turn becomes stably integrated in the cells genome, finally resulting in GFP silencing in all cells.

We have now engineered second-generation vectors by improving the shRNA expression cassette. First, shRNA coding sequences were put under control of the small nuclear promotor U6. Second, the shRNA coding sequence was flanked by microRNA-adapted sequences (miR30) to improve the intracellular processing and activity of the shRNA. To set up the system, RCR vectors encoding shRNA specific for the reporter genes green fluorescent protein (GFP) and firefly luciferase were generated. Gene suppression was monitored in the fibrosarcoma cell line HT1080 stably transduced with a single copy of GFP (HT1080-GFP) or the firefly luciferase gene (HT1080-Luc). When HT1080-Luc cells were infected with MLV-shLuc at an MOI of 1, luciferase activity was reduced by more than 90% within four days but remained unaffected when control vectors were applied. Likewise, GFP was downregulated to similar levels upon infection of HT1080-GFP cells. In general, silencing of luciferase was more rapid than GFP. Moreover, the kinetics of gene silencing, *i.e.* kinetic of shRNA spreading in cell culture depended on the dose of RCR vector applied. Even at a very low dose which resulted in an initial shRNA transfer to only 0.1% of the cells, the maximal extent of downregulation was reached. Later on, the silencing activity was also assessed upon systemic administration of MLV-shLuc into SCID mice bearing HT1080-Luc tumours. In both *in vivo* models, luciferase expression in tumor tissues was strongly reduced, whereas RCR vectors coding for control shRNA had no influence on luciferase activity. All viruses were genomically stable as demonstrated by PCR on proviral DNA.

To demonstrate the applicability of the system for genes relevant in tumor biology we targeted matrix metalloprotease 14 (MMP14), a key protease in the proteolytic activation of proMMP-2 and tumor cell invasion, as well as polo-like kinase 1 (PLK1), a key player in cell cycle progression [14, 15]. Upon infection with the respective RCR vector, PLK1 and MMP14 levels were reduced both at the mRNA and protein levels. MLV-shPLK1-infected cells were arrested in the G2-phase and underwent apoptosis. MLV-shMMP14-infected cells showed reduced MMP2 activity, as well as substantially reduced invasion and tumor growth. *In vivo*, MLV-shLuc silenced luciferase expression in HT1080-luc tumor tissue by more than 80% and MLV-shPLK1 reduced tumor growth substantially, demonstrating the therapeutic relevance of this system [8].

CONCLUSIONS

RCR vectors form a novel class of gene delivery vehicles especially relevant for gene delivery to tumor cells. We have shown that these vectors can be used as a novel RNAi transfer system allowing long-term expression and efficient delivery and distribution of shRNAs to tumor cells *in vitro* and *in vivo* combined with a strong silencing activity. In the future, it will now be possible to attack tumors *via* multiple modes of action using a variety of RNAi encoding RCR vectors. Their intrinsic tropism for mitotically-active cells can be further restricted to tumor tissue by making their cell entry dependent on the activity of tumor-associated proteases. Thus, RCR vectors hold promise both as tools for basic research in functional genomics and as novel anti-tumor agents.

ACKNOWLEDGMENTS

This work has been performed with the support of the EC-DG research through the FP6-Network of Excellence, CLINIGENE: LSHB-CT-2006-018933.

REFERENCES

1. Tai CK, Kasahara N. Replication-competent retrovirus vectors for cancer gene therapy. *Front Biosci* 2008; 13: 3083-95.

2. Tai CK, Wang WJ, Chen TC, Kasahara N. Single-shot, multicycle suicide gene therapy by replication-competent retrovirus vectors achieves long-term survival benefit in experimental glioma. *Mol Ther* 2005; 12: 842-51.

3. Hiraoka K, Kimura T, Logg CR, Tai CK, Haga K, Lawson GW, Kasahara N. Therapeutic efficacy of replication-competent retrovirus vector-mediated suicide gene therapy in a multifocal colorectal cancer metastasis model. *Cancer Res* 2007; 67: 5345-53.

4. Tai CK, Wang W, Lai YH, Logg CR, Parker WB, Li YF, *et al.* Enhanced efficiency of prodrug activation therapy by tumor-selective replicating retrovirus vectors armed with the *Escherichia coli* purine nucleoside phosphorylase gene. *Cancer Gene Ther* 2010; 17: 614-23.

5. Solly SK, Trajcevski S, Frisén C, Holzer GW, Nelson E, Clerc B. Replicative retroviral vectors for cancer gene therapy. *Cancer Gene Ther* 2003; 10: 30-9.

6. Duerner LJ, Schwantes A, Schneider IC, Cichutek K, Buchholz CJ. Cell entry targeting restricts biodistribution of replication-competent retroviruses to tumour tissue. *Gene Ther* 2008; 15: 1500-10.

7. Santilli G, Thornhill SI, Kinnon C, Thrasher AJ. Gene therapy of inherited immunodeficiencies. *Expert Opin Biol Ther* 2008; 8: 397-407.

8. Schaser T, Wrede C, Duerner L, Sliva K, Cichutek K, Schnierle B, Buchholz CJ. RNAi-mediated gene silencing in tumour tissue using replication-competent retroviral vectors. *Gene Ther* 2011; 18: 953-60

9. Buchholz CJ, Duerner LJ, Funke S, Schneider IC. Retroviral display and high throughput screening. *Comb Chem High Throughput Screen* 2008 ; 11: 99-110.

10. Hartl I, Schneider RM, Sun Y, Medvedovska J, Chadwick MP, Russell SJ, *et al.* Library-based selection of retroviruses selectively spreading through matrix metalloprotease-positive cells. *Gene Ther* 2005; 12: 918-26.

11. De Fougerolles AR. Delivery vehicles for small interfering RNA *in vivo*. *Hum Gene Ther* 2008; 19: 125-32.

12. Silva JM, Li MZ, Chang K, Ge W, Golding MC, Rickles RJ, *et al*. Second-generation shRNA libraries covering the mouse and human genomes. *Nat Genet* 2005; 37: 1281-8.

13. Sliva K, Schnierle BS. Stable integration of a functional shRNA expression cassette into the murine leukemia virus genome. *Virology* 2006; 351: 218-25.

14. Holtrich U, Wolf G, Bräuninger A, Karn T, Böhme B, Rübsamen-Waigmann H, Strebhardt K. Induction and down-regulation of PLK, a human serine/threonine kinase expressed in proliferating cells and tumors. *Proc Natl Acad Sci USA* 1994; 91: 1736-40.

15. Seiki, M. Membrane-type 1 matrix metalloproteinase: a key enzyme for tumor invasion. *Cancer Lett* 2003; 194: 1-11.

The CliniBook: Clinical gene transfer
Edited by Odile Cohen-Haguenauer – EDK, Paris © 2012, pp. 118-124

A2-4
Modular retroviral producer cell lines

ANA SOFIA COROADINHA[1]*, DAGMAR WIRTH[2], ANA F. RODRIGUES[1], LEONOR GAMA-NORTON[1,2],
CAROLINE DUROS[3], ALEXANDRE ARTUS[3], ODILE COHEN-HAGUENAUER[3],
PAULA MARQUES ALVES[1], PEDRO E. CRUZ[1,4], MANUEL J.T. CARRONDO[1,5], HANSJÖRG HAUSER[2]

[1]*Instituto de Tecnologia Química e Biológica-Universidade Nova de Lisboa/Instituto de Biologia Experimental e Tecnológica (ITQB-UNL/IBET), P-2781-901 Oeiras, Portugal.* [2]*Helmholtz Centre for Infection Research, D-38124 Braunschweig, Germany.* [3]*École Normale Supérieure de Cachan, F-94235 Cachan Cedex, France.* [4]*ECBio, S.A., P-2700-451 Amadora, Portugal.* [5]*Faculdade de Ciências e Tecnologia/Universidade Nova de Lisboa (FCT/UNL), P-2825 Monte da Caparica, Portugal.*
avalente@itqb.unl.pt
* Corresponding author

INTRODUCTION

One of the major limitations of retroviral vectors is based on the inability to produce, purify and concentrate high titers of infective virus, as required for gene therapy clinical applications. This bottleneck is mainly due to the low productivity of the packaging cell lines. Thus, robust high producer cells are required for the production of clinical grade materials. Development and screening of high titer retrovirus vector producer cell lines is time consuming. Traditionally, retroviral vector producer cell lines are established for the production of each gene vector. This is done by transfection of a packaging cell line with the gene of interest. In order to find a high titer retrovirus producer clone, exhaustive clone screening is necessary, as the random integration of the transgene gives rise to different expression levels. The viral titer is largely determined by the nature of the integration site, the influence of the neighboring chromosomal elements and its interactions with the vector control elements. This is the main reason why intensive clone screening has to be performed to identify the most stable and highly producing cell clones. Together, the identification of potent producer cell lines usually takes several months.

This issue can be overcome by the use of modular Recombinase Mediated Cassette Exchange (RMCE) packaging cell lines. This principle is outlined in *Figure 1*. Originally, two cell lines were created; Flp293A [1] and 293 FLEX [2], both derived from 293 cells, which produce retroviral vectors pseudotyped with amphotropic and GaLV envelopes, respectively.

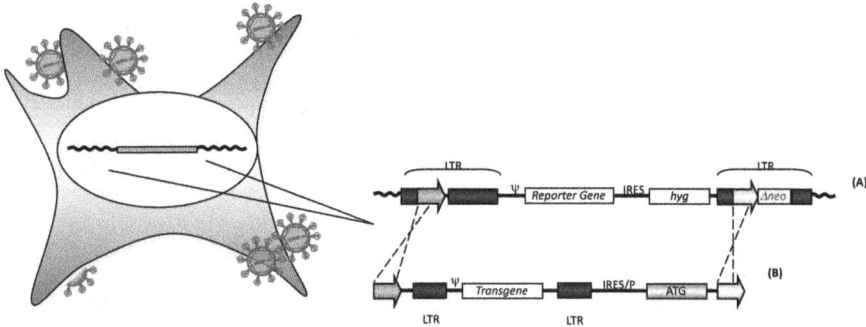

Figure 1. Principle of a modular viral producer cell line in which recombinase mediated cassette exchange (RMCE) results in targeted integration and establishment of a new retroviral producer cell line. (A) chromosomal site tagged with RMCE compatible FRT sites (arrows) and (B) recombinase mediated targeting of a retroviral vector flanked with FRT sites for the generation of a new retroviral vector producer cell.

Later, a PG13 based cell line was constructed [3]. These cell lines were developed such that a favorable chromosomal site for stable and high retroviral vector production was first identified and tagged with FRT recognition sites for the Flp recombinase. The presence of two heterologous non-compatible FRT sites flanking the tagged retroviral genome allows subsequent re-use of this defined chromosomal site by RMCE (*Figure 1*) [4]. Besides the advantageous reduction of the time required to establish each producer cell, this approach provides high predictability of the viral titers since the very same integration site is used. It also further increases safety by avoiding the generation and transfer of potentially harmful transcripts resulting from transcriptional read-through. Such modular cell lines represent a promising platform from which different retroviral vectors can be expressed. The cell lines 293 FLEX and Flp293A were characterized within the CliniGene network to assess their potential and further design an optimized manufacturing process. A summary of the major findings are described in this paper.

THE IMPORTANCE OF RETROVIRAL VECTOR COMPONENTS STOICHIOMETRY

As stated above one of the bottlenecks in the retroviral vector manufacturing are the low specific productivities of the packaging cells. The assembly of the wild type retrovirus is a complex, well regulated process controlled by a variety of mechanisms [5, 6] where the stoichiometry of the viral components is determined by both splicing of the full-length transcript to produce a specific ratio of unspliced to spliced RNA and the efficiency of translation from the resulting transcripts [7].

For the establishment of retroviral producer cell lines the three components, viral RNA genome, Gag-Pol and envelope are stably expressed in 3 separate genetic constructs, such that the possibility of generating replication competent virus is minimized. As a resulting disadvantage, the dissociation of transcription and translation of the viral components disrupts the regulatory stoichiometry of the virus and the optimal ratios of the components [7]; consequently, the cell line productivities are much reduced.

Optimal virus production will thus depend not only on a high retroviral vector transgene transcription but also on a balanced expression between the helper functions gag-

A.S. Coroadinha et al.

pol and env. The importance of the stoichiometric balance in the retroviral producer cell lines was analysed in the 293 FLEX modular cells. We could show that a low expression of either one of the components will limit the production of high titers. Moreover, we could also demonstrate that the over-expression of the *gag-pol* component can compromise retroviral production since the envelope protein or the viral RNA may become limiting [8]. It was concluded that Gag-Pol is the pivotal component around which the viral RNA and envelope stoichiometry must be optimized. A 2 fold increase in the reverse transcriptase (RT) expression led to a 10 fold improvement in the infectious particle productivity, indicating a non linear relationship, while the effects of the expression levels of transgene and envelope are shown to be linearly correlated with the infectious titer [8].

The stability of the recombinant virus was found to be independent of the viral component's stoichiometry, however, the latter has a tremendous impact in the transduction efficiency (*Table I*). An unbalanced stoichiometry results indeed in an increased production ratio of non-infectious to infectious particles.

Table I. Impact of retroviral vector components stoichiometry (different clones with different expression levels of gag-pol and env are presented).

293 FLEX Clones	Infectious Titer (10^6 i.p./mL)	Ratios I.P./RNA (10^{-3} i.p./copy)	Ratios I.P./RT (10^4 i.p./ng)	Infective per non-infective particles	Transduction Efficiency at MOI 5 (%)
#4	0.24 ± 0.09	1.02 ± 0.05	3.9 ± 0.2	1 per 490	17.5
#10	0.21 ± 0.09	1.04 ±0.05	5.7 ± 0.3	1 per 480	12.3
#3	0.74 ± 0.08	1.42 ± 0.07	3.9 ± 0.2	1 per 350	28.3
#8	2.7 ± 0.1	3.4 ± 0.2	9.6 ± 0.5	1 per 150	87.8
#17	1.6 ± 0.1	2.5 ± 0.2	6.7 ± 0.3	1 per 200	70.7
#18	3.2 ± 0.1	4.3 ± 0.2	14.0 ± 0.7	1 per 115	88.9

Both 293 FLEX and Flp293A cells were generated upon initial screening for high levels of retroviral vector expression [1, 2]. Upon integration of gag-pol it was possible to select a clone were the transgene RNA is not limiting. This allowed eliminating one important reason for low productivities. Further, the sequential transfer of the individual helper functions and screening for optimal titers addressed the need for optimal stoichiometry of the components and allowed the identification of high producer clones for both the amphotropic and the GaLV enveloped viruses.

THE ROLE OF RETROVIRAL VECTOR ELEMENTS IN TITER AND SAFETY

Modular viral producer cells provide highly predictable virus production. This speeds up the time to clinical or research application [1-3]. Moreover, the modular cell lines Flp293A and 293 FLEX constitute an excellent platform to systematically evaluate and directly compare the performance of different vector designs in a specific chromosomal locus [3, 9].

The expression of retroviral vector cassettes is dependent on chromosomal elements in the vicinity of the vector integration site. Gama-Norton *et al.* [9] showed that the nature of promoters, viral vector orientation and the nature of the integration site influence the titer in modular packaging cell lines. Importantly, for a given integration

120

site, only a combination of specific conditions will assure the production of high levels of infectious viral particles. Different commonly used 5'LTR promoters were tested in defined chromosomal sites for the generation of viral RNA and titers. High clonal homogeneity was observed in all sub-clones upon targeted integration of the same retroviral vector, as expected for this isogenic situation. However, significant differences in retroviral titers (up to 15-fold) were obtained within the five LTRs under test within the same locus. The hierarchy of performance of the 5'LTR-modified retroviral vectors was comparable in the two integration sites (ISs) of the producer cell lines. In contrast, the vector orientation had different effects in these two loci. In the 293 FLEX IS both orientations resulted in either similar titers or higher titer with anti-sense when compared to its sense counterpart. In contrast, the Flp293A cells provided a lower titer when targeting vectors were in the reverse orientation. This shows that while the integration site of 293 FLEX cells equally supports both orientations, in Flp293A cells the sense orientation is highly favored [9].

The introduction of insulator sequences in the retroviral vector cassette may introduce performance advantages, as reduced silencing in the target cell, and further enhance safety by reducing interactions with the chromosomal surroundings. The introduction of different insulator sequences within the SIN version of retroviral LTR of vectors was also tested and several vectors designed. The establishment of 293 FLEX producing SIN-insulated retroviral vectors was successfully achieved although a drop in titer was observed when compared to the control vector harbouring native LTRs. The maximal titers obtained for clones derived from this control was $4x10^6$ ip/mL while the highest titer for the insulated vectors was obtained for SIN FOCH19 construct derived clones and was $0.5x10^6$ ip/mL. In fact, SIN-gammaretrovirus vectors commonly harbour decreased titres as compared to their native LTR counterpart (as mentioned by Baum and collaborators, *ibid.*). It is thus not expected that the addition of insulator sequences inside SIN-LTRs would result in improved vector production. These lower titers could possibly be increased by the use of other 5' LTR SIN promoter such as RSV derived ones as shown in [9].

The chromosomal site of vector integration is of major importance due to the leakiness of termination of the retroviral vector transcription (poly-adenylation). The read-through activity is considered to be a mechanism that can lead to the transduction/activation of cellular oncogenes flanking viral genome IS [10, 11]. For production of recombinant retroviral vectors the adventitious transduction of cellular genes by read-through activity is thus a safety concern. Accordingly, the specific vector integration site(s) in the chromosome of packaging cells should be characterized to avoid transduction of harmful genes [9].

The retroviral vector integration site of Flp293A and 293 FLEX were mapped using a non-restrictive LAM-PCR protocol [12]. For Flp293A the tagged locus was located on the short arm of the chromosome 12, either in the first intron of DDX11 (p11.21, 31227164) or DDX12 gene (p13.31, 9600360), in reverse orientation to the endogenous gene transcription [9]. For 293 FLEX cell line, the tagged locus is positioned in an intergenic region 100Kb upstream the ARRDC3 gene on chromosome 5 (q14.3, position 90781745) [9]. Thus, the nature of the read-through transcripts produced from Flp293A and 293 FLEX cells can be fully anticipated. This provides an increased level of safety associated to these cellular producing systems.

Since the 3' elements flanking the retroviral vector integration site of the modular cell lines are known, a detailed investigation of vector-related read-through activities could be performed for different retroviral vector cassettes by assessing the transduction frequency of sequences flanking the integrated retroviral vectors. It was shown that the regulatory sequence composition of a retroviral vector and the integration site can modulate in a coordinated manner the read-through frequency on a given integrated retroviral vector cassette [3, 9].

The definition of optimal combinations of vector elements and integration sites in modular producer cell lines therefore allows the optimization of vector production while providing an improved level of safety as required in clinical trials [4].

THE INFLUENCE OF PRODUCTION MEDIA ON THE VIRAL TITER: THE SERUM

Supplementation of mammalian cell culture media with animal sera has been common practice in biomedical and biotechnological research, since it provides critical nutrients and factors that support cell growth and proliferation [13]. Nevertheless the ill-defined composition and high batch-to-batch variability of serum together with its potential source of contaminations, hinders both the bio-safety and the standardization of cell cultures. Additionally it adds further bioburden in the purification process. Retroviral vector manufacturing has been reported to rely on substantially amounts (5-10% [v/v]) of sera in the culture medium. The majority of the latest generation of packaging cell lines, particularly those derived from the HEK293, seem to require high concentrations of serum in the culture medium to support high viral titers during long term culture [14, 15]. On the other hand, HEK293-derived cells are able to grow in suspension as single cells or as small aggregates, facilitating scale-up, particularly when serum-free media are used. The production of retrovirus under serum-free media was thus tested in the modular cell lines. Several commercial serum-free media were tested, namely, EX-CELL (SAFC Biosciences/Sigma-Aldrich, St. Louis, MO), GT-3 (SAFC Biosciences/Sigma-Aldrich), HyQ (HyClone, Logan, UT), CD 293 (Invitrogen, Carlsbad, CA), and SFM2 (Invitrogen) [16]. All serum-free media supported cell growth at high cell densities in monolayer adherent cultures. In suspension cultures producer modular cells grow as single cells also at high cell densities. However, viral titers obtained in most serum-free media were low. The relationship between serum and viral production in the modular helper cell lines was further analyzed in detail for 293 FLEX [15]. It was concluded that some serum components were directly and specifically related to retroviral vector production. Although cell growth and the central energetic metabolic profile were similar at decreasing concentrations of serum, decreases in the infectious particles production were always observed [15]. The extent of the virus titer decline was proportional to serum reduction (*Table II*). Stability studies showed that production with lower percentage of serum originated a slight decrease in the vector stability, but this effect did not suffice to account for the sharp drop in infectious vector titers. Similar results were obtained both with 293 FLEX and Te Fly cells, suggesting the pattern to be independent of the producer cell line and confirming that it was vector related.

Table II. Impact of serum concentration in the production media for 293 FLEX modular cell line.

Serum (v/v) %	IP Titer (10⁶ i.p./ mL)	I.P./ TP ratio (10⁻³ i.p/RNA copy)	Vector Half-Life (h)
10	1.54 ± 0.02	5.6	9.7 ± 0.4
5	1.17 ± 0.1	5.0	8 ± 1
1	0.21 ± 0.06	0.9	6.5 ± 0.5

To identify the serum components which mostly affect viral production, a preliminary study of serum fractioning was conducted; lipoproteins were identified as the most critical parameter for the production of infectious particles. The use of de-lipidated serum confirmed that lipids are the serum components required in retrovirus production. Supplementation of culture media with fatty acids and cholesterol showed that the viral production titers could be recovered and even improved in the absence of serum when compared with the standard 10% (v/v) FBS supplementation [15]. Unless other supplements are added, serum is the only lipid source of the culture medium and, although cells should be able to sense lipid absence in the culture medium and activate biosynthetic pathways to stand up to lipid deprivation, the activation of lipid *de novo* synthesis may take hours, days, or in some cases, cells can no longer synthesize certain lipids [17].

Membrane lipids are essential players in the complex process of retroviral assembling and pseudo-typing that takes place at the host cell membrane, in which interactions of membrane lipid rafts select both envelope and core proteins, later the other viral components are recruited by cooperative interaction [13]. The production of infectious particles is known to rely on the efficiency of this process so that, changes in serum concentration will ultimately affect viral particle formation resulting in a higher production of non-infectious particles as observed for 293 FLEX (*Table II*) [15]. In fact, it has been not only demonstrated that lipids are one of the main serum components correlated with high retroviral vector infectious titers but also, that the reduction of serum concentration induces an increased production of defective particles [15].

Further studies on the effects of adapting retroviral vector packaging cell lines to serum deprivation and how it impacts infectious vector production have been performed [18]. The producer cells were analyzed for their ability to synthesize lipids using NMR and labeled glucose. Expressions of key regulatory enzymes of the lipid metabolism were also assessed. These studies showed that lipid metabolism needs to adapt to serum deprivation: cells capable of activating *de novo* lipid biosynthesis under serum withdrawal, particularly cholesterol, are able to adapt without significant loss of infectious vector titers. On the other hand, cells facing serum removal from the culture medium that are unable to activate lipid biosynthesis – such as HEK293 – lose infectious titer after a few passages [18]. Thus the culture of the modular cell lines in serum-free media requires that it contains lipids in its composition. After screening more than 13 serum-free media, high titer production of virus was observed for the modular cell lines grown in OptiPRO SFM (GIBCO; Invitrogen). Titers on the order of 1.5×10^6 IP/mL were obtained in OptiPRO SFM, and these could be further improved by the addition of lipid supplements.

IN SUMMARY

The characterization of modular producer cell lines substantiated their potential for clinical applications. They present several advantages: higher safety due to the defined integration of the vector within the packaging cell line, faster establishment of a producer cell line and of the manufacturing process since there is no need for screening and, favorable production conditions due to the possibility of pre-adaptation of the master cell line to culture conditions.

Within the CliniGene project, the advantage of these cells for optimization of retroviral vectors in defined chromosomal sites with respect to titers and safety was demonstrated. Moreover, the knowledge of media components allowed the design of better media formulations. High retroviral vector production in serum-free media was shown to be possible, as long as, adequate lipid media supplementation is performed.

Overall, therapeutic virus production from bench to bedside becomes safer, faster, and cheaper when using the RMCE modular cell lines [4, 16].

ACKNOWLEDGMENTS

This work has been performed with the support of the EC-DG research through the FP6-Network of Excellence, CLINIGENE: LSHB-CT-2006-018933.

REFERENCES

1. Schucht R, Coroadinha AS, Zanta-Boussif MA, Verhoeyen E, Carrondo MJ, Hauser H, Wirth D. A new generation of retroviral producer cells: predictable and stable virus production by Flp-mediated site-specific integration of retroviral vectors. *Mol Ther* 2006; 14: 285-92.

2. Coroadinha AS, Schucht R, Gama-Norton L, Wirth D, Hauser H, Carrondo MJ. The use of recombinase mediated cassette exchange in retroviral vector producer cell lines: predictability and efficiency by transgene exchange. *J Biotechnol* 2006; 124: 457-68.

3. Loew R, Meyer Y, Kuehlcke K, Gama-Norton L, Wirth D, Hauser H, *et al*. A new PG13-based packaging cell line for stable production of clinical-grade self-inactivating gamma-retroviral vectors using targeted integration. *Gene Ther* 2010; 17: 272-80.

4. Coroadinha AS, Gama-Norton L, Amaral AI, Hauser H, Alves PM, Cruz PE. Production of retroviral vectors: review. *Curr Gene Ther* 2010; 10: 456-73.

5. Coffin J, Hughes S, Varmus H. *Retroviruses*. Cold Spring Harbor: Cold Spring Harbor Laboratory Press, 1997.

6. Garoff H, Hewson R, Opstelten DJ. Virus maturation by budding. *Microbiol Mol Biol Rev* 1998; 62: 1171-90.

7. Yap MW, Kingsman SM, Kingsman AJ. Effects of stoichiometry of retroviral components on virus production. *J Gen Virol* 2000; 81: 2195-202.

8. Carrondo MJ, Merten OW, Haury M, Alves PM, Coroadinha AS. Impact of retroviral vector components stoichiometry on packaging cell lines: effects on productivity and vector quality. *Hum Gene Ther* 2008; 19: 199-210.

9. Gama-Norton L, Herrmann S, Schucht R, Coroadinha AS, Low R, Alves PM, *et al*. Retroviral vector performance in defined chromosomal loci of modular packaging cell lines. *Hum Gene Ther* 2010; 21: 979-91.

10. Swain A, Coffin JM. Mechanism of transduction by retroviruses. *Science* 1992; 255: 841-5.

11. Uren AG, Kool J, Berns A, van Lohuizen M. Retroviral insertional mutagenesis: past, present and future. *Oncogene* 2005; 24: 7656-72.

12. Gabriel R, Eckenberg R, Paruzynski A, Bartholomae CC, Nowrouzi A, Arens A, *et al*. Comprehensive genomic access to vector integration in clinical gene therapy. *Nat Med* 2009; 15: 1431-6.

13. Rodrigues AF, Alves PM, Coroadinha AS. Production of retroviral and lentiviral gene therapy vectors: challenges in the manufacturing of lipid enveloped virus. In: Xu K, ed. *Viral gene therapy*. InTech Publications, 2011: 15-40.

14. Pizzato M, Merten OW, Blair ED, Takeuchi Y. Development of a suspension packaging cell line for production of high titre, serum-resistant murine leukemia virus vectors. *Gene Ther* 2001; 8: 737-45.

15. Rodrigues AF, Carmo M, Alves PM, Coroadinha AS. Retroviral vector production under serum deprivation: the role of lipids. *Biotechnol Bioeng* 2009; 104: 1171-81.

16. Carrondo M, Panet A, Wirth D, Coroadinha AS, Cruz P, Falk H, *et al*. Integrated strategy for the production of therapeutic retroviral vectors. *Hum Gene Ther* 2011; 22: 370-9.

17. Seth G, Philp RJ, Denoya CD, McGrath K, Stutzman-Engwall KJ, Yap M, Hu WS. Large-scale gene expression analysis of cholesterol dependence in NS0 cells. *Biotechnol Bioeng* 2005; 90: 552-67.

18. Rodrigues AF, Amaral AI, Verissimo V, Alves PM, Coroadinha AS. Lipid biosynthetic pathways: metabolic target for improving retroviral vector titer and quality. *Biotechnol Bioeng* 2012; 109: 1269-79.

TECHNOLOGIES

Highlights on lentivirus mediated gene transfer

COORDINATED BY
MATTHIAS SCHWEIZER
AND
KLAUS CICHUTEK

The CliniBook: Clinical gene transfer
Edited by Odile Cohen-Haguenauer – EDK, Paris © 2012, pp. 127-128

A3-1
Introduction

MATTHIAS SCHWEIZER*, KLAUS CICHUTEK*

Paul-Ehrlich-Institut, Paul-Ehrlich-Straße 51-59, 63225 Langen, Germany.
matthias.schweizer@pei.de
* Corresponding authors

For many clinical gene therapy approaches, long-lasting expression of the therapeutic transgene is required. Therefore, retrovirus-derived vectors which mediate integration of the transgene into the host cell´s chromosome are frequently used. However, vectors derived from gamma-retroviruses, which have been predominantly used up to now, have several disadvantages: they are not capable of gene transfer into non-dividing cells, and they bear a risk of tumor induction as a result of insertional mutagenesis which came apparent in several patients participating in otherwise successful clinical trials for treatment of inherited immunodeficiency disorders. Lentiviral vectors are capable of stable transduction of a wide range of mammalian cell types, including dividing and non-dividing target cells. Moreover, the different integration profile of lentivectors compared to that of gammaretroviral vectors is taken as evidence for a lower risk of insertional oncogenesis. Accordingly, lentivectors are increasingly used for nonclinical gene transfer applications and also in up to now about 50 human clinical trials worldwide.

During the past five years, the lentivector platform of the European Network for the Advancement of Clinical Gene Transfer and Therapy, Clinigene, contributed to all aspects of vector development aiming at clinical applications. Main topics were the improvement of the vector design, optimization of manufacturing processes, and preclinical studies with a focus on safety aspects linked to the risk of insertional mutagenesis. Furthermore, a number of clinical trials targeting various diseases were initiated based on major contributions of platform members.

The improvement of lentivectors compassed the reduction of the potential for genotoxicity by incorporation and evaluation of a number of genetic insulators, as well as by the generation of self-inactivating vectors (SIN) and non-integrating lentivectors. For specific gene therapy approaches, e.g. for correction of Wiskott Aldrich syndrome (WAS), SCID-ADA, ZAP 70-deficiency or Fanconi's anemia vectors transferring respective transgenes controlled by optimal promoters were generated. Various approaches were developed for targeting of specific cell types, e.g. human T-cells, including modification of the envelope proteins or by use of cell-specific promoters.

The manufacturing of lentivectors is currently restrained by the lack of stable packaging cells for the generation of high-titer vectors. Thus, a great deal of work was performed to elucidate the possibility to generate stable production cell lines, the success of which may be dependent on factors such as selection of suitable chromosomal integration loci for the transfer and packaging constructs, or avoidance of RNA interference of lentiviral sequences. Using transient production, large scale production processes were optimized by testing of a number of influencing parameters such as the raw materials and ingredients used (*e.g.* cell lines or plasmids), the transfection method, the culture conditions, mode of purification and stabilization, etc. Finally, the suitability of the baculovirus system for lentivector production was evaluated. Now, several laboratories of the Clinigene lentivector platform are capable of large-scale production of lentiviral vectors in amounts sufficient for non-clinical studies and clinical trials.

Besides conventional testing of efficiency and toxicology of lentiviral vectors or lentivector-modified cells, the major issue of non-clinical testing was the elucidation of the potential risk of insertional oncogenesis which is associated with all kinds of integrating vectors. *In-vitro* assays and animal models were developed and used for comparison of this risk of vectors derived from different retroviruses (gamma-retroviruses or lentiviruses), carrying different promoters, or revealing different vector design (SIN or non-SIN). Results point to a reduced risk of tumour induction by lentiviral SIN vectors.

Several members of the Clinigene lentivector platform were involved in the preparation and initiation of gene therapy clinical trials to study new treatment options for Wiskott-Aldrich syndrome, adenosine deaminase deficiency, Parkinson´s disease or adrenoleukodystrophy. Partners also contributed to the manufacturing of investigational medicinal products, the non-clinical investigation and the implementation of the trials. A major effort included monitoring of patients for evidence of clonal cell dominance and tumour induction. Assays for this type of monitoring are up to the standard of advanced technology including next generation sequencing.

Here, some examples of the work of the Clinigene lentivector platform are illustrated. As an example for optimization of the vector design, the development of a specific lentivector derived from a simian immunodeficiency virus is described, as well as the utilization of insulators for vector improvement. In preparation of a gene therapy strategy for Huntington´s disease, lentiviral vectors targeting astrocytes by combining the usage of specific envelope proteins and miRNAs are presented. One article describes the large-scale manufacturing of lentiviruses with a focus on downstream processing, and issues arising from stable lentivector packaging cell lines are addressed.

ACKNOWLEDGMENTS

This work has been performed with the support of the EC-DG research through the FP6-Network of Excellence, CLINIGENE: LSHB-CT-2006-018933.

The CliniBook: Clinical gene transfer
Edited by Odile Cohen-Haguenauer – EDK, Paris © 2012, pp. 129-133

A3-2
MicroRNAs detargeting technology in the context of CNS applications

Angélique Colin[1,2], Mathilde Faideau[1,2], Noëlle Dufour[1,2],
Gwennaelle Auregan[1,2], Raymonde Hassig[1,2], Carole Escartin[1,2],
Philippe Hantraye[1,2], Gilles Bonvento[1,2], Nicole Déglon[1,2,3,4]*

[1]CEA, Institute of Biomedical Imaging (I2BM) and Molecular Imaging Research Center (MIRCen), Fontenay-aux-Roses, France, [2]CNRS-CEA URA2210, Fontenay-aux-Roses, France, [3]Lausanne University Hospital (CHUV), Department of Clinical Neurosciences, Laboratory of Cellular and Molecular Neurotherapies, Lausanne, Switzerland.
[4]Present address: Centre Hospitalier Universitaire Vaudois (CHUV), Département des Neurosciences Cliniques, Laboratoire de Neurothérapies Cellulaires et Moléculaires, Pavillon 3, Avenue de Beaumont, 1011 Lausanne, Suisse.
nicole.deglon@chuv.ch
* Corresponding author

SELECTIVE TRANSGENE EXPRESSION IN ASTROCYTES

The notion of a non-neuronal component of neurodegenerative disease is becoming increasingly regarded as an important aspect of the disease process [1]. However, our understanding is based mostly on data obtained *in vitro,* due to the limited existing tools for targeted expression in astrocytes *in vivo.* Current approaches are restrained to transgenic mice combining the very few astrocytic promoters available and the Cre/loxP system [2]. However, glial cell-specific promoters, such as GFAP, do not necessarily preclude transgene expression from being detected in neurons [3].
Gene transfer may therefore be valuable to target a subpopulation of cells and explore its function in experimental models. In particular, viral-mediated gene transfer provides a rapid, highly flexible and cost-effective, *in vivo* paradigm to study the impact of gene of interest during CNS development or in adult animals [4, 5]. Initial studies have shown that both adeno-associated vector type 2 and VSV-peudotyped lentiviral (LV) vector principally transduce neurons [6, 7]. However, recent studies have indicated that new AAV serotypes and lentiviral vectors pseudotyped with various envelopes infect both neurons and glial cells [8-17]. Astroglial cell-specific promoters have been proposed as a means to further restrict transgene expression. However, the low level of transcriptional activity, the difficulty of maintaining tissue-specific expression when promoters are integrated into viral vectors and the small number of characterized regulatory elements [18] currently limit this approach.
In the present program, we used the microRNA (miRNA) regulation pathway [19, 20] to develop a mokola-pseudotyped lentiviral vector (LV-MOK) specifically targeting

astroglial cells. MiRNAs are endogenous ~22-nucleotide (nt) RNAs that post-transcriptionally regulate gene expression [21]. Most miRNAs are evolutionarily conserved and regulate a variety of developmental and physiological processes. The first indication of the abundance of miRNA genes came from sequencing small RNAs from mammals, flies, and worms [22-24]. Approximately one third of the miRNAs show an expression profile with high tissue-specificity or developmental regulation and in humans, approximately 30% of all mRNAs are regulated by miRNAs. Although the precise mechanism of miRNA-mediated gene silencing remains unclear, the binding to partially complementary sites on target mRNAs promote the degradation and/or inhibit the translation [25-27]. The brain is enriched in several miRNAs, including miR124 [28, 29]. In humans and mice, miR124 is encoded by three different genes, which give rise to only one mature miR124a [28]. MiR124 is abundantly expressed in neurons but not in astrocytes [30].

We therefore inserted 4 copies of a miR124 target sequence (miR124T) at the 3' end of a transgene of interest to eliminate residual expression in neuronal cells and restrict its expression to astrocytes [31]. This highly expressed miR124 was chosen to avoid saturation/dysfunction of the miRNA regulatory pathway that may lead to deleterious effects. The first generation LVs were based on a natural and experimentally validated miR124T from the integrin-β1 gene. This partially matching sequence (miR124T) was associated with a selective silencing of the transgene in primary neurons mainly due to mRNA cleavage and not to inhibition of the translation. When combined with a mokola pseudotyping, a complete reversal of the neuron to astrocyte ratio of β-galactosidase expressing cells was observed in the striatum (6±4% vs 89±3% for the LV-MOK-miR124T; 93±1% vs 9±2% for LV-VSV) but also in the hippocampus and cerebellum. However, we noticed some species specificity, with a lower astrocytic tropism in rats than mice. To overcome this limitation we developed a second generation LV with a mir124T perfectly complementary to the mature miRNA as previously described by Brown *et al.* [19]. When injected in the striatum of adult rats, the residual transgene expression in neurons was decreased to 2.5% (Escartin *et al.*, unpublished data) (*Figure 1*).

In a subsequent work, this tool was used to evaluate the contribution of astrocytes in Huntington's disease [32]. Recent data from transgenic mice selectively expressing mutant huntingtin (Htt) in GABAergic medium-sized spiny neurons, the subpopulation of neurons that are mainly affected in the disease, suggest that cell-cell interactions are necessary for striatal pathogenesis [33]. To investigate whether astrocytes could also be involved in these pathological cell-cell interactions, we produced a LV-MOK-mutant or WT Htt-miR124T. At 4 weeks post-injection, mHtt aggregates were observed in astrocytes and not in neurons, confirming the selectivity of the vector. In adult mice, mutant Htt expression was associated with a progressive phenotype of reactive astrocytes that was characterized by a marked decreased expression of the glutamate transporters (GLAST and GLT-1) and of glutamate uptake. These impairments in glutamate transport and recycling capacity were associated with neuronal dysfunction, as observed by a reduction in DARPP-32 and NR2B expression. Moreover, expression of GLT-1 into striatal astrocytes partially rescues the phenotype. In addition, we showed that in HD patients, astrogliosis in the putamen was associated with morphological changes that increased with severity of disease. Consistent with the findings from experimental mice, there was a significant grade-dependent decrease in striatal GLT-1 expression from HD subjects. These findings suggest that the presence of mHtt in astrocytes alters glial glutamate transport capacity early in the disease process and may contribute to HD pathogenesis [32]. Thus, the ability to selectively infect non-neuronal cells may be a key component when developing gene therapy based therapeutics for neurodegenerative disease.

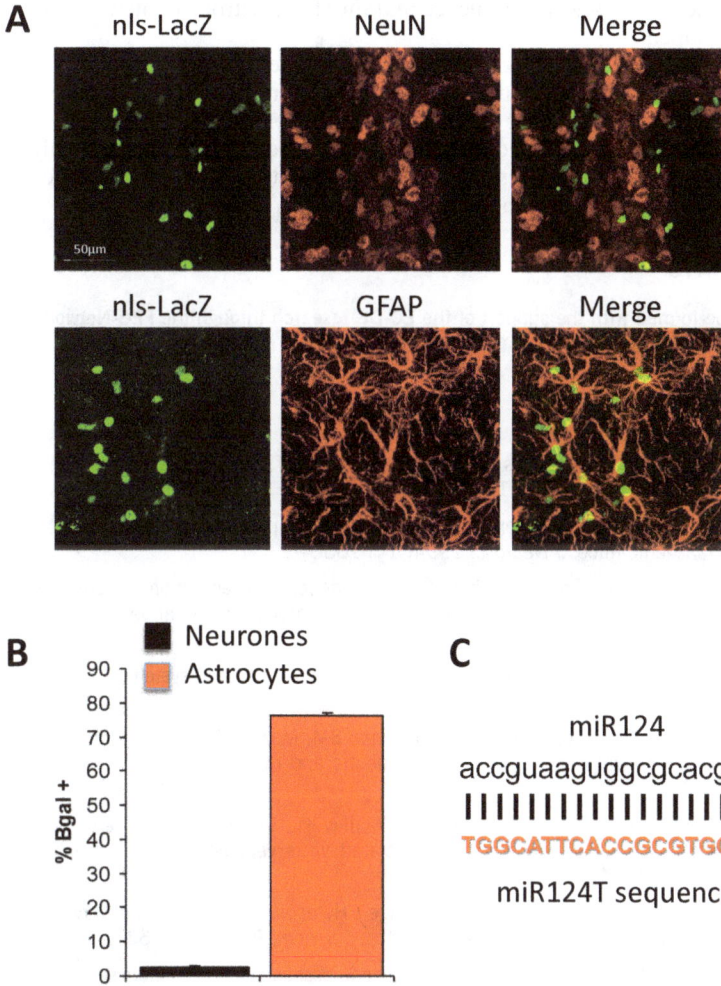

Figure 1. Targeting astrocytes *in vivo* with a combination of mokola pseudotyping and integration of four copies of fully complementary miR124 target sequence (miR124T) (C) in the 3' UTR region of a lentiviral vector. (A) Double-immunofluorescence staining of rat striatal section showing the co-localization of the transgene (nuclear beta-galactosidase) with GFAP-positive and not NeuN-positive cells. (B) Quantification of the percentage of beta-galactosidase in NeuN-and GFAP-positive cells, showing the glial tropism of the new vector in adult rats.

PERSPECTIVES

In the study of Colin *et al.* [31], we have shown that we can downregulate a glial gene (glutamate transporter GLAST; not expressed in neurons) into striatal astrocytes *in vivo*. However, this first generation vector is not suitable for an astrocyte-specific down-regulation of an ubiquitous gene. Indeed, due to the maturation/processing of siRNA, the mirRNA target sequence is cleaved during the synthesis of the siRNA. In order to solve this issue and be able to selectively silence mutant Htt in astrocytes, new LV are currently being developed.

Altogether, these results illustrate the potency of miRNA detargeting approach for cell-type specific expression in the brain. However, our current knowledge of the expression profile of miRNA in different cell subpopulations of the brain is extremely limited and additional work is needed to further extend this concept and reach highly selective and restricted transgene expression suited for dissecting the contribution of specific circuitry and pathways in pathogenic conditions.

ACKNOWLEDGMENTS

This work has been performed with the support of the EC-DG research through the FP6-Network of Excellence, CLINIGENE: LSHB-CT-2006-018933.

REFERENCES

1. Lobsiger CS, Cleveland DW. Glial cells as intrinsic components of non-cell-autonomous neurodegenerative disease. *Nat Neurosci* 2007; 10: 1355-60.

2. Brenner M, Kisseberth WC, Su Y, Besnard F, Messing A. GFAP promoter directs astrocyte-specific expression in tansgenic mice. *J Neurosci* 1994; 14: 1030-7.

3. Jakobsson J, Georgievska B, Ericson C, Lundberg C. Lesion-dependent regulation of transgene expression in the rat brain using a human glial fibrillary acidic protein-lentiviral vector. *Eur J Neurosci* 2004; 19: 761-5.

4. Jakobsson J, Lundberg C. Lentiviral vectors for use in the central nervous system. *Mol Ther* 2006; 13: 484-93.

5. Wong LF, Goodhead L, Prat C, Mitrophanous KA, Kingsman SM, Mazarakis ND. Lentivirus-mediated gene transfer to the central nervous system: therapeutic and research applications. *Hum Gene Ther* 2006: 17: 1-9.

6. Kaplitt MG, Leone P, Samulski RJ, Xiao X, Pfaff DW, O'Malley KL, During MJ. Long-term gene expression and phenotypic correction using adeno-associated virus vectors in the mammalian brain. *Nat Genet* 1994; 8: 148-54.

7. Naldini L, Blömer U, Gallay P, Ory D, Mulligan R, Gage FH, *et al. In vivo* gene delivery and stable transduction of nondividing cells by a lentiviral vector. *Science* 1996; 272: 263-7.

8. Broekman ML, Comer LA, Hyman BT, Sena-Esteves M. Adeno-associated virus vectors serotyped with AAV8 capsid are more efficient than AAV-1 or -2 serotypes for widespread gene delivery to the neonatal mouse brain. *Neuroscience* 2006; 138: 501-10.

9. Burger C, Gorbatyuk OS, Velardo MJ, Peden CS, Williams P, Zolotukhin S, *et al.* Recombinant AAV viral vectors pseudotyped with viral capsids from serotypes 1, 2, and 5 display differential efficiency and cell tropism after delivery to different regions of the central nervous system. *Mol Ther* 2004; 10: 302-17.

10. Cearley CN, Wolfe JH. Transduction characteristics of adeno-associated virus vectors expressing cap serotypes 7, 8, 9, and Rh10 in the mouse brain. *Mol Ther* 2006; 13: 528-37.

11. Desmaris N, Bosch A, Salaun C, Petit C, Prevost MC, Tordo N, *et al.* Production and neurotropism of lentivirus vectors pseudotyped with lyssavirus envelope glycoproteins. *Mol Ther* 2001; 4: 149-56.

12. Mazarakis ND, Azzouz M, Rohll JB, Ellard FM, Wilkes FJ, Olsen AL, *et al.* Rabies virus glycoprotein pseudotyping of lentiviral vectors enables retrograde axonal transport and access to the nervous system after peripheral delivery. *Hum Mol Genet* 2001; 10: 2109-21.

13. Paterna JC, Feldon J, Bueler H. Transduction profiles of recombinant adeno-associated virus vectors derived from serotypes 2 and 5 in the nigrostriatal system of rats. *J Virol* 2004: 78: 6808-17.

14. Pertusa M, Garcia-Matas S, Mammeri H, Adell A, Rodrigo T, Mallet J, *et al*. Expression of GDNF transgene in astrocytes improves cognitive deficits in aged rats. *Neurobiol Aging* 2008; 29: 1366-79.

15. Tenenbaum L, Chtarto A, Lehtonen E, Velu T, Brotchi J, Levivier M. Recombinant AAV-mediated gene delivery to the central nervous system. *J Gene Med* 2004; 6 (suppl 1): S212-22.

16. Watson DJ, Kobinger GP, Passini MA, Wilson JM, Wolfe JH. Targeted transduction patterns in the mouse brain by lentivirus vectors pseudotyped with VSV, Ebola, Mokola, LCMV, or MuLV envelope proteins. *Mol Ther* 2002; 5: 528-37.

17. Wong LF, Azzouz M, Walmsley LE, Askham Z, Wilkes FJ, Mitrophanous KA, *et al*. Transduction patterns of pseudotyped lentiviral vectors in the nervous system. *Mol Ther* 2004; 9: 101-11.

18. Xu R, Janson CG, Mastakov M, Lawlor P, Young D, Mouravlev A, *et al*. Quantitative comparison of expression with adeno-associated virus (AAV-2) brain-specific gene cassettes. *Gene Ther* 2001; 8: 1323-32.

19. Brown BD, Gentner B, Cantore A, Colleoni S, Amendola M, Zingale A, *et al*. Endogenous microRNA can be broadly exploited to regulate transgene expression according to tissue, lineage and differentiation state. *Nat Biotechnol* 2007; 25: 1457-67.

20. Brown BD, Venneri MA, Zingale A, Sergi Sergi L, Naldini L. Endogenous microRNA regulation suppresses transgene expression in hematopoietic lineages and enables stable gene transfer. *Nat Med* 2006; 12: 585-91.

21. Bartel DP, Chen CZ. Micromanagers of gene expression: the potentially widespread influence of metazoan microRNAs. *Nat Rev Genet* 2004; 5: 396-400.

22. Lagos-Quintana M, Rauhut R, Lendeckel W, Tuschl T. Identification of novel genes coding for small expressed RNAs. *Science* 2001: 294: 853-858.

23. Lau NC, Lim LP, Weinstein EG, Bartel DP. An abundant class of tiny RNAs with probable regulatory roles in *Caenorhabditis elegans*. *Science* 2001; 294: 858-62.

24. Lee RC, Ambros V. An extensive class of small RNAs in *Caenorhabditis elegans*. *Science* 2001; 294: 862-4.

25. Liu J, Valencia-Sanchez MA, Hannon GJ, Parker R. MicroRNA-dependent localization of targeted mRNAs to mammalian P-bodies. *Nat Cell Biol* 2005; 7: 719-23.

26. Wu L, Belasco JG. Micro-RNA regulation of the mammalian lin-28 gene during neuronal differentiation of embryonal carcinoma cells. *Mol Cell Biol* 2005; 25: 9198-208.

27. Yekta S, Shih IH, Bartel DP. MicroRNA-directed cleavage of HOXB8 mRNA. *Science* 2004; 304: 594-6.

28. Deo M, Yu JY, Chung KH, Tippens M, Turner DL. Detection of mammalian microRNA expression by *in situ* hybridization with RNA oligonucleotides. *Dev Dyn* 2006; 235: 2538-48.

29. Lagos-Quintana M, Rauhut R, Yalcin A, Meyer J, Lendeckel W, Tuschl T. Identification of tissue-specific microRNAs from mouse. *Curr Biol* 2002; 12: 735-9.

30. Smirnova L, Grafe A, Seiler A, Schumacher S, Nitsch R, Wulczyn FG. Regulation of miRNA expression during neural cell specification. *Eur J Neurosci* 2005; 21: 1469-77.

31. Colin A, Faideau M, Dufour N, Auregan G, Hassig R, Andrieu T, *et al*. Engineered lentiviral vector targeting astrocytes *in vivo*. *Glia* 2009; 57: 667-79.

32. Faideau M, Kim J, Cormier K, Gilmore R, Welch M, Auregan G, *et al*. *In vivo* expression of polyglutamine-expanded huntingtin by mouse striatal astrocytes impairs glutamate transport: a correlation with Huntington's disease subjects. *Hum Mol Genet* 2010; 19: 3053-67.

33. Gu X, Andre VM, Cepeda C, Li SH, Li XJ, Levine MS, Yang XW. Pathological cell-cell interactions are necessary for striatal pathogenesis in a conditional mouse model of Huntington's disease. *Mol Neurodegener* 2007; 2: 8.

The CliniBook: Clinical gene transfer
Edited by Odile Cohen-Haguenauer – EDK, Paris © 2012, pp. 134-137

A3-3
Development of SIVsmmPBj vectors for gene transfer into myeloid cells

Matthias Schweizer*, Klaus Cichutek

Paul-Ehrlich-Institut, Paul-Ehrlich-Straße 51-59, 63225 Langen, Germany.
matthias.schweizer@pei.de
* Corresponding author

Overview

To improve the target cell spectrum of lentiviral vectors, vectors were derived from SIVsmmPBj which are capable of efficient transduction of myeloid cells (monocytes, dendritic cells, and macrophages). The viral accessory gene product Vpx was identified as the factor responsible for this interesting feature. Investigation of Vpx-binding proteins led to identification of cellular HIV-1 restriction factors present in myeloid cells.

Introduction

The major advantage of viral vectors derived from retroviruses is the integration of the transferred transgene into the chromosome of the host cell, which enables long-lasting transgene expression, not only in the transduced target cell, but also in all off-spring cells after cell division. Compared to gamma-retroviral vectors, lentiviral vectors (LV) have been reported to be superior regarding safety and efficacy, especially on non-dividing target cells. Accordingly, several clinical trials using lentivectors have already been initiated. It can be expected that the use of lentiviral vectors in human gene therapy will increase in the near future, and LV may replace the use of gamma-retroviral vectors which are still predominant at present.

Lentiviral vectors are mainly derived from HIV-1, but also from non-human lentiviruses such as simian immunodeficiency viruses (SIV), feline immunodeficiency virus (FIV), or equine infectious anemia virus (EIAV). The overall vector design is very similar for all LV types. In particular, the envelope glycoprotein of the vesicular stomatitis virus (VSV) is predominantly used for pseudotyping of vector particles, which confers transduction of a wide variety of target cells.

However, although LVs are able for transduction of non-dividing cells, transduction of some primary human cells is restricted. In particular, primary human myeloid cells can only hardly be transduced by LV: whereas dendritic cells or macrophages can be transduced albeit at a comparably low efficiency, primary human monocytes are not transducible with common LV without previous stimulation. The development of LV derived from further lentivirus strains allowing monocyte transduction may be helpful not only for several gene therapy approaches targeting myeloid cells, but also for explaining the restriction for HIV-1 in these cells.

SIVsmmPBj-DERIVED VECTORS [1]

SIVsmmPBj originates from an SIV isolate from Sooty Mangabey Monkey, which had been passaged in a pig-tailed macaque [2]. Whereas the parental SIVsmm9 strain is apathogenic, the strain SIVsmmPBj14 which was isolated from the infected pig-tailed macaque causes severe pathogenicity resulting in a mortality rate of about 30 to 80% depending on the monkey species infected. This high pathogenicity of SIVsmmPBj, in contrast to SIVsmm9, is associated with the capacity of the virus to replicate in human PBMCs or unstimulated PBMCs from various monkeys [3]. This enhanced target cell spectrum of replicating SIVsmmPBj prompted us to investigate whether SIVsmmPBj-derived vectors also reveal a broader target cell spectrum than common lentiviral vectors such as HIV-1-derived ones. Actually, transduction of a wide range of target cells demonstrated that primary SIVsmmPBj vectors are capable of efficient transduction of myeloid cells. Whereas transduction using HIV-1 vectors is inefficient, although possible, for primary human dendritic cells or macrophages, it is in practice impossible for unstimulated primary human monocytes.

THE CAPACITY OF SIVsmmPBj VECTORS FOR MONOCYTE TRANSDUCTION IS DEPENDING ON THE VIRAL ACCESSORY PROTEIN Vpx [4]

To enlighten the reason for the capacity for monocyte transduction, we generated SIVsmmPBj vectors with deletions of one or more of the accessory proteins Vif, Vpx, Vpr, and Nef by introduction of stop codons into the respective genes. Extensive transduction experiments demonstrated that Vpx is the only accessory protein required for monocyte transduction. Thereby, Vpx provided in trans from a separate expression plasmid in the packaging cell was able to complement a vector in which all of the accessory proteins have been deleted (*Figure 1*).

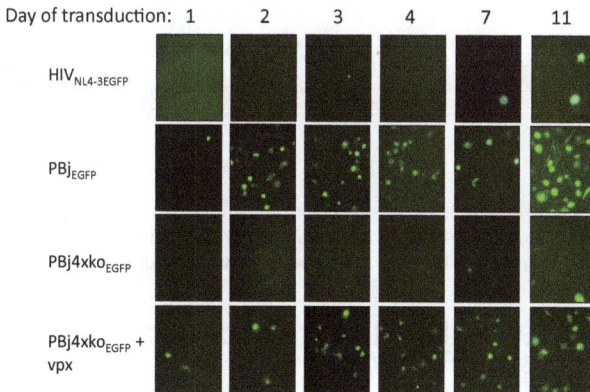

Figure 1. Transduction of primary human monocytes. Detection of gene transfer 7 days after transduction using the EGFP transferring vectors indicated on the left. Upper line: day of transduction after isolation of monocytes from PBMC. Following lines, respectively from top to bottom: HIV$_{NL4-3EGFP}$: HIV-1-derived vector. PBj: SIVsmmPBj-derived vector. PBj4xko$_{EGFP}$: SIVsmmPBj-derived vector lacking all accessory genes. PBj4xko$_{EGFP}$ + vpx: SIVsmmPBj-derived vector lacking all accessory genes, complemented with Vpx.

VPX ENABLES TRANSDUCTION OF MONOCYTES BY HIV-1 VECTORS [4, 5]

The *Vpx* gene is present in the SIVmac/SIVsmm/HIV-2 lineage of primate lentiviruses but is lacking in others, especially in HIV-1 (*Figure 2*). Actually, we found that LVs derived from all viruses encoding a *Vpx* gene are capable for monocyte transduction. Therefore, we analyzed whether supplementation of HIV-1 with *Vpx* would also allow monocyte transduction. However, in our hands complementation of HIV-1 vectors with *Vpx* by simple cotransfection of a *Vpx* expression plasmid in the packaging cells did not result in packaging of *Vpx* in vector particles. Therefore, two approaches to package *Vpx* were made: on the one hand, we inserted the *Vpx* binding site within the p6 domain of SIVsmmPBj Gag into the p6 of HIV-1 Gag. On the other hand, we generated fusion proteins of HIV-1 Vpr and SIVsmmPBj Vpx. However, although we could demonstrate packaging of *Vpx* into HIV-1 vector particles, these vectors were not able to mediate monocyte transduction.

Transduction of monocytes with HIV-1 vectors was ultimately made possible through the preincubation of target cells with *Vpx* provided via SIVsmmPBj-derived virus-like particles (VLP). VLPs were generated by cotransfection of 292T cells with SIVsmmPBj packaging plasmid, a *Vpx* expression plasmid and a plasmid encoding for the VSV-G protein. Pre-incubation of monocytes with VLPs enabled subsequent transfection with HIV-1-derived vectors, and beyond this step, the complete replication of HIV-1. We concluded that *Vpx* counteracts a cellular restriction mechanism for HIV-1 present in primary human monocytes. Beside the impact of this feature on gene therapy with the improved LV-mediated transduction of myeloid cells, this observation opened a new possibility for identification of HIV-1 restriction factors.

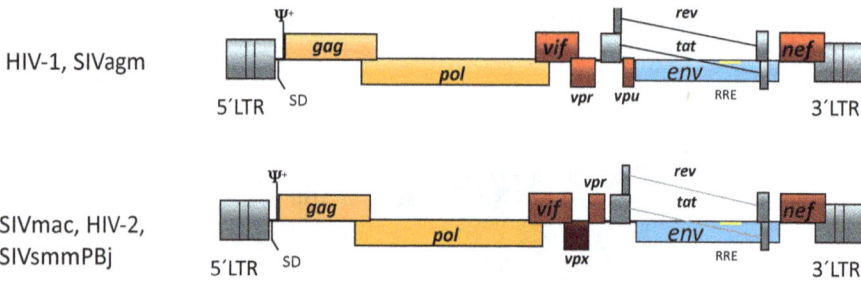

Figure 2. Genome structures of primate lentiviruses. Upper panel: viruses encoding Vpr and Vpu. Below, viruses encoding Vpx. Lower panel: SIVmac, SIVagm, or SIVsmmPBj are isolates from Rhesus macaque, African green monkey, or sooty mangabey monkey, respectively.

IDENTIFICATION OF CELLULAR HIV-1 RESTRICTION FACTORS COUNTERACTED BY SIVSMMPBJ VPX [6]

In searching for Vpx-binding proteins by co-immunoprecipitation and mass spectrometry analysis, two HIV-1 restriction factors present in myeloid cells were identified. Down-regulation of APOBEC3A and SAMHD1 enabled transduction with HIV-1 vectors in the myeloid THP1 cell line similar to results obtained with Vpx pre-incubation. Concerning SAMHD1, comparable results were recently reported by others [7, 8], underlining the relevance of these results for HIV-1 research in general.

CONSTRUCTION OF SIVSMMPBJ AND HIV-2 VECTORS [9]

High-titer state-of-the-art SIVsmmPBj and HIV-2 vectors were generated by construction of packaging and transfer vectors. Thereby, we developed a novel approach for generation of lentiviral transfer vectors, which significantly facilitates the generation of LV transfer vectors in general. Instead of conventional time-consuming cloning by gradual enhancing cloning steps, we used a highly flexible three-step fusion PCR-based approach which allowed completing the procedure, starting from the viral genome, within few days. The resulting vectors revealed titers of about 10^8 transducing units/ml and maintained the capacity for transduction of primary human monocytes.

CONCLUSION

The development of SIVsmmPBj vectors improved the application spectrum of human gene therapy by availability of LV capable of efficient transduction of myeloid cells, and led to identification of cellular HIV-1 restriction factors active in myeloid cells.

ACKNOWLEDGMENTS

This work has been performed with the support of the EC-DG research through the FP6-Network of Excellence, CLINIGENE: LSHB-CT-2006-018933.

REFERENCES

1. Muhlebach MD, Wolfrum N, Schule S, Tschulena U, Sanzenbacher R, Flory E, *et al.* Stable transduction of primary human monocytes by simian lentiviral vector PBj. *Mol Ther* 2005; 12: 1206-16.

2. Fultz PN, McClure HM, Anderson DC, Switzer WM. Identification and biologic characterization of an acutely lethal variant of simian immunodeficiency virus from sooty mangabeys (SIV/SMM). *AIDS Res Hum Retrovir* 1989; 5: 397-409.

3. Fultz PN. Replication of an acutely lethal simian immunodeficiency virus activates and induces proliferation of lymphocytes. *J Virol* 1991; 65: 4902-9.

4. Wolfrum N, Muhlebach MD, Schule S, Kaiser JK, Kloke BP, Cichutek K, Schweizer M. Impact of viral accessory proteins of SIVsmmPBj on early steps of infection of quiescent cells. *Virology* 2007; 364: 330-41.

5. Schule S, Kloke BP, Kaiser JK, Heidmeier S, Panitz S, Wolfrum N, *et al.* Restriction of HIV-1 replication in monocytes is abolished by Vpx of SIVsmmPBj. *PLoS One* 2009; 4: e7098.

6. Berger A, Munk C, Schweizer M, Cichutek K, Schule S, Flory E. Interaction of Vpx and apolipoprotein B mRNA-editing catalytic polypeptide 3 family member A (APOBEC3A) correlates with efficient lentivirus infection of monocytes. *J Biol Chem* 2010; 285: 12248-54

7. Laguette N, Sobhian B, Casartelli N, Ringeard M, Chable-Bessia C, Segeral E, *et al.* SAMHD1 is the dendritic- and myeloid-cell-specific HIV-1 restriction factor counteracted by Vpx. *Nature* 2011; 474: 654-7.

8. Hrecka K, Hao C, Gierszewska M, Swanson SK, Kesik-Brodacka M, Srivastava S, *et al.* Vpx relieves inhibition of HIV-1 infection of macrophages mediated by the SAMHD1 protein. *Nature* 2011; 474: 658-61.

9. Kloke BP, Schule S, Muhlebach MD, Wolfrum N, Cichutek K, Schweizer M. Functional HIV-2- and SIVsmmPBj- derived lentiviral vectors generated by a novel polymerase chain reaction-based approach. *J Gene Med* 2010; 12: 446-52.

The CliniBook: Clinical gene transfer
Edited by Odile Cohen-Haguenauer – EDK, Paris © 2012, pp. 138-149

A3-4
Insulated retrovirus vectors using novel synthetic genetic insulator elements to circumvent enhancer-mediated genotoxicity

CAROLINE DUROS[1]**, ALEXANDRE ARTUS[1]**, ODILE COHEN-HAGUENAUER[1,2]*

[1]*CliniGene, École Normale Supérieure de Cachan, CNRS UMR 8113, 94235 Cachan, France.*
[2]*Oncogenetics, Department of Clinical Oncology, AP-HP, Hôpital Saint-Louis, Faculté de Médecine, Université Paris7-Paris Diderot, Sorbonne Paris-Cité, Paris, France.*
odile.cohen@lbpa.ens-cachan.fr
*Corresponding author
**These authors contributed equally to the work*

INTRODUCTION

The need for better gene transfer systems, in terms of specificity, efficacy and safety has been and still remains a major challenge in the development of gene therapy, so that the risk of harm to benefit balance of treating a condition will be improved sufficiently to allow the routine use of gene therapy in patients. In otherwise successful – in terms of proof of concept for potential curative effect – gene therapy trials in patients with X-linked severe combined immunodeficiency (SCID-X1), gene therapy vector integration has resulted in six reported cases of vector induced leukaemia [1-3]. Similar effects have also been seen in several other gene therapy trials, for instance X-linked chronic granulomatous disease [4, 5] and more recently in Wiskott-Aldrich syndrome [6]. These observed side effects of gene therapy, reveal current limitations of integrative vectors for gene transfer used in clinical studies, as Self-Inactivating (SIN) vectors with strong promoters have also been shown to partially retain oncogenic potential [7]. This issue was recently considered and discussed at the international level and a report issued [8]. In response to insertional mutagenesis leading to enhancer mediated over-expression of proto-oncogenes, a number of new vector designs are being explored, including the use of modified gammaretroviral vectors and transposon based-systems as well as lentiviral vectors, which have a propensity to insert into genes rather than near transcriptional start sites.

It is all about gene transfer vector integration

Retroviral and other viral and non-viral vectors used in gene therapy often have a preference for particular chromosomal integration regions or targets. In fact, it has been shown that the integration of murine leukemia virus (MLV) based vectors is not random, as integration mainly occurs within or close to 5' regulatory regions of transcriptionnally active genes [9, 10]; lentiviral vectors do not show such preference and mostly integrate at random in the open reading frame [11]. It is also well known that chromosomal insertion of a vector can activate or inactivate genes nearby and that chromosomal regulatory sequences can affect the expression of vector encoded genes, this phenomenon being known as regulatory cross talk. Indeed, vector integration has two major functional impacts. First, *cis*-genomic sequences and chromatin structures flanking the sites of vector insertion can influence the level and pattern of expression, a phenomenon usually referred to as chromosomal position effects (CPE). This may result in either vector silencing or position effect variegation, with expression levels which greatly vary between, and even within, the progeny of transduced cells [12, 13]. Conversely, transgenic sequences can influence flanking cellular genes to induce insertional mutagenesis which leads to clonal expansion with the subsequent risk of oncogenic transformation of individual cell clones, a phenomenon referred to as vector-mediated genotoxicity: clonal outgrowth and overt malignant transformation, have been documented in both animal models and clinical trials [14, 15]. This so-called genotoxic potential of vectors may stem from the promiscuous activation of cellular genes by either endogenous and/or exogenous viral regulatory elements which drive the expression of the transgenic therapeutic sequences [16]. Vector enhancers hold the ability to activate proto-oncogenes such as genes involved in cell growth or differentiation: this may result in the expansion of rare cells bearing these vector integration sites.

Vector insertion can also affect adjacent cellular gene expression through non-enhancer mediated mechanisms. There are essentially four different alternative mechanisms, other than oncogenic activation, by which helper murine retroviruses, and more recently transposons, are known to induce cancer: (i) alternative splicing: following insertion, gene disruption can cause splicing alterations; (ii) gene inactivation: proviral integration into tumor suppressor genes might lead to tumorigenesis; (iii) truncation of cellular mRNA or protein and (iv) microRNA activation: MLV insertion in the 3' untranslated region of a gene has been shown to result in the loss of miRNAs binding sites and subsequent negative regulation of this gene, thereby increasing mRNA stability and increasing expression levels [8, 17].

Strategies to overcome enhancer-mediated insertional mutagenesis

Over the past years and following the severe adverse events directly attributable to gene transfer vectors integration, several approaches have been proposed with view to decreasing the probability of retroviral vector-mediated genotoxicity [15, 18, 19]. These include the use of vectors based on lentiviruses or other viruses that are less likely to integrate near gene promoters [20], the use of self-inactivating (SIN) vectors that delete potent enhancers and promoters in the viral long-terminal repeats (LTRs) [21], the use of lineage-restricted enhancers and promoters [19, 22, 23], and improvements to the 3' RNA processing signals [24]. However, each of these avenues has potential drawbacks.

More recently, several approaches have been pursued along distinct and potentially synergistic rationale, as follows: (i) insulating the transgenic cassette in order to prevent cross-talk in *cis* from and towards the integrated exogenous sequences: while in keeping with random integration, this strategy holds the potential to operate should integration occur at any given locus. This is providing the Genetic Insulator Elements (GIEs) under use are robust enough to act as both enhancer-blocker and boundary against potential silencing [25, 26]; (ii) inhibiting the natural integration process in knocking down in target cells LEDGF, the cell-partner of HIV integrase. This may allow to redirect integration towards defined genetic regions [27]; (iii) further along this line, the possibility to select ad hoc genetic regions for integration to take place in these safe harbors has been investigated, in particular in taking advantage of Zinc finger nucleases (ZFNs) with pre-determined specificity [28]; more recently, technologies have been developed based on meganucleases or Transcription Activator-Like Effector Nucleases (TA-LENs) which hold the potential to specifically recognize a mutation at a given gene locus (*ibid* chapters A7-3 and A7-4); (iv) investigating alternative integrative systems with a more random integration profile in human cells, such as foamy-virus vectors or non-viral vectors derived from transposons [29]; (v) constraining unwanted expression of the transgene in non-target cells is believed to add to gene transfer safety, mostly when considering a potential toxicity linked to the accumulation of the transgene product; it might also be instrumental in preventing insertional mutagenesis in the event where overstimulation of the regulatory sequences driving the transgene might be at stake [30]; however, in target cells, like would of T-cells in X-SCIDs patients, this strategy is unlikely to be of added value. Further along the way of increasing safety is targeting cell-entry of gene transfer vectors, an approach that recently met with significant success when vectors were administered *in vivo* [31]. Here, we shall focus on the use of genetic insulator elements to prevent both transgene silencing and enhancer-mediated genotoxicity following integration of a transgenic cassette into the host-cell genome.

CHROMATIN INSULATORS: ENHANCER-BLOCKING AND BARRIER GENETIC ELEMENTS

Genetic insulators are naturally occurring DNA elements that help form functional boundaries between adjacent chromatin domains [13, 32, 33] and are characterized by at least one of the following activities: enhancer-blocking and/or boundary [34, 35]. They have been reported in species as diverse as yeast and man and play a key role in genomic architecture and gene regulation since they hold the potential to limit the range of action of enhancers and silencers [36]. An insulator with enhancer-blocking properties is able to block the cross-talk between an enhancer and a promoter when interposed and thus prevent enhancer-mediated transcriptional activation of neighbouring regions that are transcriptionally quiescent or otherwise heterochromatic (*Figure 1A*). Insulators with boundary properties set the borders of neighbouring chromatin domains. Boundaries prevent the propagation of condensed chromatin structures that silence expression and counteract the effects of chromosomal position on transgene expression [37] (*Figure 1B*). Genetic insulators do not exhibit inherent transcriptional enhancing or repressing activities on their own. As such, they allow other *cis*-regulatory elements to function without interference from, or action upon, the surrounding chromatin.

A. Testing for enhancer-blocking function

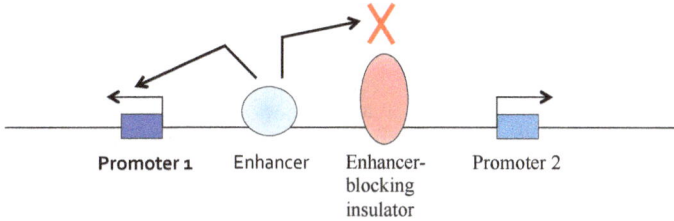

B. Testing for barrier function

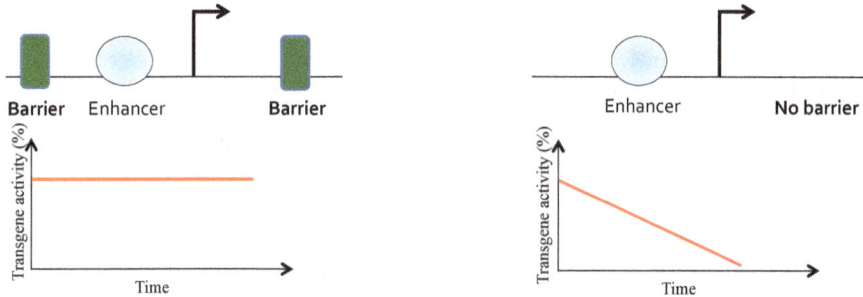

Figure 1. Testing for insulators function. A. Enhancer-blocking function: when placed between an enhancer and a promoter, an insulator with enhancer-blocking ability is expected to block enhancer-mediated transcriptional activation of neighbouring regions. B. Boundary function: Barrier insulators establish borders with neighbouring chromatin domains. They are thus able to prevent expression silencing and counteract chromosomal position effects on transgene expression.

These properties make chromatin insulators ideal elements for reducing the interaction between gene transfer vectors and the target cell genome in order to counteract both chromosomal position effect with the risk of transgene silencing on the one hand and enhancer-mediated insertional mutagenesis with the identified risk of vector-induced carcinogenesis on the other hand. Of utmost importance, chromatin insulators must be physically located between promoters and either enhancers or heterchromatin in order to provide their protective function.

Enhancer-blocking insulators

Among insulator elements identified to date, most are of the enhancer-blocking type [33, 34, 38]. In vertebrates, the function of these elements is mediated through the zinc-finger DNA-binding factor CTCF [32, 33]. In most models, these elements are thought to function through physical loop structures that are established through CTCF-mediated interactions between adjacent insulator elements or through CTCF-mediated tethering of the chromatin fiber to structural elements within the nucleus (reviewed in [38]). Such loops are thought to form functionally distinct domains, either sequestered into autonomous compartments or by blocking enhancers action along the DNA axis.

Barrier insulators

Chromosomal position effects on integrating gene transfer vectors may result in silencing with partial or complete loss of transgene expression, occurring over time or following differentiation [12, 13, 39]. Beyond retroviral vectors mediated gene transfer, this phenomenon has been reported from transposable elements in Drosophila to transgenic mice. This propensity for transgene silencing may in part result from the ability of heterochromatin to spread [32, 33]: vector silencing occurring as proviruses integrate within or near heterochromatin, or across differentiation as the genomic locus naturally becomes heterochromatinized with time.

In contrast to the enhancer-blocking insulators, much fewer barrier insulators have been reported in the literature, and less is known about their mechanisms of action [32, 33]. In the context of higher eukaryotes these elements appear to function at least in part by blocking heterochromatin spread mediated by methylation of lysine 9 on histone 3 (H3K9) and the subsequent recruitment of heterochromatin protein 1 (HP1) and other histone methyltransferases [32]. When histone acetyltransferases that competitively acetylate H3K9 are recruited, methylation is prevented at the said-site. Unlike CTCF-mediated enhancer-blocking insulators, barrier insulators may function locally, without involving higher-order chromatin structures [32, 40] which still is a matter of debate.

The prototypic insulator cHS4

Particular insulators are able to act both as enhancer-blocker and boundary, such as the well-characterized 1.2 kb fragment derived from the chicken β-globin DNase hypersensitive site-4 (cHS4)-containing insulator of the locus control region (LCR) of the chicken β-globin gene cluster [34, 41] (*Figure 2*). Initial studies with this element involved the use of a 1.2-kb fragment that contains the DNase hypersensitive site at its 5' end, and demonstrated its functionality by plasmid transfection in a murine erythroleukemia (MEL) cell line and transgenesis in Drosophila [42]. Later studies showed that the abovementioned dual activities are separable and map for their most part to distinct footprints contained within a 250-bp core fragment surrounding the DNase hypersensitive site [32, 34, 42].

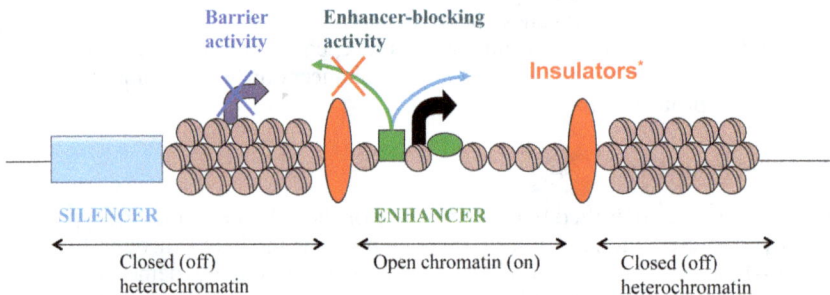

Figure 2. Insulators double function. Particular insulators harbour both an enhancer-blocking and a barrier function such as the DNase hypersensitive site-4 (cHS4)-containing insulator of the chicken β-globin gene cluster LCR [34, 41]. When placed as a pair of insulators (*pictured in red), which physically bracket the transgenic cassette, neither can the latter be silenced nor are neighbouring genes activated by the regulatory sequences shuttled by the integrating vector.

Insulated integrating gene transfer vectors

The addition of genetic insulator elements (GIE) in integrating vectors intended for gene therapy is an increasingly important avenue of research, with view to circumventing genotoxicity arising from insertional mutagenesis. Whilst the idea of insulating the vector and genome from each other so as to prevent regulatory cross talk has been known for sometime, suitable vectors have not yet been generated: therefore efficient and safe gene transfer vectors which would allow routine clinical use in human patients are still not readily available [38, 43].

When considering the mechanistic basis for insulators function, an enhancer blocking insulator must be physically located between the vector enhancer and cellular gene promoter in order to functionally separate the two; similarly, a barrier insulator must be placed between the vector expression cassette and the source of silencing heterochromatin. In the setting of an integrating gene transfer vector, it is likely that enhancer-blocking is best achieved when insulators are used in pairs each flanking the element to be insulated and physically bracket the latter, in order to separate the vector expression cassette from the surrounding genome, whether through the formation of a closed loop or by other proposed mechanisms [38]. Boundary insulators may also be used in 5' and 3' flanking pairs to secure that the progression of heterochromatin will be blocked from both sides of a transgene. Therefore genetic insulators should ideally bracket gene transfer vectors at both ends following integration. When considering the biology of retroviral vectors, this structure can be achieved when the insulator is cloned inside the 3'LTR (Long Terminal Repeat) in the plasmid construct. Upon replication and vector integration into the genome of the transduced target cell, the 3'LTR is copied to the 5'end which results in the integrated provirus insulated at both sides as represented in *Figure 3*.

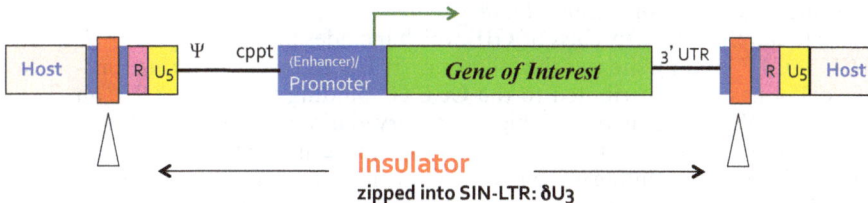

Figure 3. Structure of an insulated provirus, following integration of the retroviral vector into the host cell genome. An enhancer blocking insulator must sit in between the vector enhancer and cellular gene promoter in order to functionally separate the two; similarly, a barrier insulator must be placed between the vector expression cassette and the source of silencing heterochromatin. In the setting of an integrating gene transfer vector and considering the biology of retroviral vectors, this structure can be achieved when the insulator is cloned inside the 3'LTR in the plasmid construct.

Previous attempts to incorporate insulators in recombinant viral vectors intended for gene therapy were performed on gammaretroviral and lentiviral vectors mostly with the cHS4 insulator from chicken β-globin in various mouse and human cell types [44]; most studies lead to reduced transgene expression variegation and limited chromosomal position effect [45-49]. Implementation of the full-length 1200 bp element in gammaretroviral vectors was associated with reduced genotoxicity but also with important drop in titre of infectious particles, mainly due to the substantial size of this sequence

[43, 46, 50]. In addition, it has now been shown that the 1200 bp HS4 insulator is not genetically stable in retroviral constructs. A shorter sub-portion of the cHS4, namely the 250 bp long core sequence from this insulator was thought more suitable to fit viral vectors constraints as single or double copy cloned into the virus LTR [51], but it failed to reproduce the activity of the full-length element [22, 23, 48, 52]: when present in one or two copies it does not shield adjacent genomic neighbouring sequences against unwanted activation by the enhancer/promoter combination driving transgene expression [22, 48, 50]. In a more recent report [53], the use of core sequence dimers has also been shown to be associated with genetic instability.

There is thus a need to identify alternative sequences which: (i) harbour both properties of enhancer-blocking activity and a boundary effect, in order to also prevent silencing of the transgene; (ii) have no major effects upon virus biology and replication; (iii) remain genetically stable inside the vector at all steps following integration into the host cell genome in a sustained manner; genetic stability is essential including throughout proliferation and differentiation of gene-modified stem or progenitor cells. These considerations have formed the basis for our search towards novelty and improvement.

Previous attempts altogether have resulted in impaired vector production and/or poor insulating efficacy. In collaboration with Armelle Gaussin and Nicolas Mermod, we developed a quantitative procedure to screen insulator elements and to assess their ability to block gene activation by the strong Friend-murine leukemia virus enhancer-containing long terminal repeat (Fr-MuLV LTR). We designed novel synthetic elements acting as binding sites for CTCF and CTF/NF1 proteins which act as insulators, and mediate potent enhancer-blocking activities. Using different combinations of these elements we have established several new species of GIEs which have been shown to effectively insulate an exogenous gene in a quantitative assay from genomic regulatory interference, with both enhancer-blocking and boundary effects following integration of plasmid DNA [26].

The rationale to develop this new class of GIE which includes multiple copies of either a CTCF or CTF binding site was the following: (i) The enhancer-blocking function of the cHS4 has been attributed to the CCCTC-binding factor (CTCF), an eleven-zinc finger DNA-binding protein highly conserved in vertebrates. CTCF was implicated in diverse regulatory functions including transcriptional activation/repression, insulation and imprinting [40, 54]. CTCF organizes higher-order chromatin structures and was associated to the formation of chromatin loops that may mediate its enhancer-blocker function [55]. The boundary activity of the cHS4 element derives from the combined effect of the upstream transcription factors 1 and 2 (USF1 and USF2) [32]. In addition, the cHS4 insulator sequence was shown to be highly concentrated in the nuclear matrix fraction, suggesting that it may be involved in the topological organization of the genome [56]; (ii) CAAT box-binding transcription factor/Nuclear factor 1 (NF1, also called CTF/NF1) consists of a family of ubiquitous transcription factors that possess a barrier function [57, 58]. This family comprises NF1-A, NF1-B, NF1-C and NF1-X subtypes that share the same DNA binding domain [59, 60]. Of note, the NF1-C regulatory domain prevents transgene silencing at mammalian and yeast cells telomeres [57, 58]. NF1-C regulates DNA replication by promoting the recruitment of the DNA polymerase to the adenovirus and SV40 origins of replication, and is also involved in promoter regulation [61-63]. Thus, CTF/NF1 proteins were described as barrier elements [64, 65] that act to control DNA transcription and replication, yet a potential enhancer-blocking function had not been evidenced in previous reports.

Insulated retrovirus vectors using novel synthetic genetic insulator elements

Promising safety and efficacy improved vectors

In order to evaluate the potential of these GIEs in integrating gene transfer vectors intended for therapy, our team at ENSC has constructed SIN-insulated retrovectors with various copies of the two candidate GIEs which were compared to non-insulated SIN-LTRs counterparts. In particular, we have identified a specific combination of CTF-repeats, which has been generated through a recombination event and is genetically stable ([66], Duros *et al.*, in preparation,). When placed in the 3'SIN-LTR of both gammaretrovectors and lentivectors this insulator is functional and allows vector production at high titres. In target cells a homogenous and much less scattered expression profile is observed as compared to controls, the level of which is determined by the nature and strength of the internal promoter only. This specific GIE efficiently insulates the transgenic expression cassette, which as a result, operates autonomously from its *cis*-environment. Genotoxicity studies indicate a potentially reduced level of risk, based on both: (i) analysis of integration sites [67] and (ii) decreased tumour formation *in vivo* in cancer-prone mice as compared to genotoxic control vectors [68]. Data observed on cell-lines led us to perform experiments on human CD34+ haematopoietic cells from cord-blood: sustained expression was monitored both *in vitro* in long term liquid cultures over 10-12 weeks and *in vivo* in immunodeficient mice [65]. This holds interesting features for sustained genetic modification and expression in both HSCs and other types of stem cells with potential for clinical translation [see Bayart *et al.*, chapter A4-6, *ibid.*].

ACKNOWLEDGMENTS

This work has been performed with the support of the EC-DG research through the FP6-Network of Excellence, CLINIGENE: LSHB-CT-2006-018933. O.C.H. adresses special thanks to Emilie Bayart for critical reading of the manuscript and references.

REFERENCES

1. Hacein-Bey-Abina S, Garrigue A, Wang GP, Soulier J, Lim A, Morillon E, *et al.* Insertional onco-genesis in 4 patients after retrovirus-mediated gene therapy of SCID-X1. *J Clin Invest* 2008; 118: 3132-42.

2. Hacein-Bey-Abina S, Von Kalle C, Schmidt M, McCormack MP, Wulffraat N, Leboulch P, *et al.* LMO2-associated clonal T cell proliferation in two patients after gene therapy for SCID-X1. *Science* 2003; 302: 415-9.

3. Thrasher AJ, Gaspar HB, Baum C, Modlich U, Schambach A, Candotti F, *et al.* Gene therapy: X-SCID transgene leukaemogenicity. *Nature* 2006; 443: E5-6; discussion E6-7.

4. Ott MG, Schmidt M, Schwarzwaelder K, Stein S, Siler U, Koehl U, *et al.* Correction of X-linked chronic granulomatous disease by gene therapy, augmented by insertional activation of MDS1-EVI1, PRDM16 or SETBP1. *Nat Med* 2006; 12: 401-9.

5. Stein S, Ott MG, Schultze-Strasser S, Jauch A, Burwinkel B, Kinner A, *et al.* Genomic instability and myelodysplasia with monosomy 7 consequent to EVI1 activation after gene therapy for chronic granulomatous disease. *Nat Med* 2010; 16: 198-204.

6. Boztug K, Schmidt M, Schwarzer A, Banerjee PP, Diez IA, Dewey RA, *et al.* Stem-cell gene therapy for the Wiskott-Aldrich syndrome. *N Engl J Med* 2010; 363: 1918-27.

7. Modlich U, Navarro S, Zychlinski D, Maetzig T, Knoess S, Brugman MH, *et al*. Insertional trans-formation of hematopoietic cells by self-inactivating lentiviral and gammaretroviral vectors. *Mol Ther* 2009; 17: 1919-28.

8. Corrigan-Curay J, Cohen-Haguenauer O, O'Reilly M, Ross SR, Fan H, Rosenberg N, *et al*. Challenges in vector and trial design using retroviral vectors for long-term gene correction in hematopoietic stem cell gene therapy. *Mol Ther* 2012; 20: 1084-94.

9. Laufs S, Nagy KZ, Giordano FA, Hotz-Wagenblatt A, Zeller WJ, Fruehauf S. Insertion of retroviral vectors in NOD/SCID repopulating human peripheral blood progenitor cells occurs preferentially in the vicinity of transcription start regions and in introns. *Mol Ther* 2004; 10: 874-81.

10. Wu X, Li Y, Crise B, Burgess SM. Transcription start regions in the human genome are favored targets for MLV integration. *Science* 2003; 300: 1749-51.

11. Schroder AR, Shinn P, Chen H, Berry C, Ecker JR, Bushman F. HIV-1 integration in the human genome favors active genes and local hotspots. *Cell* 2002; 110: 521-9.

12. Ellis J. Silencing and variegation of gammaretrovirus and lentivirus vectors. *Hum Gene Ther* 2005; 16: 1241-6.

13. Emery DW, Aker M, Stamatoyannopoulos G. *Chromatin insulators and position effects, in gene transfer and expression in mammalian cells*. In: Makrides SC, ed. Norwood MA: EIC Laboratories Inc., 2003: 381-95.

14. Baum C, Kustikova O, Modlich U, Li Z, Fehse B. Mutagenesis and oncogenesis by chromosomal insertion of gene transfer vectors. *Hum Gene Ther* 2006; 17: 253-63.

15. Nienhuis AW, Dunbar CE, Sorrentino BP. Genotoxicity of retroviral integration in hematopoietic cells. *Mol Ther* 2006; 13: 1031-49.

16. Maruggi G, Porcellini S, Facchini G, Perna SK, Cattoglio C, Sartori D, *et al*. Transcriptional enhancers induce insertional gene deregulation independently from the vector type and design. *Mol Ther* 2009; 17: 851-6.

17. Dabrowska MJ, Dybkaer K, Johnsen HE, Wang B, Wabl M, Pedersen FS. Loss of MicroRNA targets in the 3' untranslated region as a mechanism of retroviral insertional activation of growth factor independence 1. *J Virol* 2009; 83: 8051-61.

18. Baum C, Schambach A, Bohne J, Galla M. Retrovirus vectors: toward the plentivirus? *Mol Ther* 2006; 13: 1050-63.

19. Chang AH, Sadelain M. The genetic engineering of hematopoietic stem cells: the rise of lentiviral vectors, the conundrum of the ltr, and the promise of lineage-restricted vectors. *Mol Ther* 2007; 15: 445-56.

20. Montini E, Cesana D, Schmidt M, Sanvito F, Ponzoni M, Bartholomae C, *et al*. Hematopoietic stem cell gene transfer in a tumor-prone mouse model uncovers low genotoxicity of lentiviral vector integration. *Nat Biotechnol* 2006; 24: 687-96.

21. Modlich U, Bohne J, Schmidt M, von Kalle C, Knoss S, Schambach A, Baum C. Cell-culture assays reveal the importance of retroviral vector design for insertional genotoxicity. *Blood* 2006; 108: 2545-53.

22. Arumugam PI, Urbinati F, Velu CS, Higashimoto T, Grimes HL, Malik P. The 3' region of the chicken hypersensitive site-4 insulator has properties similar to its core and is required for full insulator activity. *PLoS One* 2009; 4: e6995.

23. Zychlinski D, Schambach A, Modlich U, Maetzig T, Meyer J, Grassman E, Mishra A, Baum C. Physiological promoters reduce the genotoxic risk of integrating gene vectors. *Mol Ther* 2008; 16: 718-25.

24. Zaiss AK, Son S, Chang LJ. RNA 3' readthrough of oncoretrovirus and lentivirus: implications for vector safety and efficacy. *J Virol* 2002; 76: 7209-19.

25. Duros C, Artus A, Scholtz S. Insulated lentiviral vectors towards safer gene transfer to stem cells. *Mol Ther* 2011; 19: pS149.

26. Gaussin A, Modlich U, Bauche C, Niederlander NJ, Schambach A, Duros C, *et al.* CTF/NF1 transcription factors act as potent genetic insulators for integrating gene transfer vectors. *Gene Ther* 2012; 19: 15-24.

27. Marshall HM, Ronen K, Berry C, Llano M, Sutherland H, Saenz D, *et al.* Role of PSIP1/LEDGF/p75 in lentiviral infectivity and integration targeting. *PLoS One* 2007; 2: e1340.

28. Lombardo A, Cesana D, Genovese P, Di Stefano B, Provasi E, Colombo DF, *et al.* Site-specific integration and tailoring of cassette design for sustainable gene transfer. *Nat Methods* 2011; 8: 861-9.

29. Mates L, Chuah MK, Belay E, Jerchow B, Manoj N, Acosta-Sanchez A, *et al.* Molecular evolution of a novel hyperactive Sleeping Beauty transposase enables robust stable gene transfer in vertebrates. *Nat Genet* 2009; 41: 753-61.

30. Gentner B, Visigalli I, Hiramatsu H, Lechman E, Ungari S, Giustacchini A, *et al.* Identification of hematopoietic stem cell-specific miRNAs enables gene therapy of globoid cell leukodystrophy. *Sci Transl Med* 2010; 2: 58ra84.

31. Frecha C, Costa C, Negre D, Amirache F, Trono D, Rio P, *et al.* A novel lentiviral vector targets gene transfer into human hematopoietic stem cells in marrow from patients with bone marrow failure syndrome and *in vivo* in humanized mice. *Blood* 2012; 119: 1139-50.

32. Gaszner M, Felsenfeld G. Insulators: exploiting transcriptional and epigenetic mechanisms. *Nat Rev Genet* 2006; 7: 703-13.

33. Raab JR, Kamakaka RT. Insulators and promoters: closer than we think. *Nat Rev Genet* 2010; 11: 439-46.

34. West AG, Gaszner M, Felsenfeld G. Insulators: many functions, many mechanisms. *Genes Dev* 2002; 16: 271-88.

35. Bell AC, West AG, Felsenfeld G. Insulators and boundaries: versatile regulatory elements in the eukaryotic. *Science* 2001; 291: 447-50.

36. Gaussin A, Mermod N. Chromatin insulators and prospective application for gene therapy (review). *Gene Ther Rev* 2009; 1.

37. Sun FL, Elgin SC. Putting boundaries on silence. *Cell* 1999; 99: 459-62.

38. Emery DW. The use of chromatin insulators to improve the expression and safety of integrating gene transfer vectors. *Hum Gene Ther* 2011; 22: 761-74.

39. Mok HP, Javed S, Lever A. Stable gene expression occurs from a minority of integrated HIV-1-based vectors: transcriptional silencing is present in the majority. *Gene Ther* 2007; 14: 741-51.

40. Phillips JE, Corces VG. CTCF: master weaver of the genome. *Cell* 2009; 137: 1194-211.

41. Fourel G, Magdinier F, Gilson E. Insulator dynamics and the setting of chromatin domains. *Bioessays* 2004; 26: 523-32.

42. Chung JH, Bell AC, Felsenfeld G. Characterization of the chicken beta-globin insulator. *Proc Natl Acad Sci USA* 1997; 94: 575-80.

43. Li CL, Xiong D, Stamatoyannopoulos G, Emery DW. Genomic and functional assays demonstrate reduced gammaretroviral vector genotoxicity associated with use of the cHS4 chromatin insulator. *Mol Ther* 2009; 17: 716-24.

44. Bell AC, West AG, Felsenfeld G. The protein CTCF is required for the enhancer blocking activity of vertebrate insulators. *Cell* 1999; 98: 387-96.

45. Emery DW, Yannaki E, Tubb J, Nishino T, Li Q, Stamatoyannopoulos G. Development of virus vectors for gene therapy of beta chain hemoglobinopathies: flanking with a chromatin insulator reduces gamma-globin gene silencing *in vivo*. *Blood* 2002; 100: 2012-9.

46. Yannaki E, Tubb J, Aker M, Stamatoyannopoulos G, Emery DW. Topological constraints governing the use of the chicken HS4 chromatin insulator in oncoretrovirus vectors. *Mol Ther* 2002; 5: 589-98.

47. Yao S, Osborne CS, Bharadwaj RR, Pasceri P, Sukonnik T, Pannell D, *et al.* Retrovirus silencer blocking by the cHS4 insulator is CTCF independent. *Nucleic Acids Res* 2003; 31: 5317-23.

48. Aker M, Tubb J, Groth AC, Bukovsky AA, Bell AC, Felsenfeld G, *et al.* Extended core sequences from the cHS4 insulator are necessary for protecting retroviral vectors from silencing position effects. *Hum Gene Ther* 2007; 18: 333-43.

49. Nishino T, Tubb J, Emery DW. Partial correction of murine beta-thalassemia with a gammaretrovirus vector for human gamma-globin. *Blood Cells Mol Dis* 2006; 37: 1-7.

50. Urbinati F, Arumugam P, Higashimoto T, Perumbeti A, Mitts K, Xia P, Malik P. Mechanism of reduction in titers from lentivirus vectors carrying large inserts in the 3'LTR. *Mol Ther* 2009; 17: 1527-36.

51. Ye X, Liang M, Meng X, Ren X, Chen H, Li ZY, *et al.* Insulation from viral transcriptional regulatory elements enables improvement to hepatoma-specific gene expression from adenovirus vectors. *Biochem Biophys Res Commun* 2003; 307: 759-64.

52. Modin C, Pedersen FS, Duch M. Lack of shielding of primer binding site silencer-mediated repression of an internal promoter in a retrovirus vector by the putative insulators scs, BEAD-1, and HS4. *J Virol* 2000; 74: 11697-707.

53. Cavazzana-Calvo M, Payen E, Negre O, Wang G, Hehir K, Fusil F, *et al.* Transfusion independence and HMGA2 activation after gene therapy of human beta-thalassaemia. *Nature* 2010; 467: 318-22.

54. Kim TH, Abdullaev ZK, Smith AD, Ching KA, Loukinov DI, Green RD, *et al.* Analysis of the vertebrate insulator protein CTCF-binding sites in the human genome. *Cell* 2007; 128: 1231-45.

55. Splinter E, Heath H, Kooren J, Palstra RJ, Klous P, Grosveld F, Galjart N, de Laat W. CTCF mediates long-range chromatin looping and local histone modification in the beta-globin locus. *Genes Dev* 2006; 20: 2349-54.

56. Yusufzai TM, Felsenfeld G. The 5'-HS4 chicken beta-globin insulator is a CTCF-dependent nuclear matrix-associated element. *Proc Natl Acad Sci USA* 2004; 101: 8620-4.

57. Pankiewicz R, Karlen Y, Imhof MO, Mermod N. Reversal of the silencing of tetracycline-controlled genes requires the coordinate action of distinctly acting transcription factors. *J Gene Med* 2005; 7: 117-32.

58. Ferrari S, Simmen KC, Dusserre Y, Muller K, Fourel G, Gilson E, Mermod N. Chromatin domain boundaries delimited by a histone-binding protein in yeast. *J Biol Chem* 2004; 279: 55520-30.

59. Rupp RA, Kruse U, Multhaup G, Gobel U, Beyreuther K, Sippel AE. Chicken NFI/TGGCA proteins are encoded by at least three independent genes: NFI-A, NFI-B and NFI-C with homologues in mammalian genomes. *Nucleic Acids Res* 1990; 18: 2607-16.

60. Kruse U, Qian F, Sippel AE. Identification of a fourth nuclear factor I gene in chicken by cDNA cloning: NFI-X. *Nucleic Acids Res* 1991; 19: 6641.

61. Cohen RB, Sheffery M, Kim CG. Partial purification of a nuclear protein that binds to the CCAAT box of the mouse alpha 1-globin gene. *Mol Cell Biol* 1986; 6: 821-32.

62. Alevizopoulos A, Mermod N. Antagonistic regulation of a proline-rich transcription factor by transforming growth factor beta and tumor necrosis factor alpha. *J Biol Chem* 1996; 271: 29672-81.

63. Muller K, Mermod N. The histone-interacting domain of nuclear factor I activates simian virus 40 DNA replication *in vivo. J Biol Chem* 2000; 275: 1645-50.

64. Esnault G, Majocchi S, Martinet D, Besuchet-Schmutz N, Beckmann JS, Mermod N. Transcription factor CTF1 acts as a chromatin domain boundary that shields human telomeric genes from silencing. *Mol Cell Biol* 2009; 29: 2409-18.

65. Ito M, Hiramatsu H, Kobayashi K, Suzue K, Kawahata M, Hioki K, *et al*. NOD/SCID/gamma(c) (null) mouse: an excellent recipient mouse model for engraftment of human cells. *Blood* 2002; 100: 3175-82.

66. Cohen-Haguenauer O, Auclair C. *Gene transfer vectors comprising genetic insulator elements and methods to identify genetic insulator elements*. IB 2010/000950-PTC Avril 2010: USA, Europe.

67. Gabriel R, Eckenberg R, Paruzynski A, Bartholomae CC, Nowrouzi A, Arens A, *et al*. Comprehensive genomic access to vector integration in clinical gene therapy. *Nat Med* 2009; 15: 1431-6.

68. Montini E, Cesana D, Schmidt M, Sanvito F, Bartholomae CC, Ranzani M, *et al*. The genotoxic potential of retroviral vectors is strongly modulated by vector design and integration site selection in a mouse model of HSC gene therapy. *J Clin Invest* 2009; 119: 964-75.

The CliniBook: Clinical gene transfer
Edited by Odile Cohen-Haguenauer – EDK, Paris © 2012, pp. 150-155

A3-5
Facing the challenges of downstream processing of lentiviral vectors

Vanessa Bandeira[1], Cristina Peixoto[1], Ana Sofia Coroadinha[1], Pedro E. Cruz[1,2]*,
Manuel J.T. Carrondo[1], Otto-Wilhelm Merten[3], Paula Marques Alves[1,4]

*[1]IBET, Apartado 12, 2781-901 Oeiras, Portugal; [2]ECBio S.A, 2700-451 Amadora,
Portugal; [3]Généthon, F-91002 Évry-Cedex, France; [4]ITQB-UNL, Apartado 12, 2781-901
Oeiras, Portugal.*
pcruz@itqb.unl.pt
* Corresponding author

OVERVIEW

Lentiviral vectors (LVs) hold great potential in gene therapy due to their ability to
transduce both dividing and nondividing cells and their capacity to sustain long-term
transgene expression in several target cells [1]. Therefore, upscaling of these vectors
production, concentration and purification is necessary for their application in clinical
trials. Integration of membrane and chromatographic processes in downstream processing (DSP) performed in the scope of Clinigene Network allowed further improvements in large-scale production and purification of LV supernatants. An overview of
the major developments in LVs purification is herein summarized.

INTRODUCTION

Worldwide, more than 40 clinical trials are currently investigating the use of LVs for
gene delivery (http://www.wiley.com/legacy/wileychi/genmed/clinical). With this increasing use, scalable, effective and more robust LV production processes are of critical
importance. Although several stable recombinant HIV producer cell lines have already
been described [2, 3], the produced LVs are still very unstable and exhibit low titers
partially due to the fragility of the lipid membrane layer that harbors envelope glycoproteins (Env). For this reason, transient transfection approaches continue to be employed using, generally, 293T cells because of their higher productivities of LVs. Also,
several envelope glycoproteins can be used to pseudotype the viral particles produced.
The most common used is the glycoprotein from the vesicular-stomatitis virus, because
of its broad tropism, its resistance to freeze-thawing and stability to withstand concentration or purification methods [4-6].
Despite the significant progress, high quality of LV preparations with high titers is still
difficult and costly to be achieved [7]. For this reason, scalable, disposable and cost-effective technologies, involving microfiltration, anion-exchange chromatography

(AEXc) and ultrafiltration are in the front line techniques for the development of optimized purification processes for LVs, appearing as alternatives to the traditional ultracentrifugation methods and fixed bed column chromatography methodologies for gene therapy applications.

BOTTLENECKS AND CHALLENGES IN DSP OF LVS

There are several bottlenecks and challenges in the purification process of LVs. The physical-chemical properties of viral vectors and the need to maintain viral activity throughout the purification process is one of the many challenges. DSP of lentiviral vectors, especially for clinical applications, comprises a series of steps aiming to increase the potency, purity and quality of the final vector preparation, with a need for a stepwise optimization [8].

Stability of LVs

The half-life of LVs range from 5-8 hours in the cell culture supernatant [9, 10], due to their labile nature, affecting not only the titers but also the quality and efficacy of vector preparations. However, improvements to more than 100 hours have been reported [10] if DSP is performed at lower temperatures (4°C). Besides temperature, enveloped viruses are also sensible to acidic or basic pH [11], and to high salt concentrations [12]. Storage temperature is also determinant, so temperatures of -85°C should be used and freeze-thaw cycles should be avoided since it decreases the infectious titers of the viral vector samples [9]. Formulation studies performed in our laboratory showed that the combined use of lipoproteins and recombinant human serum albumin considerably improves stability of LVs at 4° and 37°C [13].

Downstream processing optimization

The main challenge facing researchers working in DSP of viral vectors is how to separate the functional viral particles from the contaminating non-functional particles, like empty capsids, and from cell membrane vesicles since, given their structure similarity, they are very difficult to separate using currently described purification procedures [8].

Current viral purification strategies mostly rely on the integration of membrane and chromatographic processes. For clarification of the LV-containing supernatant, microfiltration is the most popular technique used nowadays since centrifugation has many disadvantages (scale limitations, low efficiency in the removal of cellular debris, concentrating materials that can be toxic to target cells, and difficult to put into an GMP environment) [14, 15]. However, microfiltration also has some drawbacks because the membranes can often become obstructed by cells, and the application of high pressures to the membrane can cause losses of viral vector infectivity [16, 17]. Improved clarification systems using step filtration with decreasing pore size filters [16] may decrease these viral vector losses.

Purification techniques that remove contaminating proteins and DNA from LV-containing supernatants are achieved using several chromatographic methods, such as heparin affinity [12], gel filtration [6] and anion-exchange (AEX) chromatography (c) [18, 19]. In our lab, AEXc had already proven to be a good candidate for purification of retroviral vectors showing recovery yields of around 50% and DNA impurities removals of 90% [18].

Currently available chromatographic matrices have pore dimensions that exclude viruses, suggesting that their adsorption is restricted to the bead surface area resulting in low binding capacities [20]. This problem can be circumvented by tentacle supports, membrane chromatography and more recently by monolithic devices [21] (due to their advantages: high capacity regardless of the flow rate and size classes of the molecules they separate; mass transport by convection and low-shear fractionation environment [22, 23]).

As LVs are negatively charged, anion-exchangers bearing positively charged ligands are used for the purification of these vectors [15]. Recently, we evaluated the perform-ance of two different membrane capture matrices (Sartobind and CIM, containing DEAE ligands) [24] for baculovirus removal from lentiviral bulk and obtained an over-all higher recovery yield of 65% for CIM matrix with a 95% removal of host cell dsDNA.

Filtration approaches such as membrane ultrafiltration/diafiltration (UF/DF) are well suited and have been currently used for concentration, buffer-exchange and partial pu-rification of LVs, with 30 to 40-fold concentration factors having been reported [5]. In our experiments, we saw that tangential flow filtration (TFF) has several advantages, since it can process smaller to very large volumes in shorter times and can be used as disposable material thus facilitating GMP operations [25].

Depending on the size of the molecule to be concentrated, the molecular weight cut off (MWCO) of the membrane device has to be chosen. Since the lentiviral particle has a size ranging from 80 to 120 µm, membranes of choice need to have a pore size below this value. Thus, MWCO filters of up to 750 kDa have been tested. Membrane geometries where the retentate flows tangentially to the membrane, like hollow-fibers or flat-sheet cassettes, have been selected due to the reduced fouling under mild oper-ational conditions, allowing high permeate fluxes while maintaining viral infectivity [26]. Use of membranes with larger MWCO (500-750 kDa) allows removal of both larger MW proteins while permitting higher permeate fluxes, better purification and shorter process times [27].

A suitable downstream process backbone was also established at IBET by integration of operation units, such as clarification and ultrafiltration before intermediate purifi-cation using convective flow devices, and average yields of 44% were obtained [28].

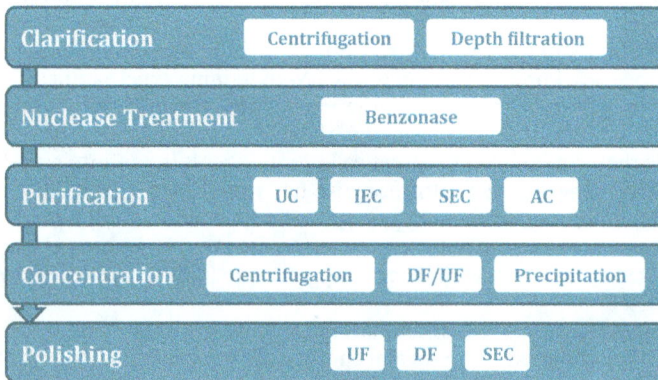

Figure 1. Overview of a general downstream purification process for LVs. UC, ultracentrifugation; IEC, ion-exchange chromatography; SEC, size-exclusion chromatography; AC, affinity chromatog-raphy; DF/UF, diafiltration/ultrafiltration.

FUTURE PERSPECTIVES

From the methods described above and taking the options for the selection of chromatography materials, *Figure 1* outlines general purification schemes for lentiviral vectors, with examples of the techniques that can be used for each step of the process. Techniques like ultracentrifugation-based methods are more suitable for laboratory scale productions. However, for large-scale purification approaches, scalable technologies, like membrane filtration and AEXc, are preferred.

Considerable progress has been achieved in the large scale manufacturing of lentiviral vectors using transient transfection methods. However, this transfection system turns out to be the main contribution of DNA impurities to the LV bulk. For this reason, advances in the field of stable producer cells will pave the way for a more efficient and safer manufacturing of large scale quantities of LVs. Also, the use of bioreactor systems and production in serum-free suspension cultures would help in the scale-up of more pure LV samples.

There is still room for improvement of each one of the purification steps of the process, especially at the capture step using AEXc, since it is not difficult to anticipate that a sensible selection of binding conditions (pH and ionic strength) should result in process performance improvements. Efficient digestion of the DNA impurities usually present in purified samples has also been described for lentiviral vector purification with the use of benzonase [7, 29] and is today used in large scale manufacturing processes despite its relatively elevated costs.

Theoretical models for DSP of LVs could also be generated, like was established in the case of baculoviruses [30], with view to serving as a useful prediction tool to determine how conditions can be altered to further improve process resolution/selectivity which will ultimately enhance final product purity and recovery yield. With this accomplishment, knowledge-based strategies could become relevant tools in streamlining the design and optimization of such purification steps.

The latest improvements in DSP protocols performed during the Clinigene Network are easy to implement and facilitate high titer LV productions at a large scale for clinical studies, by avoiding non-scalable ultracentrifugation methods.

ACKNOWLEDGMENTS

This work has been performed with the support of the EC-DG research through the FP6-Network of Excellence, CLINIGENE: LSHB-CT-2006-018933.

REFERENCES

1. Naldini L, Blomer U, Gallay P *et al*. *In vivo* gene delivery and stable transduction of nondividing cells by a lentiviral vector. *Science* 1996; 272: 263-67.

2. Ikeda Y, Takeuchi Y, Martin F, *et al*. Continuous high-titer HIV-1 vector production. *Nat Biotechnol* 2003; 21: 569-72.

3. Xu K, Ma H, McCown TJ, *et al*. Generation of a stable cell line producing high-titer self-inactivating lentiviral vectors. *Mol Ther* 2001; 3: 97-104.

4. Burns, JC, Friedmann T, Driever W, *et al*. Vesicular stomatitis virus G glycoprotein pseudotyped retroviral vectors: concentration to very high titer and efficient gene transfer into mammalian and nonmammalian cells. *Proc Natl Acad Sci USA* 1993; 90: 8033-7.

5. Slepushkin V, Chang N, Cohen R, *et al*. Large-scale purification of a lentiviral vector by size exclusion chromatography or Mustang Q ion exchange capsule. *Bioprocess J* 2003; 2: 89-95.

6. Transfiguracion J, Jaalouk DE, Ghani K, *et al*. Size-exclusion chromatography purification of high-titer vesicular stomatitis virus G glycoprotein-pseudotyped retrovectors for cell and gene therapy applications. *Hum Gene Ther* 2003; 14 : 1139-53.

7. Merten OW, Charrier S, Laroudie N, *et al*. Large-scale manufacture and characterization of a lentiviral vector produced for clinical *ex vivo* gene therapy application. *Hum Gene Ther* 2011; 22: 343-56.

8. Segura MM, Kamen AA, Garnier A. Overview of current scalable methods for purification of viral vectors. *Viral Vectors Gene Ther* 2011; 737: 89-116.

9. Higashikawa F, Chang L. Kinetic analyses of stability of simple and complex retroviral vectors. *Virology* 2001; 280: 124-31.

10. Beer C, Meyer A, Muller K, Wirth M. The temperature stability of mouse retroviruses depends on the cholesterol levels of viral lipid shell and cellular plasma membrane. *Virology* 2003; 308: 137-46.

11. Ye K, Dhiman HK, Suhan J, Schultz JS. Effect of pH on infectivity and morphology of ecotropic moloney murine leukemia virus. *Biotechnol Prog* 2003; 19: 538-43.

12. Segura MM, Kamen A, Trudel P, Garnier A. A novel purification strategy for retrovirus gene therapy vectors using heparin affinity chromatography. *Biotechnol Bioeng* 2005; 90: 391-404.

13. Carmo M, Alves A, Rodrigues AF, *et al*. Stabilization of gammaretroviral and lentiviral vectors: from production to gene transfer. *J Gene Med* 2009; 11: 670-8.

14. Reiser J. Production and concentration of pseudotyped HIV-1-based gene transfer vectors. *Gene Ther* 2000; 7: 910-3.

15. Schweizer M, Merten OW. Large-scale production means for the manufacturing of lentiviral vectors. *Curr Gene Ther* 2010; 10: 474-86.

16. Reeves L, Cornetta K. Clinical retroviral vector production: step filtration using clinically approved filters improves titers. *Gene Ther* 2000; 7: 1993-8.

17. Cruz PE, Gonçalves D, Almeida J, Moreira JL, Carrondo MJT. Modeling retrovirus production for gene therapy. 2. Integrated optimization of bioreaction and downstream processing. *Biotechnol Prog* 2000; 16: 350-7.

18. Rodrigues T, Carvalho A, Alves PM, Cruz PE. Screening anion-exchange chromatographic matrices for isolation of onco-retroviral vectors. *J Chromatogr B Analytic Technol Biomed Life Sci* 2006; 837: 59-68.

19. Yamada K, McCarty DM, Madden VJ, Walsh CE. Lentivirus vector purification using anion exchange HPLC leads to improved gene transfer. *Biotechniques* 2003; 34: 1074-8.

20. Vicente T, Peixoto C, Mota JPB, *et al*. Optimizing downstream processing of enveloped viruses. *Genetic Engineering Biotechnology News-BioProcess Tutorial* 2011; 31 (2).

21. Segura MM, Kamen A, Garnier A. Downstream processing of oncoretroviral and lentiviral gene therapy vectors. *Biotechnol Adv* 2006; 24: 321-37.

22. Gagnon P. Monoliths open the door to key growth sectors. *BioProc Int* 2010; 8: 20-3.

23. Zhou JX, Tressel T. Basic concepts in Q membrane chromatography for large-scale antibody production. *Biotechnol Prog* 2006; 22: 341-9.

24. Lesch HP, Laitinen A, Peixoto C, *et al*. Production and purification of lentiviral vectors generated in 293T suspension cells with baculoviral vectors. *Gene Ther* 2011; 18: 531-8.

25. Vicente T, Peixoto C, Carrondo MJT, Alves PM. Purification of recombinant baculoviruses for gene therapy using membrane processes. *Gene Ther* 2009; 16: 766-75.

26. Rodrigues T, Carrondo MJT, Alves PM, Cruz PE. Purification of retroviral vectors for clinical application: biological implications and technological challenges. *J Biotechnol* 2007; 127: 520-41.

27. Le Doux JM, Morgan JR, Yarmush ML. Removal of proteoglycans increases efficiency of retroviral gene transfer. *Biotechnol Bioeng* 1998; 58: 23-34.

28. Bandeira V, Peixoto C, Rodrigues AF, *et al.* Downstream processing of lentiviral vectors: releasing bottlenecks (paper in preparation).

29. Sastry L, Xu Y, Cooper R, Pollok K, Cornetta K. Evaluation of plasmid DNA removal from lentiviral vectors by benzonase treatment. *Hum Gene Ther* 2004; 15: 221-6.

30. Vicente T, Fáber R, Alves PM, *et al.* Impact of ligand density on the optimization of ion-exchange membrane chromatography for viral vector purification. *Biotechnol Bioeng* 2011; 108: 1347-59.

The CliniBook: Clinical gene transfer
Edited by Odile Cohen-Haguenauer – EDK, Paris © 2012, pp. 156-159

A3-6
Restrictions and requirements for stable lentiviral vector production in HEK293 cells

Leonor Gama-Norton[1,2], Hansjörg Hauser[1], Dagmar Wirth[1]*

[1]*Helmholtz-Zentrum für Infektionsforschung, Inhoffenstr. 7, D-38124, Braunschweig, Germany;* [2]*Instituto de Biologia Experimental e Tecnológica, Universidade Nova de Lisboa (IBET/ITQB/UNL), Oeiras, Portugal.*
dagmar.wirth@helmholtz-hzi.de
Corresponding author

HIV-based lentiviral vectors are efficient tools for stable genetic modification of cells, both for research and for clinical applications. Currently, production of lentiviral vectors is based on transient transfection protocols in 293T cells, a SV40 (T-Ag) transfected HEK293 cell line. For gene therapy applications, this protocol has two limitations: First, the transient production protocol as such cannot exclude the accidental formation of recombined vectors with altered properties; methods to detect such rare virus-derived entities are not sensitive enough. Second, the nature of the producer cell line and in particular the expression of T-Ag raises concerns with respect to safety. A clear improvement of safety conditions for gene therapy applications requires lentiviral vector production from a well characterized, stable and safe producer cell line.

Indeed, such conditions have already been achieved for production of therapeutic γ-retrovirus vectors. Well characterized γ-retrovirus producer cell lines are available that include stably integrated helper genes as well as the therapeutic vector. Moreover, the targeting of therapeutic vectors into defined genomic sites can predict the structure of the packaged RNA and exclude the generation and transfer of harmful RNAs that would arise from readthrough of viral vector transcripts into cellular genes with oncogenic potential [1-3]. In addition, this technology allows to evaluate and optimize viral vectors to the specific requirements of the given integration site [3]. Conceptually, safe *i.e.*, defined and genetically stable production systems for γ-retroviral and lentiviral vectors would profit from a single vector copy integrated into the producer cell genome.

While several γ-retroviral packaging cells are available, the experience of the last decades shows that the construction of lentiviral packaging cells is not straight forward. Due to the cytotoxic properties of helper proteins such as protease, Rev and VSV-G envelope, one of the major obstacles to the successful generation of a stable packaging cell line is the need for controlled expression systems that allow accurate adjustment of protein expression. Exploitation of novel gene switcher systems [4] or strategies that circumvent or reduce the need for gene regulation [5] resulted in the generation of lentiviral helper cell lines with reasonable stability and titer. So far, the copy number of the therapeutic vector has not been considered. Protocols used in these studies commonly allow integration of increased numbers of integrated vector copies. For example, satisfactory titers were achieved upon introduction of hundreds of concatemerized lentiviral vector copies into the cellular genome [6, 10].

INTEGRATION OF SINGLE COPY LENTIVIRAL VECTORS IN CHROMOSOMAL SITES

Within the Clinigene program, we investigated if single copy integration of lentiviral vectors can provide titers sufficient for production processes. We applied various strategies to identify single chromosomal sites supporting high titer virus production of lentiviral vectors. These strategies were designed to ensure high transcription rates resulting in sufficient amounts of viral RNA. This included both conventional SIN-lentiviral vectors and a Tat-dependent non-SIN lentiviral vector. Also, to exclude any bias from the gene transfer method, both plasmid transfection and lentiviral transduction of screening vectors were applied.

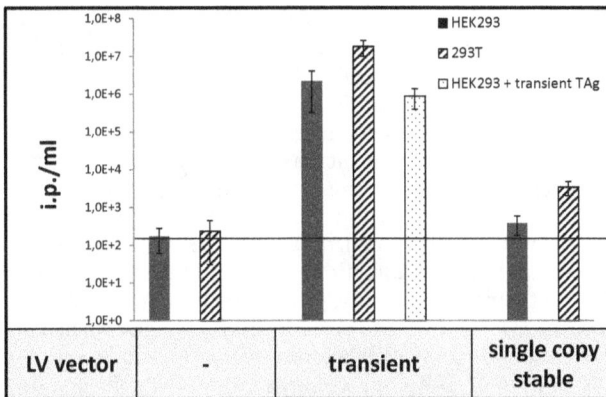

Figure 1. Summary of lentiviral vector production from HEK293 cells and 293T cells. HEK293 and 293T derived cell lines were analyzed for their capacity to produce lentiviral infectious particles. The impact of the state of the lentiviral vector was evaluated.

LV vector transient:
In this experiment HEK293 cells (black) and 293 T cells (hatched) were (transiently) co-transfected with the lentiviral vector and the helper functions (gagpol, rev and VSV-G); this represents the classical virus production procedure. The stippled bar represents the titer obtained upon co-transfection of the helper function, the lentiviral vector and SV40 T-antigen. The arrow bars represent the mean of four independent transient transfection assays.

LV vector stable:
Virus production was evaluated from HEK293 and 293T cells into which single copies of lentiviral vector genomes have previously been integrated. The virus production capacity of these individual clones was determined upon transient transfection of the helper functions (gagpol, rev and VSV-G). The mean titer and the variation is given from more than 40 individual clones of single copy HEK293 and 293T cells, respectively.

More than 60 individual HEK293 chromosomal sites with a single copy integration of a given lentiviral vector have been evaluated for virus production in this study. However, among these cell clones not a single clone was able to produce more than 10^3 infectious lentiviral particles per ml (*Figure 1*, "single copy stable", black bar; see [7]). We also evaluated the efficiency of lentiviral vector expression in two chromosomal loci in HEK293 cells that were previously identified for their capacity to support high titer retroviral expression [2, 3]. For this purpose, the retroviral tagging vector was exchanged for the lentiviral cassette by means of recombinase mediated cassette exchange, RMCE [8]. However, while high level expression of the internal promoter could be confirmed, lentiviral particle production upon transient transfer of the helper plasmids was in the same range as reported for the randomly integrated vectors [7]. Thus, we conclude that lentiviral vectors both after random chromosomal integration and after targeting into established high expression sites for γ-retrovectors do not support high titer vector production.

THE PRODUCTION OF LENTIVIRAL VECTORS FROM SINGLE COPY INTEGRATION SITES IS ENHANCED IN SV40 T-AG TRANSFECTED CELLS

The standard cell line for production of lentiviral vectors is 293T. These cells have been derived from HEK293 cells upon stable integration of SV40 T-Ag and allow high titer production of lentiviral vectors in transient production protocols. We evaluated the impact of SV40 T-Ag expression for production of episomal (*i.e.* transiently transfected) and stably integrated lentiviral vectors. For this purpose, we first compared virus production upon transient transfection of 293T cells and 293 cells. Indeed, we could confirm that 293T cells allow a 10 fold higher production of viral vectors if compared to HEK293 cells (*Figure 1*; "transient"). Thus, we investigated if virus production from integrated lentiviral vectors would be similarly increased. According to the strategy described above, single copy lentiviral vectors were integrated at random chromosomal sites in 293T cells. Transduced cell clones, harbouring one or few copies of the lentiviral vector were identified on the basis of GFP reporter gene expression. More than 40 independent cell clones were analysed for infectious virus production upon transient transfection of the helper functions. Importantly, production of lentiviral vectors upon chromosomal integration in 293T was found to be about 10-fold higher when compared to titers obtained from corresponding HEK293 clones (*Figure 1*, "single copy stable"). This suggests that the expression of T-Ag in these cells improves the formation of infectious lentivirus particles from integrated vector copies to a certain extent.

T-Ag has been shown to be a pleiotropic protein that interacts with many cellular proteins [9] and deregulates about 5% of cellular genes [10]. Moreover, T-Ag is known to exert non-reversible effects, often as a result of increased genome instability but possibly also by other mechanisms. We tried to enlighten the mechanism by which T-Ag improves virus production. We investigated if transient transfection of T-Ag would be sufficient to improve virus production from 293 cells. Interestingly, upon transient co-transfection of the lentiviral vectors together with T-Ag in HEK293 cells, we could not increase virus titers (*Figure 1*; "transient"). This indicates that the increase of virus titers is not directly mediated by T-Ag protein. Rather, it suggests that an indirect effect of T-Ag might be responsible. Interestingly, a comparable increase in expression from integrated lentiviral vectors was observed upon stable expression of the ras oncogene (not shown). This suggests that the increase of virus production is an indirect effect triggered by both ras or SV40 T-Ag.

We anticipate that global effects are triggered by T-Ag and ras expression and are necessary to convert a non-productive cell system towards a cell with capacity for lentiviral production. We hypothesize that pleiotropic effects are achieved upon long term expression of these oncogenes and are necessary to promote lentiviral production from a single integrated copy of the viral genome. The notion that only multi-copy integrants lead to higher lentiviral titers has been implied in several reports *e.g.* [6, 10]. It remains to be elucidated if higher titers achieved upon multi-copy integration are due to the increased number of vector genomes transcribed. This approach might augment the chances of hitting a rare chromosomal locus that supports high levels of lentiviral genome expression *per se* or by another not anticipated scenario.

Data presented here point towards the need for multiple copy integration of lentiviral vectors in order to bypass a still non-defined bottleneck for lentiviral vector generation imposed by the producer cell. The observation that both T-Ag and ras expression improve this blockade potentially opens a way to overcome this bottleneck. Strategies based on non-oncogenic approaches instead of T-Ag and ras should preferably be followed to achieve significant improvement of lentivector production.

ACKNOWLEDGMENTS

This work has been performed with the support of the EC-DG research through the FP6-Network of Excellence, CLINIGENE: LSHB-CT-2006-018933.

REFERENCES

1. Schucht R, Coroadinha AS, Zanta-Boussif MA, Verhoeyen E, Carrondo MJ, Hauser H, Wirth D. A new generation of retroviral producer cells: predictable and stable virus production by Flp-mediated site-specific integration of retroviral vectors. *Mol Ther* 2009; 14: 285-92.

2. Coroadinha AS, Schucht R, Gama-Norton L, Wirth D, Hauser H, Carrondo MJ. The use of recombinase mediated cassette exchange in retroviral vector producer cell lines: predictability and efficiency by transgene exchange. *J Biotechnol* 2006; 124: 457-68.

3. Gama-Norton L, Herrmann S, Schucht R, Coroadinha AS, Low R, Alves P, *et al.* Retroviral vector performance upon integration in to defined chromosomal loci of modular packaging cell lines. *Hum Gene Ther* 2010; 21: 979-91.

4. Broussau S, Jabbour N, Lachapelle G, Durocher Y, Tom R, Transfiguracion J, *et al.* Inducible packaging cells for large-scale production of lentiviral vectors in serum-free suspension culture. *Mol Ther* 2008; 16: 500-7.

5. Ikeda Y, Takeuchi Y, Martin F, Cosset FL, Mitrophanous K, Collins M. Continuous high-titer HIV-1 vector production. *Nat Biotechnol* 2003; 21: 569-72.

6. Wirth D, Gama-Norton L, Riemer P, Sandhu U, Schucht R, Hauser H. Road to precision: recombinase-based targeting technologies for genome engineering. *Curr Opin Biotechnol* 2007; 18: 411-9.

7. Gama-Norton L, Botezatu L, Herrmann S, Schweizer M, Alves PM, Hauser H, Wirth D. Lentivirus production is influenced by SV40 large T antigen and chromosomal integration of the vector in HEK293 cells. *Hum Gene Ther* 2012 (in press).

8. Ahuja D, Saenz-Robles MT, Pipas JM. SV40 large T antigen targets multiple cellular pathways to elicit cellular transformation. *Oncogene* 2005; 24: 7729-45.

9. May T, Hauser H, Wirth D. Transcriptional control of SV40 T-antigen expression allows a complete reversion of immortalization. *Nucleic Acids Res* 2004; 32: 5529-38.

10. Throm RE, Ouma AA, Zhou S, Chandrasekaran A, Lockey T, Greene M, *et al.* Efficient construction of producer cell lines for a sin lentiviral vector for SCID-X1 gene therapy by concatemeric array transfection. *Blood* 2009; 113: 5104-10.

The CliniBook: Clinical gene transfer
Edited by Odile Cohen-Haguenauer – EDK, Paris © 2012, pp. 160-181

A3-7
Novel lentiviral vector pseudotypes for stable gene transfer into resting hematopoietic cells

ELS VERHOEYEN*, FRANÇOIS-LOÏC COSSET

Université de Lyon, F69007; Inserm, EVIR, U758, Human Virology Department, F-69007; École Normale Supérieure de Lyon, F-69007; Université Lyon 1, F-69007, Lyon, France.
els.verhoeyen@ens-lyon.fr
* Corresponding author

INTRODUCTION

It is now clear that lentiviral vectors can transduce many non-dividing cell types. However, some important gene therapy target cells such as T and B cells and hematopoietic stem cells (HSCs), which are for the vast majority resting cells *in vivo* are not efficiently transduced by classical lentiviral vectors pseudotyped with the vesicular stomatitis virus G (VSV-G) protein, although this envelope glycoprotein confers a large tropism to these vectors. The last years, though, the field has moved forward and new transduction protocols, as also new lentiviral vector pseudotypes have been developed that now allow very efficient transduction of these resting hematopoietic cells. Here, we report on the importance of gene transfer into these resting cells for gene therapy and the new tools and protocols developed that allow efficient lentiviral mediated gene transfer into resting T and B lymphocytes and HSCs.

LENTIVIRAL VECTOR-MEDIATED TRANSDUCTION OF RESTING T AND B LYMPHOCYTES

T and B lymphocytes are important gene therapy target cells

T cells as targets for gene therapy and immunotherapy
One of the major advantages of using peripheral blood T cells is that they are more easily accessible for genetic modification than other targets such as HSCs. Moreover, they can be isolated in high amounts. T cells most likely have a lower risk of transformation, as up to now a leukaemia was not observed in T cell-based gene therapies [1-4]. Recently, it was also shown that retroviral vector integration deregulates gene expression in T cells to some extent. But this had no consequences on the function and biology of the transplanted T cells [5]. Of importance, the naive T-cell subset, which

responds to a novel antigen, has a long-term life span and persists over years in the patients so at least a long term-correction can be envisaged by T-cell gene therapy. Moreover, gene transfer into T cells enormously improved in the last years thanks to the engineering of new gene transfer vehicles, the lentiviral vectors (LVs). These new vehicles enable to obtain highly efficient T cell transduction without changing neither their phenotype nor their functional characteristics.

Gene transfer into T lymphocytes may allow the treatment of several genetic dysfunctions of the hematopoietic system, such as severe combined immunodeficiency [1, 2], and the development of novel therapeutic strategies for diseases such as cancers and for acquired diseases such as AIDS [6].

ADA deficient SCID was the first inherited disease investigated for T cell gene therapy because of a postulated survival advantage for gene corrected T lymphocytes. Indeed, in an allogenic BM transplantation normal ADA expressing T lymphocytes have a selective advantage in SCID patients and develop a protective immune system of donor-derived T lymphocytes [7-9]. Aiuti *et al.* showed immune reconstitution in ADA-SCID patients after T-cell gene therapy [10]. Patients received multiple infusions of autologous retroviral vector transduced peripheral blood lymphocytes (PBLs). Discontinuation of ADA replacement therapy led then to a selective growth of the infused ADA expressing lymphocytes, which eventually replaced the non-transduced T-cell population up to nearly 100%. These ADA corrected T cells were capable of responding to novel antigens and represented a new polyclonal T-cell repertoire. Thus PBL-ADA gene therapy leads to sustained T-cell functions in the absence of enzyme therapy. T cells of Wiskott-Aldrich Syndrome (WAS) patients were also functionally corrected by transduction with a lentiviral vector encoding for the WAS protein [11].

In the treatment of several blood T-cell malignancies, gene therapy has now proven to correct severe side effects of bone marrow transplantation (Allo-BMT). Allo-BMT is widely used as a curative approach to many hematologic malignancies [12, 13]. Treatment with allogenic T cells, either as a part of an allo-BMT or as and infusion of isolated allogenic lymphocytes, offers the possibility of cure for patients with chronic myelogenous leukemia (CML) [14]. The specificity of this effect, called graft versus leukemia effect (GVL) is not fully understood. Frequently, but not always, GVL is associated with graft versus host disease (GVHD). The latter is a very severe side effect of allogenic bone marrow transplantation, mediated by allospecific T cells within the graft. A strategy for the prevention of GVHD, now starting to be implemented, is the *in vivo* depletion of donor T cells following infusion into the recipient in cases where GVHD becomes severe. This can be achieved by gene transfer of a suicide gene such as herpes simplex virus thymidine kinase (HSV-tk) into T cells before infusion. Should the need for eradication of these cells arise, the administration of the drug ganciclovir will induce apoptotic death of HSV-tk transduced T cells. This has already proven to be effective in the treatment of GVHD in clinical trials [15-17].

An important anti-cancer strategy based on the transfer of tumor-specific T cell receptor (TCR) genes into patients' T cells has proved successful in the clinic [18]. More recently, a quite different strategy which consists of introducing a coding sequence for a chimeric antigen receptor (CAR), allowed to confer to T cells the desired specificity for a cancer antigen. Recent case reports from on-going clinical trials have described durable rejection of previously refractory B-cell malignancy in patients after CD19-directed CAR therapy [19, 20].

When addressing acquired diseases such as AIDS where novel treatments are required, T-cell gene therapy might be an important option. While the treatment of HIV infected individuals has been greatly improved by the development of Highly Active Anti-Retroviral Therapy (HAART) several problems remain. Limitations of HAART such as appearance of drug-resistant HIV variants and toxicity show that patients need novel additional immune therapies [21, 22]. Here, anti-HIV T-cell gene therapy is an interesting option since it could allow to protect both CD4⁺ T cells as the main virus reservoir, against HIV infection and specific memory T cells, which are preferentially attacked by HIV.

The first clinical gene therapy trials used genes that inhibit HIV RNA and protein production (*e.g.* Transdominant rev and tat) which led to poor antiviral activity in treated patients. Indeed, genes that inhibit the production of both viral RNA and protein, but still allow the provirus to integrate are expected to mediate selection of cells containing a suppressed HIV provirus [23, 24].

An HIV-1 based lentiviral vector was engineered expressing an HIV envelope antisense that could efficiently protect T cells from healthy and infected patients against HIV infection [25, 26]. A phase I clinical trial including patients with chronic HIV infection was performed using this strategy, which improved immune function in 4 out of 5 patients [27]. Recently, an antiviral gene was developed that encodes for a membrane-anchored peptide, which inhibits HIV entry at the level of virus-cell fusion with great efficacy [28]. Efficacy was also shown against several primary isolates in primary lymphocytes from different donors [29]. Genes with a inhibitory capacity prior to provirus integration are expected to to result in the preferential selection of non-infected, gene-protected T cells. This type of therapies offer a solution for patients who do not respond any more to anti-retroviral therapy. It becomes clear that T-cell based gene therapy will offer a valuable alternative for treating patients.

B-cell based gene therapy and immunotherapy

B-cell gene therapy or immunotherapy has long been hampered due to the lack of an efficient LV ensuring stable long term transgene expression in these cells but, as reported below, a novel LV pseudotype may allow many applications from now on.

Transgene expression in B cells is of particular interest as B cells have the potential to mediate specific immune activation and tolerance, which could improve genetic vaccination against cancer or autoimmune diseases [30-33]. One of the major goals of cancer immunotherapy is to increase the immunogenicity of tumor cells. Although several surface molecules play a role in T-B cell collaborations, the role of the CD40 receptor appears to be crucial [34, 35]. Thus, to overcome the immunological defect against malignant B cells, several groups induced forced ectopic expression of CD40L or other stimulatory factors [33, 36, 37]. Thus, vaccination strategies using autologous tumor cells manipulated *ex vivo* might be considered as a new approach for patients with B-cell malignancies, especially for those patients who are not responding to current treatment regimen [38].

Autoimmune diseases represent failure of self-tolerance in populations of circulating B and T cells [31, 32, 39]. Current treatments include long-term drug-induced immunosuppression and immune deviation, which bring along deleterious effects. Thus novel approaches that can induce tolerance are required. B-cell gene therapy is an important option towards induction of potent tolerogenic APCs. Scott and colleagues have shown that peptide-IgG fusion proteins, delivered *via* retroviral vectors into mouse B cells render these cells highly tolerogenic for the epitopes present in the peptide associated with the IgG *in vitro* and *in vivo* [40-42]. Mouse B cells can in this way efficiently express multiple antigenic epitopes presented in a tolerogenic manner on class II MHC, which results in tolerance induction in both naive and already primed immunocompetent animals. The clinical relevance of this B-cell gene therapy approach has been demonstrated by tolerance induction for targeted antigens in experimental models of several autoimmune disease [42-44]. In these models, this gene therapy induced protection, was shown to delay both the onset and even reversed the ongoing course of the disease [42-44].

Of importance, primary B cells are the most potent antibody producing cells. Indeed, B-cell programming to make a predefined protective antibody would provide a continuous supply of antibodies *in vivo* that might reduce the viral load in patients [45]. Recently, a B cell based anti-HIV strategy was proposed. LVs were used to introduce anti-HIV antibody coding regions into HSCs: differentiation of the transduced cells into antibody-secreting autologous B cells was successfully achieved [45]. Alternatively, lentiviral transduction and reinfusion of autologous B cells would allow a quick and continuous supply of HIV neutralizing antibodies *in vivo*. Of note, in the context of B-cell immunotherapy, traditional methods used to generate human mAbs include screening Epstein-Bar virus (EBV-) transformed human B-cell clones [46, 47] or antibody phage display libraries [48]. These methods are often time-consuming and may result in low yields of pathogen-specific mAbs. A novel strategy may facilitate production and the identification of monoclonal neutralizing antibodies which requires efficient transduction of primary patient memory B cells with BCL6 and BCL-XL genes inducing immortalization [49].

Stable gene transfer in human B cells may thus allow to design improved genetic vaccination strategies against cancer, infectious or autoimmune diseases [50, 51].

Restrictions of LV-mediated gene transfer in human T cells and B cells

Several studies have now established the capacity of VSVG-pseudotyped HIV-1-derived vectors to transduce various types of non-proliferating cells both *in vitro* and *in vivo* [52]. However, some cell types that are important gene therapy targets are refractory to gene transfer with lentiviral vectors. These include, in particular resting T lymphocytes [53]. That the parental virus, HIV-1, can enter into resting T-lymphocytes but does not replicate, has been attributed to multiple post-entry blocks as well as several cellular restriction factors [54]. Focusing on LVs, restrictions encountered include in particular, i) defects in initiation and completion of the reverse-transcription process [55-57], ii) lack of ATP-dependent nuclear import [58], and iii) lack of integration of the proviral genome. Indeed, activation of these cells, causing G_0 to G_{1b} transition of the cell cycle, is required to relieve the blocks in gene delivery [53, 59]. It has been reported that inducing the resting T cells to enter into the G_{1b} phase of the cell cycle without triggering cell division could render them permissive to transduction with HIV-1-vectors [59-62].

As mentioned above achieving long-term gene transfer into primary human B cells has been notoriously difficult [63-65] and LV transduction of truly quiescent B cells had not yet been reported. In T cells IL-7 stimulation leads to transition from G_0/G_{1a} to G_{1b} thus enabling gene delivery with high efficiency. However, this is not the case for human B cells. Serafini *et al.* showed that conventional VSV-G-LVs could mediate only low transduction efficiency in anti-CD40-triggered B cells [65]. It has been demonstrated that VSV-G-LVs can indeed enter into a very small subset of B cells, to undergo reverse transcription (RT) and further proviral integration into the B-cell genome. It is worth pointing out though, that VSV-G-LV cell entry, RT and nuclear entry occur in proliferating B cells but are very inefficient as compared to proliferating T cells [65]. Cellular factors obviously either facilitate or counteract different steps of lentiviral transduction in T cells, but B cell-specific putative blocking factors remain to be identified which makes unkown obstacles difficult to overcome.

E. Verhoeyen, F.-L. Cosset

Overcoming restrictions in quiescent T and B cell lentiviral gene transfer

Survival-cytokine stimulation of resting T cells overcomes lentiviral vector restrictions
The mature adult T cell population can be divided into two different subsets namely memory and naive T cells. Naive T cells are especially important as gene therapy target cells since they maintain the capacity to respond to novel antigens. It is also of utmost importance that T cell responses to antigens are not dramatically altered by the gene transfer protocol. We and others have reported that inducing cell cycle entry into G_{1b} via stimulation through the TCR allows efficient transduction of adult naive T cells by HIV-1-based vectors [59, 60]. However, TCR-stimulation of T cells alters their half-life and immune-competence, results in an inversion of the CD4/CD8 ratio, and is associated with loss of naive T cell subsets and a skewed TCR repertoire [66-68]. Of note, up to now T cell gene therapy trials were based on TCR-mediated stimulation of T cells. However, transduction of naive T cells is a pre-requisite for any T cell mediated gene therapy trial aimed at providing long-lasting immune reconstitution in patients. Therefore, protocols were developed which allow LV transduction of T cells in the absence of TCR triggering. It was shown that IL-7, but also IL-2 promoted long-term survival of T lymphocytes [69, 70]. Interestingly, exposure of adult T cells to the cytokines IL-2 and IL-7 renders them permissive to lentiviral transduction in the absence of TCR activation [53, 62, 68, 71, 72]. These cytokine-treated T cells move out of G_0 into the G_{1b} phase of the cell cycle, a phase in which T cells are susceptible to LV transduction, but do not yet proliferate. Clearly, IL-2 and IL-7 stimulation allowing lentiviral T-cell transduction could preserve a functional T-cell repertoire and maintain an appropriate proportion of naive and memory CD4+ and CD8+ T cells [71]. Naive and memory T-cell responses to rIL-7 stimulation are different [73]. Accordingly, naive adult T cells need longer IL-7 stimulation than memory cells to allow efficient LV transduction [68, 74]. In conclusion, IL-2 or IL-7 T-cell stimulation overcomes the limitation of TCR-mediated LV gene transfer.
We developed a strategy for LV-targeting by specific vector-mediated target cell activation. Our strategy consists of the interaction of a ligand which is displayed on the vector surface, with its specific receptor, thereby inducing signalling and stimulation of the target cells. As a consequence of the specific stimulation, gene transfer into the target cell is significantly enhanced. Upgraded lentiviral vector have therefore been engineered in order to overcome their inability to transduce non-activated T cells: a T cell activating polypeptide is displayed on HIV-1 vector particles in order to target and stimulate T cells precisely at the time of infection. A single-chain antibody variable fragment (scFv) which derives from the anti-CD3 OKT3 monoclonal antibody and both recognises and activates the T cell receptor, was fused to the SU subunit amino-terminus of MLV envelope glycoprotein. This chimeric CD3-targeted MLV glycoprotein demonstrated reduced infectivity. Co-expression of an "escorting" wild type VSV-G envelope protein was necessary to render lentiviral particles fully infectious. Stimulation by this vector was sufficient to allow gene transfer in up to 48% of the lymphocytes, *i.e.*, which represents a 100-fold increase compared to the performance of unmodified lentiviral vectors in non-activated T cells [60]. However, as a result, the phenotype of transduced naive T cells was modified to memory cells. Therefore, in a further step and in order to transduce resting T cells while conserving their phenotype [75, 76], the human IL-7 gene was fused to the amino-terminus of the MLV envelope glycoprotein. IL-7 displaying lenti-vectors could mediate efficient transduction, up to 40%, of naive CD4+ T cells as well as memory CD4+ T cells while allowing to maintain the functional characteristics of naive T cells [68].

Efficient transduction of IL-7 stimulated resting T cells under physiological in vivo *like* oxygen conditions

We and others have previously shown that naive as well as memory human CD4 and CD8 T lymphocytes respond to IL-7 stimulation *ex vivo*, as monitored by the activation of proximal signaling molecules, anti-apoptotic effectors, and cell cycle entry [53, 71, 73, 75]. Nevertheless, all previously mentioned studies were performed in atmospheric oxygen conditions (20-21% O_2) whereas the oxygen tensions *in vivo* are <6% (excepting lung alveoli which are approximately 14%). Indeed, direct measurement of oxygen tensions in murine lymphoid organs *in vivo* have revealed partial pressures of 0.5-4.5% [77]. Peripheral blood T cells are exposed to higher oxygen conditions in the range of 5%, but these cells account for only 2% of T lymphocytes in the body [78, 79]. Although lymphocytes will encounter fluctuations in oxygen levels, the conditions to which they are exposed *in vivo* thus dramatically differ from the 20-21% oxygen tension in standard incubators.

We assessed how naive and memory T cells respond to IL-7 under oxygen pressures to which they are exposed *in vivo* and further assessed their susceptibility to HIV-1 vector transduction. We recently reported that proximal IL-7 signaling, monitored as a function of IL-7R downregulation and STAT5 phosphorylation, is preserved at 2.5% oxygen, but cell cycle entry is significantly decreased (*Figure 1*; [80]). Intriguingly though, HIV-1 vector transduction, which generally requires a transition into cell cycle, is maintained. We found that under 2.5% oxygen conditions, there is an enhanced cell surface expression of the Glut1 glucose transporter (*Figure 1*) and a 3-fold increase in glucose uptake. HIV-1 vector transduction is notably concordant with Glut1 surface expression and is abrogated by inhibition of the PI3K pathway or with Glut1-specific siRNAs [80]. Thus, Glut1 induction by IL-7 and concomitant glucose uptake positively regulate lentiviral vector transduction of T cells under low oxygen *in vivo* like conditions [80].

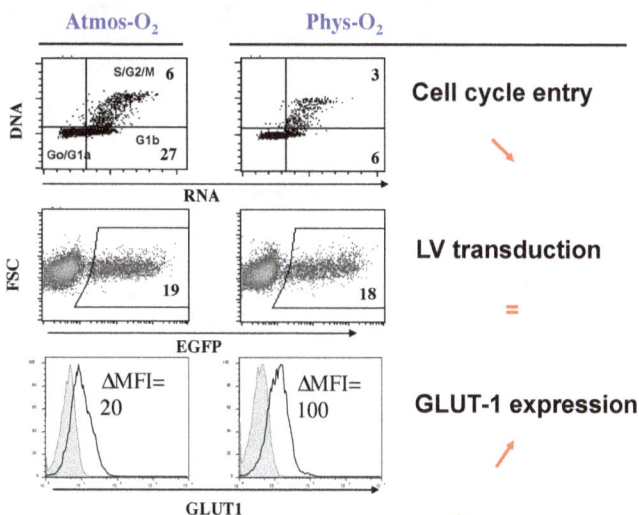

Figure 1. Permissivity of IL-7-stimulated CD4+ T lymphocytes to infection by VSV-G-pseudotyped HIV-1 vectors does not correlate with cell cycle kinetics under physiological O_2 concentrations. T cells were stimulated for 9 days with IL-7 (10 ng/ml) under 20% (Atmos-O_2) or 2.5% (Phys-O_2) conditions and then infected with a VSV-G envelope-pseudotyped HIV-1 vector expressing EGFP. The percentages of EGFP+ cells are indicated (middle panels). The corresponding level of cell cycle entry, assessed at the time of infection by PY(RNA)/7AAD(DNA) staining, is shown. The percentages of cells in the G1b and S/G2/M phases of the cell cycle are indicated (upper panels). Data are representative of 3 independent experiments. Glut1 expression was monitored at the time of infection. Representative histograms showing specific Glut1 staining (open) relative to control staining (filled) are shown (lower pannels). Mean fluorescence intensities (MFIs) are indicated.

Co-culture conditions that overcome lentiviral vector restrictions for gene transfer into primary resting B cells

Different B-cell activation/stimulation protocols have been set up in order to achieve stable gene transfer into human B cells. One way of inducing B-cell activation is *via* addition of both antiCD40-crosslinking antibodies and IL-4 that induces proliferation and entry into S/G$_2$/M phase of the cell cycle. Under these conditions VSV-G-LVs nevertheless allow only very poor transduction of B cells while similar vector doses allow the transduction of almost 100% of PHA-stimulated T cells as was reported in three independent studies [63-65]. Bovia *et al.* [63] reported efficient VSV-G-LV mediated transduction of human B cells only upon activation and proliferation in a coculture system using murine thymoma cells as helper T cells in the presence of a cytokines cocktail. In addition, infection of B cells by Epstein-Barr Virus (EBV) or stimulation with CpG DNA and cytokines can lead to efficient transduction [81, 82]. More sophisticated approaches use LVs that display an anti-CD20 scFv to target gene transfer to B cells [83-85]. However, all these protocols that render B cells permissive to LV transduction have a serious drawback since they induce B cell differentiation [86, 87]. In our view, it is of the utmost importance for many applications and fundamental studies that both the primitive characteristics of target B cell are preserved upon transduction, and the vector does not induce itself any activation and/or differentiation as a secondary effect.

A novel lentiviral vector pseudotyped with measles virus gps allows quiescent T- and B-lymphocyte transduction without affecting their cell cycle status

As mentioned above a major limitation of current LVs such as the widely used VSVG-LVs is their inability to govern efficient gene transfer into quiescent cells such as primary T cells and B cells, which hampers their application for gene therapy and immunotherapy. To overcome this limitation, we engineered a novel lentiviral vector pseudotype which incorporates measles virus (MV) glycoproteins H and F on their surface (MV-LVs) with the objective to conserve measles virus known tropism for T and B cells (*Figure 2*). Indeed, these MV-LVs allowed efficient transduction through the MV receptors SLAM and CD46, which are both present on blood T and B lymphocytes [88, 89].

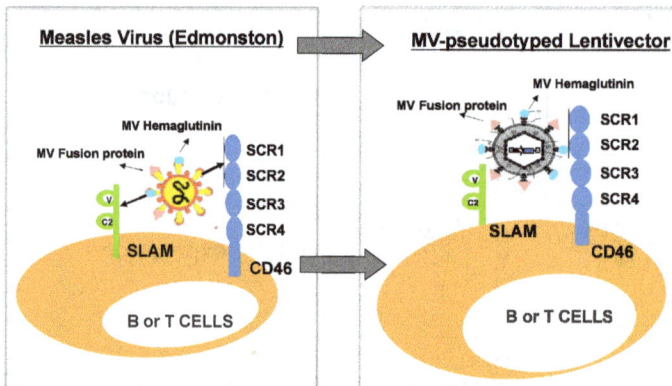

Figure 2. Design of lentiviral vectors that conserve measles virus tropism for lymphocytes. Edmonston strain of measles virus is a vaccine strain that has gained, next to entry trough the signaling lymphocyte activation molecule (SLAM), entry through the complement protein, the CD46 receptor present on all nucleated cells. In contrast, SLAM is mainly present on subpopulations of T and B cells and is upregulated after lymphocyte activation. The measles virus (MV) propagates mainly *via* a cell-to-cell fusion mechanism, using its two surface glycoproteins: haemaglutinin (H) that binds to the cellular receptor of the host cell and fusion protein (F) that mediates fusion of the viral and the cellular membranes. The strategy exist in the display of these glycoproteins H and F on lentiviral vector cores in a way that they conserved the measles virus parental tropism.

Efficient incorporation of the measles virus gps, H and F was achieved by a 24 amino-acids (aa) and 30 aa truncation of their cytoplasmic tail, respectively (*Figure 3A*). Importantly, a single exposure to these MV-LVs allowed efficient stable gene transfer to quiescent T cells, which are not permissive for classical VSVG-LVs. Indeed, high-level transduction was achieved in both resting memory (50%) and naive T cells (11%) with MV-LVs (*Figure 3B*; [90]). Especially the naive T cell population is of great interest since it represents *in vivo* the long-lived cell pool which may mediate a long-term gene correction. Resting $CD4^+$ and $CD8^+$ T cells were both efficiently transduced by MV-LVs with a preference for $CD4^+$ cells (*Figure 3B*). Surprisingly, B cells were transduced up to 50% in their resting state whereas they remained refractory to VSV-G-LVs (*Figure 3C*; [91]). Unexpectedly, although classical lentiviral transduction demands at least cell-cycle entry into the G_{1b} phase of the cell cycle, MV-LVs did not even induce cell-cycle entry upon transduction in either quiescent T or B cells [90, 91]. Importantly, MV-LV-mediated gene transfer conserved the naive and memory phenotypes of transduced resting T and B cells.

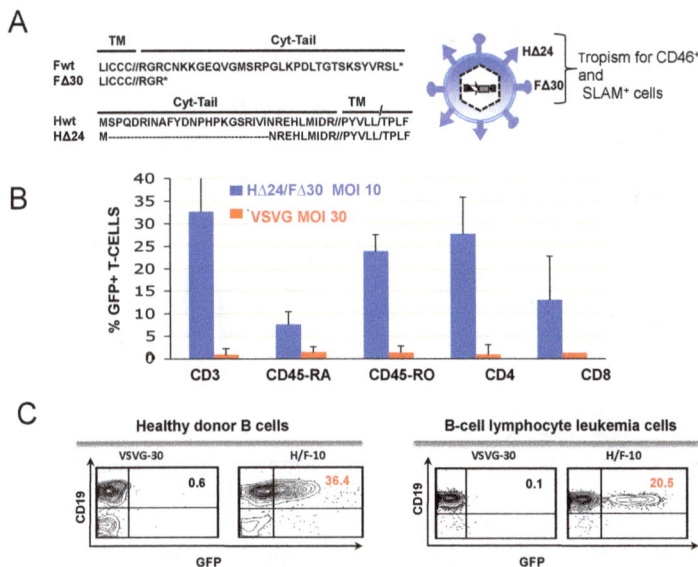

Figure 3. The measles virus gp-displaying lentiviral vectors efficiently transduce quiescent T cells and healthy and cancer B cells. (A) Schematic representation of the lentiviral vectors (LVs) displaying Hemaglutinin (H) and Fusion (F) glycoproteins derived from Edmonston strain measles virus (MV). The combination of the cytoplasmic-tail mutants of MV gps, HΔ24 and FΔ30, allowed efficient co-incorporation on the LV surface resulting in high-titer HIV vectors. (B) Resting hT-cells were transduced with HΔ24/FΔ30- or VSV-G-pseudotyped LVs at an MOI of 10 or 30 in the absence of exogenous stimuli. Surface staining for naive and memory subsets was performed by anti-CD45RA/anti-CD45RO double staining. In parallel, surface staining for the $CD3^+$, $CD4^+$ and $CD8^+$ T-cells subsets was performed and the % GFP expression for each of these T-cell subsets was analysed by FACS 3 days post-transduction (means ± SD, n = 5). (C) Resting B cells and chronic lymphocyte leukemic B cells (B-CLLs) were transduced with HΔ24/FΔ30- or VSV-G-pseudotyped LVs at an MOI of 10 or 30 in the absence of exogenous stimuli. Three days post-transduction the % GFP expression for each of these B-cell types was analysed by FACS. Data are representative of 5 experiments.

Of utmost importance, the MV-LVs are the first tools to allow stable transduction of B-CLL cells, one of the most prominent B-cell malignancies with cell cycle arrested in the G_0/G_{1a} phase (*Figure 3C*; [91, 92]). In addition, MV-LVs were able to efficiently transduce unstimulated marginal zone lymphoma (MZL) B cells, another less recurrent B-cell malignancy [92]. Overall these data suggest that MV-LVs may represent a new important tool for the genetic modification of quiescent primary lymphocytes.

Unraveling the entry pathway into quiescent T and B lymphocytes of measles virus gp pseudotyped LVs

As mentioned above, it is generally accepted that truly quiescent cells in G_0/G_{1a} phase are known to be resistant to classical VSVG-LV transduction. MV-LVs are an exception since the presence of H and F gps on the lentiviral surface turns the vector into a potent transduction tool for quiescent lymphocytes. Indeed, in contrast to VSV-G-LVs, these new pseudotypes perform all transduction steps into resting T cells: entry, fusion, reverse transcription and integration (*Figure 4A*). The MV-LVs induced high levels of reverse transcription in contrast to VSV-G-LVs early upon infection (*Figure 4C*), followed by nuclear import and stable integration into the host genome as demonstrated by Alu-PCR (*Figure 4A* and *D*).

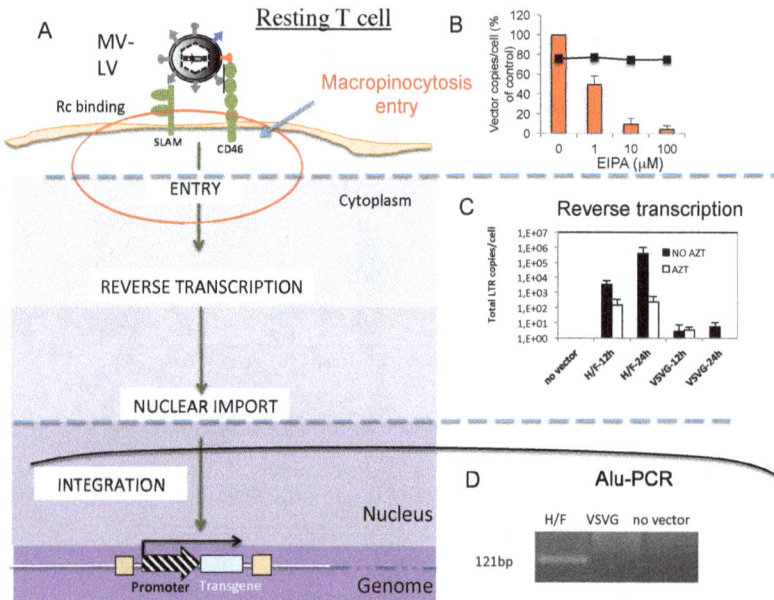

Figure 4. Schematic presentation of the important steps in lentiviral transduction of quiescent lymphocytes by MVgp-LVs. (A) MVgp-LVs absolutely require the binding through the CD46 and SLAM receptors for entry into quiescent T- and B-cells. Subsequently, they efficiently perform the different steps (reverse transcription, nuclear import) up to proviral integration, whereas for VSV-G-LVs all these steps are very inefficient. (B) Incubation with the drug IEPA suggested that the entry mechanism of MV-LVs into resting T cells relies on macropinocytosis. (C) Upon entry, very rapidly a much more efficient RT activity was detected for the MV-LVs as compared to VSV-G-LVs in these quiescent T cells without affecting their quiescent state. VSV-G-LVs show very low reverse transcription activity. (D) Finally nuclear import resulted in low proviral integration efficiency for VSV-G-LVs, whereas following nuclear import efficient proviral integration is achieved in quiescent T cells for the MV-LVs as detected by Alu-PCR.

We sought to determine the roles of MV receptors in MV-LV transduction process into quiescent lymphocytes. By using CD46-tropic MV-LVs and receptor blocking assays we found that vector-T cell binding, fusion and reverse transcription can occur by unique interaction through CD46; however, this did not result in final proviral integration. Indeed, in addition to CD46, SLAM engagement was needed for vector integration into the host cell genome of resting T and B cells. Moreover, an efficient transduction only occurs if the SLAM and CD46 receptor binding residues are both present in *cis* in the MV-H gp [93]. In addition, we found that high transduction efficiency is observed only when CD46 and SLAM are appropriatly engaged which triggers an entry mechanism that strongly resembles macropinocytosis. Micropinocytosis causes cytoskeletal rearrangements to occur in cells that lead to ruffling and blebbing at the plasma membrane. These changes in actin polymerisation are induced through tyrosine kinases receptor signaling which can be directly or indirectly activated by virus binding to a receptor or protein on the plasma membrane. When the blebs that are formed retract into the plasma membrane they engulf the virus into a macropinosome [94]. Multiple lines of evidence strongly suggest that MV-LVs enter into quiescent T cells *via* macropinocytosis [93]: 1) the micropinocytosis inhibiting drug, IEPA, blocked MV-LV entry into T cells (*Figure 4B*), 2) MV-LV vector entry was shown to be dependent on the actin cytoskeleton and microtubule formation as it was inhibited by both Cytochalasin and Nocodazole inhibitors, 3) Blebbistatin that prevents membrane blebbing, also decreased MV-LV entry, 4) the PI(3)K inhibitor LY (LY294002) completely inhibited MV-LV T cell entry, 5) Genistein, also affected MV-LV entry suggesting that tyrosine kinase activity plays a role in quiescent T cells. This entry pathway through SLAM/CD46 may also alter trafficking of the particles through cellular compartments and protect them from proteasome degradation [95] or induce the uncoating process. In using this alternative cell entry mechanism MV-LVs, might in addition avoid interaction with post-entry restriction factors. In conclusion, our results suggest that even if vector entry can occur through the CD46 receptor, SLAM-binding and signal triggering is needed for efficient LV transduction of quiescent lymphocytes and that these vectors use an alternative pathway of entry in quiescent lymphocytes that strongly resembles macropinocytosis.

LENTIVIRAL VECTOR MEDIATED TRANSDUCTION OF RESTING HEMATOPOIETIC STEM CELLS

Hematopoietic stem cells (HSCs) as important targets for gene therapy

Indeed, HSC-based gene therapy has proven over the past years to be a therapeutic option for several inherited diseases such as severe combined immunodeficiency (SCID-X1) [96, 97], adenosine deaminase deficiency (ADA- SCID) [98] and hemophilia [99] with clinical success in trials. A gene therapy trial for chronic granulomatous disease (CGD) resulteded in successful functional recovery in the myeloid compartment [100]. Most trials, however, consisted of stem cell based gene therapy using retroviral murine leukemia virus derived vectors. Next, two clinical trials have been reported for the treatment of adrenoleukodystrophy and β-thalassemia using lentiviral vectors for the first time which resulted in encouraging data [101, 102]. Indeed a successful outcome is achieved in patients suffering from X-linked adrenoleukodystrophy (ALD) using lentiviral vector HSC-based gene therapy which was able to stop disease progression in two patients suffering from this fatal demyelating disease of the central nervous system.

Importantly, when addressing the genetic correction of defects of the hematopoietic system, the therapeutic gene must be delivered to cells which are able to both self-renew and differentiate into all hematopoietic lineages. Since HSCs answer to these criteria they represent one of the most attractive candidates for gene therapy applications.

Restriction of LV-mediated gene transfer in quiescent HSCs

To allow functional recovery in all hematopoietic lineages, the correcting gene needs to be stably integrated into the hematopoietic stem cell (HSC). Although classical VSV-G pseudotyped HIV-derived LVs can transduce non-dividing cells, fully quiescent G_0 cells such as T cells and HSCs are poorly transduced [59, 90, 103]. A major barrier to LV transduction of HSCs is that 75% of HSCs reside in the G_0 phase of the cell cycle [103]. Only the use of cytokine cocktails inducing cell cycle entry has resulted in efficient VSV-G-LV based transduction [104-108].

Cytokine-cocktail stimulation overcomes LV-mediated gene transfer of resting HSCs

Lentiviral vectors (LV) have been shown to transduce CD34+/CD38- cells upon a short *ex vivo* incubation, in the absence of fibronectin (FN) or cytokine stimulation while conserving their engraftment and long-term differentiation potential as well as long-term transgene expression [109]. However, the HSC population contains many cells with different degrees of restriction to LVs. Indeed, the majority of HSCs (residing in G0 phase of the cell cycle) remain refractory even when LVs are added at high doses [110]. To increase transduction rates the addition of early-acting cytokine cocktails containing IL-6, SCF, TPO and Flt3 ligand (Flt3L) are needed. Mechanistically, culture of hCD34+ cells in the presence of these cytokines promotes cell cycle progression from G0 to G1, a pre-requisite for LV transduction not only of T cells but also of HSCs [103]. Additionally, this causes the down-regulation of the proteasome, which otherwise acts as a restrictive factor for LV transduction, resulting in enhanced gene transfer efficiency [95]. LVs allow to reach higher levels of gene marking than oncoretroviral vectors with a shorter *ex vivo* manipulation resulting in long-term persistence of transduced cells *in vivo*, as assessed with primary and secondary transplants into immunodeficient mice. However, *ex-vivo* manipulation of HSC may have negative effects on this population. First, stemness and function of HSC might be affected by cell cycle entry induced by cytokine cocktails. Second, the cell fate homing and extravasation ability may also be affected by cytokines used in *ex-vivo* culture since circulating CD34+ cells need BM cytokine activation to extravasate and home [111]. With a few exceptions cytokine stimulation is mostly inducing cell cycle entry followed by both proliferation and promotion of differentiation rather than expansion of the HSC pool [112]. Of note, thus far, the proper mixture of growth factors that would retain HSC stemness while allowing high LV transduction remains to be established.

Early-acting-cytokine-displaying lentiviral vectors to target gene transfer in resting HSCs

Engineering of SCF/TPO-displaying lentivectors for gene transfer in resting HSCs
Two HSC-specific cytokines that have shown to promote HSC survival without inducing loss of homing and engraftment are stem cell factor (SCF) and thrombopoietin (TPO). Their cellular receptors are c-Kit and Mpl, respectively. Trombopoietin (TPO) is a unique cytokine, which induces survival on its own, renewal and slight proliferation of hematopoietic progenitor cells. TPO also synergizes with stem cell factor (SCF) to induce *in vitro* and *in vivo* expansion of these cells. Therefore, we identified TPO and SCF as the most attractive candidates for surface-display on lentiviral vectors to achieve minimal and specific stimulation of CD34+ HSCs in order to improve gene transfer while preserving their stem cell character. To achieve an efficient functional presentation on the vector surface, the cytokines were fused to the N-terminus of the

haemaglutinin influenza glycoprotein (gp) HA (TPOHA and SCFHA; *Figure 5*). However, these gps resulted in a strongly reduced vector-cell fusion capacity next to a functional ligand-receptor binding. Thus, both HA-chimeric cytokines had to be displayed at the LV surface, together with an escorting fusion partner gp, VSV-G, to allow fusion of the vector with the target cell (*Figure 5*).

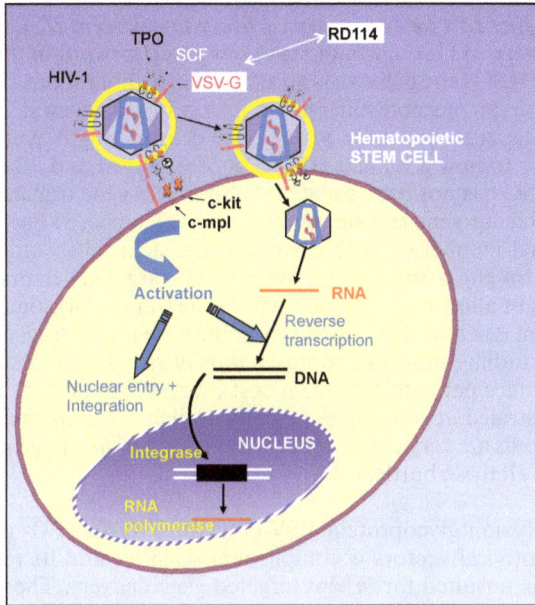

Figure 5. Lentiviral vectors displaying stem cell factor (SCF) and thrombopoietin (TPO) to target gene transfer to hematopietic stem cells. SCF and TPO were displayed on lentiviral vector by fusion to the N-terminus of the influenza envelope glycoprotein. This allows specific targeting of the vector particles to HSCs expressing c-Kit and c-Mpl, the receptors for SCF and TPO, respectively. Since the chimeric cytokine displaying vectors showed a reduced vector-cell fusion capacity, an escort envelope glycoprotein, VSV-G gp or RDTR gp, needs to be co-expressed on the vector surface to allow efficient vector-cell fusion. After binding to the c-Kit or/and Mpl receptors, the cells get slightly activated, allowing all the steps of lentiviral transduction (reverse transcription of viral RNA into DNA, nuclear proviral DNA entry and provirus integration into the host genome) to occur, resulting in productive transduction.

Indeed, TPO-, SCF- or TPO/SCF-codisplaying LVs dramatically improved gene transfer into quiescent cord blood CD34[+] cells, a population highly enriched in HSCs, as compared to conventional lentiviral vectors [108]. Our data showed that following vector exposure and after *in vitro* myeloid and lymphoid differentiation of hCD34[+] cells, the level of transduced cells was consistently much higher for the TPO-, SCF-, and TPO/SCF-displaying LVs as compared to unmodified LVs in the presence of recombinant TPO and/or SCF. Most importantly, these vectors capacity to promote selective transduction of CD34[+] cell was demonstrated by both an *in vitro* readout in long-term culture initiating cell colonies (LTC-ICs) and long-term NOD/SCID repopulation of mice with these cells (SRCs) [108]. Thus, these novel LVs allow superior gene transfer to HSCs *ex vivo* as compared to conventional LVs in the presence of high concentration of recombinant cytokines used up to now. It is speculated that the superior performance of TPO-, SCF-, and TPO/SCF-displaying LVs might be due to increased specific activity of the cytokines when presented on the viral surface as multivalent tri-mers or to an increased targeting of HSCs. Moreover, the improved transduction speci-ficity within the CD34$^+$ cell population allowed us to decrease vector doses; thus reducing the number of genomic insertion sites per cell without decreasing gene trans-fer efficacy, a feature which makes this system safer vectors for gene therapy.

Upgraded cytokine displaying LVs for in vivo *gene delivery to quiescent HSCs*

In vivo targeted gene delivery to HSCs, would mean a big step forward in the field of gene therapy since *ex vivo* HSC gene delivery is accompanied by limitations: 1) *Ex vivo* stimulation protocols in use can promote differentiation, loss of self-renewal, and affect the homing/engraftment capacity of HSCs. *In vivo* gene delivery might avoid or help reduce these effects; 2) Up to now a human HSC is poorly defined and "the genuine auto-replicating stem" HSC has not been isolated. In an *in vivo* gene transfer setting, all HSCs would be available for gene transfer in their stem cell niche; 3) For gene the-rapy to perform a minimal number of gene-corrected true stem cells would already allow an efficient long-term engraftment. The use of HSC-targeted vectors injected into the bone marrow might allow high local lentiviral gene transfer; 4) some patients *e.g.* suffering from Fanconi Anemia BM failure syndrome have a very fragile hCD34$^+$ population and *ex vivo* handling induces apoptosis: thus *in vivo* gene transfer would bring a solution; 5) To reduce patients' treatment costs, we need to provide therapies that can be easily administrated *in vivo*, since currently available *ex vivo* gene transfer procedures into hCD34$^+$-cells are very costly. Indeed, the option of *in vivo* gene transfer might bring a solution to all these bottlenecks.

However, given that the fusion glycoprotein VSV-G in the VSV-G/TPO- and VSV-G/SCF- co-displaying lentiviral vectors is complement sensitive and its receptor is present on all tissues, it is unsuited for *in vivo* targeted gene delivery. Therefore, we exchanged it for another fusion partner, a feline endogenous glycoprotein, RD114 (*Figure 5*). RD114 is an attractive candidate as fusion partner for *in vivo* use because of multiple reasons: First, RD114 gp is resistant to human complement-mediated de-gradation. Second, RD114-pseudotyped oncoretroviral vectors (MLV) are known to transduce CD34$^+$ HSCs efficiently. Finally, high glycoprotein incorporation onto len-tiviral vectors has been achieved by exchanging the RD114 cytoplasmic tail with that of MLV-gp, hereafter called RDTR [113]. Of importance, RDTR single pseudotyped LVs allow high CD34$^+$ cell transduction only in the presence of retronectin. The latter mediates, on the one hand binding of the cells *via* VLA-4 and VLA-5 receptors and on the other hand binding of envelope gp displayed on the vector. In this way both vectors and cells are connected to allow efficient virus-cell binding and fusion. In fur-ther experiments we showed that, in the absence of retronectin, the resulting RDTR/SCF- and RDTR/SCF/TPO-displaying lenti-vectors were far more efficient in transducing hCD34$^+$ cells (up to 40%) than RDTR vectors in the presence of cy-tokines (< 0.5%; [114]). Of importance, these novel cytokine-displaying LVs are thus completely independent of retronectin. In addition, vector doses can be decreased which also reduces the risk for insertional mutagenesis while high transduction effi-ciency is maintained.

With the prospect of *in vivo* gene therapy LVs need to be able to distinguish between target cells of interest and other cells. Indeed, we showed that the novel RDTR/SCF-displaying lentiviral vectors could mediate selective targeted transduction to 30-40% of hCD34$^+$-cells among cord blood (CB) mononuclear cells and in unfractionated BM of healthy and Fanconi anemia donors [114]. Moreover, this new LV pseudotype per-mitted efficient *FANCA* gene correction of hCD34$^+$ cells from Fanconi Anemia patients [114]. Next, we sought to mimic as close as possible an *in vivo* setting to target gene transfer to CD34$^+$ cells by transducing fresh cord blood samples which consist of only 0,001% CD34$^+$ cells. Importantly, RDTR/SCF-pseudotyped LVs efficiently targeted transduction to CD34$^+$ cells with 95-fold selectivity for CD34$^+$ cells as compared to T cells in the sample. In contrast, SCF-vectors transduced also the non-target T-cell population resulting in only 1.8-fold selectivity for CD34$^+$ cells transduction. We evaluated the capacity of these LVs to allow *in vivo* gene transfer into hHSCs using humanized *rag2$^{-/-}$, γc$^{-/-}$* Balbc mice, in which hCD34$^+$ cells were transplanted 13 weeks prior to intrafemural LV inoculation. We injected 2x10^5-1x10^6 infectious units of the RDTR/SCFHA-LVs or the RDTR-LVs locally into both femurs of the humanized mice (*Figure 6A*; [114]).

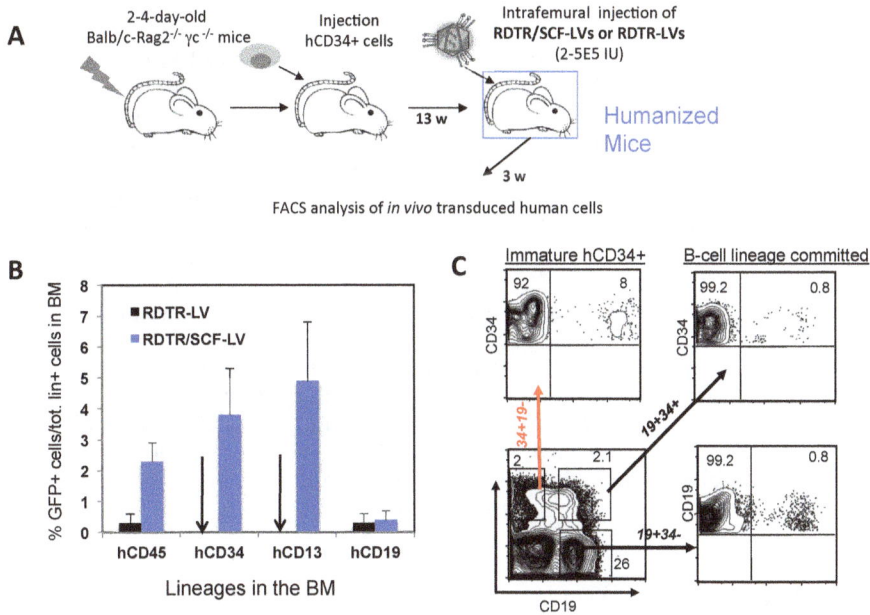

Figure 6. RDTR/SCFHA-displaying LVs allow *in vivo* gene transfer into very immature hCD34$^+$-cells in humanized mice. (A) Newborn Balbc *rag2$^{-/-}$, γc$^{-/-}$* mice received sub-lethal irradiation (2 x 1.5G) and subsequently 2x10^5 hCD34$^+$ CB cells were injected into the fetal liver at day 2 to 4 after birth. After 13 weeks of reconstitution, RDTR/SCF-LVs or RDTR-LVs were injected into the femurs of the humanized mice. Three weeks after injection we sacrificed the mice and analyzed transduction of the different cell lineages in the bone marrow. (B) The percentage of total transduced human cells (hCD45$^+$GFP$^+$), immature progenitors (hCD34$^+$GFP$^+$), myeloid progenitors (hCD13$^+$GFP$^+$) and B cells (hCD19$^+$ GFP$^+$) in the BM was analyzed by FACS. (C) Evaluation of transduction of different BM subpopulations in humanized mice by CD34/CD19 double staining, 3 weeks after RDTR/SCF-LV injection. Transduction is shown for very immature not lineage committed CD34$^+$-cells (CD34$^+$CD19$^-$), for pre- and pro-B cells (CD34$^+$CD19$^+$) and further differentiated B cells (CD34$^-$CD19$^+$).

Three weeks post-injection with these RDTR/SCFHA-LVs, on average 2.3% transduction revealed in human cells (hCD45$^+$) that had colonized the mice marrow (*Figure 6B*). Interestingly, in the BM a transduction of 2.1-6.6% of early human progenitors (CD34$^+$) and 2.9-7.3% of total myeloid progenitors (CD13$^+$) was detected whereas non-target cells, like pre- and pro-B cells (CD19$^+$) were transduced to a much lower extent (*Figure 6B*; [114]). In sharp contrast, RDTR-LV intra-marrow injection resulted in low transduction of hBM without any transduction of hCD34+-cells (*Figure 6B*). To confirm that RDTR/SCFHA-LVs transduced immature hCD34+-cells *in vivo*, a CD34+/CD19+-double-staining was performed. Of utmost importance, a 10-fold higher transduction of hCD34+CD19-cells, not yet showing B-cell commitment, was repeatedly detected as compared to both early B-cell progenitors (CD34+CD19+) and more committed B cells (CD34-CD19+; *Figure 6C*).

In summary, this new LV will facilitate HSC-based gene therapy by direct targeting of these primitive cells in BM aspirates or total CB. Most importantly, RDTR/SCF-LVs might completely suppress the need for *ex vivo* handling and through a direct *in vivo* inoculation thereby simplify gene therapy for many hematopoietic defects in the future.

CONCLUSION

Most T and B lymphocytes in the human blood stream are quiescent cells; therefore efficient transduction of quiescent lymphocytes is in itself an important goal for many applications. Basic biological studies on cell differentiation and oncogenic onset of lymphocytes as well as the development of gene therapy strategies would benefit from stable quiescent T and B cell transduction. This would avoid long-term *ex vivo* culture and phenotypic loss, which is essential for the long-term persistence of naive cells in the human body. Finally, a new lentiviral vector allowing high and stable gene transfer of primary quiescent B cells, T cells and cancer B cells, will now make it possible and easier to study gene functions in these cells. These lentiviral tools may open the way to improved genetic vaccination strategies against cancer, infectious or autoimmune diseases as well as gene therapy of genetic diseases.

The newly engineered generation of HSC-targeted-LVs should already simplify and improve current gene therapy protocols through transduction of primitive HSCs directly in the BM of patients with genetic diseases. In the future, this new tool could make all *ex vivo* handling tedious steps purposeless and allow gene-correction of numerous hematopoietic diseases *via* a direct intra-marrow inoculum *in vivo*.

ACKNOWLEDGMENTS

We would like to thank all lab members (Inserm U758, Lyon, France) that contributed to the experimental work presented here: Cecilia Frecha, Camille Lévy, Caroline Costa, Fouzia Amirache, Didier Nègre, and Robin Buckland. We would also like to express our thanks to Naomi Taylor, Séverine Loisel-Meyer and Louise Swainson and all other lab member of the Taylor lab (IGM, Montpellier, France) for the longstanding collaboration and of course all other dear collaborators that contributed to these exciting results. This work was supported by grants from the «Agence Nationale pour la Recherche contre le Sida et les Hépatites Virales» (ANRS), the "Agence Nationale de la Recherche" (ANR), the European Research Council (ERC-2008-AdG-233130 "HEPCENT") and the European Community (FP7-HEALTH-2007-B/222878 «PERSIST» and FP7-E-Rare "GENTHALTHER").

REFERENCES

1. Blaese RM, Culver KW, Miller AD, Carter CS, Fleisher T, Clerici M, Shearer G, Chang L, *et al.* T lymphocyte-directed gene therapy for ADA-SCID: initial trial results after 4 years. *Science* 1995; 270: 475-80.

2. Bordignon C, Notarangelo LD, Nobili N, Ferrari G, Casorati G, Panina P, Mazzolari E, Maggioni D, *et al.* Gene therapy in peripheral blood lymphocytes and bone marrow for ADA-immunodeficient patients. *Science* 1995; 270: 470-5.

3. Deeks SG, Wagner B, Anton PA, Mitsuyasu RT, Scadden DT, Huang C, Macken C, Richman DD, *et al.* A phase II randomized study of HIV-specific T-cell gene therapy in subjects with undetectable plasma viremia on combination antiretroviral therapy. *Mol Ther* 2002; 5: 788-97.

4. Mitsuyasu RT, Anton PA, Deeks SG, Scadden DT, Connick E, Downs MT, Bakker A, Roberts MR, *et al.* Prolonged survival and tissue trafficking following adoptive transfer of CD4zeta gene-modified autologous CD4+ and CD8+ T cells in human immunodeficiency virus-infected subjects. *Blood* 2000; 96: 785-93.

5. Recchia A, Bonini C, Magnani Z, Urbinati F, Sartori D, Muraro S, Tagliafico E, Bondanza A, *et al.* Retroviral vector integration deregulates gene expression but has no consequence on the biology and function of transplanted T cells. *Proc Natl Acad Sci USA* 2006; 103: 1457-62.

6. Buchschacher GL Jr, Wong-Staal F. Approaches to gene therapy for human immunodeficiency virus infection. *Hum Gene Ther* 2001; 12: 1013-9.

7. Hirschhorn R, Yang DR, Puck JM, Huie ML, Jiang CK, Kurlandsky LE. Spontaneous *in vivo* reversion to normal of an inherited mutation in a patient with adenosine deaminase deficiency. *Nat Genet* 1996; 13: 290-5.

8. Stephan V, Wahn V, Le Deist F, Dirksen U, Broker B, Muller-Fleckenstein I, Horneff G, Schroten H, *et al.* Atypical X-linked severe combined immunodeficiency due to possible spontaneous reversion of the genetic defect in T cells. *N Engl J Med* 1996; 335: 1563-7.

9. Tjonnfjord GE, Steen R, Veiby OP, Friedrich W, Egeland T. Evidence for engraftment of donor-type multipotent CD34+ cells in a patient with selective T-lymphocyte reconstitution after bone marrow transplantation for B-SCID. *Blood* 1994; 84: 3584-9.

10. Aiuti A, Vai S, Mortellaro A, Casorati G, Ficara F, Andolfi G, Ferrari G, Tabucchi A, *et al.* Immune reconstitution in ADA-SCID after PBL gene therapy and discontinuation of enzyme replacement. *Nat Med* 2002; 8: 423-5.

11. Dupre L, Trifari S, Follenzi A, Marangoni F, Lain de Lera T, Bernad A, Martino S, Tsuchiya S, *et al.* Lentiviral vector-mediated gene transfer in T cells from Wiskott-Aldrich syndrome patients leads to functional correction. *Mol Ther* 2004; 10: 903-15.

12. Szydlo R, Goldman JM, Klein JP, Gale RP, Ash RC, Bach FH, *et al.* Results of allogeneic bone marrow transplants for leukemia using donors other than HLA-identical siblings. *J Clin Oncol* 1997; 15: 1767-77.

13. Vigorito AC, Azevedo WM, Marques JF, Azevedo AM, Eid KA, Aranha FJ, *et al.* A randomised, prospective comparison of allogeneic bone marrow and peripheral blood progenitor cell transplantation in the treatment of haematological malignancies. *Bone Marrow Transplant* 1998; 22: 1145-51.

14. Horowitz MM, Gale RP, Sondel PM, Goldman JM, Kersey J, Kolb HJ, *et al.* Graft-versus-leukemia reactions after bone marrow transplantation. *Blood* 1990; 75: 555-62.

15. Bondanza A, Valtolina V, Magnani Z, Ponzoni M, Fleischhauer K, Bonyhadi M, *et al.* Suicide gene therapy of graft-versus-host disease induced by central memory human T lymphocytes. *Blood* 2006; 107: 1828-36.

16. Bonini C, Ferrari G, Verzeletti S, Servida P, Zappone E, Ruggieri L, *et al.* HSV-TK gene transfer into donor lymphocytes for control of allogeneic graft-versus-leukemia. *Science* 1997; 276: 1719-24.

17. Tiberghien P, Ferrand C, Lioure B, Milpied N, Angonin R, Deconinck E, *et al*. Administration of herpes simplex-thymidine kinase-expressing donor T cells with a T-cell-depleted allogeneic marrow graft. *Blood* 2001; 97: 63-72.

18. Morgan RA, Dudley ME, Wunderlich JR, Hughes MS, Yang JC, Sherry RM, *et al*. Cancer regression in patients after transfer of genetically engineered lymphocytes. *Science* 2006; 314: 126-9.

19. Kalos M, Levine BL, Porter DL, Katz S, Grupp SA, Bagg A, June CH. T cells with chimeric antigen receptors have potent antitumor effects and can establish memory in patients with advanced leukemia. *Sci Transl Med* 2011; 3: 95ra73.

20. Kochenderfer JN, Wilson WH, Janik JE, Dudley ME, Stetler-Stevenson M, Feldman SA, *et al*. Eradication of B-lineage cells and regression of lymphoma in a patient treated with autologous T cells genetically engineered to recognize CD19. *Blood* 2010; 116: 4099-102.

21. Chun TW, Stuyver L, Mizell SB, Ehler LA, Mican JA, Baseler M, *et al*. Presence of an inducible HIV-1 latent reservoir during highly active antiretroviral therapy. *Proc Natl Acad Sci USA* 1997; 94: 13193-7.

22. Finzi D, Hermankova M, Pierson T, Carruth LM, Buck C, Chaisson RE, *et al*. Identification of a reservoir for HIV-1 in patients on highly active antiretroviral therapy. *Science* 1997; 278: 1295-300.

23. Ranga U, Woffendin C, Verma S, Xu L, June CH, Bishop DK, Nabel GJ. Enhanced T cell engraftment after retroviral delivery of an antiviral gene in HIV-infected individuals. *Proc Natl Acad Sci USA* 1998; 95: 1201-6.

24. Woffendin C, Ranga U, Yang Z, Xu L, Nabel GJ. Expression of a protective gene-prolongs survival of T cells in human immunodeficiency virus-infected patients. *Proc Natl Acad Sci USA* 1996; 93: 2889-94.

25. Braun SE, Wong FE, Connole M, Qiu G, Lee L, Gillis J, *et al*. Inhibition of simian/human immunodeficiency virus replication in CD4$^+$ T cells derived from lentiviral-transduced CD34$^+$ hematopoietic cells. *Mol Ther* 2005; 12: 1157-67.

26. Humeau LM, Binder GK, Lu X, Slepushkin V, Merling R, Echeagaray P, *et al*. Efficient lentiviral vector-mediated control of HIV-1 replication in CD4 lymphocytes from diverse HIV+ infected patients grouped according to CD4 count and viral load. *Mol Ther* 2004; 9: 902-13.

27. Levine BL, Humeau LM, Boyer J, MacGregor RR, Rebello T, Lu X, *et al*. Gene transfer in humans using a conditionally replicating lentiviral vector. *Proc Natl Acad Sci USA* 2006; 103: 17372-7.

28. Hildinger M, Dittmar MT, Schult-Dietrich P, Fehse B, Schnierle BS, Thaler S, *et al*. Membrane-anchored peptide inhibits human immunodeficiency virus entry. *J Virol* 2001; 75: 3038-42.

29. Egelhofer M, Brandenburg G, Martinius H, Schult-Dietrich P, Melikyan G, Kunert R, *et al*. Inhibition of human immunodeficiency virus type 1 entry in cells expressing gp41-derived peptides. *J Virol* 2004; 78: 568-75.

30. Lei TC, Scott DW. Induction of tolerance to factor VIII inhibitors by gene therapy with immunodominant A2 and C2 domains presented by B cells as Ig fusion proteins. *Blood* 2005; 105: 4865-70.

31. Melo ME, Qian J, El-Amine M, Agarwal RK, Soukhareva N, Kang Y, Scott DW. Gene transfer of Ig-fusion proteins into B cells prevents and treats autoimmune diseases. *J Immunol* 2002; 168: 4788-95.

32. Scott DW, Venkataraman M, Jandinski JJ. Multiple pathways of B lymphocyte tolerance. *Immunol Rev* 1979; 43: 241-80.

33. Stripecke R, Cardoso AA, Pepper KA, Skelton DC, Yu XJ, Mascarenhas L, *et al*. Lentiviral vectors for efficient delivery of CD80 and granulocyte-macrophage-colony-stimulating factor in human acute lymphoblastic leukemia and acute myeloid leukemia cells to induce antileukemic immune responses. *Blood* 2000; 96: 1317-26.

34. Aruffo A, Farrington M, Hollenbaugh D, Li X, Milatovich A, Nonoyama S, *et al*. The CD40 ligand, gp39, is defective in activated T cells from patients with X-linked hyper-IgM syndrome. *Cell* 1993; 72: 291-300.

35. Fuleihan R, Ramesh N, Loh R, Jabara H, Rosen RS, Chatila T, *et al*. Defective expression of the CD40 ligand in X chromosome-linked immunoglobulin deficiency with normal or elevated IgM. *Proc Natl Acad Sci USA* 1993; 90: 2170-3.

36. Cantwell M, Hua T, Pappas J, Kipps TJ. Acquired CD40-ligand deficiency in chronic lymphocytic leukemia. *Nat Med* 1997; 3: 984-9.

37. Cantwell MJ, Sharma S, Friedmann T, Kipps TJ. Adenovirus vector infection of chronic lymphocytic leukemia B cells. *Blood* 1996; 88: 4676-83.

38. Moskowitz CH. Pretreatment prognostic factors and outcome in patients with relapsed or primary-refractory diffuse large B-cell lymphoma treated with second-line chemotherapy and autologous stem cell transplantation. *Ann Oncol* 2006; 17 (suppl 4): iv37-9.

39. Lei TC, Su Y, Scott DW. Tolerance induction via a B-cell delivered gene therapy-based protocol: optimization and role of the Ig scaffold. *Cell Immunol* 2005; 235: 12-20.

40. El-Amine M, Melo M, Kang Y, Nguyen H, Qian J, Scott DW. Mechanisms of tolerance induction by a gene-transferred peptide-IgG fusion protein expressed in B lineage cells. *J Immunol* 2000; 165: 5631-6.

41. Gourley TS, Patel DR, Nickerson K, Hong SC, Chang CH. Aberrant expression of Fas ligand in mice deficient for the MHC class II transactivator. *J Immunol* 2002; 168: 4414-9.

42. Xu B, Scott DW. A novel retroviral gene therapy approach to inhibit specific antibody production and suppress experimental autoimmune encephalomyelitis induced by MOG and MBP. *Clin Immunol* 2004; 111: 47-52.

43. Agarwal RK, Kang Y, Zambidis E, Scott DW, Chan CC, Caspi RR. Retroviral gene therapy with an immunoglobulin-antigen fusion construct protects from experimental autoimmune uveitis. *J Clin Invest* 2000; 106: 245-52.

44. Song L, Wang J, Wang R, Yu M, Sun Y, Han G, *et al*. Retroviral delivery of GAD-IgG fusion construct induces tolerance and modulates diabetes: a role for CD4+ regulatory T cells and TGF-beta? *Gene Ther* 2004; 11: 1487-96.

45. Luo XM, Maarschalk E, O'Connell RM, Wang P, Yang L, Baltimore D. Engineering human hematopoietic stem/progenitor cells to produce a broadly neutralizing anti-HIV antibody after in vitro maturation to human B lymphocytes. *Blood* 2009; 113: 1422-31.

46. Cole SP, Campling BG, Atlaw T, Kozbor D, Roder JC. Human monoclonal antibodies. *Mol Cell Biochem* 1984; 62: 109-20.

47. Liao HX, Levesque MC, Nagel A, Dixon A, Zhang R, Walter E, *et al*. High-throughput isolation of immunoglobulin genes from single human B cells and expression as monoclonal antibodies. *J Virol Methods* 2009; 158: 171-9.

48. Garet E, Cabado AG, Vieites JM, Gonzalez-Fernandez A. Rapid isolation of single-chain antibodies by phage display technology directed against one of the most potent marine toxins: Palytoxin. *Toxicon* 2010; 55: 1519-26.

49. Kwakkenbos MJ, Diehl SA, Yasuda E, Bakker AQ, van Geelen CM, Lukens MV, *et al*. Generation of stable monoclonal antibody-producing B cell receptor-positive human memory B cells by genetic programming. *Nat Med* 16: 123-8.

50. Li LH, Biagi E, Allen C, Shivakumar R, Weiss JM, Feller S, *et al*. Rapid and efficient nonviral gene delivery of CD154 to primary chronic lymphocytic leukemia cells. *Cancer Gene Ther* 2006; 13: 215-24.

51. White H, Thrasher A, Veys P, Kinnon C, Gaspar HB. Intrinsic defects of B cell function in X-linked severe combined immunodeficiency. *Eur J Immunol* 2000; 30: 732-7.

52. Vigna E, Naldini L. Lentiviral vectors: excellent tools for experimental gene transfer and promising candidates for gene therapy. *J Gene Med* 2000; 2: 308-16.

53. Dardalhon V, Jaleco S, Kinet S, Herpers B, Steinberg M, Ferrand C, *et al*. IL-7 differentially regulates cell cycle progression and HIV-1-based vector infection in neonatal and adult CD4+ T cells. *Proc Natl Acad Sci USA* 2001; 98: 9277-82.

54. Strebel K, Luban J, Jeang KT. Human cellular restriction factors that target HIV-1 replication. *BMC Med* 2009; 7: 48.

55. Stevenson M, Stanwick TL, Dempsey MP, Lamonica CA. HIV-1 replication is controlled at the level of T cell activation and proviral integration. *EMBO J* 1990; 9: 1551-60.

56. Zack JA. The role of the cell cycle in HIV-1 infection. *Adv Exp Med Biol* 1995; 374: 27-31.

57. Zack JA, Haislip AM, Krogstad P, Chen IS. Incompletely reverse-transcribed human immunodeficiency virus type 1 genomes in quiescent cells can function as intermediates in the retroviral life cycle. *J Virol* 1992; 66: 1717-25.

58. Bukrinsky MI, Sharova N, Dempsey MP, Stanwick TL, Bukrinskaya AG, Haggerty S, Stevenson M. Active nuclear import of human immunodeficiency virus type 1 preintegration complexes. *Proc Natl Acad Sci USA* 1992; 89: 6580-4.

59. Korin YD, Zack JA. Progression to the G1b phase of the cell cycle is required for completion of human immunodeficiency virus type 1 reverse transcription in T cells. *J Virol* 1998; 72: 3161-8.

60. Maurice M, Verhoeyen E, Salmon P, Trono D, Russell SJ, Cosset FL. Efficient gene transfer into human primary blood lymphocytes by surface-engineered lentiviral vectors that display a T cell-activating polypeptide. *Blood* 2002; 99: 2342-50.

61. Sun Y, Pinchuk LM, Agy MB, Clark EA. Nuclear import of HIV-1 DNA in resting CD4+ T cells requires a cyclosporin A-sensitive pathway. *J Immunol* 1997; 158: 512-7.

62. Unutmaz D, KewalRamani VN, Marmon S, Littman DR. Cytokine signals are sufficient for HIV-1 infection of resting human T lymphocytes. *J Exp Med* 1999; 189: 1735-46.

63. Bovia F, Salmon P, Matthes T, Kvell K, Nguyen TH, Werner-Favre C, *et al*. Efficient transduction of primary human B lymphocytes and nondividing myeloma B cells with HIV-1-derived lentiviral vectors. *Blood* 2003; 101: 1727-33.

64. Janssens W, Chuah MK, Naldini L, Follenzi A, Collen D, Saint-Remy JM, VandenDriessche T. Efficiency of onco-retroviral and lentiviral gene transfer into primary mouse and human B-lymphocytes is pseudotype dependent. *Hum Gene Ther* 2003; 14: 263-76.

65. Serafini M, Naldini L, Introna M. Molecular evidence of inefficient transduction of proliferating human B lymphocytes by VSV-pseudotyped HIV-1-derived lentivectors. *Virology* 2004; 325: 413-24.

66. Ferrand C, Robinet E, Contassot E, Certoux JM, Lim A, Herve P, Tiberghien P. Retrovirus-mediated gene transfer in primary T lymphocytes: influence of the transduction/selection process and of ex vivo expansion on the T cell receptor beta chain hypervariable region repertoire. *Hum Gene Ther* 2000; 11: 1151-64.

67. Marktel S, Magnani Z, Ciceri F, Cazzaniga S, Riddell SR, Traversari C, Bordignon C, Bonini C. Immunologic potential of donor lymphocytes expressing a suicide gene for early immune reconstitution after hematopoietic T-cell-depleted stem cell transplantation. *Blood* 2003; 101: 1290-8.

68. Verhoeyen E, Dardalhon V, Ducrey-Rundquist O, Trono D, Taylor N, Cosset FL. IL-7 surface-engineered lentiviral vectors promote survival and efficient gene transfer in resting primary T lymphocytes. *Blood* 2003; 101: 2167-74.

69. Fry TJ, Mackall CL. Interleukin-7: master regulator of peripheral T-cell homeostasis? *Trends Immunol* 2001; 22: 564-71.

70. Geiselhart LA, Humphries CA, Gregorio TA, Mou S, Subleski J, Komschlies KL. IL-7 administration alters the CD4: CD8 ratio, increases T cell numbers, and increases T cell function in the absence of activation. *J Immunol* 2001; 166: 3019-27.

71. Cavalieri S, Cazzaniga S, Geuna M, Magnani Z, Bordignon C, Naldini L, Bonini C. Human T lymphocytes transduced by lentiviral vectors in the absence of TCR activation maintain an intact immune competence. *Blood* 2003; 102: 497-505.

72. Ducrey-Rundquist O, Guyader M, Trono D. Modalities of interleukin-7-induced human immunodeficiency virus permissiveness in quiescent T lymphocytes. *J Virol* 2002; 76: 9103-11.

73. Swainson L, Verhoeyen E, Cosset FL, Taylor N. IL-7R alpha gene expression is inversely correlated with cell cycle progression in IL-7-stimulated T lymphocytes. *J Immunol* 2006; 176: 6702-8.

74. Verhoeyen E. CCaCF-L: lentiviral vector gene transfer into human T cells. In: Baum C, ed. *Genetic modification of hematopoietic stem cells. Methods and protocols.* [Walker JM (Series Editor): Methods in molecular biology, vol. 506]. New York: Humana Press, 2009: 97-114.

75. Soares MV, Borthwick NJ, Maini MK, Janossy G, Salmon M, Akbar AN. IL-7-dependent extrathymic expansion of CD45RA+ T cells enables preservation of a naive repertoire. *J Immunol* 1998; 161: 5909-17.

76. Webb LM, Foxwell BM, Feldmann M. Putative role for interleukin-7 in the maintenance of the recirculating naive CD4+ T-cell pool. *Immunology* 1999; 98: 400-5.

77. Caldwell CC, Kojima H, Lukashev D, Armstrong J, Farber M, Apasov SG, Sitkovsky MV. Differential effects of physiologically relevant hypoxic conditions on T lymphocyte development and effector functions. *J Immunol* 2001; 167: 6140-9.

78. Sopper S, Nierwetberg D, Halbach A, Sauer U, Scheller C, Stahl-Hennig C, *et al.* Impact of simian immunodeficiency virus (SIV) infection on lymphocyte numbers and T-cell turnover in different organs of rhesus monkeys. *Blood* 2003; 101: 1213-9.

79. Westermann J, Pabst R. Distribution of lymphocyte subsets and natural killer cells in the human body. *Clin Invest* 1992; 70: 539-44.

80. Loisel-Meyer S, Swainson L, Craveiro M, Oburoglu L, Mongellaz C, Costa C, *et al.* Glut-1 mediated glucose transport regulates HIV infection. *Proc Natl Acad Sci USA* 2012; 109: 2549-54.

81. Kvell K, Nguyen TH, Salmon P, Glauser F, Werner-Favre C, Barnet M, *et al.* Transduction of CpG DNA-stimulated primary human B cells with bicistronic lentivectors. *Mol Ther* 2005; 12: 892-9.

82. Lizee G, Gonzales MI, Topalian SL. Lentivirus vector-mediated expression of tumor-associated epitopes by human antigen presenting cells. *Hum Gene Ther* 2004; 15: 393-404.

83. Funke S, Maisner A, Muhlebach MD, Koehl U, Grez M, Cattaneo R, Cichutek K, Buchholz CJ. Targeted cell entry of lentiviral vectors. *Mol Ther* 2008; 16: 1427-36.

84. Yang L, Bailey L, Baltimore D, Wang P. Targeting lentiviral vectors to specific cell types *in vivo*. *Proc Natl Acad Sci USA* 2006; 103: 11479-84.

85. Ziegler L, Yang L, Joo K, Yang H, Baltimore D, Wang P. Targeting lentiviral vectors to antigen-specific immunoglobulins. *Hum Gene Ther* 2008; 19: 861-72.

86. Buchholz CJ, Muhlebach MD, Cichutek K. Lentiviral vectors with measles virus glycoproteins: dream team for gene transfer? *Trends Biotechnol* 2009; 27: 259-65.

87. Fecteau JF, Roy A, Neron S. Peripheral blood CD27+ IgG+ B cells rapidly proliferate and differentiate into immunoglobulin-secreting cells after exposure to low CD154 interaction. *Immunology* 2009; 128: e353-65.

88. Dorig RE, Marcil A, Chopra A, Richardson CD. The human CD46 molecule is a receptor for measles virus (Edmonston strain). *Cell* 1993; 75: 295-305.

89. Tatsuo H, Ono N, Tanaka K, Yanagi Y. SLAM (CDw150) is a cellular receptor for measles virus. *Nature* 2000; 406: 893-7.

90. Frecha C, Costa C, Negre D, Gauthier E, Russell SJ, Cosset FL, Verhoeyen E. Stable transduction of quiescent T cells without induction of cycle progression by a novel lentiviral vector pseudotyped with measles virus glycoproteins. *Blood* 2008; 112: 4843-52.

91. Frecha C, Costa C, Levy C, Negre D, Russell SJ, Maisner A, *et al*. Efficient and stable trans-duction of resting B lymphocytes and primary chronic lymphocyte leukemia cells using measles virus gp displaying lentiviral vectors. *Blood* 2009; 114: 3173-80.

92. Levy C, Frecha C, Costa C, Rachinel N, Salles G, Cosset FL, Verhoeyen E. Lentiviral vectors and transduction of human cancer B cells. *Blood* 2010; 116: 498-500 (author reply 500).

93. Frecha C, Levy C, Costa C, Negre D, Amirache F, Buckland R, *et al*. Measles virus glycoprotein-pseudotyped lentiviral vector-mediated gene transfer into quiescent lymphocytes requires binding to both SLAM and CD46 entry receptors. *J Virol* 2011; 85: 5975-85.

94. Mercer J, Helenius A. Virus entry by macropinocytosis. *Nat Cell Biol* 2009; 11: 510-20.

95. Santoni de Sio FR, Cascio P, Zingale A, Gasparini M, Naldini L. Proteasome activity restricts lentiviral gene transfer into hematopoietic stem cells and is down-regulated by cytokines that en-hance transduction. *Blood* 2006; 107: 4257-65.

96. Cavazzana-Calvo M, Fischer A. Efficacy of gene therapy for SCID is being confirmed. *Lancet* 2004; 364: 2155-6.

97. Hacein-Bey-Abina S, Le Deist F, Carlier F, Bouneaud C, Hue C, De Villartay JP, *et al*. Sustained correction of X-linked severe combined immunodeficiency by *ex vivo* gene therapy. *N Engl J Med* 2002; 346: 1185-93.

98. Aiuti A, Slavin S, Aker M, Ficara F, Deola S, Mortellaro A, *et al*. Correction of ADA-SCID by stem cell gene therapy combined with nonmyeloablative conditioning. *Science* 2002; 296: 2410-3.

99. Powell JS, Ragni MV, White GC 2nd, Lusher JM, Hillman-Wiseman C, Moon TE, *et al*. Phase 1 trial of FVIII gene transfer for severe hemophilia A using a retroviral construct administered by pe-ripheral intravenous infusion. *Blood* 2003; 102: 2038-45.

100. Ott MG, Schmidt M, Schwarzwaelder K, Stein S, Siler U, Koehl U, *et al*. Correction of X-linked chronic granulomatous disease by gene therapy, augmented by insertional activation of MDS1-EVI1, PRDM16 or SETBP1. *Nat Med* 2006; 12: 401-9.

101. Cartier N, Hacein-Bey-Abina S, Bartholomae CC, Veres G, Schmidt M, Kutschera I, *et al*. Hematopoietic stem cell gene therapy with a lentiviral vector in X-linked adrenoleukodystrophy. *Science* 2009; 326: 818-23.

102. Cavazzana-Calvo M, Payen E, Negre O, Wang G, Hehir K, Fusil F, *et al*. Transfusion independ-ence and HMGA2 activation after gene therapy of human beta-thalassaemia. *Nature* 2010; 467: 318-22.

103. Sutton RE, Reitsma MJ, Uchida N, Brown PO. Transduction of human progenitor hematopoietic stem cells by human immunodeficiency virus type 1-based vectors is cell cycle dependent. *J Virol* 1999; 73: 3649-60.

104. Hanawa H, Hematti P, Keyvanfar K, Metzger ME, Krouse A, Donahue RE, *et al*. Efficient gene transfer into rhesus repopulating hematopoietic stem cells using a simian immunodeficiency virus-based lentiviral vector system. *Blood* 2004; 103: 4062-9.

105. Horn PA, Morris JC, Bukovsky AA, Andrews RG, Naldini L, Kurre P, Kiem HP. Lentivirus-medi-ated gene transfer into hematopoietic repopulating cells in baboons. *Gene Ther* 2002; 9: 1464-71.

106. Horn PA, Topp MS, Morris JC, Riddell SR, Kiem HP. Highly efficient gene transfer into baboon marrow repopulating cells using GALV-pseudotype oncoretroviral vectors produced by human packaging cells. *Blood* 2002; 100: 3960-7.

107. Trobridge GD, Beard BC, Gooch C, Wohlfahrt M, Olsen P, Fletcher J, Malik P, Kiem HP. Efficient transduction of pigtailed macaque hematopoietic repopulating cells with HIV-based lentiviral vectors. *Blood* 2008; 111: 5537-43.

108. Verhoeyen E, Wiznerowicz M, Olivier D, Izac B, Trono D, Dubart-Kupperschmitt A, Cosset FL. Novel lentiviral vectors displaying early-acting cytokines selectively promote survival and transduction of NOD/SCID repopulating human hematopoietic stem cells. *Blood* 2005; 106: 3386-95.

109. Ailles L, Schmidt M, Santoni de Sio FR, Glimm H, Cavalieri S, Bruno S, *et al*. Molecular evidence of lentiviral vector-mediated gene transfer into human self-renewing, multi-potent, long-term NOD/SCID repopulating hematopoietic cells. *Mol Ther* 2002; 6: 615-26.

110. Guenechea G, Gan OI, Inamitsu T, Dorrell C, Pereira DS, Kelly M, Naldini L, Dick JE. Transduction of human CD34+ CD38- bone marrow and cord blood-derived SCID-repopulating cells with third-generation lentiviral vectors. *Mol Ther* 2000; 1: 566-73.

111. Ahmed F, Ings SJ, Pizzey AR, Blundell MP, Thrasher AJ, Ye HT, *et al*. Impaired bone marrow homing of cytokine-activated CD34+ cells in the NOD/SCID model. *Blood* 2004; 103: 2079-87.

112. Sorrentino BP. Clinical strategies for expansion of haematopoietic stem cells. *Nat Rev Immunol* 2004; 4: 878-88.

113. Sandrin V, Boson B, Salmon P, Gay W, Negre D, Le Grand R, Trono D, Cosset FL. Lentiviral vectors pseudotyped with a modified RD114 envelope glycoprotein show increased stability in sera and augmented transduction of primary lymphocytes and CD34+ cells derived from human and nonhuman primates. *Blood* 2002; 100: 823-32.

114. Frecha C, Costa C, Negre D, Amirache F, Trono D, Rio P, *et al*. A novel lentivector targets gene transfer into hHSC in marrow from patients with BM-failure-syndrome and *in vivo* in humanized mice. *Blood* 2012; 119: 1139-50.

Highlights on gene-modified cell therapy

COORDINATED BY
GÖSTA GAHRTON

The CliniBook: Clinical gene transfer
Edited by Odile Cohen-Haguenauer – EDK, Paris © 2012, pp. 185-186

A4-1
Cell therapy
Introduction

Gösta Gahrton

Karolinska Institutet, Department of Medicine, Karolinska University Hospital, Huddinge, SE 14186 Stockholm, Sweden.
gosta.gahrton@ki.se

The Cell Therapy platform in Clinigene has focused on a selected number of projects – both basic science related and clinical trials. Here we report on projects that delineate methods to produce cells, gene transduced or in other ways manipulated, aimed to eventually be used in clinical trials. In another section (Part II) of this book, three clinical trials in the Clinigene Cell Therapy platform are described, *i.e.* treatment of patients with Alzheimer's disease with encapsulated human nerve growth factor (NGF) transduced immortalized retinal pigmental epithelial cells (Eriksdotter-Jönhagen *et al.*) (See chapter C1-4), treatment of ADA deficiency with ADA gene transduced hematopoietic stem cells (Aiuti *et al.*) (See chapter C1-3) and Adrenoleukodystrophy (ALD) as the first clinical success reported with lentivirus-vector transduced haematopoietic cells (Cartier *et al.*) (See chapter C1-2).

The production of cells for clinical use is hampered by numerous difficulties. The product should be GMP-compliant. The cells should be effective and targeted to specific diseases. They should be non-toxic or have acceptable toxicity in view of the severity of the disease and related favourable risk/benefit ratio. The cells often have to be expanded either for efficient transduction with the candidate gene or else with view to obtaining the desired efficacy.

An important aim for the Cell Therapy platform has been to develop methods for production of various cell types for clinical use. We describe here how NK cells can be effectively expanded with increased efficacy in experimental systems (Alici and Gahrton) (See chapter A4-4). Transduction of expanded NK cells with specific genes seems to make them even more effective for malignant cell killing.

Other cells have shown importance for immunologic suppression. Mesenchymal stem cell (MSC) are important immune suppressor cells. Currently they are being tested with view to treating and preventing graft versus host disease (GVHD) associated with allogeneic stem cell transplantation. Large numbers of cells are frequently needed. Cruz *et al.* (See chapter A4-2) and Lindenmaier *et al.* (See chapter A4-3) describe methods for their expansion and production in large quantities.

Other cells of therapeutic importance are dendritic cells (DC:s) that are used for various vaccination strategies. Lindenmaier *et al.* describe a completely closed bag system for the generation of human monocyte derived DC:s. Using sterile docking, all steps from cell isolation by leukapheresis to cryo-conservation of adenovirally modified DC:s are performed without opening the system. In another project efficacy of vaccination of mice with dendritic cells transduced with IL-12 has been documented in HPV16-associated tumours [1].

Regulatory T-cells are important immune regulators. They can be used to suppress immune reaction and are tried to treat various immunological disorders. On the other hand they can also be depleted to enhance a graft versus tumor effect in association with allogeneic stem cell transplantation. Methods have been developed for their effective production as well as procedures to obtain clinical grade Treg depleted products which are described in this section (Klatzmann *et al.*) (See chapter A4-5). Their potential in cancer treatment is emphasized which includes first evidence of clinical efficacy in leukemia.

Fanconi anemia (FA) is a rare inherited genomic instability syndrome representing one of the best examples of hematopoietic stem cell deficiency. Here we describe (Cohen-Haguenauer *et al.*) (See chapter A4-6) how unselected bone marrow cells, that are retrovirally tranduced with the main complementation group FANCA-cDNA, could achieve long-term reconstitution of the stem cell compartment both *in vitro* and *in vivo*. Further on-going studies make use of novel lentivirus vectors. Taking from iPS cells as models, the ultimate goal would consist in expanding the gene-corrected cells to serve as an unlimited source for the treatment of FA aplastic anemia syndrome.

Cells transduced with therapeutic genes or manipulated in other ways to make them more effective for treatment of specific disorders will certainly be more important in the future. Hematopoietic stem cell transplantation was first performed in humans in 1957 and its therapeutic importance was not acknowledged until many years later. Therapy with gene manipulated stem cells or other cells types like NK cells, MSC:s and dendritic cells is only in its beginning.

ACKNOWLEDGMENTS

This work has been performed with the support of the EC-DG research through the FP6-Network of Excellence, CLINIGENE: LSHB-CT-2006-018933.

REFERENCE

1. Indrová M, Símová J, Bieblová J, Bubeník J, Reinis M. NK1.1+ cells are important for the development of protective immunity against MHC I-deficient, HPV16-associated tumours. *Oncol Rep* 2011; 25: 281-8.

The CliniBook: Clinical gene transfer
Edited by Odile Cohen-Haguenauer – EDK, Paris © 2012, pp. 187-193

A4-2
Ex-vivo expansion of human mesenchymal stem cells

Pedro E. Cruz[1,2]*, Helder J.S. Cruz[1], Rita N. Bárcia[1], Jorge M. Santos[1], Susanne Pohl[3], Mari Gilljam[4], Kurt E.J. Dittmar[3], Werner Lindenmaier[3], Evren Alici[4]

[1]ECBio, S.A., R. Henrique Paiva Couceiro, 27, 2700-451 Amadora, Portugal.
[2]IBET, Apartado 12, 2781-901 Oeiras, Portugal.
[3]Helmholtz-Centre for Infection Research, Inhoffenstr. 7, D-38124 Braunschweig, Germany.
[4]Cell and gene therapy center, department of medicine, divison of hematology, Karolinska Institutet, Karolinska University Hospital, Huddinge, Sweden.
pcruz@itqb.unl.pt
* Corresponding author

INTRODUCTION

Mesenchymal stem cells, or MSCs, were first isolated from bone marrow in the 1960's. MSCs are nonhematopoietic stem cells that have an inherent ability both to self-renew and to differentiate into multiple lineages including osteoblasts, chondrocytes and adipocytes [1]. MSCs adhere to plastic and are phenotypically characterized as CD73[+], CD90[+], CD105[+], CD14[-], CD34[-], CD19[-], HLA-DR[-] and CD45[-] [2].

Several sources of MSCs have been described and used in the clinic [3]. Most applications to date focus on the use of MSCs derived from bone marrow and adipose tissue [4]. The reason for this is that the tissues are available and collection is done by standardised, though very invasive, procedures. These cells are of adult origin and thus their expansion potential is low given that the clinical applications have to be performed at early passages (typically around 3) [5].

Other sources of MSCs for clinical applications are related to fetal or neonatal tissues namely umbilical cord blood and Wharton's jelly. Interest in these sources relates to the yields with more primitive MSCs allowing a larger expansion. Nevertheless, in the case of cord blood, the MSCs isolation success is below 50% and is highly dependent on the time between collection and processing, the volume of blood collected, and the nucleated cell content [6]. In contrast, the Wharton's jelly contains a much larger population of MSCs and the isolation success is close to 100%. The umbilical cord MSCs have more primitive properties than any other adult MSCs obtained later in life, which make them a useful source for clinical applications [5]. In Clinigene most of the work was done with MSCs derived from the Wharton's jelly, also named umbilical cord matrix - ucmMSCs.

BOTTLENECKS AND CHALLENGES

There are three major bottlenecks and challenges in the *ex vivo* expansion of MSCs for cellular therapy, which are related to the increasing requirements for cell expansion under GMP conditions: the definition of the culture medium and its supplements, the establishment of robust production systems and the standardisation of quality and safety assays.

Culture medium

Different isolation methods, culture conditions and media additives are known to affect cell yield and phenotype of the expanded cell product [7]. Consequently, the medium composition is crucial for both efficacy and safety of the final MSC product. Furthermore, the need for greater cell expansion demands that the media used maintain the phenotype, genotypic stability, and therapeutic activity of MSCs for several passages. The common use of fetal bovine serum (FBS) as a supplement poses several concerns. First, FBS shows significant batch-to-batch variability, which can result in negative effects on production yields. Second, it has been shown that MSCs can retain in their cytoplasm proteins present in FBS, which may thus be responsible for the transmission of prions or other zoonoses; these proteins may also cause immune reactions in the host - sensitization -, especially in the context of repeated injection protocols, ultimately leading to the rejection of the transplanted cells.

A logical approach to help solve these issues is the development of serum-free media, appropriate for cell expansion and devoid of risks associated to xenoproducts. Several media providers have developed serum-free media for MSC culture but since they lack adhesion molecules the process involves the coating of the culture surface. The fact that the coating is done with undisclosed composition formulations severely hampers their use in clinical trials [8].

As alternative supplements, human serum (HS) and platelet lysate (hPL) have shown good results with cell expansion. Although a higher percentage is necessary (20% in comparison with 10% for FBS) and the costs are significantly higher, some authors report increased proliferative capacity [7]. However, MSCs expanded in hPL containing medium showed impaired inhibitory capacity on T-cell proliferation to alloantigen and NK-cell proliferation and cytotoxicity, thus limiting their application as immunomodulators in clinical applications [9].

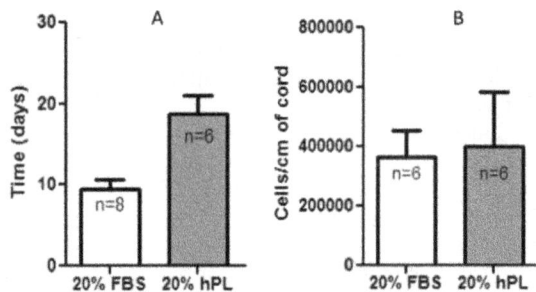

Figure 1. Comparison of the performance of fetal bovine serum (FBS) *versus* human platelet lysate (hPL) in umbilical cord matrix MSCs initial expansion: time to confluence until P0 (A) and cells per cm of cord at the end of P0 (B).

Also the replacement of FBS by HS or hPL may change processing yields. In the case of ucmMSCs the time to reach confluency in P0 is higher when hPL is used in comparison with FBS at the same percentage, although the final cell yield is the same (*Figure 1*). Nevertheless, after passage 1 the growth rates are very similar when FBS of hPL are used. The phenotypical characterization further showed the presence of CD31 expressing subpopulations that, although being a minority, confirm the influence of medium additives in cell characteristics.

Culture techniques

For GMP production of MSCs, as for any other cellular products involving long term cell culture, the establishment and validation of aseptic conditions are required [10]. Since the validation of aseptic techniques is an important part of the validation process for MSC production, closed systems have advantages over classic T-flasks. In fact, for a typical therapeutic dose of 10^6 cells/kg the necessary dosing will consist in almost 10^8 MSCs, which corresponds to over ten 175cm^2 flasks. The increase in the number of required flasks significantly increases the risk of contamination, in particular as it is preferable to avoid the use of antibiotics. Some suppliers have nevertheless developed multilayered systems that can be stacked in incubators. These culture devices can be used to expand MSCs with savings in personnel costs, contamination risk, culture medium volume, incubator space and the number of flasks in a quasi-closed system. However, cell harvest is a more complicated step and may need complex optimisation. Using the CellSTACKs (Corning) or culture bags (Macopharma) it is possible to produce more than 10^8 cells in 3 weeks [11].

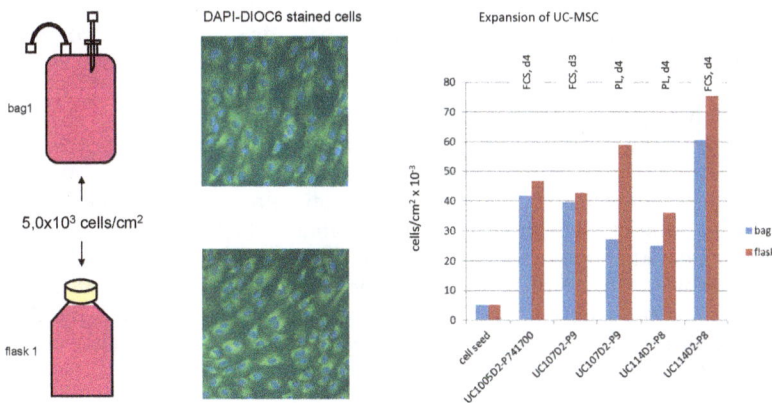

Figure 2. ucmMSC grown in αMEM-supplemented with 20%FCS or 10% hPL were seeded in parallel in cell culture flasks and APTMS-coated bags at a density of 5x10^3 cells/ cm^2 . Staining with DAPI/DIOC6 shows adherent growth in the coated bag comparable to growth on the flask surface. After expansion for 3 or 4 days cell yields were determined.

At ECBio, a new protocol has been developed for the isolation of ucmMSCs which is safe, robust, greatly efficient in terms of cell number/tissue mass, and effective against microbiological contaminations often found in umbilical cord samples obtained from non caesarean births. Both technical aspects and main applications of the method are protected by patent (PCT/IB2008/054067). The high yields obtained permit to initiate differentiation at very early passages and allow a great expansion potential compatible with the clinical demand for high cell numbers at low passages in order to meet safety requirements. Such characteristics make this protocol ideal for working under GMP and broadly expanding the scope of clinical applications. In order to meet the *ex-vivo* expansion challenges, a closed bag system that has been tested for bone marrow-derived MSCs was evaluated for ucmMSCs. The inner surface of the cultivation bag is modified by dielectric barrier discharge (DBD) to allow adherent cell growth [12]. The modified bags have been tested for cell expansion and *in situ* cryopreservation in a completely closed system (Patent application No. EP10165451.1). Comparison of bag cultivated bone marrow derived MSC with ucmMSCs with respect to surface markers, transduction efficiency and expression profile did not show significant differences (*Figure 2*).

Expanded ucmMSCs were successfully transduced in closed bags using GFP encoding AdV vectors. Furthermore, genetic modification of ucmMSCs was also performed with a clinical grade lentiviral vector coding for TK.007-IRES-OuaS. Despite the low titer yields with transient production, it was possible to satisfactorily transduce MSCs with this vector. *In vivo* analysis of transduced and selected cells and further *ex vivo* transduction protocol are currently ongoing.

Safety issues

One of the most critical issues in MSC culture is the culture duration. Adult MSCs may acquire karyotypic abnormalities during long-term culture. Thus, to further broaden MSC application as an immunosuppressive therapeutic option, different sources with richer seeding populations are needed. For this purpose, umbilical cord matrix MSCs (ucmMSCs) seem to be one of the prime candidates to test. Genomic stability remains a major safety concern that needs to be addressed using karyotype and comparative genomic hybridization. Tarte and colleagues (2010) showed that clinical grade-cultured human MSCs reached senescence and never transformed, in spite of the presence of aneuploidy (mainly duplication of chromosomes 5 and 8) [11].

In order to evidence any potential for malignant proliferation, a significant effort was made to analyse clonality of ucmMSCs at different passages. In short, all karyotype analysis samples gave good quality after overnight activation with colchicine for metaphasic fixing. A total of 20 metaphases and 400 bands were analysed.

The latest passage that is analysed so far is passage 15 where no clonal aberrations were found. The analyses were confirmed by two independent specialists at different time points from the same culture samples. A typical karyotypic overview is shown in *Figure 3*. *In vivo* assays were also performed for ucmMSCs. Cells were introduced in testicular capsules of SCID-Beige mice where no teratoma formation was observed.

Quality control and criteria for cell release

The existence of validated quality controls are of germane importance in GMP to ensure the safety and efficacy of the MSCs. For microbiological safety, controls are well described and standardized. As in the case of the established microbiological tests, other assays need to be standardised including the evaluation of the risks related to transformation and senescence and MSC immunomodulatory properties and differentiation potential. These protocols will have to be used as quality controls of GMP-grade MSCs to test their characteristics before their clinical use.

We have spent significant effort to set-up a GMP certified phenotypic characterization of freshly isolated as well as long-term cultured and gene modified MSCs. A multi-parameter flow cytometric panel is now established using the following mon-oclonal antibodies: CD31 (WM59,BD), CD34 (581,BD), CD73 (AD2,BD), CD90 (eBio5E10,eBioscience), CD44(G44-26,BD), CD14 (MoP9,BD), CD19 (HIB19,BD), HLA-DR (Tu36,Invitrogen), CD45 (HI30,Invitrogen), CCR1(53504,R&D), CCR2(48607,R&D), CCR3(5E8,BD), CCR7(3D12,BD), CCR9(112509,BD), CCR10(314305,R&D), CX3CR1(2A9-1,BioLegend), CXCR4(12G5,BD), CXCR5(RF8B2,BD), CXCR6(56811,R&D), C3aR(hC3aRZ8,BD), C5aR(D53-1473,BD), CCR4(1G1,BD), CCR5(2D7,BD), and CXCR3(1C6,BD). The estab-lished panel has been tested and validated with MSCs from umbilical cord matrix, adipose tissue, bone marrow and foetal sources.

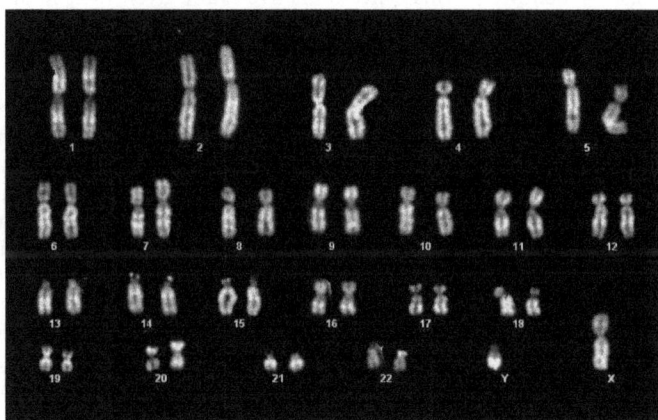

Figure 3. Typical result of karyotype analysis of ucmMSCs at passage 7. No chromosomal abnor-malities were observed.

FUTURE DIRECTIONS

As the use of MSCs becomes more and more widespread and the knowledge about the cells' properties consolidates, new challenges arise. The possibility of allogeneic use for a number of conditions raises the bar for *ex-vivo* expansion of MSCs, more specifically with safety aspects. Donor selection criteria and quality and safety assays will have to be standardised in order to establish the full potential of these cells.

Allogeneic application

The clinical potential of MSCs is far from being limited to their differentiation poten-tial and applications in regenerative medicine. Due to their low immunogenicity, MSCs may be transplanted in HLA-unmatched individuals [13]. An international phase II trial showed a 68% response rate to BM-MSC infusion in therapy-refractory GvHD patients [14]. Indeed, resident MSCs suppress both transient and continuous immune surveillance, which aims at facilitating the healing process [15]. These observations make undifferentiated MSCs important agents to treat both autoimmune and/or in-flammation-related disorders particularly in the allogeneic context.

For the current applications, MSCs are already greatly expanded *ex vivo* before use [2]. The allogeneic use of MSCs will put pressure on the *ex-vivo* expansion processes having impact in a number of areas related to clinical grade MSC production, namely the selection of donors and the standardisation of quality and safety assays.

Donor selection

Apart from the usual donor eligibility criteria including the absence of HIV1, HIV2, HepB and syphilis the criteria for a good allogeneic MSC donor are not easy to establish. For some specific sources such as bone marrow, age is relevant due to the decrease in MSC cell numbers and proliferation rates with the donor's age. Also, the existence of abnormalities or risk of abnormalities is likely to increase with the age of the donor. In contrast, in the case of ucmMSCs this criterion is irrelevant given their neonatal nature.

Standardisation of quality and safety assays

As mentioned above, the use of different isolation methods and culture conditions may lead to distinct MSC populations with slightly different immunophenotypical and functional properties. This fact emphasizes the need for the establishment and validation of isolation and expansion protocols supported by the use of immunophenotypic, functional and genetic stability assays. These assays should be performed before *in vivo* infusion in order to ensure that the MSCs remain suitable for clinical application after *ex vivo* expansion. A thorough analysis of surface markers and functional assays is required and recommended in order to specifically identify subpopulations of MSCs that should be further investigated. Furthermore, the use of microarray analysis can shed some light on the MSC expression profile and its relation to certain functional properties.

By addressing these challenges in MSC *ex vivo* expansion it is likely that in a near future MSCs will become a main therapeutic option in an allogeneic context in several areas, particularly as modulators of the immune response in hematopoietic stem cell transplantation, inflammatory and autoimmune diseases.

ACKNOWLEDGMENTS

This work has been performed with the support of the EC-DG research through the FP6-Network of Excellence, CLINIGENE: LSHB-CT-2006-018933.

REFERENCES

1. Pittenger MF, Mackay AM, Beck SC, Jaiswal RK, Douglas R, Mosca JD, *et al.* Multilineage potential of adult human mesenchymal stem cells. *Science* 1999; 284:143-7.

2. Horwitz EM, Le Blanc K, Dominici M, Mueller I, Slaper-Cortenbach I, Marini FC, *et al.* Clarification of the nomenclature for MSC: the International society for cellular therapy position statement. *Cytotherapy* 2005; 7: 393-5.

3. Barry FP, Murphy JM. Mesenchymal stem cells: clinical applications and biological characterization. *Int J Biochem Cell Biol* 2004; 36: 568-84.

4. Sensebe L, Bourin P, Tarte K. Good manufacturing practices production of mesenchymal stem/stromal cells. *Hum Gene Ther* 2011; 22: 19-26.

5. Troyer DL, Weiss ML. Wharton's jelly-derived cells are a primitive stromal cell population. *Stem Cells* 2008; 26: 591-9.

6. Bieback K, Kern S, Kluter H, Eichler H. Critical parameters for the isolation of mesenchymal stem cells from umbilical cord blood. *Stem Cells* 2004; 22: 625-34.

7. Bernardo ME, Cometa AM, Pagliara D, Vinti L, Rossi F, Cristantielli R, *et al. Ex vivo* expansion of mesenchymal stromal cells. *Best Pract Res Clin Haematol* 2011; 24: 73-81.

8. Philippe B, Luc S, Valerie PB, Jerome R, Alessandra BR, Louis C. Culture and use of mesenchymal stromal cells in phase I and II clinical trials. *Stem Cells Int* 2010; 2010: 503-93.

9. Abdelrazik H, Spaggiari GM, Chiossone L, Moretta L. Mesenchymal stem cells expanded in human platelet lysate display a decreased inhibitory capacity on T and NK-cell proliferation and function. *Eur J Immunol* 2011; 41: 3281-90.

10. Alici E, Blomberg P. GMP facilities for manufacturing of advanced therapy medicinal products for clinical trials: an overview for clinical researchers. *Curr Gene Ther* 2010; 10:508-15.

11. Tarte K, Gaillard J, Lataillade JJ, Fouillard L, Becker M, Mossafa H, *et al.* Clinical-grade production of human mesenchymal stromal cells: occurrence of aneuploidy without transformation. *Blood* 2010; 115: 1549-53.

12. Lachmann K, Dohse A, Thomas M, Pohl S, Meyring W, Dittmar KEJ, *et al.* Surface modification of closed plastic bags for adherent cell cultivation. *Eur Phys J Appl Phys* 2011; 55: 533-7.

13. Le Blanc K, Ringden O. Immunomodulation by mesenchymal stem cells and clinical experience. *J Intern Med* 2007; 262: 509-25.

14. Le Blanc K, Frassoni F, Ball L, Locatelli F, Roelofs H, Lewis I, *et al.* Mesenchymal stem cells for treatment of steroid-resistant, severe, acute graft-versus-host disease: a phase II study. *Lancet* 2008; 371: 1579-86.

15. Petrie Aronin CE, Tuan RS. Therapeutic potential of the immunomodulatory activities of adult mesenchymal stem cells. *Birth Defects Res C Embryo Today* 2010; 90: 67-74.

The CliniBook: Clinical gene transfer
Edited by Odile Cohen-Haguenauer – EDK, Paris © 2012, pp. 194-200

A4-3
Closed bag cultivation systems for the production of gene modified dendritic cells and MSC for clinical use

WERNER LINDENMAIER[1]*, LARS MACKE[1,2], WILHELM MEYRING[1,2], HENK S.P. GARRITSEN[2], KURT E.J. DITTMAR[1], KRISTINA LACHMANN[3], MICHAEL THOMAS[3]

[1] *Department of Molecular Biotechnology, Helmholtz Centre for Infection Research (HZI), Inhoffenstr. 7, D-38124 Braunschweig, Germany.* [2] *Institute for Clinical Transfusion Medicine, Städtisches Klinikum Braunschweig gGmbH, Braunschweig, Germany.*
[3] *Fraunhofer-Institut für Schicht- und Oberflächentechnik (IST), Braunschweig, Germany.*
werner.lindenmaier@helmholtz-hzi.de
* Corresponding author

INTRODUCTION

The new insights and developments in the areas of genetics and cell biology open up a plethora of cell based new treatment options for inherited and acquired diseases. A major drawback of such cell therapeutic approaches is the fact that in general it requires the isolated cultivation and genetic modification of autologous cells. This is, however, not an insurmountable obstacle. Well established examples of cell therapies are transplantation of haematopoietic stem cells (HSCs), adoptive T-cells transfer and the correction of immune-deficiencies [1]. The potential of this approach is intensively investigated in connection with the availability of pluripotent stem cells. Until now, however, more widespread application of cell therapies is prevented by the limited availability and the difficulties in the cultivation and modification of the primary human cells. Moreover, standardisation and GMP compliant cultivation, which is required for advanced therapies medicinal products (ATMP) represent a major unsolved challenge [2].
The aim of this project was to contribute to the development cGMP-compliant standardized cultivation systems for the generation of dendritic cells (DC) and mesenchymal stromal cells (MSC) for immunotherapies. Dendritic cells are the antigen presenting cells that can initiate an effective immune response by stimulating naive T-cells. But also in secondary responses they represent the most effective immune stimulators [3]. Vaccination with dendritic cells (DC) therefore is an appealing strategy to induce effective immune responses to tumours and persistent infections. Standardized *ex vivo* generation of genetically modified APC is an important prerequisite of DC vaccine development. It allows optimising and testing the stimulatory properties in advance. Mesenchymal stromal cells (MSC), on the other hand, represent multipotent

adult stem cells with the capacity to differentiate into different cell types, *e.g.* into osteogenic, adipogenic and chondrogenic lineages [4]. In the context of immunotherapies they have the potential to control immune reactions. The immunomodulatory properties of mesenchymal stem cells have been demonstrated in therapies for several inflammatory and immune related disorders [5, 6].

For the development of a standardized, cGMP-compliant production system for the therapeutic cells a modular bag system has many advantages with respect to handling, safety, and flexibility. Therefore we developed a completely closed bag system for the generation of human monocyte derived dendritic cells. Using sterile docking, all steps starting from cell isolation by leukapheresis up to the final formulation and cryo-conservation of adenovirally modified DC can be performed without opening the system. For the cultivation of the adherently growing MSC the system was adapted by coating of the bag surface using dielectric barrier discharge. Quality controls and a scrutinized, detailed comparison of bag and flask generated cells demonstrated the feasibility of closed bag cultivation for both cell types.

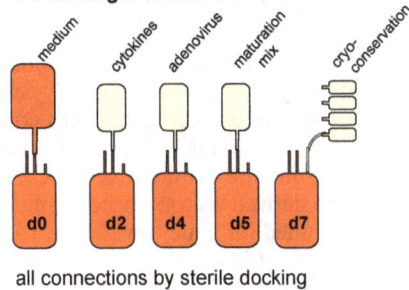

RESULTS

Closed bag dendritic cell cultivation

Major efforts of the project were directed towards the development of a cultivation system for the safe, GMP-compliant generation of human dendritic cells for therapeutic application in collaboration with the academic and industrial partners. For this purpose the reproducible generation of sufficient numbers of well defined pure APC is required. With the objective of efficient, long term, antigen presentation in the context of diverse MHC haplotypes these cells should be modified for endogenous expression of multiple defined antigens. Therefore, a safe and standardised, GMP compliant integrated completely closed bag cultivation system had to be developed (*Figure 1*).

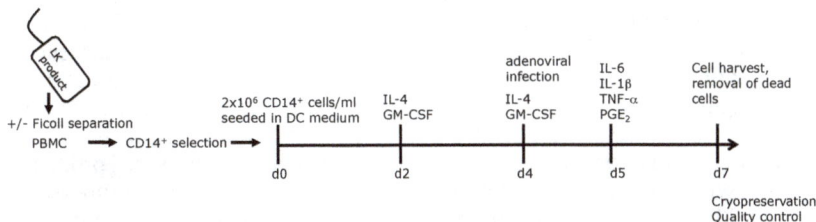

Figure 1. Completely closed bag system for DC by combination. A. Commercial closed bag systems, leukapheresis for cell isolation and the CliniMacs system for precursor cell purification, were combined with a bag-cultivation system, in which all steps including differentiation, genetic modification, maturation and cryo-conservation are included. The time schedule for DC cultivation and QC is given in B.

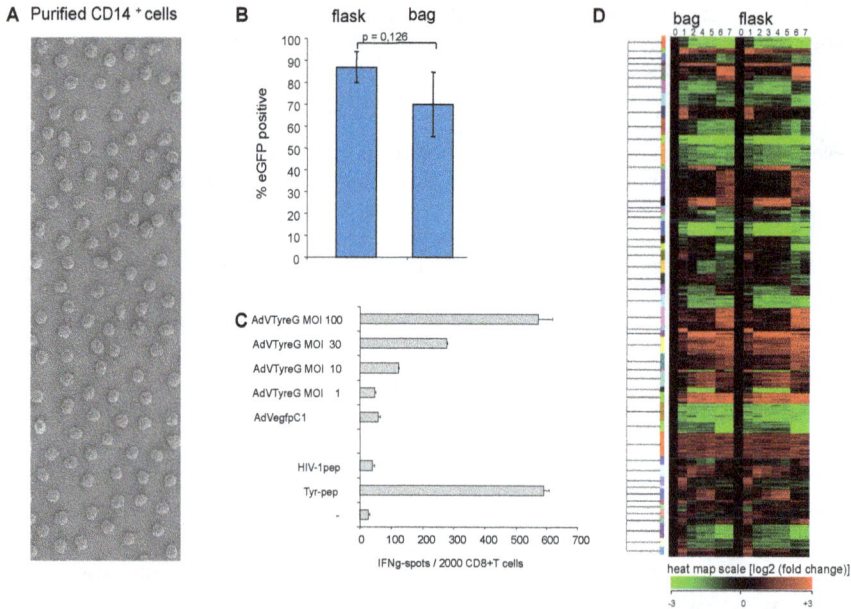

Figure 2. Characterisation of bag and flask cultivated dendritic cells. A. Electron micrograph of CliniMacs-sorted CD14 positive cells shows a homogenous monocyte population (purity >90% according to flow cytometry). B. Transduction efficacy by adenoviral vectors was determined as gfp-positive cells after infection with AdVeGFP. C. Antigen presentation of adenovirally infected cells. Stimulation of a tyrosinase specific T-cell line was determined as a function of m.o.i. used for adenoviral gene transfer by AdTyreG, a recombinant adenovirus encoding tyrosinase and eGFP. The transduced gene product is processed and presented efficiently to antigen specific T-cells after the 7 day cultivation period. The stimulatory efficacy is comparable to DC loaded with the specific peptide in this *in vitro* assay. D. The expression profiles of flask DC were indistinguishable from the profiles of the bag DC, as shown here by k-means clustering of the 1547 genes regulated during the cultivation period. No significant difference between bag and flask culture was detected.

Toward implementation of this concept monocytes isolated by leukapheresis were positively selected using magnetic cell sorting yielding about 1.2×10^9 CD14+-cells which represent about 10% of altogether 10^{10} cells collected by leukapheresis [7]. Serum-free cultivation conditions and GMP-grade cytokines were used to generate immature dendritic cells. The immature dendritic cells were genetically modified with recombinant adenovirus type 5 derived vectors encoding multiple defined protein antigens [8]. These vectors are well suited for gene transfer into a variety of primary cells with high efficacy, have a low risk of insertional mutagenesis and do not significantly interfere with cellular functions. The adenocosmid system allows simple construction of recombinant viral genomes. By insertion of multicistronic expression cassettes into the E1 or the E3 loci a collection of vectors has been created, which express a variety of transgenes encoding for *e.g.*: tumour or viral antigens, co-stimulatory molecules or cytokines, reporter genes or regulatory functions [7, 9, 10]. They are also able to efficiently transduce non-proliferating cells like immature dendritic cells (DC) since up to 99% of the latter could be transduced at an m.o.i. of 30 pfu/cell [8]. After DC maturation the cell product could be cryopreserved. Final yield of DC was about 18% of the isolated monocytes, of which about 80% were CD83+ mature dendritic cells. The quality of the product was controlled by biochemical and functional assays (*Figure 2*). All steps from cell isolation by leukapheresis up to the final formulation of the cryopreserved gene-modified cell product were performed in the closed bag system using sterile docking. Stringent comparison of closed bag cultivated DC with DC cultivated in conventional cell culture flasks confirmed that bag-DC characteristics prove as good as the "golden standard" [7, 8]. A master batch protocol for GMP compliant generation of modified DC at the GBF-GMP facility based on clinical grade materials and standard operating procedures (SOP's) was established. Quality control for cell products included tests for genetic identity and stability, global expression profiling and functional assays of stimulatory capacity [11].

Modified closed bag cell cultivation system for MSC

The closed process for the generation of adenovirus- modified dendritic cells was developed with the DC generation bag (Miltenyi). When exploiting the advantages of the closed bag system for the cultivation of mesenchymal stromal cells, however, available cell culture bags did not support growth of adherent cells like MSC. To overcome these limitations we investigated the possibility to modify the inner surface of the bag. A possible solution is provided by the application of dielectric barrier discharge (*Figure 3*). This technique allows the modification of plastic surfaces in a flexible and defined way, as suitable precursor molecules are introduced into the bag together with the carrier gas (He) during plasma treatment [12]. The inner surface and possible 3D objects included are then coated according to the precursors added. A number of materials and modifications were tested for biocombatibility and support of adherent cell growth. Polyolefine or Teflon bags coated with precursors providing amino functions (APTMS – aminopropyltrimethoxysilane, DACH – diaminocyclohexane) proved to be especially well suited. Established MSC lines could be expanded on these surfaces (*Figure 4A*) also under "animal free" cultivation conditions. Bag cultivated cells retained osteogenic and adipogenic differentiation potential (*Figure 4B*). In addition we have shown that mesenchymal stromal cells can also be efficiently modified with adenoviral vectors [13] with view to influencing their regenerative and immune-modulatory functions. Addition of adenoviral vectors to the bag cultures allowed genetic modification of MSC with an efficacy comparable to standard flask cultivated MSC. Furthermore, direct *in situ* cryoconservation of adherent cell onto the modified surfaces is possible [14]. These surface modified bags therefore provide a basis for the development of a closed bag system for adherent cells. Through variations in both physicochemical and biological properties of the surfaces further optimisation is possible.

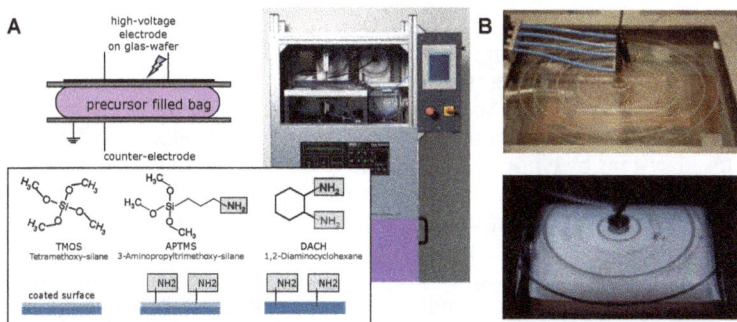

Figure 3. Surface modification by dielectric barrier discharge. A. Scheme of the modification of the inner surface of the bags by plasma treatment. The bag is filled with carrier gas and precursor molecules of choice. Three of the precursors tested are shown here. APTMS and DACH coated bags supported growth of adherent primary human cells, *e.g.* mesenchymal stem cell. A prototype apparatus (M. Thomas, FhG IST) with automatic filling station and ITO electrode is shown on the right. B. Bag between electrodes. After application of high voltage the ignited plasma lights up.

For quality control of MSC flow cytometry analysis of relevant cell surface markers (CD73, CD90, CD105), differentiation assays and expression profiling (*Figure 4C*) to describe the global status of cell activity were established. In addition, authenticity and chromosomal integrity are becoming important issues especially for cells like MSC, which require extensive expansion [11]. The necessity of such controls is underscored by the observation that up to 30 per cent of cell lines are misidentified. Short tandem repeat (STR)-, microsatellite instability (MSI)- and mtDNA-analysis as well as karyotyping were used to control identity and euploidy. Even though available techniques are not yet sensitive enough to exclude oncogenic alterations in single cells and potential selection of oncogenic variants, they allow a thorough quality control in verifying that the conditions of isolation, modification, and expansion do not strongly select mutated genotypes.

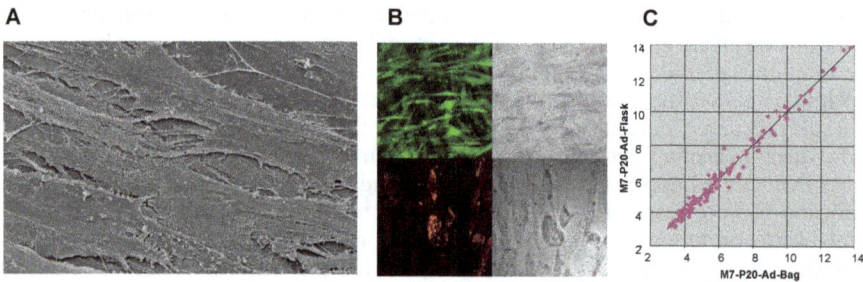

Figure 4. Characterisation of bag cultivated mesenchymal stem cells. A. Electron micrograph shows adherent growth of bone derived MSC on APTMS coated bag surface. B. Osteogenic and adipogenic differentiation of bag-cultivated MSC. For osteogenic differentiation (top) cells were stimulated for 28 days with β-glycerophosphate, ascorbic acid and dexamethasone. Confocal micrographs of calcein staining in APTMS modified bags are shown. Adipogenic differentiation (bottom) was stimulated by IBMX, insulin and hydrocortisone supplemented basal medium. Adipogenic potential was demonstrated by Nile Red staining of lipid droplets. C. Expression profiling of adenovirally modified MSC cultivated in parallel in bags and flasks was done using Affymetrix HG-U133_Plus_2 arrays. Expression signals for genes involved in lineage definition and immunoregulation were extracted for pairwise comparison of bag and flask cultures. No significant difference between bag and flask cultivated MSC was detected also when all 54,676 probesets were compared.

CONCLUSIONS

The goal of this project was to develop a cultivation system for standardized reproducible, cGMP-compliant production of autologous human cells for immunotherapies, especially dendritic cells and mesenchymal stem cells. Bag systems, widely used in clinical applications, were used as the basis for the development of these cultivation systems. For the generation of monocyte derived dendritic cells we could realise a completely closed system by combining leukapheresis, CliniMacs cell separation, and bag cultivation. In this system all manipulations including cell isolation, separation, cultivation, genetic modification up to the final conservation step in bags were done using sterile docking. Using this system, it will be possible to produce cellular vaccines in a standardized procedure adapted to low-cost GMP requirements. Genetic modification of the immature dendritic cells is easily achieved using recombinant adenoviruses. Simultaneous transfer and expression of multiple target genes allows the presentation of multiple epitopes by different HLA alleles and reduces the risk of immune escape. Cryo-conservation of the final gene modified DC vaccine is a prerequisite of relevant quality control before therapeutic application. Quality control of DC by flow cytometry allowed determining homogeneity and viability and the efficiency of adenoviral gene transfer. Tests for genetic integrity and authenticity in addition to functional assays are included for a well-defined cell product. The modular nature facilitates upgrading and adaptation of transduction, cultivation and cryopreservation protocols.

Toward further translating the system to MSC, the bags had to be modified because they did not support adherent cell growth necessary for the expansion of MSC. For the generation of MSC-compatible surfaces we took advantage of a newly developed efficient atmospheric-pressure plasma process. By dielectric barrier discharge it was feasible to modify the inner surface of the cell culture bags at will, depending on the choice of the chemical precursors which were used to modify the surface. The use of hydrophilic and positively charged precursors most efficiently supported the attachment and growth of adherence-dependent cells. Cultivation of adherent cell lines, epithelial progenitor cells and mesenchymal stem cells proved successful on each dedicated modified bag surface only. MSC expanded in APTMS-modified bags retained their growth characteristics, expression profile and differentiation potential. In addition, MSC could be cultured under FCS-free conditions, genetically modified by direct addition of recombinant adenoviral vectors and finally cryo-preserved as the adherent cell layer on the modified surface.

Given data presented here, we believe that a bag based, easy to use, closed system technology is especially well suited for clinical applications. These bag based systems may advance the technology for cultivating and manipulating cells from various sources for routine use in therapeutic application or cell expansion. The flexibility of the surface modification and the modular nature allow easy adaptation to the specific requirements of each application. In parallel to cultivation technologies, methods for structural and especially functional characterisation of the different cells have to be developed further as part of quality control and as diagnostic tool. By providing reproducible, standardized culture conditions for the generation of defined cell products the bag cultivation systems hopefully can contribute to easier and more widespread successful application of cells- and gene-modified cells- based therapeutic products.

ACKNOWLEDGEMENTS

Thanks for excellent technical assistance are due to J. Draheim, K. Littmann-Janßen, and S. Pohl. We are grateful for cells and advice to N. Zghoul and B. Wörmann, to W. Dirks, DSMZ, Braunschweig and H. Hannig, Klinikum Braunschweig, for genetic analysis, to K. Miller, MHH, Hannover, for karyotyping, to A. Dohse for surface coating and to R. Geffers, HZI-Array facility, for help with expression profiling.

This work has been performed with the support of the EC-DG research through the FP6-Network of Excellence, CLINIGENE: LSHB-CT-2006-018933 and by grants from the Federal Ministry of Economics and Technology (Innonet projects 16IN170 and 16IN0546), the German Research Foudation (DFG) through the Excellence Cluster Rebirth.

REFERENCES

1. Naldini L. *Ex vivo* gene transfer and correction for cell-based therapies. *Nat Rev Genet* 2011; 12: 301-15.

2. Committee for Advanced Therapies (CAT) and CAT scientific secretariat. Challenges with advanced therapy medicinal products and how to meet them. *Nat Rev Drug Discov* 2010; 9: 195-201.

3. Banchereau J, Steinman RM. Dendritic cells and the control of immunity. *Nature* 1998; 392: 245-52.

4. Dominici M, Le Blanc K, Mueller I, Slaper-Cortenbach I, Marini F, Krause D, *et al*. Minimal criteria for defining multipotent mesenchymal stromal cells. The International Society for Cellular Therapy position statement. *Cytotherapy* 2006; 8: 315-7.

5. Le Blanc K, Frassoni F, Ball L, Locatelli F, Roelofs H, Lewis I, *et al*. Mesenchymal stem cells for treatment of steroid-resistant, severe, acute graft-versus-host disease: a phase II study. *Lancet* 2008; 371: 1579-86.

6. Barry FP, Murphy JM. Mesenchymal stem cells: clinical applications and biological characteri-zation. *Int J Biochem Cell Biol* 2004; 36: 568-84.

7. Macke L, Garritsen HS, Meyring W, Hannig H, Pagelow U, Wormann B, *et al*. Evaluating matu-ration and genetic modification of human dendritic cells in a new polyolefin cell culture bag system. *Transfusion* 2010; 50: 843-55.

8. Garritsen HS, Macke L, Meyring W, Hannig H, Pagelow U, Wormann B, *et al*. Efficient generation of clinical-grade genetically modified dendritic cells for presentation of multiple tumor-associated proteins. *Transfusion* 2010; 50: 831-42.

9. Wiethe C, Dittmar K, Doan T, Lindenmaier W, Tindle R. Provision of 4-1BB ligand enhances ef-fector and memory CTL responses generated by immunization with dendritic cells expressing a hu-man tumor-associated antigen. *J Immunol* 2003; 170: 2912-22.

10. Wiethe C, Dittmar K, Doan T, Lindenmaier W, Tindle R. Enhanced effector and memory CTL responses generated by incorporation of receptor activator of NF-kappaB (RANK)/RANK ligand costimulatory molecules into dendritic cell immunogens expressing a human tumor-specific antigen. *J Immunol* 2003; 171: 4121-30.

11. Dittmar KE, Simann M, Zghoul N, Schon O, Meyring W, Hannig H, *et al*. Quality of cell products: authenticity, identity, genomic stability and status of differentiation. *Transfus Med He-mother* 2010; 37: 57-64.

12. Lachmann K, Dohse A, Thomas M, Pohl S, Meyring W, Dittmar KE, *et al*. Surface modification of closed plastic bags for adherent cell cultivation. In: Hakone XII, *12th International Symposium on High Pressure Low Temperature Plasma Chemistry*. Trencianske Teplice, Slovakia, 2010: 533-7.

13. Mayer H, Bertram H, Lindenmaier W, Korff T, Weber H, Weich H. Vascular endothelial growth factor (VEGF-A) expression in human mesenchymal stem cells: autocrine and paracrine role on os-teoblastic and endothelial differentiation. *J Cell Biochem* 2005; 95 :827-39.

14. Dittmar KEJ, Lindenmaier W, Zghoul N, Just L, Garritsen H, Thomas M, *et al*. Process for cell cultivation and for cyropreservation. *Patent filed EP09162323* 2010.

The CliniBook: Clinical gene transfer
Edited by Odile Cohen-Haguenauer – EDK, Paris © 2012, pp. 201-207

A4-4
Genetically modified NK cells for cancer treatment: facts and visions

Evren Alici, Gösta Gahrton*

Karolinska Institutet, Department of Medicine, Karolinska University Hospital, Huddinge, SE 14186 Stockholm, Sweden.
gosta.gahrton@ki.se
* Corresponding author

BACKGROUND

Natural killer (NK) cells are innate lymphocytes with an immediate response capability and are a part of the interface of the adaptive and innate immune systems. NK cell recognition of target cells is a tightly regulated process that involves a balance of signals from various activating and inhibitory receptors that dictate their overall response [1]. Owing to their immune stimulatory and direct cytotoxic functions, NK cells are appealing to be exploited for immunotherapy especially in the hematopoietic stem cell transplantation (HSCT) setting where they are shown to improve leukemia treatment [2]. Despite its significant promise, clinical implementation of NK cell-based therapy is currently limited due to the lack of robust isolation and expansion techniques for generating clinical-grade NK cell products. The obvious route for acquiring NK cells is their enrichment from leukapheresis products under GMP conditions. However, low NK cell yield, and poor activation status are issues that have not been solved so far. The main obstacle originates from the fact that they are normally present only in low numbers in peripheral blood mononuclear cells (PBMCs) and effector cell preparations such as LAK cells. Thus, a significant challenge to the development of successful NK cell adoptive transfer protocols has been the difficulty to obtain sufficient number of active cells [1].

SELECTIVE EXPANSION OF NATURAL KILLER CELLS

Our group has described a novel method using GMP quality media and culture components that allows us to expand high numbers of polyclonal NK cells using PBMCs from healthy donors [3], as well as patients with hematological malignancies [4, 5] (*Figure 1*). These cells have been shown to exert specific cytotoxic activity against fresh human tumor cells *in vitro* [5] and in experimental models of human tumors [6] which opened up the possibility of their use in clinical settings. A phase I/II clinical trial where we administered allogeneic donor derived *ex vivo* expanded NK cells in patients with solid tumors and chronic leukemia has recently been completed [7]. No severe side effects, or signs of GVHD developed. Infusion of the *ex vivo* expanded cells were found to be safe, whether administered alone or with IL-2. Furthermore, a phase I clinical trial for the use of such expanded cells following autologous transplantation in multiple myeloma is now approved by the Swedish medicinal products agency as an investigational ATMP.

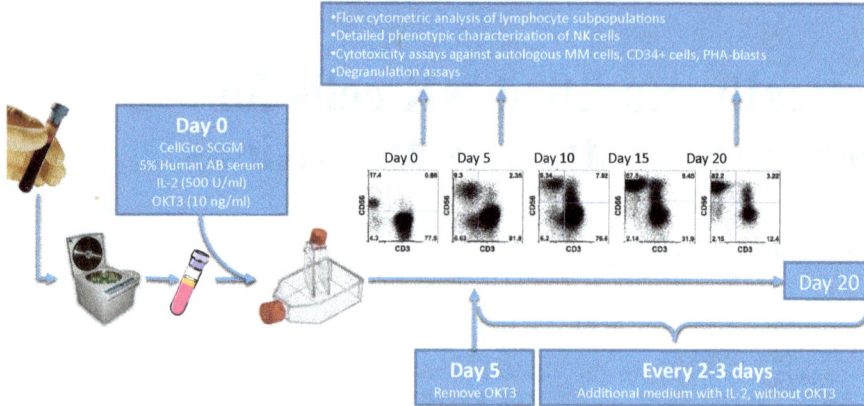

Figure 1. The NK cell expansion process and established release criteria. NK cells preferentially take over the culture reaching up to 90% purity at the end of expansion process. A representative flow cytometric read-out is presented.

Although applied in the clinic and well tolerated in general, there are disadvantages that render previous protocols suboptimal and unfeasible for large-scale clinical studies. An optimal procedure for the expansion of effector cells should be cost-effective, easy to handle and must include well-defined cGMP quality components, as well as a preferably dynamic closed culture system free of animal products and feeder cells. Unfortunately, previous studies that fulfill these criteria report relatively low levels of cell expansion, which may be sufficient in some cases but still needs improvement (*Figure 2*).

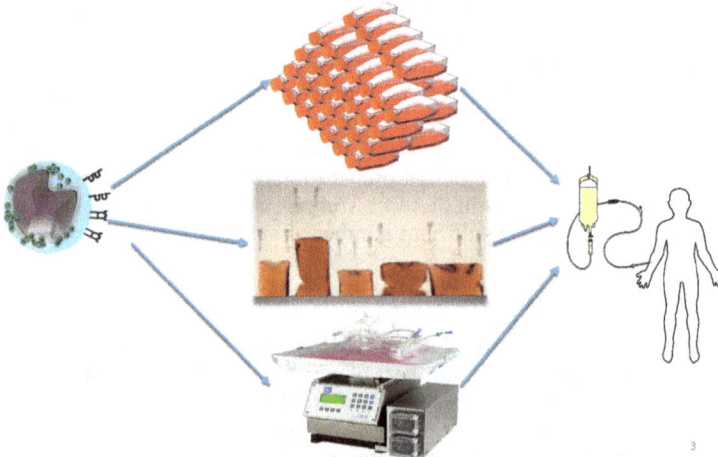

Figure 2. Current NK cell expansion strategies. Expansions in cell culture flasks are tedious, infection-prone and costly. Thus, alternative expansion systems are needed. The figure shows expansions in static bags and bioreactor systems. Expansion yield and purity in bioreactor systems proved to be comparable to flask based expansions.

We have demonstrated that both the Wave Bioreactor and Vuelife bags provide expansion of NK cells with the latter having higher fold expansion at the expense of decreased purity. An overall comparison of the expansion rates and end product purity between the two closed systems utilized in this study reveals that the Bioreactor system provides sufficient amount of NK cells with higher purity and moreover comprises much less remaining T cells in the final product when compared to Vuelife bags.

Regardless of which expansion protocol was used, the final products had very similar phenotype and cytotoxic capacity. This suggests that although the expansion rates and distribution of subpopulations may vary, the cells reach a phenotype and activation status at the end of the 21 day culture period.

We have observed that all systems under consideration have certain practical advantages and disadvantages. Overall, the expansion of NK cells in cell culture flasks shows better yields than the closed systems but has the inherent risk of exposure to external agents and contamination. Although this risk is minimized in GMP laboratory environments, the use of closed automated systems is preferred as long as it supplies sufficient amounts of cells. Having optimized the procedure for NK cell expansion in a closed-automated bioreactor using clinical grade components, we are currently in the process of translating this research into the clinic.

GENETIC MODIFICATION OF NATURAL KILLER CELLS

Another approach for NK cell applications in immunotherapy is through gene modification to improve their anti-tumoral activity and specificity, or provide them additional capabilities. An important issue for gene-modified NK cells towards translation into patients is the ability to achieve efficient transgene expression. Historically, primary NK cells have been difficult to gene modify. Also, unlike T cells, the generation of sufficient numbers of gene-modified autologous NK cells has been problematic. As the active division of cells is a prerequisite for efficient retroviral insertion, the high rate of expansion in the abovementioned protocol provides more efficient transduction by retroviral vectors. Based on this system, we have optimized a simple and efficient retroviral vector based gene-transfer protocol for such *ex vivo* cultured primary human NK cells [8].

Gene transfer into NK cells may open new possibilities for the immunotherapy of cancer in both autologous and allogeneic settings. Applications of genetic modification could include various approaches from induction of proliferation/survival *via* gene transfer mediated cytokine therapy to specific targeting of NK cells to certain tissues or malignant cells. Such investigations have primarily began from proof-of-principle studies that resulted in the optimization of NK cell genetic modification *via* various methods including electroporation, nucleofection, transduction by chimeric adenoviral, chimeric EBV/retroviral, retroviral and lentiviral vectors.

Transfection of the *CD18* gene into a clone of the NK cell line YT-1, that lacks functional CD18 expression, has been reported previously. In this study, it was demonstrated that upon genetic modification, the cell line restores its cytotoxic capacity against a B cell lymphoma line [9]. It has also been shown that the delivery of *IL-15* gene to NK cell lines increases their proliferative rate and cytotoxic capacity [10]. Likewise, the delivery of the *IL-12* gene to mouse NK cells has increased their survival rate and *in vivo* anti-tumour activity [11].

It has been well defined that interleukin-2 (IL-2) activation of NK cells can result in cytotoxic activity against targets that were previously NK cell-resistant. Reports of IL-2 based treatment in clinical trials have established a basis for efficiency of this approach for cancer immunotherapy in different settings.

Systemic IL-2 administration frequently causes undesirable side effects [12, 13], *e.g.* the activation of other immune cell populations. More specifically, activated T cells increase the risk of GvHD [14], while the stimulation of immunosuppressive T_{reg} cells hampers the antitumoral effect of cytotoxic T-lymphocytes [15]. In settings where IL-2 is given primarily to enhance NK activity, administration in a form that stimulates NK cells, without unwanted side effects, would be ideal. There have been various reports on *IL-2* gene delivery *via* retroviral transduction or particle mediated transfection to the IL-2 dependent NK cell line NK-92. Stable transduction of the *IL-2* gene increased cytotoxic activity against tumour cell lines *in vitro*. Such a modification enabled the secretion of IL-2 by the NK92 cells and saved the cells from the dependency on exogenous IL-2 supplementation. Moreover, the IL-2 transduced cells showed greater *in vivo* antitumour activity in mice. Similarly, Miller *et al.* have reported that IL-2 transduced mouse NK cells sustained proliferation in the absence of exogenously supplied IL-2 [16]. However, the secretion of IL-2 by NK cells may affect neighbouring cells or have the potential to cause a systemic IL-2 effect in patients. This risk prompted us to investigate alternative approaches for IL-2 delivery retained in NK cells in a controlled and localized manner. Our group has constructed an endoplasmic reticulum-retained *IL-2* gene that is not secreted but still confines autocrine growth stimulation to NK-92 cells [17]. Such an approach may be useful for future applications where secretion of high levels of IL-2 by the adoptively transferred NK cells could otherwise have caused side effects.

Another approach to genetic modification of NK cells for cancer immunotherapy is retargeting NK cells to tumour cells *via* the expression of a chimeric antigen specific receptor using a single-chain variable fragment receptor specific for a certain tumour-associated antigen fused to the intracellular portion of the signalling molecule CD3z. Such receptors have been used by different groups and proved to be operating in NK cells. Chimeric receptors against various antigens have been successfully delivered to NK cell lines and were shown to increase antigen specific cytotoxic activity of NK cells both *in vitro* and *in vivo*.

These improvements have rapidly been translated to the use of primary NK cells in experimental models. Adoptive transfer of genetically modified primary mouse NK cells to express a chimeric receptor against Her2/neu to mice bearing Her2+ tumours inhibits tumour progression *in vivo* [18]. Likewise, Kruschinski *et al.* have modified primary NK cells from human donors to express a chimeric receptor against Her2/neu and observed high level of cytotoxic activity against Her2+ cell lines both *in vitro* and in xenograft models with *RAG2*-/- mice [19]. Moreover, Imai *et al.* have successfully demonstrated that NK cells from B-lineage ALL patients genetically modified to express a chimeric receptor against CD19 efficiently kill autologous leukemic cells *in vitro* [20]. Taken together, these data indicate that the adoptive transfer of chimeric antigen-specific bearing NK cells might be an efficient approach in cancer immunotherapy.

NATURAL KILLER CELL - TUMOR INTERACTIONS

The development of any malignancy is under close surveillance by NK cells as well as other members of the immune system. Nevertheless, malignant cells escape from the immune system and proliferate without control. General mechanisms include saturation of the immune system by the rapid growth of the tumour, inaccessibility of the tumour owing to defective vascularisation, its large dimension or its localization in immune-privileged sites and resistance to the Fas- or perforin-mediated apoptosis. Additionally, defective expression activation receptors and various intracellular signalling molecules of both T cells and NK cells was observed in cancer patients and reported to correlate with disease progression [21]. It has also been shown that malignant cells secrete immunosuppressive factors that inhibit NK cell proliferation [22]. As a result of all these events, defective immunity secondary to tumour development has been a well-established phenomenon [23].

In order to effectively use autologous NK cells for tumour immunotherapy, the reversal of phenotypic and functional defects is of paramount importance. Unfortunately, most of the earlier clinical studies did not include a detailed phenotypic and functional characterization of NK cells at the time of harvest or before infusion to the patient. Future studies should provide better insights into the characterization of the defects in the NK cell compartment and provide answers to whether these defects have been overcome after *ex vivo* manipulation of the cells. Although testing NK cell cytotoxicity against cell lines and allogeneic targets gives an estimation about the functional capacity of the cells, the analysis of cytotoxicity against fresh autologous tumour cells would be more informative.

Today, we know that NK cell cytotoxicity is the result of a complex balance between the inhibitory and activating receptors [24] (*Figure 3*). Upon recognition of the ligands on the target cell surface by activating NK cell receptors, various intracellular signalling pathways drive NK cells towards cytotoxic action and this results in target cell cytolysis. However, these processes are tightly controlled by a group of inhibitory receptors. These receptors act as negative regulators of NK cytotoxicity and inhibit the action of NK cells against "self" targets. A main group of this type of receptors is KIRs, which are mainly specific for self MHC Class-I molecules. If the target cell is recognized by inhibitory KIRs, according to the expression of self MHC Class-I molecules on the cell surface, sufficient amount of inhibitory signal from KIRs stops the action of cytotoxic pathways triggered by activating receptors [25, 26].

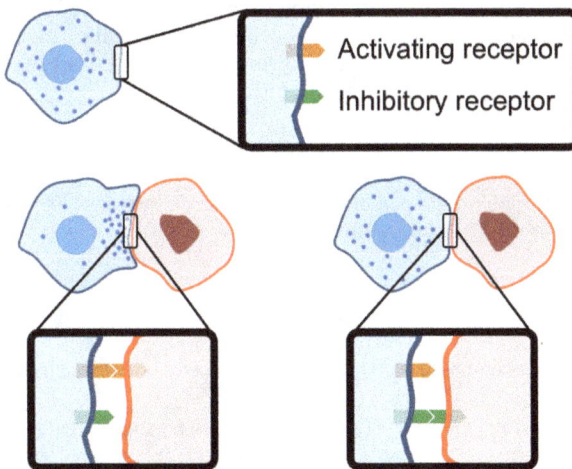

Figure 3. Tumor cell recognition is achieved by two receptor groups. Inhibitory receptors recognize self whereas activating receptors will recognize ligands on virally infected or malignant cells and induce granule polarization eventually leading to cytotoxicity of the target cell.

The activating side of the balance also includes a series of different receptors. The main activating receptor group is called natural cytotoxicity receptors (NCRs) [27], and it is believed that the main control over the NK cell activating pathways is regulated by these receptors. Currently there are three different NCRs identified: NKp30, NKp44 and NKp46. NKp30 and NKp46 are expressed both in activated and non-activated NK cells whereas NKp44 expression is restricted to activated NK cells. Unfortunately, the ligands for numerous NK cell receptors (including the NCRs) are yet to be identified. This lack of knowledge, often presents an obstacle in identification of interactions between NK cells and tumor cells. Current approaches to the characterization of such interactions include the phenotyping of tumor cells for a limited number of identified ligands as well as carrying out cytotoxicity assays in the presence of blocking antibodies against NK cell receptors. Although widely used, both approaches harbour significant defects in picking up targets that could be relevant for NK cell-mediated cytotoxicity. Phenotyping the identified ligands often results in detection of one or more NK cell ligands on the tumor targets, while being restricted to only those ligands that are well-established with available antibodies. On the other hand, blocking the NK cell receptors gives a more functional readout, but relies on the presence of expression for that receptor prior to blocking, which is not always the case, especially in cases of tumor-induced defects of receptor expression.

CONCLUSIONS

The phenotypic diversity of responses between patient and donor NK cells and the corresponding variety in response against different target cells warrants further analysis of the roles of different activating and inhibitory receptors in the encounter between NK cells and target cells. In order to address this issue, we have undertaken an comprehensive effort to upregulate or downregulate different receptors on NK cells one-at-a-time and evaluate functional readouts such as NK cell degranulation and cytotoxic activity against tumor cell lines or primary tumor targets. Such dissection and fine-tuning of the complex interaction between the NK cell and target cell by means of genetic modification will potentially be of value towards prognostic and therapeutic approaches in NK cell-based immunotherapy of cancer.

ACKNOWLEDGMENTS

This work has been performed with the support of the EC-DG research through the FP6-Network of Excellence, CLINIGENE: LSHB-CT-2006-018933.

REFERENCES

1. Sutlu T, Alici E. Natural killer cell-based immunotherapy in cancer: current insights and future prospects. *J Intern Med* 2009; 266: 154-81.

2. Ruggeri L, Capanni M, Urbani E, *et al*. Effectiveness of donor natural killer cell alloreactivity in mismatched hematopoietic transplants. *Science* 2002; 295: 2097-100.

3. Carlens S, Gilljam M, Chambers BJ, *et al*. A new method for in vitro expansion of cytotoxic human CD3-CD56+ natural killer cells. *Hum Immunol* 2001; 62: 1092-8.

4. Guven H, Gilljam M, Chambers BJ, *et al*. Expansion of natural killer (NK) and natural killer-like T (NKT)-cell populations derived from patients with B-chronic lymphocytic leukemia (B-CLL): a potential source for cellular immunotherapy. *Leukemia* 2003; 17: 1973-80.

5. Alici E, Sutlu T, Bjorkstrand B, *et al*. Autologous antitumor activity by NK cells expanded from myeloma patients using GMP-compliant components. *Blood* 2008; 111: 3155-62.

6. Guimaraes F, Guven H, Donati D, *et al*. Evaluation of ex vivo expanded human NK cells on antileukemia activity in SCID-beige mice. *Leukemia* 2006; 20: 833-9.

7. Barkholt L, Alici E, Conrad R, *et al.* Safety analysis of ex vivo-expanded NK and NK-like T cells administered to cancer patients: a phase I clinical study. *Immunotherapy* 2009; 1: 753-64.

8. Alici E, Sutlu T, Dilber MS. Retroviral gene transfer into primary human natural killer cells. *Methods Mol Biol* 2009; 506: 127-37.

9. Liu JH, Wei S, Blanchard DK, Djeu JY. Restoration of lytic function in a human natural killer cell line by gene transfection. *Cell Immunol* 1994; 156: 24-35.

10. Zhang J, Sun R, Wei H, Tian Z. Characterization of interleukin-15 gene-modified human natural killer cells: implications for adoptive cellular immunotherapy. *Haematologica* 2004; 89: 338-47.

11. Goding SR, Yang Q, Knudsen KB, Potter DM, Basse PH. Cytokine gene therapy using adenovirally transduced, tumor-seeking activated natural killer cells. *Hum Gene Ther* 2007; 18: 701-11.

12. Maas RA, Dullens HF, Den Otter W. Interleukin-2 in cancer treatment: disappointing or (still) promising? A review. *Cancer Immunol Immunother* 1993; 36: 141-8.

13. Ardizzoni A, Bonavia M, Viale M, *et al.* Biologic and clinical effects of continuous infusion interleukin-2 in patients with non-small cell lung cancer. *Cancer* 1994; 73: 1353-60.

14. Roychowdhury S, Blaser BW, Freud AG, *et al.* IL-15 but not IL-2 rapidly induces lethal xenogeneic graft-versus-host disease. *Blood* 2005; 106: 2433-5.

15. Malek TR, Bayer AL. Tolerance, not immunity, crucially depends on IL-2. *Nat Rev Immunol* 2004; 4: 665-74.

16. Miller JS, Tessmer-Tuck J, Blake N, *et al.* Endogenous IL-2 production by natural killer cells maintains cytotoxic and proliferative capacity following retroviral-mediated gene transfer. *Exp Hematol* 1997; 25: 1140-8.

17. Konstantinidis KV, Alici E, Aints A, Christensson B, Ljunggren HG, Dilber MS. Targeting IL-2 to the endoplasmic reticulum confines autocrine growth stimulation to NK-92 cells. *Exp Hematol* 2005; 33: 159-64.

18. Pegram HJ, Jackson JT, Smyth MJ, Kershaw MH, Darcy PK. Adoptive transfer of gene-modified primary NK cells can specifically inhibit tumor progression *in vivo. J Immunol* 2008; 181: 3449-55.

19. Kruschinski A, Moosmann A, Poschke I, *et al.* Engineering antigen-specific primary human NK cells against HER-2 positive carcinomas. *Proc Natl Acad Sci USA* 2008; 105: 17481-6.

20. Imai C, Iwamoto S, Campana D. Genetic modification of primary natural killer cells overcomes inhibitory signals and induces specific killing of leukemic cells. *Blood* 2005; 106: 376-83.

21. Matsuda M, Petersson M, Lenkei R, *et al.* Alterations in the signal-transducing molecules of T cells and NK cells in colorectal tumor-infiltrating, gut mucosal and peripheral lymphocytes: correlation with the stage of the disease. *Int J Cancer* 1995; 61: 765-72.

22. Orleans-Lindsay JK, Barber LD, Prentice HG, Lowdell MW. Acute myeloid leukaemia cells secrete a soluble factor that inhibits T and NK cell proliferation but not cytolytic function: implications for the adoptive immunotherapy of leukaemia. *Clin Exp Immunol* 2001; 126: 403-11.

23. Kiessling R, Wasserman K, Horiguchi S, *et al.* Tumor-induced immune dysfunction. *Cancer Immunol Immunother* 1999; 48: 353-62.

24. Lanier LL. Natural killer cell receptor signaling. *Curr Opin Immunol* 2003; 15: 308-14.

25. Veillette A, Latour S, Davidson D. Negative regulation of immunoreceptor signaling. *Annu Rev Immunol* 2002; 20: 669-707.

26. Long EO. Negative signaling by inhibitory receptors: the NK cell paradigm. *Immunol Rev* 2008; 224: 70-84.

27. Moretta A, Bottino C, Vitale M, *et al.* Activating receptors and coreceptors involved in human natural killer cell-mediated cytolysis. *Annu Rev Immunol* 2001; 19: 197-223.

The CliniBook: Clinical gene transfer
Edited by Odile Cohen-Haguenauer – EDK, Paris © 2012, pp. 208-215

A4-5
Regulatory T lymphocyte depletion for cancer immunotherapies

MICHELLE ROSENZWAJG[1,2], FRANÇOIS LEMOINE[1,2], DAVID KLATZMANN[1,2]*

[1]*Université Pierre et Marie Curie, UPMC Université Paris 06, CNRS UMR7211, Inserm U959, Hôpital Pitié-Salpêtrière, 83, boulevard de l'Hôpital, 75013 Paris, France.*
[2]*Clinical Investigation Center in Biotherapy, AP-HP, Hôpital Pitié-Salpêtrière, F-75651, Paris 13, France.*
david.klatzmann@upmc.fr
* *Corresponding author*

THE REGULATORY/EFFECTOR T CELL BALANCE IN PHYSIOLOGY AND PATHOPHYSIOLOGY

The existence of suppressor T cells that could negatively regulate immune responses was postulated in the 1970s [1]. However, doubts were cast on their existence because of the inability to identify them with specific markers. The field was reborn with the discovery that, in mice, the absence of CD25+CD4+ T lymphocytes led to the appearance of severe multi-organ autoimmunity. This defined a population of cells, called natural regulatory T cells (Tregs), the main function of which was thought to be the maintenance of self-tolerance, and likewise the prevention/control of autoimmune diseases [2]. In mice, these Tregs constitute 5-10% of the CD4+ T cell pool [3]; in humans, Tregs are currently characterized as CD4+CD25hiCD127- cells and represent around 5% of CD4+ T cells [4]. Both mouse and human Tregs express the transcription factor Forkhead box P3 (FOXP3) which regulates Treg development and correlates with suppressor activity [5-7]. The highest levels of suppression are mediated by Tregs that express FOXP3 and high levels of CD25 [8]. This Treg population is of considerable physiological importance since its absence in genetically FOXP3-deficient IPEX patients leads to lymphoproliferation, massive autoimmunity and death [5, 6].

In fact, the discovery of Tregs rapidly revealed that all immune responses are regulated (*Figure 1*) and that a balance between effector (Teff) and Treg responses is constantly at work [9]. The Treg/Teff balance appears critical for maintaining a healthy immune status. Uncontrolled activation of Teffs could lead to chronic inflammation and autoimmune diseases. Conversely, uncontrolled Treg-mediated suppression, for example in the context of infectious tissue damage, could lead to poor anti-infectious immune responses.

Treg are involved all immune responses

BENEFICIAL EFFECTS

DELETERIOUS EFFECTS

Prevention of auto-immune diseases

Prevention of fetus rejection

Control of inflammation

Inhibition of antitumor immune responses

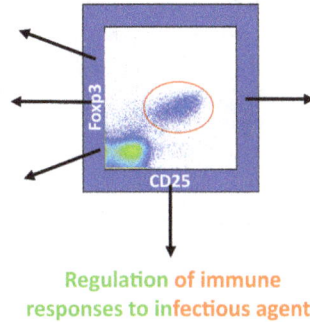

Regulation of immune responses to infectious agents

Figure 1. Tregs are involved in the regulation all immune responses.

Tregs, shown here in mice as CD25^{high}, FOXP3+ cells, have beneficial and deleterious effects:

- They prevent autoimmune disease development [9, 46].
- They prevent allogeneic fetus rejection [39].
- They control inflammation [47].
- They prevent an excessive acute immune response that could be deleterious [9].
- They control alloreactivity [33, 34].
- They inhibit antitumor effector immune responses [15, 19].
- They can favor the establishment of chronic infection [48].

There are various described factors involved in the maintenance of a proper Treg/Teff balance. For example, a feedback regulatory loop controlled by Treg and dendritic cell (DC) numbers has just been identified [10]. An increase in DC numbers induces an expansion of Tregs (Teffs varying oppositely), which in turn decreases DC numbers and then Treg numbers, and so forth [10]. Moreover, in the context of Type 1 diabetes, Teffs have been shown to boost Treg activity, contributing to reduction in autoimmunity [11]. There seems to be a feedback regulatory loop that dynamically tunes the size of the Treg population to that of the Teff population.

In cancer, several lines of evidence suggest that Tregs are partly responsible for immune tolerance to cancer cells, which impairs the development of effector immune responses directed against tumor antigens [9]. In cancer patients, an increased pool of blood Tregs has been reported [12]. At the tumor site as well as in draining lymph nodes, a large number of Tregs with potent immunosuppressive functions accumulates [13, 14] and their number correlates with poor prognosis [15-17].

Thus, cancer and autoimmune diseases appear to develop from opposite disturbance of the Treg/Teff balance. Recent data show that emergent cancer cells are rapidly recognized as self by Tregs, which then imprint a tolerant dominant environment that prevents the proper activation and function of otherwise efficient antitumor Teffs [18, 19]. Autoimmune diseases represent a mirror setting in which Tregs fail to control Teffs which in turn are activated too much and destroy normal tissues. Schematically, autoimmune diseases result from not enough Treg activation and too much Teff activation, while cancer develops when there is too much Treg activation and not enough Teff activation.

Treg depletion for improving cancer immunotherapies

The notion that immune responses can control cancer led to the development of various approaches to immunotherapy (or to immunotherapeutics). However, after years of clinical trials in humans, results have been quite disappointing [20]. Despite the fact that many vaccination strategies were shown to induce substantial antigen-specific responses, they led to little or no clinical benefits [21]. Complex cell therapies based on the *ex vivo* expansion of tumor-specific lymphocytes or on injecting DCs sensitized with tumor antigens did not achieve better results [22]. However, the likely main explanation for the poor efficacy of cancer immunotherapy came from the identification of Tregs [2]. Treg depletion has been proposed as a relevant strategy for cancer immunotherapy [23] and numerous preclinical models have strengthened the concept (*Figure 2*).

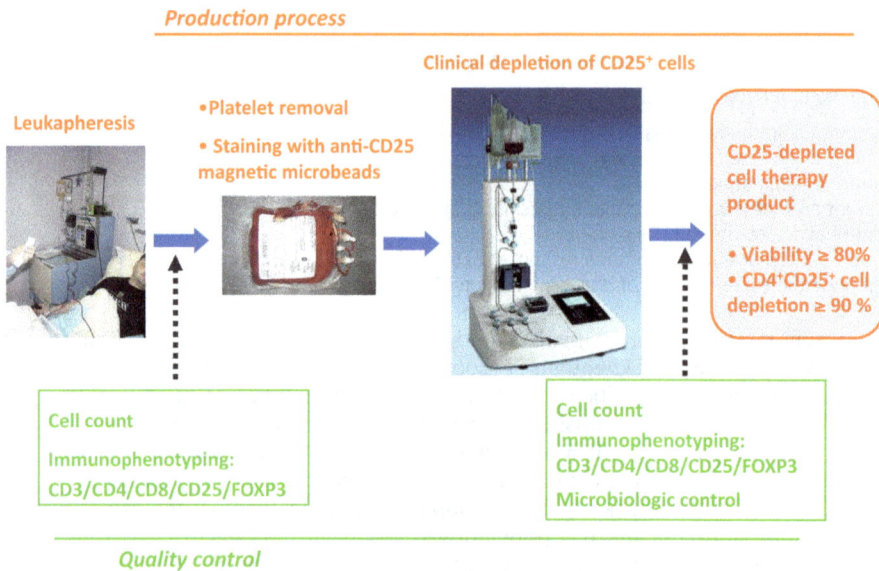

Figure 2. Schematic representation of the *ex vivo* Treg depletion process.

Although the field is still in its infancy, evidence is emerging that inhibition of Tregs may help in tumor containment, especially when combined with appropriate immunotherapies that activate Teffs. In many mouse tumor models, Treg ablation before tumor implantation leads to antigen-specific T cell-mediated tumor rejection and induces an immunological memory that protects mice against a tumor challenge [19, 24]. When combined with immunogenic stimulation of intratumoral immune effector cells, Treg depletion resulted in cure of 90% of animals who had large and weakly immunogenic sarcomas [25]. In metastatic melanoma patients, transient systemic Treg depletion allows the expansion of Teffs with specificity against neoplastic cells [26].

Altogether, it appears that approaches to the immunotherapy of cancer will likely be effective only if Tregs are controlled or eliminated (*Figure 3*)

Several therapeutics that have the potential to deplete Tregs are clinically available. Most Treg-depletion strategies have focused on monoclonal antibodies or ligand-directed toxins targeted to cell-surface receptors, such as CD25. Daclizumab and basiliximab are anti-CD25 antibodies that cause cell death by IL-2 deprivation and by triggering antibody-dependent cell-mediated cytotoxicity or complement-dependent cytotoxicity. Results from an ongoing clinical trial have shown that daclizumab reduces Tregs and, thereby, enhances cytotoxic T lymphocyte responses to tumor antigen induced by vaccination [27]. However, it appears that the Treg depletion achieved with these treatments is not clinically significant for cancer immunotherapies. We reasoned that, pending the magic bullet that will allow proper *in vivo* Treg control, *ex vivo* Treg depletion could prove useful, and explored this strategy first in the context of leukemia relapse after hematopoietic stem cell transplantation (HSCT).

Tregs cancer immunotherapy

1. Treg depletion
- Specific Ab
- Chemotherapy
- Radiation therapy
- Ex vivo...

3. Active Immunization

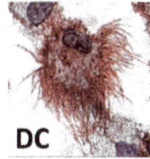

DC   vector

2. Tumor destruction
(for the release of tumor antigens)
- Radiofrequency ablation
- Chemotherapy
- Radiation therapy
- Gene Therapy/Virotherapy

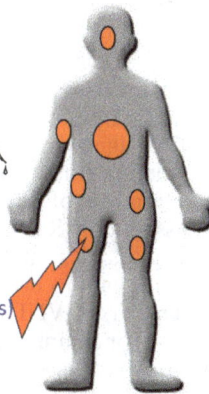

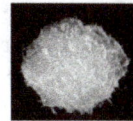

Effector cells

Figure 3. Treg control or depletion is essential for the development of efficient immune responses. Effective cancer immunotherapies will likely combine enhancement of effector immune response by active immunization or passive cell transfer, tumor destruction to debulk the tumor mass and release tumor antigens, and Treg depletion.

ALLOREACTIVITY AND CANCER

HSCT is a treatment of choice for several hematological disorders, including leukemia and lymphoma [28]. Its major complication is life-threatening graft-versus-host disease (GVHD) [29] due to donor T cells. Alloreactive T cells represent 5-10% of a normal T cell repertoire [30]. When infused into an allogeneic recipient, these cells are activated in response to host antigen-presenting cells [31], expand and differentiate into cytokine-producing and cytotoxic effector cells that cause tissue damage in target organs [29]. In order to prevent GVHD, grafted patients receive an immunosuppressive regimen, but this treatment is only partially effective. Ultimately, 20 to 40% of patients die from complications associated with GVHD, the incidence being higher when donor marrow is not from an HLA-identical sibling.

Since alloreactive donor T cells are at the center of the graft-versus-tumor (GVT) effect, donor lymphocyte infusion (DLI) is routinely used to induce such an effect in patients with relapsing malignancies after allogeneic HSCT [32].

It now is clear that Tregs also play a key role in the control of alloreactive responses. In mice, accelerated GVHD is observed when the transplant is Treg-depleted [33, 34] and protection against GVHD is achieved using Tregs [35-38]. Moreover, Treg depletion before mating is associated with allogeneic fetus rejection in mice [39].

Thus, modulating the immune response in the field of allogeneic HSCT is a key issue if it can maintain the required graft-versus-tumor effect without GVHD [40]. Acute GVHD may be attenuated or prevented by increasing the ratio of Tregs in the transplant and, alternatively, Treg depletion may improve the graft-versus-tumor effect of donor lymphocytes [41].

GRAFT-VERSUS-TUMOR EFFECT BY DONOR REGULATORY T-CELL DEPLETION BEFORE DONOR LYMPHOCYTE INFUSION

From preclinical models showing that Treg depletion is a viable strategy to increase allogeneic response, we inferred that Tregs present in the DLI might limit their alloreactivity and likewise the graft-versus-tumor effect.

This hypothesis was tested in a phase I/II clinical trial in which a Treg-depleted donor lymphocyte infusion (d-DLI) was given to patients refractory to standard DLI (std-DLI) for treatment of relapse after HSCT [42]. Tregs were removed from donor lymphocytes after leukapheresis using anti-CD25 magnetic microbeads with a CliniMACS device (Mylteni Biotec) (*Figure 2*). Treg depletion efficacy was confirmed by flow cytometry with a CD4+CD25hiFoxP3+ depletion rate of 98±5% in accordance with a FOXP3 expression decrease by 92±5% as assessed by RTq-PCR.

Seventeen adult patients with relapsing hematological malignancies after allogeneic HSCT, and who never displayed GVHD manifestations before, received a d-DLI. Two of the 17 developed GVHD after d-DLI. This first GVHD occurrence in their transplant history was associated with a partial (n=1) or complete (n=1) long-term remission of their malignancy. No such remission was observed in the other 15 patients. This positive yet unsatisfactory result could be explained by the presence of endogenous Tregs in the recipient, which would limit the alloreactivity induced by d-DLI.

Four of the 17 patients in whom the first treatment failed were given lymphodepleting chemotherapy combining cyclophosphamide with fludarabine, to eliminate endogenous Tregs before infusion, followed immediately by d-DLI [43]. They all developed acute GVHD that could be controlled by classic immunosuppressive regimens. GVHD induction was associated with transient (n=2) or lasting (n=2) control of the malignancy.

This clinical trial is the first demonstration that Treg depletion improves antitumor immune responses.

REGULATORY T-CELL DEPLETION TO BREAK IMMUNE TOLERANCE IN COLORECTAL CANCER

Ex vivo Treg depletion could also be useful for the treatment of solid tumors. We started a phase I/II clinical trial investigating ex vivo Treg depletion for patients with advanced metastatic colorectal cancer who are not eligible for surgery [44]. The goal of the proposed clinical trial is to create temporarily a Treg-depleted environment that promotes an efficient immune antitumor response. Patients undergo blood cytapheresis to collect circulating lymphocytes. *Ex vivo* Treg depletion is achieved as described above, and autologous Treg-depleted lymphocytes are administered to the patient following a 5-day reduced intensity chemotherapeutic conditioning [43] to deplete endogenous Tregs. We further hypothesize that Treg depletion associated with transient lymphodepletion will induce a homeostatic expansion of the infused Teffs, thereby enhancing the specific immune antitumor response [45]. This trial is ongoing and could represent a preliminary step toward future trials that combine Treg depletion and vaccine-based strategies.

CONCLUSION

There is now a robust set of experimental and clinical data to support the notion that any cancer immunotherapy will have to deal with the control of Tregs. Intense efforts notably based on various omics may provide drugs that can do this. Meanwhile, the *ex vivo* depletion of Tregs remains an alternative to the temporary creation of a Treg-depleted environment.

ACKNOWLEDGMENTS

This work has been performed with the support of the EC-DG research through the FP6-Network of Excellence, CLINIGENE: LSHB-CT-2006-018933.

REFERENCES

1. Gershon RK, Cohen P, Hencin R, Liebhaber SA. Suppressor T cells. *J Immunol* 1972; 108: 586-90.

2. Sakaguchi S, Sakaguchi N, Asano M, Itoh M, Toda M. Immunologic self-tolerance maintained by activated T cells expressing IL-2 receptor alpha-chains (CD25). Breakdown of a single mechanism of self-tolerance causes various autoimmune diseases. *J Immunol* 1995; 155: 1151-64.

3. Viglietta V, Baecher-Allan C, Weiner HL, Hafler DA. Loss of functional suppression by CD4+CD25+ regulatory T cells in patients with multiple sclerosis. *J Exp Med* 2004; 199: 971-9.

4. Riley JL, June CH, Blazar BR. Human T regulatory cell therapy: take a billion or so and call me in the morning. *Immunity* 2009; 30: 656-65.

5. Fontenot JD, Gavin MA, Rudensky AY. Foxp3 programs the development and function of CD4+CD25+ regulatory T cells. *Nat Immunol* 2003; 4: 330-6.

6. Hori S, Takahashi T, Sakaguchi S. Control of autoimmunity by naturally arising regulatory CD4+ T cells. *Adv Immunol* 2003; 81: 331-71.

7. Ziegler SF. FOXP3: of mice and men. *Annu Rev Immunol* 2006; 24: 209-26.

8. Liu W, Putnam AL, Xu-Yu Z, *et al.* CD127 expression inversely correlates with FoxP3 and suppressive function of human CD4+ T reg cells. *J Exp Med* 2006; 203: 1701-11.

9. Sakaguchi S, Yamaguchi T, Nomura T, Ono M. Regulatory T cells and immune tolerance. *Cell* 2008; 133: 775-87.

10. Darrasse-Jeze G, Deroubaix S, Mouquet H, *et al.* Feedback control of regulatory T cell homeostasis by dendritic cells *in vivo*. *J Exp Med* 2009; 206: 1853-62.

11. Grinberg-Bleyer Y, Saadoun D, Baeyens A, *et al.* Pathogenic T cells have a paradoxical protective effect in murine autoimmune diabetes by boosting Tregs. *J Clin Invest* 2010; 120: 4558-68.

12. Wolf AM, Wolf D, Steurer M, Gastl G, Gunsilius E, Grubeck-Loebenstein B. Increase of regulatory T cells in the peripheral blood of cancer patients. *Clin Cancer Res* 2003; 9: 606-12.

13. Liyanage UK, Moore TT, Joo HG, *et al.* Prevalence of regulatory T cells is increased in peripheral blood and tumor microenvironment of patients with pancreas or breast adenocarcinoma. *J Immunol* 2002; 169: 2756-61.

14. Bates GJ, Fox SB, Han C, *et al.* Quantification of regulatory T cells enables the identification of high-risk breast cancer patients and those at risk of late relapse. *J Clin Oncol* 2006; 24: 5373-80.

15. Curiel TJ, Coukos G, Zou L, *et al.* Specific recruitment of regulatory T cells in ovarian carcinoma fosters immune privilege and predicts reduced survival. *Nat Med* 2004; 10: 942-9.

16. Wolf AM, Rumpold H, Wolf D, *et al.* Role of forkhead box protein 3 expression in invasive breast cancer. *J Clin Oncol* 2007; 25: 4499-500.

17. Merlo A, Casalini P, Carcangiu ML, *et al.* FOXP3 expression and overall survival in breast cancer. *J Clin Oncol* 2009; 27: 1746-52.

18. Bergot AS, Durgeau A, Levacher B, Colombo BM, Cohen JL, Klatzmann D. Antigen quality determines the efficiency of antitumor immune responses generated in the absence of regulatory T cells. *Cancer Gene Ther* 2010; 17: 645-54.

19. Darrasse-Jeze G, Bergot AS, Durgeau A, *et al.* Tumor emergence is sensed by self-specific CD44hi memory Tregs that create a dominant tolerogenic environment for tumors in mice. *J Clin Invest* 2009; 119: 2648-62.

20. Lesterhuis WJ, Haanen JB, Punt CJ. Cancer immunotherapy revisited. *Nat Rev Drug Discov* 2011; 10: 591-600.

21. Dillman RO. Cancer immunotherapy. *Cancer Biother Radiopharm* 2011; 26: 1-64.

22. Paulos CM, Kaiser A, Wrzesinski C, *et al.* Toll-like receptors in tumor immunotherapy. *Clin Cancer Res* 2007; 13: 5280-9.

23. Zou W. Immunosuppressive networks in the tumour environment and their therapeutic relevance. *Nat Rev Cancer* 2005; 5: 263-74.

24. Chaput N, Darrasse-Jeze G, Bergot AS, *et al.* Regulatory T cells prevent CD8 T cell maturation by inhibiting CD4 Th cells at tumor sites. *J Immunol* 2007; 179: 4969-78.

25. Whelan MC, Casey G, MacConmara M, *et al.* Effective immunotherapy of weakly immunogenic solid tumours using a combined immunogene therapy and regulatory T-cell inactivation. *Cancer Gene Ther* 2010; 17: 501-11.

26. Rasku MA, Clem AL, Telang S, *et al.* Transient T cell depletion causes regression of melanoma metastases. *J Transl Med* 2008; 6: 12.

27. Rech AJ, Vonderheide RH. Clinical use of anti-CD25 antibody daclizumab to enhance immune responses to tumor antigen vaccination by targeting regulatory T cells. *Ann NY Acad Sci* 2009; 1174: 99-106.

28. Welniak LA, Blazar BR, Murphy WJ. Immunobiology of allogeneic hematopoietic stem cell transplantation. *Annu Rev Immunol* 2007; 25: 139-70.

29. Ferrara JL, Levine JE, Reddy P, Holler E. Graft-versus-host disease. *Lancet* 2009; 373: 1550-61.

30. Suchin EJ, Langmuir PB, Palmer E, Sayegh MH, Wells AD, Turka LA. Quantifying the frequency of alloreactive T cells *in vivo*: new answers to an old question. *J Immunol* 2001; 166: 973-81.

31. Teshima T, Ordemann R, Reddy P, *et al.* Acute graft-versus-host disease does not require alloantigen expression on host epithelium. *Nat Med* 2002; 8: 575-81.

32. Kolb HJ. Graft-versus-leukemia effects of transplantation and donor lymphocytes. *Blood* 2008; 112: 4371-83.

33. Cohen JL, Trenado A, Vasey D, Klatzmann D, Salomon BL. CD4+CD25+ immunoregulatory T Cells: new therapeutics for graft-versus-host disease. *J Exp Med* 2002; 196: 401-6.

34. Taylor PA, Lees CJ, Blazar BR. The infusion of *ex vivo* activated and expanded CD4+CD25+ immune regulatory cells inhibits graft-versus-host disease lethality. *Blood* 2002; 99: 3493-39.

35. Edinger M, Hoffmann P, Ermann J, *et al*. CD4+CD25+ regulatory T cells preserve graft-versus-tumor activity while inhibiting graft-versus-host disease after bone marrow transplantation. *Nat Med* 2003; 9: 1144-50.

36. Hoffmann P, Ermann J, Edinger M, Fathman CG, Strober S. Donor-type CD4+CD25+ regulatory T cells suppress lethal acute graft-versus-host disease after allogeneic bone marrow transplantation. *J Exp Med* 2002; 196: 389-99.

37. Trenado A, Charlotte F, Fisson S, *et al*. Recipient-type specific CD4+CD25+ regulatory T cells favor immune reconstitution and control graft-versus-host disease while maintaining graft-versus-leukemia. *J Clin Invest* 2003; 112: 1688-96.

38. Fisson S, Djelti F, Trenado A, *et al*. Therapeutic potential of self-antigen-specific CD4+ CD25+ regulatory T cells selected *in vitro* from a polyclonal repertoire. *Eur J Immunol* 2006; 36: 817-27.

39. Darrasse-Jeze G, Klatzmann D, Charlotte F, Salomon BL, Cohen JL. CD4+CD25+ regulatory/suppressor T cells prevent allogeneic fetus rejection in mice. *Immunol Lett* 2006; 102: 106-9.

40. Cohen JL, Boyer O. The role of CD4+CD25hi regulatory T cells in the physiopathogeny of graft-versus-host disease. *Curr Opin Immunol* 2006; 18: 580-585.

41. Hicheri Y, Bouchekioua A, Hamel Y, *et al*. Donor regulatory T cells identified by FoxP3 expression but also by the membranous CD4+CD127low/neg phenotype influence graft-versus-tumor effect after donor lymphocyte infusion. *J Immunother* 2008; 31: 806-11.

42. ClinicalTrials.gov NCT00987987. Amplifying graft-versus-tumor effect by donor regulatory T-cell depletion before donor lymphocytes infusion (ILD-Treg), 2009.

43. Dudley ME, Wunderlich JR, Robbins PF, *et al*. Cancer regression and autoimmunity in patients after clonal repopulation with antitumor lymphocytes. *Science* 2002; 298: 850-4.

44. Maury S, Lemoine FM, Hicheri Y, *et al*. CD4+CD25+ regulatory T cell depletion improves the graft-versus-tumor effect of donor lymphocytes after allogeneic hematopoietic stem cell transplantation. *Sci Transl Med* 2010; 2: 41ra52.

45. ClinicalTrials.gov NCT00986518. T regulatory lymphocytes (Treg) depletion for cancer treatment efficacy and safety study (STARTREK), 2011.

46. Rudensky AY. Regulatory T cells and Foxp3. *Immunol Rev* 2011; 241: 260-8.

47. Ait-Oufella H, Salomon BL, Potteaux S, *et al*. Natural regulatory T cells control the development of atherosclerosis in mice. *Nat Med* 2006; 12: 178-80.

48. Mills KH. Regulatory T cells: friend or foe in immunity to infection? *Nat Rev Immunol* 2004; 4: 841-55.

The CliniBook: Clinical gene transfer
Edited by Odile Cohen-Haguenauer – EDK, Paris © 2012, pp. 216-225

A4-6
Gene therapy of Fanconi's anaemia aplastic syndrome

ÉMILIE BAYART[1], CAROLINE DUROS[1], ALEXANDRE ARTUS[1], STÉPHANIE LEMAIRE[1],
ODILE COHEN-HAGUENAUER[1,2*]

[1]*CliniGene, École Normale Supérieure de Cachan, CNRS UMR 8113, 94235 Cachan,
France and* [2]*Department of Medical Oncology, Hopital Saint-Louis and Faculté de
Médecine, Université Paris-Diderot, Sorbonne-Paris-Cité, 75475 Paris Cedex 10, France.*
* *Corresponding author*
odile.cohen@lbpa.ens-cachan.fr

INTRODUCTION

Fanconi anemia (FA) is a rare autosomal recessive disease that results in early bone
marrow (BM) failure [1]. Aplastic anemia develops at an average age of 7 years. Other
features of the disease include abnormal skin pigmentation, growth retardation, skeletal malformations, abnormalities in the kidney and heart together with an increased
risk for the development of leukemia and squamous cell carcinoma [2-4]. The prevalence of Fanconi's anemia is 1 to 5 cases per 1 million persons. There are 15 distinct
genes known to carry mutations resulting in FA. FANC proteins are involved in DNA
repair/cell cycle checkpoints [5], redox metabolism and differentiation processes [6, 7].
Cells cultured from FA patients exhibit increased spontaneous chromosomal aberrations and hypersensitivity to DNA cross-linking agents such as Mitomycin C (MMC)
or Diepoxybutane (DEB) [8, 9]. This *in vitro* phenotype has become the basis for including FA as one of the genomic instability syndromes [10].
Pancytopenia is associated with reduced bone marrow cellularity, with a profound
deficiency in the erythroid compartment. In addition to aplastic anemia, at least 20%
of FA-patients are at high risk of developing malignancies, in particular, squamous-
cell carcinomas of the head and neck as well as gynecologic, esophageal carcinoma,
and tumours of the liver, brain, skin, colon and kidney together with secondary acute
myeloid leukemia. The discovery that FANCD1 is identical to BRCA2 merged two
previously unrelated fields of medical research that had in common the mechanisms
involved in DNA repair [11]. To emphasize the connection between Fanconi's anemia
and breast cancer, the pathway was renamed the FA-BRCA pathway [5, 12]. Carriers
of mutations in BRCA2/FANCD1 have an elevated lifetime risk of breast cancer
[13, 14]. The tumours in heterozygotes result from loss of the second (wild-type)
BRCA2 allele, resulting in biallelic extinction of BRCA2. The *BRCA2-/-* cells undergo
chromosome breakage when exposed to DNA cross-linkers and exhibit triradial
chromosomes, which are the hallmark of FA-cells [15]. To date, three Fanconi's ane-

mia genes (FANCD1, FANCN, and FANCJ) have been shown to be bona fide breast-cancer-susceptibility genes: biallelic mutations in BRIP1/BACH1 (FANCJ) and PALB2 (FANCN) [16, 17] cause rare subtypes of Fanconi's anemia.

The primary therapeutic option available for FA-aplastic anaemia is allogeneic hematopoietic stem cell, from BM or cord-blood, transplantation (HSCT), which carry significant side effects due to the disease background and as a consequence of increased sensitivity to the cytotoxic conditioning [2, 18, 19] needed to facilitate allogeneic stem cell engraftment and graft versus host disease (GVHD) whether acute or chronic. Despite progress over the ten past years partially due to improvement of pre-transplantation conditioning [20-23], HSCT still results in significant early or long-term morbidity/mortality with late appearance of secondary epithelia-derived tumours of either the oral cavity or female genitals [2, 24]. The goal of our research is to establish a gene and cell-based therapy for Fanconi's aneamia (FA) aplastic syndrome in order to substitute bone-marrow or cord-blood allogeneic transplantation significant burden of side-effects. Although FA might in theory have been regarded as a good candidate for BM genetic correction *ex vivo*, gene therapy attempts in FA patients have failed [25, 26]. Several obstacles need to be overcome for this approach to become successful including (i) the scarcity of FA primary BM cells in hypoplastic or aplastic marrow; (ii) their extraordinary fragility and (iii) limitations of current gene transfer technology. We have recently demonstrated that the BM cell dysfunction associated with FA, can be ameliorated protecting cells from oxidative stress. By coupling (i) specific culture conditions involving low-oxygen pressure and addition of N-Acetyl Cystein as the best performing anti-oxydative agent with (ii) retroviral-mediated gene transfer of the main complementation group FANCA, we have achieved the long-term reconstitution of the stem cell compartment both *in vitro* and *in vivo* [27].

Within the next five years, we have designed and developed a new generation of genetically stable insulated vectors in order to prevent gene transfer induced malignancies in a cancer-prone disorder [28-30] because in SCID [31], CGD [32] and WAS [33] patients, secondary leukemia have been induced in retrovirus gene-modified cells. Therefore, current limitations and bottlenecks in this life-threatening and cancer-prone disease need to be addressed which form the basis of our research developed along two main lines: (i) challenging the most recent gene transfer technologies that we have developed with improved safety and efficacy properties, to treat FA aplastic syndrome, and (ii) generation of FA-induced pluripotent stem cells (iPS) as an improved model of this fascinating disease - since rodent animal models do not compare the human phenotype – in order to provide an unlimited source of cells as a pre-clinical model of gene transfer in an ideal ethical context: indeed, this is in avoiding to retrieve part of patients' poor hematopoietic resource which would otherwise shorten their life-span. Gene therapy intervention consisting into stable gene transfer of a functional FANC-gene (or cDNA) in patients' haematopoietic progenitors should be beneficial. *In vivo* selective growth advantage of successfully transduced cells is expected. This is likely to help genetically engineered haematopoietic progenitors settle and reconstitute host without prior myeloablation. In particular, the potential addition of a functional FA-gene into genuine haematopoietic stem cells should translate into a major improvement of patients' condition.

OVERCOMING THE CELL CATASTROPHE IN FA-BM CELLS

In FA BM-cells are extremely fragile: cell-density decreases with the condition. Although FA might in theory have been regarded as a good candidate for BM genetic correction *ex vivo*, gene therapy attempts in FA-patients so far have proved rather disappointing, as neither permanent hematopoietic stem cell correction nor even sustained *in vitro* culture of FA blood-forming cells have been observed to date [25, 26, 34] KO-animal models are not accurate since the phenotype does not compare the human situation and haematopoiesis becomes impaired only following the administration of a three-month low-dose MMC regimen [35].

Beginning with the biology of target cells, we focused on controlling cell-fragility and early death [27], before improving gene transfer in a next step. In order to avoid any unnecessary manipulation of the cells that might cause additional cell injury and loss we used unfractionated FA-patients' bone marrow with their informed consent. Of necessity for ethical reasons relating to the disease features themselves and the paucity of the samples available from each patient, experiments were performed on a limited number of cells, *i.e.* $2x10^5$ nucleated BM cells. When cells were incubated under low oxygen pressure (5%) and in the presence of the anti-oxidative agent, NAC (N-acetyl cysteine), by day 8 of culture, a statistically significant improvement (p = 0,045) in BM cell viability and survival was seen with the combination of hypoxia and NAC (*Figure 1*). CFU-assays proved to be even more discriminating, since 9 out of 9 FA-A samples tested were able to generate CFU, of which 8 contained erythroid and 4 mixed (CFU-GEMM) colonies. Without antioxidant conditions, only 3 of 9 bone marrow samples gave rise to a few myeloid clusters, and only one to erythroid clusters. Under no circumstances were either BFU-E or GEMM-CFUs observed when cells were cultured under "standard conditions" (p values - erythroid: 0,027 and global: 0,009). All experiments have been conducted with an extremely limited amount of patient's primary BM cells. Despite this limitation, our data clearly demonstrate that bone marrow cells from the majority of patients with FANCA can be successfully grown under special conditions which reduce unnecessary physical manipulation and provide for anti-oxidant growth conditions.

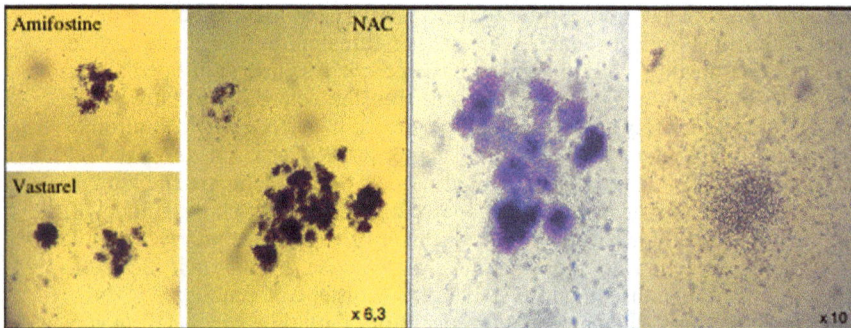

Figure 1. Effects of the antioxidants conditioning on the clonogenicity of FA patients' BM cells (left) 1 and 2 small colonies obtained with Amifostine or Vastarel; with 55 large colonies with NAC ($50x10^3$ cells were seeded maintained under 5%O2; unconditioned cells not represented: no colony); (right) NAC conditioned BM cells differentiate into different lineages BFU-E (left) and CFU-GM (right). Reproduced from Cohen-Haguenauer *et al.* [27].

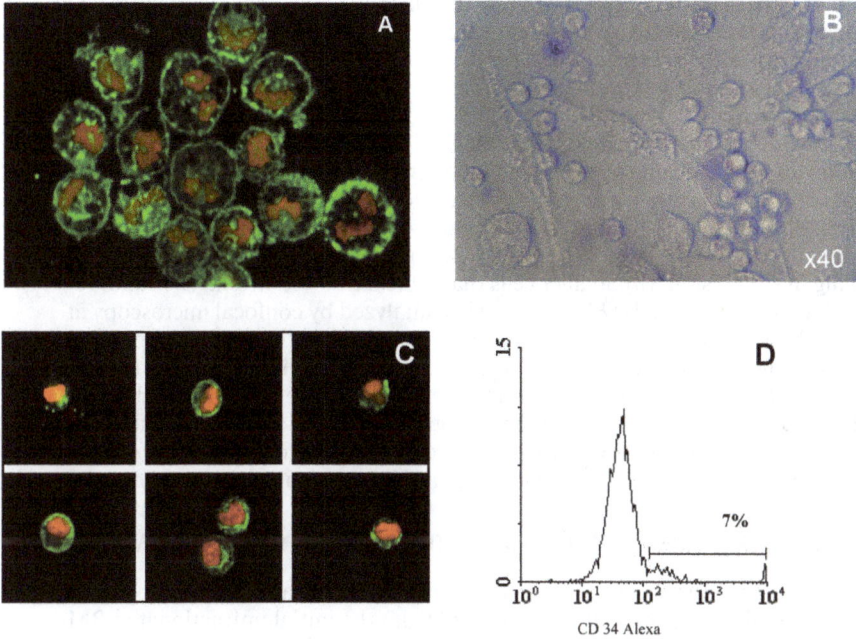

Figure 2. FICD-mediated reconstitution of a haematopoietic stem/progenitor cells compartment (day 60). A. Analysis of CD24 expression by confocal microscopy at day 65: a positive signal is present in all cells alive as a marker of FICD- transduction (nuclei coloured in red). B. Refringent, smaller semi-adherent cells growing on the autologous stroma. At day 70, these cells were analyzed by (C) confocal microscopy confirming CD34 positivity and a high nucleo-cytoplasmic ratio, (D) FACS showing 7% CD34+ cells (relative to the whole cell population, whether growing in suspension or adherent). Reproduced from Cohen-Haguenauer *et al.* [27].

GENE ADDITION RESULTS IN FUNCTIONAL RESTORATION OF FA PATIENT'S PRIMARY BM CELLS

Using this procedure, FA patients' primary BM cells could be maintained in culture long enough to match the minimal conditions needed for retrovirus-mediated gene transfer. We chose to focus on FA-A patients, the most common FA complementation group (over 70%). A bicistronic retrovirus vector was designed, FOCHA-*FANCA*-IRES-CD24 (FOCHA-FICD). This original vector was derived from the FB29-Fr-MuLV strain as a high-titer (10^6cfu/ml) GALV producer clone [36]. We used NAC-hypoxia cultured BM samples from 10 different patients (2×10^5 cells per patient), among which 9 were of A (FA-A) complementation group and 1 from complementation group C as control. Within 15 days of culture, untransduced FA-A cells and the FA-C cells disappeared from culture dishes. By contrast, FOCHA-FICD transduced hematopoietic cells from all FA-A patients were able to develop into Long Term Cultures (LTCs). A layer of autologous stroma spontaneously developed since un-fractionated BM was used to establish the cultures. LTCs could be maintained for over five weeks under minimal cytokine regimen. Interestingly, cultures established from transduced cells could be (i) returned under normal oxygen pressure after 4 weeks (but not earlier) and (ii) exposed to low-dose MMC over 15 days (from day 28 to 43) without noticeable impairment of either morphology, growth rate or cell counts as compared to untreated controls. Evidence for a selective growth advantage of transduced cells was the observation that a subset of cells began to regenerate the culture beginning around day 20-30. Progressive increase in erythroid progenitors up to 30-50% over 28 days accounts for a striking improvement since the absence of erythroid progenitors is the primary hallmark of FA. It is of interest to note that the FACS analysis also had to be adjusted to account for dramatic changes in cell diameters from 5-7 μm in starting material to 10-15μm at day 70; accordingly, the gain was changed from 30 to 10. At day 60, hematopoietic cells all stained positive for CD24 (*Figure 2A*) and could clearly be subdivided into two subsets: (i) A majority of larger cells (12-15 μm) with a low nucleus/cytoplasm ratio growing in suspension; (ii) Smaller cells that attached to the stroma as round, refringent and semi-adherent cells (*Figure 2B*): when analyzed by confocal microscopy at day 70 of the LTC, these cells had a high nucleus/cytoplasm ratio and tested positive for CD34 expression (*Figure 2C*) a feature further confirmed by FACS-analysis (*Figure 2D*). Among the 9 FA-A patients that we tested, similar data have been observed in cultured BM samples from eight (thus, with the exception of one) and are clearly the result of functional complementation resulting from successful introduction of the FANCA transgene, as confirmed by PCR assays evidencing its integration in all outgrowing cells.

LONG TERM ENGRAFTMENT OF FA HAEMATOPOIETIC STEM CELLS *IN VIVO*

Encouraging data from the above-mentioned *in vitro* assays indicate that hematopoietic cells with myeloid lineage potential have emerged from the initial unfractionated BM sample following gene-addition of a functional cDNA. Therefore, a contingent of less differentiated cells might carry potential for hematopoietic reconstitution, a potential that required *in vivo* challenge to be conclusively demonstrated. We thus chose to first expand transduced cells in long-term culture, in order for gene-corrected cells to emerge from a bulk of diseased cells, then to transplant cultured cells into NOD/SCID mice as a secondary assay. In order to evaluate this potential, BM cells were taken from 3 FA-A patients at distinct phases of the disease: patient #1: early diagnosis; patient #2: initial phase of leukemic transformation and patient #3: terminal aplastic anaemia. With each sample, $2x10^5$ unfractionated BM cells were transduced and grown for 9 weeks in LTC after which they were infused in NOD-SCID mice. 12 weeks after *in vivo* infusion, human cells were detected by FACS in the bone-marrow from mice injected with the early diagnosed patient only. These data demonstrate, despite the limited numbers of cells available for analysis, that gene-corrected primary BM cells from FA patients selectively grow in culture and sustain hematopoietic potential that translates into a positive engraftment *in vivo* in NOD/SCID mice. By comparison, untransduced cells died in culture by 15 days.

In this study, we showed that in overcoming the initial cell catastrophe caused by oxidative stress and DNA-damage, we were able to restore the long term ability of retro-virally- transduced stem cells to proliferate and differentiate both *in vitro* and *in vivo* in a stem cell disorder where cells can otherwise not replicate and die. Of interest, these data have been obtained using unfractionated BM cells so that autologous gene-corrected stromal/mesenchymal cells provide natural support for the patient's hematopoietic stem cells growth. Our data clearly demonstrate that bone marrow cells from patients with FANCA can be successfully grown and will differentiate along myeloid lineages under special conditions which reduce unnecessary physical manipulation, provide for anti-oxidant growth conditions, secure natural environment in using autologous stromal support and restore gene function *via* retrovirus-mediated gene transfer. In addition, our procedures meet criteria matching regulatory bodies most stringent requirements with the use of unfractionated autologous BM cells, serum-free media, market-approved anti-oxidative agents, minimal cytokine-regimen.

SAFETY AND EFFICACY IMPROVED INTEGRATIVE VECTORS

While long-term reconstitution of the stem cell compartment both *in vitro* and *in vivo* has been achieved in our lab with retroviral-mediated gene transfer of the main complementation group FANCA, in SCID [31], CGD [32] and WAS [33] patients however, secondary leukemia have been induced in retrovirus gene modified cells as a direct consequence of MLV-vector integration which is not random. We have thus designed and developed a new generation of genetically stable insulated vectors in order to help prevent gene transfer induced malignancies. Indeed new vectors backbones have been generated in our lab which incorporate new synthetic Genetic Insulator Elements (GIEs) which are capable of both preventing insertional mutagenesis and the extinction of transgene expression [30], in a lentivector context (see chapter A3-4, *ibid.*). Genotoxicity evaluation have been validated with constructs shuttling the EGFP1 cDNA as reporter, based on: (i) high throughput analysis of integration sites in collaboration with Christof von Kalle (National Center for Tumor Diseases, Heidelberg, Germany) and (ii) in cancer prone mice with Eugenio Montini (Fondazione Centro San Raffaele del Monte Tabor, Milano, Italy).

Moving to gene transfer of the FANCA cDNA, we have made use of our best new insulated vectors to encode for it and tested for the phenotypic correction of FA under the control of either one of three different promoters: the strong Fr-MuLV-U3, the housekeeping hPGK and the newly cloned FANCA homologous promoter that we have engineered. Phenotypic correction of FA cells is functionally assessed by (i) loss of sensitivity to chronic treatment with low-dose Mitomycin C; (ii) overcoming cell-cycle G2M block induced by high-dose Mitomycin C treatment and (iii) restoring FANCD2 monoubiquitination. By coupling specific culture conditions and this novel lentivirus constructs, we have also genetically corrected mesenchymal cells from three different *FANCA$^{-/-}$* patients' bone marrow (BM). Other studies have shown that the very weak vav promoter as well as the strong viral spleen focus-forming virus (SFFV) [37] corrects FANCA cellular phenotype; we report first evidence that the FANCA gene placed under the control of its own promoter performs at best. In fact, an intensive and permanent expression of FANCA - as would result from a strong viral promoter-driven expression - could be unsuitable for cell cycle regulation, and translate into noticeable toxicity in primary cells likely to compromise long-term genetic correction.

ENDOGENESIS

Finally, given that FA HSCs are especially fragile, their targeted *in vivo* transduction would represent a major advance. A further goal could consist of *in vivo* activation of stem cells. The direct regeneration of a stem cell pool from endogenous cells residing in their bone-marrow niche, where they remain preserved from oxidative stress, would by far the best option in FA-patients rather than potentially compromising their survival following *ex vivo* manipulation. In addition, vectors for in vivo HSC transduction must be specific for the target cell, to avoid vector spreading while enhancing transduction efficiency. Specific pseudotypes engineered by Verhoyen and Cosset hold major promises in that regard. Recently they have reported on successful *in vivo* transduction of human haematopoietic progenitors with a novel LV displaying SCF and a mutant cat endogenous retroviral glycoprotein, RDTR ([38]; see chapter A3-7, *ibid.*). The rationale for using SCF-display is the following: *in vivo*, a majority of HSCs are residing in the G0 phase of the cell cycle and are not quite permissive to classical VSV-G pseudotyped LVs. In contrast, vector particles displaying early-acti-vating-cytokine (SCF or/and TPO) allow a slight and transient stimulation of hCD34+ cells which results in efficient gene transfer to these target cells. First, these RDTR/SCF-LVs outperformed RDTR-LVs for transduction of human CD34+ cells *in vitro* since 30%-40% of these cells could be readily transduced from cord blood mo-nonuclear cells and in the unfractionated BM of healthy and Fanconi anaemia's do-nors; subsequent correction of patients' cells was achieved. Then, and most interestingly *in vivo*, these novel RDTR/SCF-displaying LVs were shown to be able to distinguish between the target hCD34+ cells of interest and nontarget cells, when the vector was directly injected into the BM cavity of humanized BALB/c Rag2-null/IL2rgc-null (BALB/c RAGA) mice. This resulted in the highly selective trans-duction of candidate hCD34(+)Lin(-) HSCs. Indeed, in the future, these RDTR/SCF lentiviral vectors might completely alleviate *ex vivo* handling and target cells loss re-lated to *ex-vivo* manipulations, with the combined risk of cell death, differentiation, loss of stemness characteristics and homing/engraftment potential along with the *ex-vivo* procedures for culture, transduction and/or expansion. This is likely to simplify gene therapy for other hematopoietic defects, should direct *in vivo* inoculation of the vector off the shell become a clinical reality.

SPECULATIONS ON MECHANISMS OF FA-PATHOGENESIS

A speculative model of how FA-associated proteins repair interstrand crosslinks during DNA replication had been strengthened by the identification of two FA genes [39]. In our long-term functional correction study [27], we could monitor full recovery of cell-growth and proliferation with each patient's sample from day 28 post-transduction. At that time, cells were brought back to normoxia and addition of NAC was stopped. Based on these observations, passed a necessary lag-time of several weeks where cells still need to be preserved, gene-corrected cells are capable of both proliferation and differentiation, which may account for an improved capacity for DNA to replicate. Another striking empiric observation is the delayed functional recovery of cell-mem-brane resistance and cell-diameter. Prior studies have hypothesized the role of abnor-mal redox status that may account for FA-related membrane fragility [8, 9, 40]. Interestingly, our data show that cell-membrane fragility would not recover before day 60 of culture *in vitro*, the time by which cell diameter would also normalize, as per FACS analysis. Thus, cells might recover from the ability to sustain oxidative stress at a much later stage where DNA can supposedly already replicate. Analysing the se-quential phases of human primary stem cells recovery might provide insights into the molecular mechanisms involved in FA: this unique model carries potential to better delineate the combined role of both DNA-repair deficiency and oxidative stress in the pathogenesis of Fanconi's anaemia. Obviously, a diseased FA-iPS cell-line would re-present a significant added value in order to investigate and dissect in depth the precise mechanisms involved. Altogether, increasing knowledge in this fascinating disease is likely to improve our understanding of other genetic, DNA-repair, cancer or haema-topoietic related conditions.

CONCLUSION

Gene transfer intended as a treatment is conceptually simple, as it involves the delivery of highly-defined nucleic acid sequences in order to mediate therapy providing a suf-ficient number of target cells can express the gene of interest. Up until recently, safer gene transfer systems with improved specificity, efficacy and safety towards clinical translation have remained a major bottleneck in the development of gene therapy, so that the risk of harm/benefit balance will be improved for patients. With significant improvements now at reach, in Fanconi's anaemia, the clinical challenge remains to efficiently correct through gene transfer, a sufficient number of patients' cells to sustain a prolonged hematopoietic reservoir able to (i) reconstitute a human BM and (ii) produce good quality and accurate amounts of peripheral blood cells without developing clonality or increasing the risk of malignancy in cancer-prone patients. In order to circumvent the risk of harm and in particular, insertional mutagenesis, we have pursued a synergistic approach with preliminary but robust hints of success, based on the combination of new synthetic elements which result in long term expression of integrative gene transfer systems, including when and if landing in heterochromatin. Clinical prospects might be considered, making use of those safety-improved vectors that we are currently developing, providing all pre-clinical steps will be conclusive and reassuring as compared to former attempts which failed.

Gene therapy intervention consisting into the stable transfer of a functional *FANC*-gene in patients' hematopoietic progenitors should be beneficial: *in vivo* selective growth advantage of transduced cells is expected. This is likely to help genetically engineered hematopoietic progenitors settle and reconstitute host without prior myeloablation alleviating the potential side effects of conditioning in these fragile patients. In particular, the potential addition of a functional FA-gene into genuine hematopoietic stem cells should translate into a pivotal improvement of patients' condition. Our data provide strong evidence that this potential varies widely from one patient to the next: therefore, clinical success of gene therapy will be possible only in those patients diagnosed early enough in the course of the disease, where a hematopoietic stem cell pool might be spared and appropriate for gene correction, as demonstrated by our *in vivo* data. In this context, a first-in-human clinical study might be considered, since in the event where the gene therapy protocol would fail, blood stem cells transplantation could still be considered and performed: indeed, without prior conditioning, haplo-identical HSCT transplantation remains an option without any loss of chance.

ACKNOWLEDGMENTS

This work has been performed with the support of the EC-DG research through the FP6-Network of Excellence, CLINIGENE: LSHB-CT-2006-018933.
E.B. received a post-doctoral grant of Région Île-de-France DIM Stem-Pole.
O.C.H. addresses special thanks to Eliane Gluckman.

REFERENCES

1. Butturini A, Gale RP, Verlander PC, Adler-Brecher B, Gillio AP, Auerbach AD. Hematologic abnormalities in Fanconi anemia: an international Fanconi anemia registry study. *Blood* 1994; 84: 1650-5.

2. Alter BP. Cancer in Fanconi anemia, 1927-2001. *Cancer* 2003; 97: 425-40.

3. Alter BP, Giri N, Savage SA, Peters JA, Loud JT, Leathwood L, *et al*. Malignancies and survival patterns in the National Cancer Institute inherited bone marrow failure syndromes cohort study. *Br J Haematol* 2010; 150: 179-88.

4. Auerbach AD, Allen RG. Leukemia and preleukemia in Fanconi anemia patients. A review of the literature and report of the international Fanconi anemia registry. *Cancer Genet Cytogenet* 1991; 51: 1-12.

5. D'Andrea AD. Susceptibility pathways in Fanconi's anemia and breast cancer. *N Engl J Med* 2010; 362: 1909-19.

6. Mace G, Bogliolo M, Guervilly JH, Dugas du Villard JA, Rosselli F. 3R coordination by Fanconi anemia proteins. *Biochimie* 2005; 87: 647-58.

7. Pagano G, Youssoufian H. Fanconi anaemia proteins: major roles in cell protection against oxidative damage. Bioessays 2003; 25: 589-95.

8. Cumming RC, Lightfoot J, Beard K, Youssoufian H, O'Brien PJ, Buchwald M. Fanconi anemia group C protein prevents apoptosis in hematopoietic cells through redox regulation of GSTP1. *Nat Med* 2001; 7: 814-20.

9. Joenje H, Arwert F, Eriksson AW, de Koning H, Oostra AB. Oxygen-dependence of chromosomal aberrations in Fanconi's anaemia. *Nature* 1981; 290: 142-3.

10. Ishida R, Buchwald M. Susceptibility of Fanconi's anemia lymphoblasts to DNA-cross-linking and alkylating agents. *Cancer Res* 1982; 42: 4000-6.

11. Stewart G, Elledge SJ. The two faces of BRCA2, a FANCtastic discovery. *Mol Cell* 2002; 10: 2-4.

12. D'Andrea AD, Grompe M. The Fanconi anaemia/BRCA pathway. *Nat Rev Cancer* 2003; 3: 23-34.

13. Chen S, Parmigiani G. Meta-analysis of BRCA1 and BRCA2 penetrance. *J Clin Oncol* 2007; 25: 1329-33.

14. King MC, Marks JH, Mandell JB. Breast and ovarian cancer risks due to inherited mutations in BRCA1 and BRCA2. *Science* 2003; 302: 643-6.

15. Patel KJ, Yu VP, Lee H, Corcoran A, Thistlethwaite FC, Evans MJ, *et al.* Involvement of Brca2 in DNA repair. *Mol Cell* 1998; 1: 347-57.

16. Reid S, Schindler D, Hanenberg H, Barker K, Hanks S, Kalb R, *et al.* Biallelic mutations in PALB2 cause Fanconi anemia subtype FA-N and predispose to childhood cancer. *Nat Genet* 2007; 39: 162-4.

17. Xia B, Dorsman JC, Ameziane N, de Vries Y, Rooimans MA, Sheng Q, *et al.* Fanconi anemia is associated with a defect in the BRCA2 partner PALB2. *Nat Genet* 2007; 39: 159-61.

18. Gluckman E, Auerbach AD, Horowitz MM, Sobocinski KA, Ash RC, Bortin MM, *et al.* Bone marrow transplantation for Fanconi anemia. *Blood* 1995; 86: 2856-62.

19. Gluckman E, Rocha V, Ionescu I, Bierings M, Harris RE, Wagner J, *et al.* Results of unrelated cord blood transplant in fanconi anemia patients: risk factor analysis for engraftment and survival. *Biol Blood Marrow Transplant* 2007; 13: 1073-82.

20. Chaudhury S, Auerbach AD, Kernan NA, Small TN, Prockop SE, Scaradavou A, *et al.* Fludarabine-based cytoreductive regimen and T-cell-depleted grafts from alternative donors for the treatment of high-risk patients with Fanconi anaemia. *Br J Haematol* 2008; 140: 644-55.

21. MacMillan ML, Hughes MR, Agarwal S, Daley GQ. Cellular therapy for fanconi anemia: the past, present, and future. *Biol Blood Marrow Transplant* 2011; 17 (1 suppl): S109-14.

22. Pasquini R, Carreras J, Pasquini MC, Camitta BM, Fasth AL, Hale GA, *et al.* HLA-matched sibling hematopoietic stem cell transplantation for fanconi anemia: comparison of irradiation and nonirradiation containing conditioning regimens. *Biol Blood Marrow Transplant* 2008; 14: 1141-7.

23. Wagner JE, Eapen M, MacMillan ML, Harris RE, Pasquini R, Boulad F, Zhang MJ, Auerbach AD. Unrelated donor bone marrow transplantation for the treatment of Fanconi anemia. *Blood* 2007; 109: 2256-62.

24. Alter BP. Fanconi's anemia, transplantation, and cancer. *Pediatr Transplant* 2005; 9 (suppl 7): 81-6.

25. Kelly PF, Radtke S, von Kalle C, Balcik B, Bohn K, Mueller R, *et al*. Stem cell collection and gene transfer in Fanconi anemia. *Mol Ther* 2007; 15: 211-9.

26. Liu JM, Kim S, Read EJ, Futaki M, Dokal I, Carter CS, *et al*. Engraftment of hematopoietic progenitor cells transduced with the Fanconi anemia group C gene (FANCC). *Hum Gene Ther* 1999; 10: 2337-46.

27. Cohen-Haguenauer O, Peault B, Bauche C, Daniel MT, Casal I, Levy V, *et al. In vivo* repopulation ability of genetically corrected bone marrow cells from Fanconi anemia patients. *Proc Natl Acad Sci USA* 2006; 103: 2340-5.

28. Duros C, Artus A, Scholtz S. Insulated lentiviral vectors towards safer gene transfer to stem cells. *Mol Ther* 2011; 19: pS149.

29. Duros C, Artus A, Scholz S, Ragon I, Cesana D, Paruzynski A, *et al*. Stability and safety improved retroviral and lentiviral vectors comprising CTF/NF1 genetic insulator elements efficiently reconstitute hu-CD34+ cord blood cells. 2012 ; Submission pending.

30. Gaussin A, Modlich U, Bauche C, Niederlander NJ, Schambach A, Duros C, *et al*. CTF/NF1 transcription factors act as potent genetic insulators for integrating gene transfer vectors. *Gene Ther* 2011; 19: 15-24.

31. Hacein-Bey-Abina S, Garrigue A, Wang GP, Soulier J, Lim A, Morillon E, *et al. Insertional oncogenesis in 4 patients after retrovirus-mediated gene therapy of SCID-X1. J Clin Invest* 2008; 118: 3132-42.

32. Stein S, Ott MG, Schultze-Strasser S, Jauch A, Burwinkel B, Kinner A, *et al*. Genomic instability and myelodysplasia with monosomy 7 consequent to EVI1 activation after gene therapy for chronic granulomatous disease. *Nat Med* 2010; 16: 198-204.

33. Boztug K, Schmidt M, Schwarzer A, Banerjee PP, Diez IA, Dewey RA, *et al*. Stem-cell gene therapy for the Wiskott-Aldrich syndrome. *N Engl J Med* 2010; 363: 1918-27.

34. Liu JM, Young NS, Walsh CE, Cottler-Fox M, Carter C, Dunbar C, Barrett AJ, Emmons R. Retroviral mediated gene transfer of the Fanconi anemia complementation group C gene to hematopoietic progenitors of group C patients. *Hum Gene Ther* 1997; 8: 1715-30.

35. Galimi F, Noll M, Kanazawa Y, Lax T, Chen C, Grompe M, Verma IM. Gene therapy of Fanconi anemia: preclinical efficacy using lentiviral vectors. *Blood* 2002; 100: 2732-6.

36. Cohen-Haguenauer O, Restrepo LM, Masset M, Bayer J, Dal Cortivo L, Marolleau JP, *et al*. Efficient transduction of hemopoietic CD34+ progenitors of human origin using an original retroviral vector derived from Fr-MuLV-FB29: *in vitro* assessment. *Hum Gene Ther* 1998; 9: 207-16.

37. Gonzalez-Murillo A, Lozano ML, Alvarez L, Jacome A, Almarza E, Navarro S, *et al*. Development of lentiviral vectors with optimized transcriptional activity for the gene therapy of patients with Fanconi anemia. *Hum Gene Ther* 2010; 21: 623-30.

38. Frecha C, Costa C, Negre D, Amirache F, Trono D, Rio P, *et al*. A novel lentiviral vector targets gene transfer into human hematopoietic stem cells in marrow from patients with bone marrow failure syndrome and *in vivo* in humanized mice. *Blood* 2012; 119: 1139-50.

39. Thompson LH. Unraveling the Fanconi anemia-DNA repair connection. *Nat Genet* 2005; 37: 921-2.

40. Leurs C, Jansen M, Pollok KE, Heinkelein M, Schmidt M, Wissler M, *et al*. Comparison of three retroviral vector systems for transduction of nonobese diabetic/severe combined immunodeficiency mice repopulating human CD34+ cord blood cells. *Hum Gene Ther* 2003; 14: 509-19.

TECHNOLOGIES

Adenovirus mediated gene transfer: current developments

COORDINATED BY
STEFAN KOCHANEK

The CliniBook: Clinical gene transfer
Edited by Odile Cohen-Haguenauer – EDK, Paris © 2012, pp. 229-231

A5-1
Overview on adenovirus vectors

STEFAN KOCHANEK

Department of Gene Therapy, University of Ulm, Helmholtz Str. 8/1, 89081 Ulm, Germany.
stefan.kochanek@uni-ulm.de

INTRODUCTION TO ADENOVIRUS

Adenovirus has been an important model used by many researchers to study basic mechanisms in molecular and cell biology including RNA transcription, RNA splicing (Nobel Prize in Physiology/Medicine 1993 to Roberts and Sharp), cell transformation, cell-cycle control and many others.

Adenoviruses have been identified and isolated in many vertebrates including mammals, reptiles, birds, amphibia and fish. The virus family of Adenoviridae consists of 5 genera. Within the genus mastadenovirus more than 50 human adenovirus types, currently grouped in species A to G, are distinguished based on sequence information and, more in the past than today, immunological typing.

Briefly, adenovirus is a non-enveloped virus with a diameter of about 100 nm, a molecular weight of about 150 MDa, and the form of an icosahedron, carrying a linear, double-stranded genome with a size of about 30 to 40 kb, depending on the specific adenovirus type. The adenovirus genome carries about 30 genes, all (except one or two) coding for proteins. The mature particle, in addition to the DNA genome, consists of 11 structural proteins, of which 7 form the capsid and 4 are packaged inside the capsid. Uptake of the virus (and vector) particle occurs by receptor-mediated endocytosis via capsid interaction with cell surface receptors as the first step. *In vitro*, most human Ad types bind to the Coxsackie and Adenovirus Receptor (CAR), through binding of the knob part of the homotrimeric fiber to CAR, although some types are rather taken up into cells after primary interaction with CD46, CD80/86 or DSG-2.

Today mainly three Adenovirus (Ad) vector types can be distinguished that are used for different and partly overlapping applications: ΔE1 Ad vectors, HC-Ad vectors and replicating Ad vectors (*Figure 1*).

ΔE1 AD VECTORS

ΔE1 Ad vectors (also called first-generation or E1-deleted Ad vectors, respectively) are the most frequently used Ad vector type. Mostly they are based on human Ad type 5 (hAd5), but more recently Ad vectors have been generated that are derived from other human Ad types (*e.g.* hAd6, hAd26, hAd35) or from other species such as chimpanzee. This vector type retains most of the viral genes except the *E1A* and *E1B* genes. Since the *E1A* gene is the first viral gene to be expressed after virus entry into a cell, and because the *E1A* gene products stimulate expression of most other viral genes and also interact with many different cellular factors as a precondition for a viral infectious cycle to occur, ΔE1 Ad vectors are replication deficient in normal human cells. Nowadays this vector type is mainly used as delivery vehicle for genetic vaccines, either for prophylactic vaccination in the case of infectious diseases and for tumor vaccination. Production of this vector type follows standard procedures and GMP processes have been established. In general this vector type is not suitable for long-term gene therapy: in immunocompetent hosts, cellular immune responses against adenoviral proteins are observed resulting in removal of vector-transduced cells due to leaky expression of viral proteins encoded on the vector genome despite deletion of the *E1* genes.

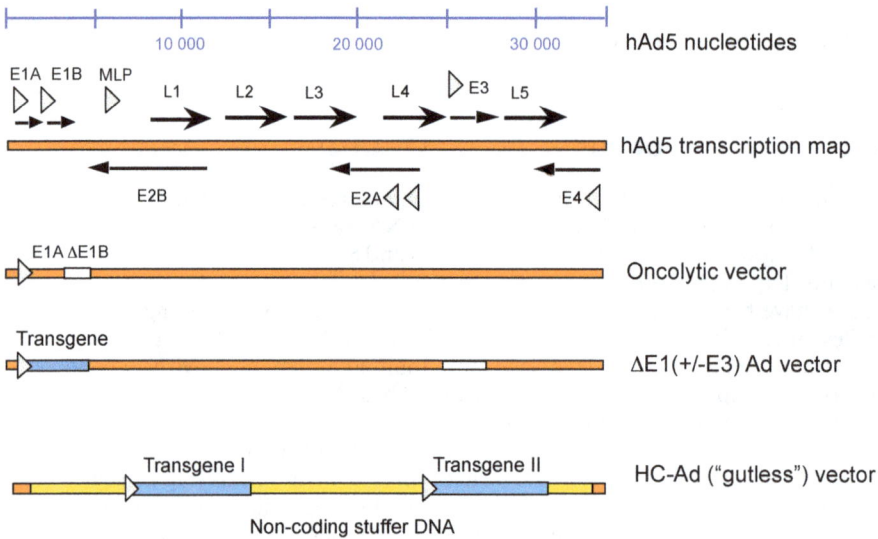

Figure 1. Overview on frequently used Adenovirus vectors.

HIGH-CAPACITY ADENOVIRUS VECTORS

High-capacity adenovirus (HC-Ad) vectors are also called helper-dependent or "gutless" Ad vectors. In this vector type all the viral genes are deleted so that an increased uptake capacity for foreign DNA of about 35 kb results. This vector is produced with a helper virus that is removed, to a large degree, during the production process, by Cre-recombinase mediated excision of the packaging signal of the helper virus. Use of this vector results in long-term expression in cells replicating slowly or not at all, even in an immunocompetent host. While this vector type has several principal advantages over ΔE1 Ad vectors, clinical introduction so far has not been possible due to a complicated production process that is difficult to standardize.

REPLICATING ADENOVIRUS VECTORS

While ΔE1 Ad vectors may efficiently transduce tumor cells they are not able to spread within solid tumors. With the aim to improve anti-tumor activity Ad vectors have been developed that selectively replicate in tumor cells but not in non-neoplastic normal cells. Therefore, these vectors are also called conditionally replicating adenovirus vectors (CRADs). Different principles, alone or in combination, are followed to achieve tumor cell selective replication and amplification: (i) Either these vectors have mutations in the ΔE1A and/or ΔE1B region, thereby preventing interaction with their cellular binding partners, *e.g.* p53 or Rb; although the mechanisms are not totally clear, as a result such recombinant Ad-vectors will not amplify in untransformed cells, while still replicate in tumor cells, in which the p53 and/or Rb systems are inactivated; (ii) Or the *E1A* gene (potentially also additional other virus genes) is under the control of a tumour-specific promoter.

Examples of the current use of the Adenovirus system mostly in tumour gene therapy are exposed in the following chapters (Lucas and Kochanek, Gänsbacher and Anton, Ylä-Herttuala, respectively) which also include Marques-Alves and co-workers' contribution on the production and purification of recombinant Ad-derived vectors.

ACKNOWLEDGMENTS

This work has been performed with the support of the EC-DG research through the FP6-Network of Excellence, CLINIGENE: LSHB-CT-2006-018933.

REFERENCES

1. Imperiale MJ, Kochanek S. Adenovirus vectors: biology, design, and production. *Curr Top Microbiol Immunol* 2004; 273: 335-57.

2. Silva AC, Peixoto C, Lucas T, Küppers C, Cruz PE, Alves PM, Kochanek S. Adenovirus vector production and purification. *Curr Gene Ther* 2010; 10: 437-55.

The CliniBook: Clinical gene transfer
Edited by Odile Cohen-Haguenauer – EDK, Paris © 2012, pp. 232-237

A5-2
Tumour barriers influencing adenovirus vector delivery and therapeutic efficacy

TANJA LUCAS, STEFAN KOCHANEK*

Department of Gene Therapy, University of Ulm, Helmholtz Str. 8/1, 89081 Ulm, Germany.
stefan.kochanek@uni-ulm.de
* Corresponding author

Adenovirus-based gene transfer vectors (Ad vectors) have been used so far in more than 400 clinical trials worldwide and in several thousand patients (http://www.wiley.com//legacy/wileychi/genmed/clinical/). Most of the studies have been performed in patients with solid cancers. Both ΔE1 Ad vectors and replicating Ad vectors (CRADs) have been used in these studies, either given as intratumoural or as systemic injection. Two Ad vectors, one expressing p53, the other being a replicating "oncolytic" adenovirus, have been approved (*i.e.*: marketing authorisation being granted) and are in use in China for tumour therapy. None of these two or other vectors have been market-approved in Western countries.

Altogether, clinical studies have demonstrated safety of Ad vectors after intratumoural injection. Even after intravascular delivery of high vector doses vector-related death cases in clinical tumour therapy studies have not been reported. In general, vector-related side effects, if present, have been mild (increased temperature, change in blood chemistry, etc.) and limited. While safety has been demonstrated, therapeutic efficacy either as monotherapy or in combination with radio- or chemotherapy has overall been very low to the degree that only few companies in Europe or the USA have sustained their investments in the further development of Ad vector-based anti-tumour drugs. What are the reasons for this slow progression in the clinical development of a conceptually intriguing biological therapy such as a Thymidine kinase-expressing ΔE1 Ad vector or an Ad vector that selectively replicates in tumour cells? Why do Ad vectors not work as well as one would have hoped?

Adenoviruses like other viruses have coevolved with their vertebrate hosts over millions of years. In general, a fine-tuned balance exists between the ability of a virus to infect, to multiply, to spread to another host (*e.g.* by shedding in the stool) and/or to persist, and the host counteracting virus infection in different ways to avoid an overwhelming infection and disease. Thus, viruses are not "made" for an efficient and safe delivery of their cargo (their genome) to target cells. *In vivo* many factors function as natural barriers for adenovirus infection, many of which have only been identified in recent years.

In this general overview we will not analyse all known virus-host interaction barriers in comprehensive details. A relevant overview is presented in Strauss and Lieber [1].

Rather, we elect to expose the identified bottlenecks along general categories, as follows: (i) Some of the barriers will be significant for any disease that is addressed by gene therapy; (ii) others are tissue and disease specific; and (iii) again some are unique to solid tumours, the latter being the focus of this overview. Of course, whether barriers are relevant for certain applications or not, is a question that may also depend on practical issues such as the route of vector delivery, *i.e.* by intra-tumoural injection or by systemic delivery.

TRANSPORT OF VECTOR PARTICLES THROUGH THE VASCULAR SPACE

When an adenoviral vector is delivered to a person by intravascular injection, it is transported in the blood through the vascular space. Here it will interact with both the non-cellular and the cellular compartment. The non-cellular compartment consists mainly of proteins such as blood coagulation factors, complement factors and anti-adenoviral antibodies, the latter being present in about 60% of individuals. Recently, it has been demonstrated that, in addition to the well-known anti-adenovirus neutralizing activity of pre-existing antibodies, and to activation of the complement system [2], Ad5-based vector may bind to the complement receptor 1 (CR1) in the presence of complement and anti-adenoviral antibodies [3]. Interestingly, CR1 is present on human erythrocytes but not on erythrocytes from mice. It has also been shown in recent years, as a very interesting finding, that the hexon protein of adenovirus interacts with blood coagulation factor X and that this interaction mediates adenovirus entry into hepatocytes [4-6] and not the receptor CAR.

Interaction of adenovirus vectors with the cellular compartment is a second and quite significant reason for low efficacy of cells and tumour transduction after systemic delivery. Besides interacting with platelets [7], direct interaction of the adenovirus particle with erythrocytes [2] *via* binding of the fiber knob domain to CAR [3] (again present on human but not on murine erythrocytes), will likely reduce the vector amount that is available for intended *in vivo* transduction of cells/tumour cells. Resident macrophages, particularly Kupffer cells, located in the liver sinusoids and the spleen, represent another very important barrier for systemic Ad vector delivery. Although hAd5 based vectors stand as one of the most efficient vehicles for *in vivo* delivery to hepatocytes, data from animal experimentation indicate that only 1 of about 10^3 or 10^4 hAd5 particles will in fact express its cargo in hepatocytes, the vast majority of particles being removed from the circulation by Kupffer cells. Interestingly, it has recently been shown that at least part of the observed toxicity that has been following i.v. injection in mice is due to release of platelet activation factor (PAF) from Kupffer cells [9] resulting from the interaction of hAd5 with Kupffer cells which triggers an endothelial cell activation and a hemodynamic response [10].

VECTOR PARTICLES REACHING OUT TO THE TUMOUR

A third important aspect for vector delivery to tumours relates to the vascular morphology, which is highly abnormal in tumours. Tumour vessels are characterized by a high degree of heterogeneity, the presence of discontinuous capillaries and arterio-venous anastomoses, resulting in inhomogenous blood supply negatively affects intra-tumoural vector distribution.

Following vector arrival at the tumour, the further transport of vector particles (and macromolecules) across the microvascular wall and through interstitial space is influenced by both physical and chemical parameters which will greatly impact on vector particle delivery to and distribution within a solid tumour. Transport across the microvascular wall within a tumour depends on properties of the vessel wall (morphology, absence or presence of endothelial fenestrae), properties of the vector particle (size, charge, etc.) and on transport parameters (diffusion and convection) [11]. Movement within the interstitial space depends on: (i) diffusion which is influenced by concentration gradients, properties of both interstitial space and the vector; (ii) convection which is influenced by pressure gradients and properties of the interstitial space and the vector, both of these parameters are being unfavourable in tumours; and finally (iii) on intercellular distances, the latter being increased in tumours *versus* normal tissues [11]. As a result extravasation and intra-tumoural distribution of Ad vectors (as would be the same with other vectors) is very limited.

COMPLEX COMPOSITION OF TUMOURS PREVENT SPREADING OF VECTORS

Following delivery to the tumour either after intravascular or intra-tumoural injection, two major blocks can be distinguished: the complex composition of solid tumours and the frequent absence of natural receptors on tumour cells.

In contrast to models of tumour transplantation in mice, solid epithelial cancers consist of both tumour cells and many additional cell types. In some cancers, like for example of the pancreas, a strong stromal component will prevent the spreading of both replicating and non-replicating vectors. In addition, the spreading of Ad vectors which specifically replicate in tumour cells is strongly inhibited by the stromal tumour compartment [12]. Further, CAR, the natural receptor for several Ad vector types including hAd5 is only poorly expressed on neoplastic cells, contributing to the low anti-tumour efficiency of ΔE1 and replicating Ad vectors [13, 14].

Altogether, barriers exist at different levels that can explain the low efficacy of current Ad vector-mediated tumour therapy; some of the barriers can be considered as common to all or most macromolecules, such as heterogenous vascular morphology and physical parameters when related to diffusion and convection issues. Others are likely relevant for different viral or non-viral vector types, such as interaction with macrophages and Kupffer cells. Finally, others will likely be specific to Ad vectors such as hexon-specific interaction with coagulation factor X and fiber-knob interaction with CAR present on erythrocytes.

CURRENT STRATEGIES TO OVERCOME BARRIERS FOR ADENOVIRUS-MEDIATED TUMOUR THERAPY

Only some of the research strategies to overcome recognized barriers are discussed in this paper.

Since most neoplastic cells express only low levels of CAR, retargeting strategies represent a logical approach. Different tropisms can be achieved by either introducing targeting peptides into the knob domain of the adenoviral fiber or replacing the fiber or the fiber knob with the corresponding part from another adenovirus type which targets a different attachment site. Quite promising strategies include the targeting of CD46, a surface molecule with increased expression levels in many tumour types; this can be performed by generating chimeric hAd5-based Ad vectors carrying for example the fiber of hAd35 [15] or the fiber knob of hAd3 [16].

Another potentially promising strategy is based on the manipulation of solvent-exposed hexon part(s) that are known to interact with blood coagulation factor X. Introducing a targeting epitope into the hexon may also lead to detargeting from hepatocytes, besides providing a new uptake mechanism and tropism [17], which is likely to increase the biosafety of this vector type. A difficulty in the rationale design and development of new targeting/retargeting strategies is the lack of good animal models fitted to most approaches. For example and as discussed above, mice do not carry CAR or CR1 on the erythrocytes, while they are present on human erythrocytes. Also, regular xenotransplantation models, performed in mice, do not recapitulate the complex tumour composition observed in human primary tumours most of which are developing slowly.

A different approach based on bioselection of replicating Ad vectors may be an attractive alternative for the identification of Ad vectors with improved growth properties in tumours [18-21].

As mentioned above, an important barrier in solid tumours, which limits the spreading of replicating Ad vectors is a prominent stromal cell component which is frequently surrounding tumour cell nests in some cancers such as from the pancreas. It might thus be necessary to "re-restrict" replicating Ad vectors in order to allow their penetration also into the tumour stroma [22, 23].

Finally, a completely different approach to achieve improved delivery to tumours is based on coating the adenoviral surface by covalent attachment of a polymer shield. This approach has the potential advantages to both be suitable for different adenoviral vector types and to address unwanted interactions of Ad vector particles with either already well identified or so far still unknown soluble components or surfaces. Two polymer coating strategies are currently being developed, either based on chemical capsid surface modification with poly-N-(2-hydroxylpropyl) methacrylamide (poly-HPMA) or polyethylene glycol (PEG) [24, 25]. The attachment of synthetic polymers to the adenoviral surface promises to prevent many unwanted interactions of the viral capsid with cellular and non-cellular compartments discussed above, such as binding to blood components [26, 27]; they can additionnally be combined with targeting approaches [28-30]. An approach under current development involves the specific modification of Ad vectors capsid *via* attachment of PEG or other molecules to a cysteine residue which has been introduced by the genetic engineering of solvent exposed areas of the hexon or other capsid proteins [31] allowing, for example, the detargeting of hepatocytes after i.v. injection in mice [32].

Taken together, these strategies hold promise for increased specificity and safety towards Adenovirus vector delivery to tumours with improved therapeutic efficacy.

ACKNOWLEDGMENTS

This work has been performed with the support of the EC-DG research through the FP6-Network of Excellence, CLINIGENE: LSHB-CT-2006-018933.

REFERENCES

1. Strauss R, Lieber A. Anatomical and physical barriers to tumour targeting with oncolytic adenoviruses *in vivo. Curr Opin Mol Ther* 2009; 11: 513-22.

2. Cichon G, Boeckh-Herwig S, Schmidt HH, Wehnes E, Muller T, Pring-Akerblom P, Burger R. Complement activation by recombinant adenoviruses. *Gene Ther* 2001; 8: 1794-800.

3. Carlisle RC, Di Y, Cerny AM, Sonnen AF, Sim RB, Green NK, *et al.* Human erythrocytes bind and inactivate type 5 adenovirus by presenting Coxsackie virus-adenovirus receptor and complement receptor 1. *Blood* 2009; 113: 1909-18.

4. Kalyuzhniy O, Di Paolo NC, Silvestry M, Hofherr SE, Barry MA, Stewart PL, Shayakhmetov DM. Adenovirus serotype 5 hexon is critical for virus infection of hepatocytes *in vivo. Proc Natl Acad Sci USA* 2008; 105: 5483-8.

5. Waddington SN, McVey JH, Bhella D, Parker AL, Barker K, Atoda H, *et al.* Adenovirus serotype 5 hexon mediates liver gene transfer. *Cell* 2008; 132: 397-409.

6. Vigant F, Descamps D, Jullienne B, Esselin S, Connault E, Opolon P, *et al.* Substitution of hexon hypervariable region 5 of adenovirus serotype 5 abrogates blood factor binding and limits gene transfer to liver. *Mol Ther* 2008; 16: 1474-80.

7. Shimony N, Elkin G, Kolodkin-Gal D, Krasny L, Urieli-Shoval S, Haviv YS. Analysis of adenoviral attachment to human platelets. *Virol J* 2009; 6: 25.

8. Cichon G, Boeckh-Herwig S, Kuemin D, Hoffmann C, Schmidt HH, Wehnes E, *et al.* Titer determination of Ad5 in blood: a cautionary note. *Gene Ther* 2003; 10: 1012-7.

9. Schiedner G, Bloch W, Hertel S, Johnston M, Molojavyi A, Dries V, *et al.* A hemodynamic response to intravenous adenovirus vector particles is caused by systemic Kupffer cell-mediated activation of endothelial cells. *Hum Gene Ther* 2003; 14: 1631-41.

10. Xu Z, Smith JS, Tian J, Byrnes AP. Induction of shock after intravenous injection of adenovirus vectors: a critical role for platelet-activating factor. *Mol Ther* 2010; 18: 609-16

11. Jain RK. Vascular and interstitial barriers to delivery of therapeutic agents in tumours. *Cancer Metast Rev* 1990; 9: 253-66.

12. Kuppen PJ, van der Eb MM, Jonges LE, Hagenaars M, Hokland ME, Nannmark U, *et al.* Tumour structure and extracellular matrix as a possible barrier for therapeutic approaches using immune cells or adenoviruses in colorectal cancer. *Histochem Cell Biol* 2001; 115: 67-72.

13. Li Y, Pong RC, Bergelson JM, Hall MC, Sagalowsky AI, Tseng CP, *et al.* Loss of adenoviral receptor expression in human bladder cancer cells: a potential impact on the efficacy of gene therapy. *Cancer Res* 1999; 59: 325-30.

14. Okegawa T, Li Y, Pong RC, Bergelson JM, Zhou J, Hsieh JT. The dual impact of coxsackie and adenovirus receptor expression on human prostate cancer gene therapy. *Cancer Res* 2000; 60: 5031-6.

15. Ni S, Gaggar A, Di Paolo N, Li ZY, Liu Y, Strauss R, *et al.* Evaluation of adenovirus vectors containing serotype 35 fibers for tumour targeting. *Cancer Gene Ther* 2006; 13: 1072-81.

16. Kanerva A, Mikheeva GV, Krasnykh V, Coolidge CJ, Lam JT, Mahasreshti PJ, *et al.* Targeting adenovirus to the serotype 3 receptor increases gene transfer efficiency to ovarian cancer cells. *Clin Cancer Res* 2002; 8: 275-80.

17. Jullienne B, Vigant F, Muth E, Chaligne R, Bouquet C, Giraudier S, *et al.* Efficient delivery of angiostatin K1-5 into tumours following insertion of an NGR peptide into adenovirus capsid. *Gene Ther* 2009; 16: 1405-15.

18. Gros A, Martinez-Quintanilla J, Puig C, Guedan S, Mollevi DG, Alemany R, Cascallo M. Bioselection of a gain of function mutation that enhances adenovirus 5 release and improves its antitumoural potency. *Cancer Res* 2008; 68: 8928-37.

19. Uil TG, Vellinga J, de Vrij J, van den Hengel SK, Rabelink MJ, Cramer SJ, *et al*. Directed adenovirus evolution using engineered mutator viral polymerases. *Nucleic Acids Res* 2011; 39: e30.

20. Yan W, Kitzes G, Dormishian F, Hawkins L, Sampson-Johannes A, Watanabe J, *et al*. Developing novel oncolytic adenoviruses through bioselection. *J Virol* 2003; 77: 2640-50.

21. Kuhn I, Harden P, Bauzon M, Chartier C, Nye J, Thorne S, *et al*. Directed evolution generates a novel oncolytic virus for the treatment of colon cancer. *PLoS One* 2008; 3: e2409.

22. Hsieh CL, Gardner TA, Miao L, Balian G, Chung LW. Cotargeting tumour and stroma in a novel chimeric tumour model involving the growth of both human prostate cancer and bone stromal cells. *Cancer Gene Ther* 2004; 11: 148-55.

23. Puig-Saus C, Gros A, Alemany R, Cascallo M. Adenovirus i-leader truncation bioselected against cancer-associated fibroblasts to overcome tumour stromal barriers. *Mol Ther* 2011; August 23 (*online*).

24. Fisher KD, Seymour LW. HPMA copolymers for masking and retargeting of therapeutic viruses. *Adv Drug Deliv Rev* 2010; 62: 240-5.

25. Kreppel F, Kochanek S. Modification of adenovirus gene transfer vectors with synthetic polymers: a scientific review and technical guide. *Mol Ther* 2008; 16: 16-29.

26. Subr V, Kostka L, Selby-Milic T, Fisher K, Ulbrich K, Seymour LW, Carlisle RC. Coating of adenovirus type 5 with polymers containing quaternary amines prevents binding to blood components. *J Control Release* 2009; 135: 152-8.

27. Hofherr SE, Mok H, Gushiken FC, Lopez JA, Barry MA. Polyethylene glycol modification of adenovirus reduces platelet activation, endothelial cell activation, and thrombocytopenia. *Hum Gene Ther* 2007; 18: 837-48.

28. Morrison J, Briggs SS, Green NK, Thoma C, Fisher KD, Kehoe S, Seymour LW. Cetuximab retargeting of adenovirus via the epidermal growth factor receptor for treatment of intraperitoneal ovarian cancer. *Hum Gene Ther* 2009; 20: 239-51.

29. Green NK, Morrison J, Hale S, Briggs SS, Stevenson M, Subr V, *et al*. Retargeting polymer-coated adenovirus to the FGF receptor allows productive infection and mediates efficacy in a peritoneal model of human ovarian cancer. *J Gene Med* 2008; 10: 280-9.

30. Corjon S, Wortmann A, Engler T, van Rooijen N, Kochanek S, Kreppel F. Targeting of adenovirus vectors to the LRP receptor family with the high-affinity ligand RAP via combined genetic and chemical modification of the pIX capsomere. *Mol Ther* 2008; 16: 1813-24.

31. Kreppel F, Gackowski J, Schmidt E, Kochanek S. Combined genetic and chemical capsid modifications enable flexible and efficient de- and retargeting of adenovirus vectors. *Mol Ther* 2005; 12: 107-17.

32. Prill JM, Espenlaub S, Samen U, Engler T, Schmidt E, Vetrini F, *et al*. Modifications of adenovirus hexon allow for either hepatocyte detargeting or targeting with potential evasion from Kupffer cells. *Mol Ther* 2011; 19: 83-92.

The CliniBook: Clinical gene transfer
Edited by Odile Cohen-Haguenauer – EDK, Paris © 2012, pp. 238-241

A5-3
Tumor imaging with adenoviral vectors

MARTINA ANTON, BERND GÄNSBACHER*

Institute of Experimental Oncology and Therapy Research, Klinikum rechts der Isar der Technischen Universität München, Munich, Germany.
bernd.gansbacher@lrz.tum.de
* Corresponding author

Imaging of gene transfer was first established in 1995 [1]. Since early on non-invasive methods of gene imaging have been of special interest with view to following the fate of gene transfer vectors *in vivo*, since it was assumed that they can help to detect and measure gene transfer efficacy and follow the fate of vectors/gene expression over time and over space, as an alternative method of biodistribution analysis.

IMAGING MODALITIES

There are several available modalities of imaging that comprise different optical methods as well as methods relying on nuclear imaging techniques and magnetic resonance. Optical imaging, *e.g.* detection of fluorescence or bioluminescence stands as a well suited method for both *in vitro* analyses and detection in small animals, the latter two methods allow for detection of gene transfer in larger animals and humans. While fluorescence, like that of the commonly used enhanced green fluorescent protein (eGFP) is only suitable for surface detection, firefly luciferase can be detected in small animals without need of surface exposure, thus allowing repeated measurements. One of the more recent techniques that have been adopted for imaging of gene transfer is the application of near-infrared imaging [2]: Filanov and colleagues were able to detect an AdV that expresses iRFP in mouse liver after i.v. injection.

The nuclear imaging techniques like position emission tomography (PET), gamma camera or single photon emission computed tomography (SPECT) rely on the detection of selectively accumulated radioisotopes. Whereas gamma-camera and SPECT detect gamma-decay which occurs when ^{131}I, ^{99m}Tc, are used; PET will detect positrons emission, which is produced during decay of ^{18}F, ^{11}C, ^{124}I and others. Since normal clinical scanners have only a limited resolution, dedicated small animal scanners have been developed that allow for higher resolution. Magnetic resonance imaging (MRI) is a method that allows for detailed morphological information depending on the spin of hydrogen atoms and thus water within the body or of contrast agents, based on *e.g.* iron oxide or gadolinium. This imaging method has been used as accompanying technique for monitoring progress of gene therapy.

One of the advantages of PET over MRI is that signals correlate with function: accumulation of PET probes only occurs in live cells, that express the reporter gene, whereas MRI is usually not specific for a reporter. According to the current state-of-the art the sensitivity of the former method is higher than MRI, although spatial resolution of MRI is better.

REPORTER GENES FOR ADENOVIRAL GENE TRANSFER IMAGING

Over time all of these modalities have been applied for imaging in conjunction with adenoviral gene transfer (ADV-GT), not only in the setting of tumor imaging, but also for assessing gene transfer *e.g.*: to muscle and heart.

Imaging can be used in at least two different ways: either to detect a vector that is directly labeled with a *e.g.* fluorescence or radioactive marker or to monitor gene transfer, mediated by a vector expressing a reporter gene, which can in turn be detected by one of the above mentioned imaging techniques. In this case the functionality of the AdV will be monitored indirectly. Next to the optical reporter genes, alternative markers can be *e.g.* herpes virus type-1 thymidine kinase (HSV-TK) or sodium iodide symporter (NIS) amongst others, that allows for accumulation of radioactively labelled substrate or radioactively labeled iodine or meta-stable technetium, which can be detected by position emission tomography (PET), gamma camera or single photon emission computed tomography (SPECT), depending on the isotope used. Finally – not using radioisotopes – the bioluminescence of luciferase can be detected with optical systems after application of the substrate luciferin. To this extent we and others have used tumor cells stably expressing luciferase to monitor reduction of tumor mass after application of an YB-1 dependent oncolytic adenovirus [3]. The imaging of enhanced fluorescent protein (eGFP) is not well suited in *in vivo* models, since there is only limited penetration of light into/from the tissue.

COMBINING IMAGING AND THERAPY MEDIATED BY ADENOVIRAL GENE TRANSFER

Our group has experience is in the use of monitoring gene transfer to the heart *via* adenoviral nuclear reporter gene transfer such as HSV-TK or NIS [4] and co-delivery of reporter genes and therapeutically active VEGF [5]. These analyses also demonstrated that non-invasive imaging of adenoviral gene transfer is feasible in large animals such as pigs [6, 7]. In addition we have used adenoviral vectors expressing VEGF to enhance the survival of endothelial progenitor cells and thus allow for improved detection of transplanted cells by PET imaging [8]. More recently we have used a transcriptionally targeted liver specific AdV expressing NIS for combined imaging and treatment of hepatic carcinoma. This vector resulted in improved target over background expression in a HCC xenograft model and thus better - tumor specific - gamma camera imaging, slowed down tumor growth and mediated prolonged survival of mice [9].

As mentioned above the indirect effects of (adeno)viral vectors in tumor treatment have been monitored by MRI and PET early on in clinical trials. Additionally HSV-TK reporter gene transfer by replication defective adenoviral vector has been imaged by PET and PET-CT in liver cancer patients using [^{18}F]FHBG [10]. However recently NIS has gained more attention since it can serve as imaging as well as therapeutic gene in conjunction with ^{131}I radioiodine therapy. Feasibility of imaging and therapy of oncolytic adenovirus expressing CD and mutHSV-TK as well as NIS as reporter gene has been shown in first clinical trials of prostate cancer patients [11, 12].

M. Anton, B. Gänsbacher

FUTURE PROSPECTS

While the use of optical imaging certainly results in import information on tumor behavior and fate of adenoviral vector, requiring relatively "simple" technology and being relatively inexpensive, it is mainly suited for small animal models. The main advantage of nuclear imaging with its high end technology, expensive time on instruments and drawback of radioactive exposure might nevertheless be considered advantageous, especially if it can be combined with tumor therapy. This is already obvious with the fact that first clinical trials have been conducted using NIS as both the reporter and the therapeutic gene. It can thus be speculated, that imaging of successful gene transfer and therapy might gain even more relevance and might contribute to the development of safer vectors in the near future.

ACKNOWLEDGMENTS

This work has been performed with the support of the EC-DG research through the FP6-Network of Excellence, CLINIGENE: LSHB-CT-2006-018933.

REFERENCES

1. Tjuvajev JG, Stockhammer G, Desai R, Uehara H, Watanabe K, Gansbacher B, Blasberg RG. Imaging the expression of transfected genes *in vivo. Cancer Res* 1995; 55: 6126-32.

2. Filonov GS, Piatkevich KD, Ting LM, Zhang J, Kim K, Verkhusha VV. Bright and stable near-infrared fluorescent protein for *in vivo* imaging. *Nat Biotechnol* 2011; 29: 757-61.

3. Holzmüller R, Mantwill K, Haczek C, Rognoni E, Anton M, Kasajima A, *et al*. YB-1 dependent virotherapy in combination with temozolomide as a multimodal therapy approach to eradicate malignant glioma. *Int J Cancer* 2011; 129: 1265-76.

4. Miyagawa M, Anton M, Wagner B, Haubner R, Souvatzoglou M, Gansbacher B, *et al*. Non-invasive imaging of cardiac transgene expression with PET: comparison of the human sodium/iodide symporter gene and HSV1-tk as the reporter gene. *Eur J Nucl Med Mol Imaging* 2005; 32: 1108-14.

5. Anton M, Wittermann C, Haubner R, Simoes M, Reder S, Essien B, *et al*. Coexpression of herpesviral thymidine kinase reporter gene and VEGF gene for noninvasive monitoring of therapeutic gene transfer: an *in vitro* evaluation. *J Nucl Med* 2004; 45: 1743-6.

6. Bengel FM, Anton M, Richter T, Simoes MV, Haubner R, Henke J, *et al*. Noninvasive imaging of transgene expression by use of positron emission tomography in a pig model of myocardial gene transfer. *Circulation* 2003; 108: 2127-33.

7. Wagner B, Anton M, Nekolla SG, Reder S, Henke J, Seidl S, *et al*. Noninvasive characterization of myocardial molecular interventions by integrated positron emission tomography and computed tomography. *J Am Coll Cardiol* 2006; 48: 2107-15.

8. Higuchi T, Anton M, Saraste A, Dumler K, Pelisek J, Nekolla SG, *et al*. Reporter gene PET for monitoring survival of transplanted endothelial progenitor cells in the rat heart after pretreatment with VEGF and atorvastatin. *J Nucl Med* 2009; 50: 1881-6.

9. Klutz K, Willhauck MJ, Wunderlich N, Zach C, Anton M, Senekowitsch-Schmidtke R, *et al*. Sodium iodide symporter (NIS)-mediated radionuclide (^{131}I, [188]Re) therapy of liver cancer after transcriptionally targeted intratumoral *in vivo* NIS gene delivery. *Hum Gene Ther* 2011; 22: 1403-12.

10. Peñuelas I, Mazzolini G, Boán JF, Sangro B, Martí-Climent J, Ruiz M, *et al*. Positron emission tomography imaging of adenoviral-mediated transgene expression in liver cancer patients. *Gastroenterology* 2005; 128: 1787-95.

11. Barton KN, Stricker H, Brown SL, Elshaikh M, Aref I, Lu M, *et al.* Phase I study of noninvasive imaging of adenovirus-mediated gene expression in the human prostate. *Mol Ther* 2008; 16: 1761-9.

12. Barton KN, Stricker H, Elshaikh MA, Pegg J, Cheng J, Zhang Y, *et al.* Feasibility of adenovirus-mediated hNIS gene transfer and 131I radioiodine therapy as a definitive treatment for localized prostate cancer. *Mol Ther* 2011; 19: 1353-9.

The CliniBook: Clinical gene transfer
Edited by Odile Cohen-Haguenauer – EDK, Paris © 2012, pp. 242-244

A5-4
Treatment of brain tumors with adenoviruses: preclinical development

SEPPO YLÄ-HERTTUALA

A.I. Virtanen Institute, University of Eastern Finland, P.O. Box 1627, FI-70211 Kuopio, Finland.
seppo.ylaherttuala@uef.fi

INTRODUCTION

Gene therapy has evolved as a new option for the therapy of malignant gliomas. Most brain tumors are localized lesions of dividing cancer cells in a background of non-dividing neurons, and they usually do not metastasize outside of the central nervous system (CNS). Recurrence of malignant glioma also usually occurs at the site of the original lesion. Therefore, malignant glioma is an excellent target for local gene therapy [1]. Herpes simplex virus thymidine kinase (HSV-tk) suicide gene therapy has been among the first gene therapy systems that have been developed for malignant glioma. Early clinical success with this approach using adenoviral therapy has also been reported [2, 3]. Other systems developed for the treatment of brain tumors include *E. coli* cytosine deaminase and cytochrome P450/CYP2B1 systems. HSV-tk was cloned already in 1980 [4]. Its potential for cancer therapy was first suggested by Frederick Moolten [5]. The first proof-of-principle experiments were done already in 1990, when *in vivo* efficacy of the treatment was demonstrated. Initially, retrovirus was used to transfect packaging cells with *HSV-tk* gene and the treatment included inoculation into the brain of retrovirus packaging cells producing HSV-tk viruses. However, this therapy was not successful in phase III trial [6]. Therefore, adenoviral vectors have been used after that for the development of HSV-tk gene therapy. In this chapter preclinical development of HSV-tk system will be discussed.

HSV-TK/GANCICLOVIR THERAPY AND MECHANISM OF ACTION

Ganciclovir is a synthetic nucleoside analogue that was originally designed to be an antiviral drug. It is currently used for the treatment and prevention of cytomegalovirus infection especially in newborns and immunocompromised patients. In cytotoxic gene therapy ganciclovir is converted to ganciclovir monophosphate by HSV-tk, which is approximately 100 times more efficient in phosphorylating ganciclovir than any human enzymes [1]. Thereafter cellular kinases convert the monophosphate to a ganciclovir 3 phosphate which can stop continuous DNA elongation in nucleus, since it lacks 3'hydroxyl group that is needed for the phosphodiester bond formation during DNA synthesis. The resulting fragmented non-functional DNA induces apoptosis in cancer cells. HSV-tk/ganciclovir therapy also induces p53 accumulation and expression of death receptors, which ultimately leads to mitochondrial membrane potential disturbances and release of cytochrome C. Thus, destruction of cancer cells is also cell-cycle dependent, where only dividing cells will be affected. In CNS this is an advantage, since rapidly dividing tumor cells are usually surrounded by non-dividing neurons. HSV-tk/ganciclovir therapy has also a bystander effect whereby phosphorylated ganciclovir can be transported to the neighboring cells thus increasing significantly the efficacy of the treatment. It has been shown that approximately 10 % of the tumor cells need to be transduced with HSV-tk in order to achieve significant tumor regression in animal models [7]. Cellular gap junctions are believed to be associated to the bystander effect. Additionally, HSV-tk probably induces antitumoral immune responses against non-transduced cells. It is likely that both local and systemic immune responses contribute to the HSV-tk/ganciclovir antitumor effect.

PRECLINICAL STUDIES

Tumor regression has been demonstrated in several studies [1]. Apart from brain tumors, HSV-tk/ganciclovir approach has been also evaluated in many other types of cancers including prostate cancer, sarcomas and breast cancer. HSV-tk treatment effect could be seen already in 3-4 days after gene transfer of adenoviral vectors expressing HSV-tk, followed by ganciclovir administration. Gene delivery has been achieved usually with intratumoral injections in rodent models.

In the studies by Sandmair *et al.* [7] safety of adenovirus-HSV-tk/ganciclovir gene therapy was thoroughly evaluated including MRI evaluation of the shrinking tumors and thoroughful histology to demonstrate both regression of the tumor and potential effects on neurons. No necrosis, demyelination or loss of neurons were detected. Dose finding studies indicated that doses ranging from 5×10^6 to 5×10^7 pfu were well tolerated in conjunction with 20 mg/kg ganciclovir treatment given for two weeks after the gene therapy. No clinical signs of illness could be detected, although increases in liver enzymes were detected in some animals 2-3 days – 1 week after the therapy. Also, increases in anti-adenovirus antibodies were detected in most animals. As a late-state finding, enlargement of brain ventricles were detected in some long-term surviving animals. Overall, approximately 20 % of the treated rats could be rescued from malignant glioma with local adenovirus-mediated HSV-tk/ganciclovir therapy [8]. Inflammatory reactions, as detected by histological stainings were present around tumor area, including infiltration of chronic inflammatory cells, macrophages and T-cells. These inflammatory reactions probably contribute to the therapeutic effect in rodent models.

CLINICAL TRIALS

Most recent HSV-tk/ganciclovir applications have relied on adenoviruses, since their production systems and ability to lead to a strong expression of transgene were seen most suitable for these purposes. Even though positive results with improved survival and positive primary endpoints have been reported in phase II trials [2, 3], phase III studies have not yet given uniformly significant survival advantage, although certain patient groups significantly benefit from the therapy. In the future, HSV-tk/ganciclovir gene therapy will be given in combination with both radiation therapy, surgery and temozolomide chemotherapy. Phase III randomized, controlled clinical trials will be needed to evaluate the final efficacy of the HSV-tk/ganciclovir gene therapy in human patients with malignant glioma.

ACKNOWLEDGEMENTS

This study was supported by grants from the Academy of Finland, Tekes (the Finnish Funding Agency for Technology and Innovation), EC-DG research through the FP6-Network of Excellence (Clinigene LSHB-CT-2006-018933) and Ark Therapeutics Ltd.

REFERENCES

1. Pulkkanen KJ, Ylä-Herttuala S. Gene therapy for malignant glioma: current clinical status. *Mol Ther* 2005; 12: 585-98.

2. Sandmair AM, Loimas S, Puranen P, Immonen A, Kossila M, Puranen M, *et al.* Thymidine kinase gene therapy for human malignant glioma, using replication-deficient retroviruses or adenoviruses. *Hum Gene Ther* 2000; 11: 2197-205.

3. Immonen A, Vapalahti M, Tyynelä K, Hurskainen H, Sandmair A, Vanninen R, *et al.* AdvHSV-tk gene therapy with intravenous ganciclovir improves survival in human malignant glioma: a randomised, controlled study. *Mol Ther* 2004; 10: 967-72.

4. McKnight SL. The nucleotide sequence and transcript map of the herpes simplex virus thymidine kinase gene. *Nucleic Acids Res* 1980; 8: 5949-64.

5. Moolten FL. Tumor chemosensitivity conferred by inserted herpes thymidine kinase genes: paradigm for a prospective cancer control strategy. *Cancer Res* 1986; 46: 5276-81.

6. Rainov NG. A phase III clinical evaluation of herpes simplex virus type 1 thymidine kinase and ganciclovir gene therapy as an adjuvant to surgical resection and radiation in adults with previously untreated glioblastoma multiforme. *Hum Gene Ther* 2000; 11: 2389-401.

7. Sandmair AM, Turunen M, Tyynelä K, Loimas S, Vainio P, Vanninen R, *et al.* Herpes simplex virus thymidine kinase gene therapy in experimental rat BT4C glioma model: effect of the percentage of thymidine kinase-positive glioma cells on treatment effect, survival time, and tissue reactions. *Cancer Gene Ther* 2000; 7: 413-21.

8. Tyynelä K, Sandmair AM, Turunen M, Vanninen R, Vainio P, Kauppinen RA, *et al.* Adenovirus-mediated herpes simplex virus thymidine kinase gene therapy in BT4C rat glioma model. *Cancer Gene Ther* 2002; 9: 917-24.

The CliniBook: Clinical gene transfer
Edited by Odile Cohen-Haguenauer – EDK, Paris © 2012, pp. 245-250

A5-5
Production and purification of Ad vectors: current status and future needs for adenovirus vector production

Ana Carina Silva[1,2], Daniel Simão[1], Marcos F.Q. Sousa[1], Cristina Peixoto[1], Pedro E. Cruz[1,3*], Manuel J.T. Carrondo[1], Paula Marques Alves[1,2]

[1]*IBET, Apartado 12, 2781-901 Oeiras, Portugal.*
[2]*ITQB-UNL, Apartado 12, 2781-901 Oeiras, Portugal.*
[3]*ECBio, S.A., R. Henrique Paiva Couceiro, 27, 2700-451 Amadora, Portugal.*
pcruz@itqb.unl.pt
*Corresponding author

During the last two decades, remarkable progress has been made in the development of Ad vectors and in the understanding of the toxicity related to the Ad vector system. Ad vector has certain advantages such as high transduction efficiency for different quiescent and dividing cell types and high levels of short-term expression to provide therapeutic benefits. However, researchers are facing the challenges associated with tissue-specific targeting of vectors, vector-mediated immunogenicity, low degree of tumor spread/distribution in the case of E1-deleted and also oncolytic vectors.

The increasing importance of Ad vectors for gene therapy, cancer therapy, and the development of vaccines have led to worldwide efforts toward scalable process development suitable for commercial manufacturing. However, there are still some bottlenecks that need to be addressed concerning Ad vectors production. These include the lack of standardized high yield production systems and safety issues namely the production of replication-competent adenoviruses (RCA).

AD VECTORS PRODUCTION

The production of Ad vectors contains several bioengineering challenges that must be carefully dealt with in order to improve up- and downstream processing with the final goal of maximizing performance and reducing production costs. In general, all Ad vectors culture processes start by growing the cell line of choice to the desired cell concentration for infection followed by infection with an adenovirus stock to start the virus production cycle.

The most common packaging cell line for Ad vectors production is the Human Embryonic Kidney 293 cell line, which contains the E1 region of the adenovirus [1]. Since the work of Garnier *et al.* [2] concerning the use of 293 suspension cells and adenovirus vectors system several efforts have been made to improve the vector yields. Several variables affecting the virus production were evaluated from temperature, pH, cell concentration at infection (CCI), time of infection (TOI), multiplicity of infection (MOI), time of harvesting (TOH), culture medium used (serum containing versus serum free media), cell culture system (adherent, aggregated and suspension cells from small culture flasks to high volume bioreactors) among others. Studies on the cell environment have permitted to enhance specific Ad vectors productivity through better cell culture environment control (medium formulation and feeding strategies). These strategies have also been developed to increase the cell concentration at infection to ultimately enhance volumetric productivity. The challenge has been to keep the specific productivity obtained at low cell density constant without feeding. The cell density effect describes a drop in the specific virus production when the cell density is above 0.5×10^6 cells/ml [3]. The major hypothesis behind the cell density effect is that nutrient depletion and metabolite accumulation affect cell metabolism to support viral production at high cell densities. Therefore, in order to improve substrate renewal and metabolite removal, production modes have increased in complexity from batch to perfusion system. Several strategies have been applied to try to unravel the so called "cell density effect" from a 293 cell cycle evaluation for better Ad vectors production [4] to a better characterization of the cell metabolic state using isotopomer analysis [5] however, none of them have resulted in a complete understanding of this phenomenon.

Even with all these efforts for the production of Ad vectors (mostly for ΔE1) in 293 cells, homologous recombination between the left terminus of first-generation Ad vector or helper-virus DNA and partially overlapping E1 sequences in the genome of 293 cells may lead to the emergence of RCA, which contain E1 genes [6]. To overcome this problem, alternative host cell lines have been developed by reducing these overlapping sequences, as for 911 cells, or by eliminating any overlap, as for N52.E6 [7] or PER.C6 [8] cells. More recently, another human cell line derived also from human amniocyte cells containing the Ad5 E1A and E1B genes plus sequences from the pIX gene, and with only little overlap between vector and cellular DNA has been described as being a good producer cell for Ad vectors at higher cell concentration than 293 cells (*Table I*) [9].

Table I. Ad vectors productivities in human amniocyte cells and 293 cells growing in different culture systems.

Culture System	Human amniocyte cells			293 cells		
	Static	Shake Flask	Bioreactor	Static	Shake Flask	Bioreactor
rAdV$_{max}$ (ip/mL)	1×10^9	7×10^8 (CCI 1)	7×10^9 (CCI 3)	3×10^9	1×10^9 (CCI 1)	2×10^9 (CCI 1)

rAdV$_{max}$ – Maximal adenoviral productivity; ip – infectious particles; CCI - cell concentration at infection; CCI 1 - 1×10^6 cells/mL; CCI 3 – 3×10^6 cells/mL.

The PER.C6 cells have been the most used and some of the strategies for Ad vectors production applied for 293 cells have been applied for this alternative cell line. The new generation of Ad vectors namely the HC-Ad and CRADs have been produced using other cell lines based on A549, 116 or HeLa cells and much more work need to be done to achieve better production results.

For a more detailed assessment of the adenovirus production processes described in the literature we recommend the reading of published reviews [10,11].

AD VECTORS PURIFICATION

The development of fast and efficient purification procedures that permit high recovery of infectious particles, removal of host cell proteins and DNA, clearance of unpackaged viral DNA and also concentration of virus formulations is essential for their use in gene and cancer therapy. The scalability of the process is important and necessary for large-scale production of adenoviral particles needed for clinical trials and final accomplishment of adenoviral vectors as therapeutics.

The first efforts in Ad vectors purification date back to the late 1950s using anion exchange chromatography and two-phase extraction [12] however resulted in relatively low yields and infectivity assays difficult to handle in order to monitor fractionation. This was improved by the development of CsCl-density gradient ultracentrifugation for adenovirus in 1962, which enabled rapid purification of adenovirus in sufficient quantities for research purposes based solely on visible band collection. Nevertheless this method has not been adopted by the manufacturers due to difficulties of scaling up, costs and toxicity of cesium chloride.

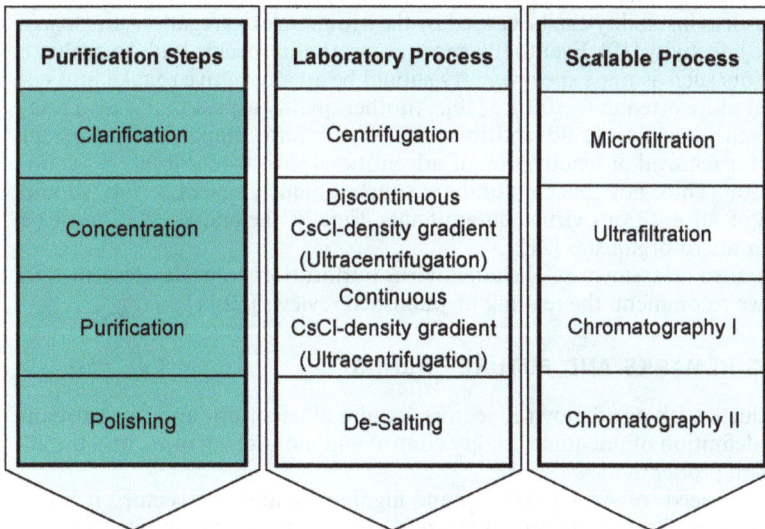

Purification Steps	Laboratory Process	Scalable Process
Clarification	Centrifugation	Microfiltration
Concentration	Discontinuous CsCl-density gradient (Ultracentrifugation)	Ultrafiltration
Purification	Continuous CsCl-density gradient (Ultracentrifugation)	Chromatography I
Polishing	De-Salting	Chromatography II

Figure 1. General purification process flowcharts for Ad vectors.

There were no further improvements in the purification of Ad vectors since density-gradient ultracentrifugation separates empty capsids, until the 1990s when these vectors started to be used in gene therapy. After that chromatographic-based processes have been exploited and the chromatographic resins have been improved, enabling adenovirus particles to be bound and eluted with higher recoveries; chromatographic purification of adenovirus mainly exploit their size, surface charge or specific receptor binding properties (*Figure 1*). In most processes described in the literature, at relevant conferences, in patents, and in patent applications, anion exchange chromatography is the "heart" of the process. However, increasing demands on Ad vectors created a bottleneck in downstream processing, especially since chromatography offers high resolution but low throughput at larger scales. In the literature it is possible to find a detailed comparative review of all chromatographic methods explored for Ad vectors purification [13] and also, a comprehensive study combining anion exchange and size exclusion chromatography is now available [14]. The use of membrane chromatography was also applied for adenoviruses purification [15]. Another alternative to overcome the disadvantages of using traditional column chromatography could be the use of monolithic columns, a technology that is still in its infancy, but promising preliminary results for virus detection are described in literature [16]. Furthermore, it was already reported as a tool for adenovirus analysis in crude samples [17].

The use of Ad vectors as a gene therapy product not only depends on the availability of efficient and robust downstream processes but also on the establishment of analytical tools that are able to track the bioprocess and to characterize the final Ad vector [18]. The presence of contaminants must be quantified, namely, the host cell protein, DNA and contaminants from culture media. Ad vectors infectivity should be used as a process performance indicator, with ratios between infectious and total vector particles for the final product being often required by the authorities. FDA requires that the ratio of total to infectious particles be lower than 30. The absence of replication competent adenovirus (RCA) [6] is always part of the quality control for E1-deleted adenovirus vectors. Ad vectors aggregation is another parameter that should be evaluated because virus instability can be caused by the irreversible aggregation and consequent losses of infectivity [19]. Eventually, more accurate and specific tools to evaluate quality of vectors such as mass spectrometry should be an alternative to take into account and used more often in the future [20]. Another quality aspect that is also a safety concern is the detection of adventitious virus from vector preparations. Current methods used for removal or inactivation of adventitious virus would result in adenovirus inactivation. Thus, possible contaminant sources, namely raw materials, should be shown free of adventitious virus contaminants. Finally, the end-product must be tested for other micro-organisms [21].

For a more detailed assessment of the adenovirus purification processes described in the literature we recommend the reading of published reviews [10,11].

CONCLUDING REMARKS AND FUTURE TRENDS

Complex products such as adenoviral vectors require efficient up- and downstream strategies, the definition of adequate quality control and monitoring tools, and the attainment of high productivities.

Since the growing needs of Ad vectors demand highly pure and safe vectors, it is important for all proceedings designing, analyzing, and controlling manufacturing as early as possible in the development phase to increase the information and follow the process analytical technologies (PAT) initiative. This will be accomplished by the use of modern optical sensors like oxygen sensors in shake flasks [22] and bioprocess monitoring devices like optical fiber technology for 2D fluorymetry that allows the simultaneous monitoring of several compounds present outside (envirome) and inside (metabolome) of the cells [23] will help to improve Ad vector productivities.

The production of a different generation of Ad vectors and the use of safer cell lines available could help in increase substantially the vectors' applications facilitating the strategies to achieve the quantity demands of these type of vectors. For all new processes it is necessary to interplay between all the process-related parameters such as MOI, TOI, TOH and CCI. In order to avoid repeating all experimentation done for example for the 293 cells for the new cells and vectors available mathematical models and design of experiments could be applied. These tools have been successfully used for other viral systems like production of virus-like particles using the baculovirus/insect cell system [24].

In order to continuously gain knowledge in the metabolic requirements for cell growth and viral production by metabolic flux analysis techniques combined with non-invasive and high information techniques like NMR will allow the improvement in viral productivities and surpass the "cell density effect" by the manipulation of energy metabolism as already obtained for other systems [25].

An improved knowledge and use of disposable culture and purification ware will also allow increased flexibility and cost-effectiveness especially since the vectors need to be produced and purified under GMP conditions.

Being a complex product, adenoviruses require a battery of analytic assays during and at the end of the downstream process. Moreover, the use of different serotypes or helper-dependent adenovirus vectors provide new challenges in the purification process making downstream processing of adenovirus vectors to continue being an important area of research in the future.

In the end a better integration between up- and downstream following the new tendencies in Ad vectors process development (*Table II*) will help in having more standardized and integrated high yield productions processes giving higher quality products.

Table II. Some new tendencies for Ad vectors process development.

Production	Monitoring/quality control	Purification
- Disposable ware	- Optical sensors	- Disposables ware
- Safer cell lines	- 2D fluorometry	- Monolithic columns
- Safer vectors	- Metabolic flux analysis	- ...
- Mathematical models	- NMR	
- ...	- Mass spectroscopy	
	- ...	

ACKNOWLEDGMENTS

This work has been performed with the support of the EC-DG research through the FP6-Network of Excellence, CLINIGENE: LSHB-CT-2006-018933.

REFERENCES

1. Graham FL, Smiley J, Russell WC, Nairn R. Characteristics of a human cell line transformed by DNA from human adenovirus type 5. *J Gen Virol* 1977; 36: 59-74.

2. Garnier A, Cote J, Nadeau I, Kamen A, Massie B. Scale-up of the adenovirus expression system for the production of recombinant protein in human 293S cells. *Cytotechnology* 1994; 15: 145-55.

3. Kamen A, Henry O. Development and optimization of an adenovirus production process. *J Gene Med* 2004; 6 (suppl 1): S184-92.

4. Ferreira TB, Perdigao R, Silva AC, *et al.* 293 cell cycle synchronisation adenovirus vector production. *Biotechnol Prog* 2009; 25: 235-43.

5. Henry O, Jolicoeur M, Kamen A. Unraveling the metabolism of HEK-293 cells using lactate isotopomer analysis. *Bioprocess Biosyst Eng* 2011; 34: 263-73.

6. Lochmuller H, Jani A, Huard J, *et al.* Emergence of early region 1-containing replication-competent adenovirus in stocks of replication-defective adenovirus recombinants (delta E1 + delta E3) during multiple passages in 293 cells. *Hum Gene Ther* 1994; 5: 1485-91.

7. Schiedner G, Hertel S, Kochanek S. Efficient transformation of primary human amniocytes by E1 functions of Ad5: generation of new cell lines for adenoviral vector production. *Hum Gene Ther* 2000; 11: 2105-16.

8. Fallaux FJ, Kranenburg O, Cramer SJ, *et al.* Characterization of 911: a new helper cell line for the titration and propagation of early region 1-deleted adenoviral vectors. *Hum Gene Ther* 1996; 7: 215-22.

9. Silva AC, Simão D, Sousa MFQ, *et al.* Human amniocyte-derived cells for production of adenovirus vectors for gene therapy. In *21th ESACT meeting-European society for animal cell technology.* Vienna, Austria, 2011.

10. Dormond E, Kamen AA. Manufacturing of adenovirus vectors: production and purification of helper dependent adenovirus. *Methods Mol Biol* 2011; 737: 139-56.

11. Silva AC, Peixoto C, Lucas T, *et al.* Adenovirus vector production and purification. *Curr Gene Ther* 2010; 10: 437-55.

12. Green M, Pina M. Biochemical studies on adenovirus multiplication. IV. Isolation, purification, and chemical analysis of adenovirus. *Virology* 1963; 20: 199-207.

13. Segura MM, Alba R, Bosch A, Chillon M. Advances in helper-dependent adenoviral vector research. *Curr Gene Ther* 2008; 8: 222-35.

14. Charcosset C. Membrane processes in biotechnology: an overview. *Biotechnol Adv* 2006; 24: 482-92.

15. Peixoto C, Ferreira TB, Sousa MF, Carrondo MJ, Alves PM. Towards purification of adenoviral vectors based on membrane technology. *Biotechnol Prog* 2008; 24: 1290-6.

16. Branovic K, Forcic D, Ivancic J, *et al.* Application of short monolithic columns for improved detection of viruses. *J Virol Methods* 2003; 110: 163-71.

17. Whitfield RJ, Battom SE, Barut M, Gilham DE, Ball PD. Rapid high-performance liquid chromatographic analysis of adenovirus type 5 particles with a prototype anion-exchange analytical monolith column. *J Chromatogr A* 2009; 1216: 2725-9.

18. Roitsch C, Achstetter T, Benchaibi M, *et al.* Characterization and quality control of recombinant adenovirus vectors for gene therapy. *J Chromatogr B Biomed Sci Appl* 2001; 752: 263-80.

19. Konz JO, Lee AL, Lewis JA, Sagar SL. Development of a purification process for adenovirus: controlling virus aggregation to improve the clearance of host cell DNA. *Biotechnol Prog* 2005; 21: 466-72.

20. Mirza UA, Liu YH, Tang JT, *et al.* Extraction and characterization of adenovirus proteins from sodium dodecylsulfate polyacrylamide gel electrophoresis by matrix-assisted laser desorption/ionization mass spectrometry. *J Am Soc Mass Spectrom* 2000; 11: 356-61.

21. Darling A. Validation of biopharmaceutical purification processes for virus clearance evaluation. *Mol Biotechnol* 2002; 21: 57-83.

22. Gupta A, Rao G. A study of oxygen transfer in shake flasks using a non-invasive oxygen sensor. *Biotechnol Bioeng* 2003; 84: 351-8.

23. Teixeira AP, Oliveira R, Alves PM, Carrondo MJ. Advances in on-line monitoring and control of mammalian cell cultures: supporting the PAT initiative. *Biotechnol Adv* 2009; 27: 726-32.

24. Roldao A, Vieira HL, Charpilienne A, *et al.* Modeling rotavirus-like particles production in a baculovirus expression vector system: Infection kinetics, baculovirus DNA replication, mRNA synthesis and protein production. *J Biotechnol* 2007; 128: 875-94.

25. Carinhas N, Bernal V, Monteiro F, Carrondo MJ, Oliveira R, Alves PM. Improving baculovirus production at high cell density through manipulation of energy metabolism. *Metab Eng* 2010; 12: 39-52.

TECHNOLOGIES

Non-viral based gene transfer: a new era

COORDINATED BY
GEORGE DICKSON

The CliniBook: Clinical gene transfer
Edited by Odile Cohen-Haguenauer – EDK, Paris © 2012, pp. 253-265

A6-1
Non viral plasmid delivery and imaging of transgene expression

Pascal Bigey, Michel-Francis Bureau, Gonzalo Cordova, Virginie Escriou, Antoine Kichler, Nathalie Mignet, Daniel Scherman*

CNRS, UMR8151, Paris, F-75006 France; Inserm, U1022, Paris, F-75006 France; Université Paris Descartes, Sorbonne Paris Cité, Faculté de Pharmacie, Chemical and Genetic Pharmacology and Imaging Laboratory, Paris, F-75270 France; École Nationale Supérieure de Chimie de Paris, Chimie ParisTech, Paris, F-75005, France.
daniel.scherman@parisdescartes.fr
* Corresponding author

The principle of gene therapy drugs is based on the Watson-Crick recognition of genetically encoded material. The molecular structure of "non viral" gene therapy vectors can be very diverse. It can be composed of either a small synthetic oligonucleotide (*i.e.* an oligodeoxyribonucleotide for an antisense or exon-skipping strategy, or a small interfering RNA). Alternatively, a "non viral gene therapy" agent can consist of a biochemically produced messenger RNA, or even of a large size double-brand circular plasmid DNA.

Whatever their diversity, all non viral gene therapy agents are hydrophilic compounds, which are confronted to the same obstacle: the crossing of the plasmatic membrane in order to access their intracellular target. Several chemical and physical strategies have been developed to overcome this barrier: (1) self-assembling cationic lipidic vectors, which form *"lipoplexes"* with the nucleotidic agent; (2) polymeric cationic vectors forming *"polyplexes"* with the nucleotidic agent; and (3) a physical membrane permeabilizing technique mediated either by electric pulses (designated as electroporation, electrotransfer and electro-gene transfer) or by hydrodynamic forces.

This chapter will present several of the most recent progresses obtained on these different delivery techniques, *i.e.*: new cationic lipid formulations for siRNA delivery, a new non cationic lipothiourea based formulation, and innovative polymeric and peptidic vectors for gene delivery. In addition, the use of electrotransfer for genetic vaccination is illustrated, as well as the imaging of plasmid delivered to muscle and joints by this physical technique.

LIPIDIC VECTORS FOR SIRNA DELIVERY

Whether applying siRNA technology to fundamental research or potential therapeutic ends, success hinges largely on the development of a delivery vehicle that can vectorise biologically competent siRNA to target cells. As in all *in vivo* gene delivery paradigms there will be a need for optimization of delivery according to the route of administration, the tissue or cell type expressing the target gene and whether long- or short-term effects are required. The misadventures of gene therapy speak in favor of the siRNA solution (direct delivery of siRNAs rather than plasmid DNA), where smaller, easily diffusible molecules have only to be delivered to the cytoplasm.

Recently, we have developed an efficient formulation of siRNA, based on a three-component delivery system (1) the cationic lipid 2-{3-[Bis-(3-amino-propyl)-amino]-propylamino}-N-ditetradecyl carbamoyl methyl-acetamide, which we termed DMAPAP (synthesized as described [1]), (2) the neutral lipid 1,2-dioleoyl-sn-glycero-3-phosphoethanolamine or DOPE and (3) a nucleic acid used as an anionic cargo (*Figure 1*).

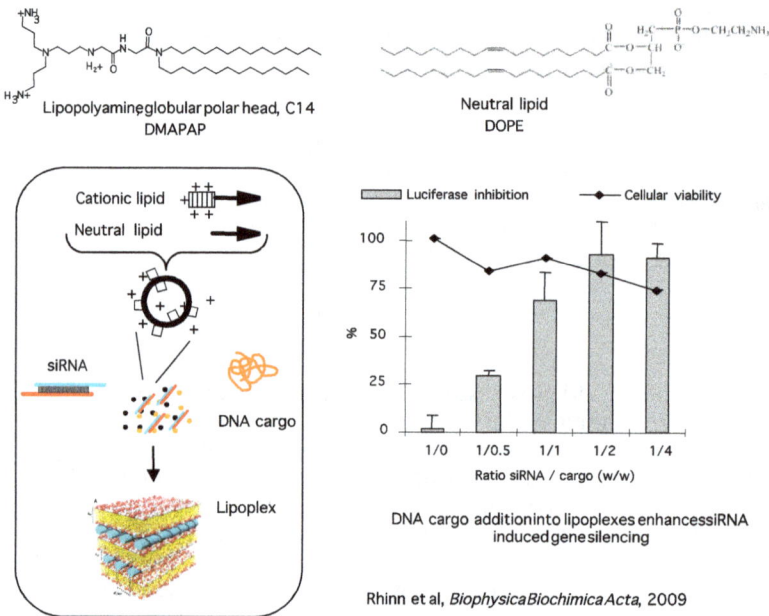

Figure 1. Addition of a nucleic acid cargo into siRNA lipoplexes enhanced siRNA induced gene silencing in cell cultures (H. Rhinn *et al.* [2]).

We have shown that the addition of anionic cargo to siRNA prior to form the complex with cationic liposome leads to enhanced gene silencing efficiency with diminished siRNA concentrations [2]. However, we suspected that the addition of a DNA molecule in siRNA lipoplexes will not be acceptable in a clinical application since pDNA is a biomolecule that contains potentially expressible coding sequences. The incorporation of anionic polymers presented several advantages because it increased the gene silencing efficiency of the vectors in cell culture, it decreased their cellular toxicity and it increased siRNA recovery in organs after intravenous application of the vectors. The polymer used to design these siRNA vectors is biodegradable and FDA-approved for use in humans. Other polymers can be used with the same efficiency in cell culture [3]. We applied our new siRNA vector in a mouse arthritis model to target TNFα. Following intravenous injection this siRNA lipoplex proved to be efficient in restoring immunological balance in a collagen-induced arthritis mouse model [4]. We next applied these formulations to test other siRNA targeted to various genes candidates [5-7]. We showed that weekly injections of siRNAs targeted to IL-1, IL-6 or IL-18, delivered in combination and formulated with cationic liposomes significantly reduced all pathological rheumatoid arthritis features including inflammation, joint destruction and Th1 response [5] (*Figure 2*).

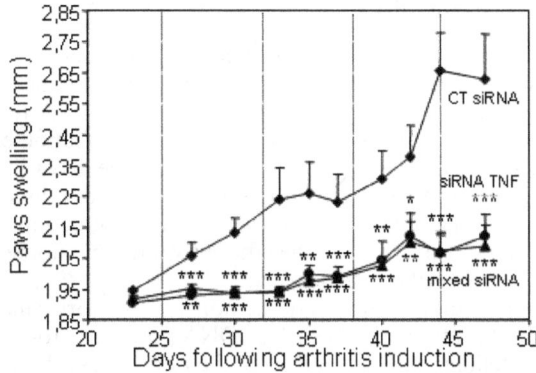

Figure 2. Weekly injections of siRNAs targeted to IL-1, IL-6 and IL-18, delivered in combination and formulated with cationic liposomes significantly reduced the progression of the disease in a mouse collagen-induced arthritis model.

The active siRNA complexes exhibited a multi-organ tropism, with strong silencing in lymphoid organs, and we determined that the preferential immune cell type targeted by the siRNA complexes was macrophage, the main inflammatory cytokine producer cell in rheumatoid arthritis. Indeed, the physico-chemical characteristics of the siRNA complexes we designed provide cell type-specific delivery upon intravenous administration with preferential targeting of monocyte/macrophage cells that naturally internalize large particles. We thus have with this technique a promising novel anti-inflammatory therapy in rheumatoid arthritis, as well as a useful and simple tool for understanding rheumatoid arthritis pathophysiology and for evaluating new therapeutic candidates.

This siRNA vector has next been used for specific siRNA-mediated gene silencing in osteosarcoma models by targeting luciferase expression [8]. We have thus defined a siRNA injection protocol efficient to downregulate a target gene and associated with no unspecific inhibition of the osteosarcoma growth when the targeted gene is not implicated in cell proliferation. Next we have investigated the effects of siRNA which were designed to target mouse and rat *Rankl* transcripts and formulated with DMA-PAP/DOPE liposome in two models of murine osteosarcoma: a syngenic osteolytic POS-1 model induced in immunocompetent mice and a xenograft osteocondensant model of rat OSRGA in athymic mice [9].

The decrease of Rankl in serum and at tumor site following *Rankl*-directed siRNA (*Rankl*- siRNA] injections protected bone from osteolysis but had no significant effect on tumor growth. In contrast when associated to conventional chemotherapy (ifosfamide], *Rankl*-siRNAs were more efficient to inhibit osteosarcoma growth than chemotherapy alone. Moreover, tumor relapse observed after the last ifosfamide course was delayed by *Rankl*-siRNA injections as compared to control-siRNA ones. Our study demonstrated the relevance of using a new methology for specific inhibition of Rankl production in bone tumor microenvironment. Indeed, our results validated a designed siRNA sequence wich was efficient to decrease local and systemic Rankl production respectively in osteolytic POS-1 and osteogenic OSRGA osteosarcoma models. This inhibition was associated to a decrease of Rankl function as revealed by the decrease of osteolytic lesions and osteoclasts at the bone-tumor interface [9].

NON VIRAL VECTORS: LIPOTHIOUREA

Among non-viral vectors for gene delivery, cationic lipids and polymers are the main studied systems. Cationic nanoparticles formed between DNA and cationic liposomes or polymers forming lipoplexes or polyplexes respectively, protect DNA from enzymatic degradation, improve its cellular uptake, increasing its transfection efficiency [10]. Clinical trials have been, and are currently performed by the means of lipofection in cystic fibrosis indication. The intranasal and intrabronchial routes of administration chosen reflect the interests and the limits of these vectors based on cationic charges which are, on one side needed to transfer the gene efficiently and, on another side, to avoid for their high risk of non-specific gene delivery.

In this context, we aimed at developing non cationic non-viral vectors which would maintain the advantages of the cationic lipids such as DNA protection towards enzymatic degradation and intracellular delivery, and avoid their hurdles, such as non-specific interactions with proteins.

Taking a closer look at bio-macromolecular structures, we developed bio-inspired vectors based on hydrogen bonds interactions. We conceived lipids bearing strong hydrogen bond donor chemical functions, called thiourea, and hypothesized that structures between these lipids and DNA could be formed thanks to hydrogen bond interaction between the lipid thiourea and the DNA phosphates. These vectors could lead to DNA protection, increased circulation time *in vivo* and targeting feasibility (*Figure 3*).

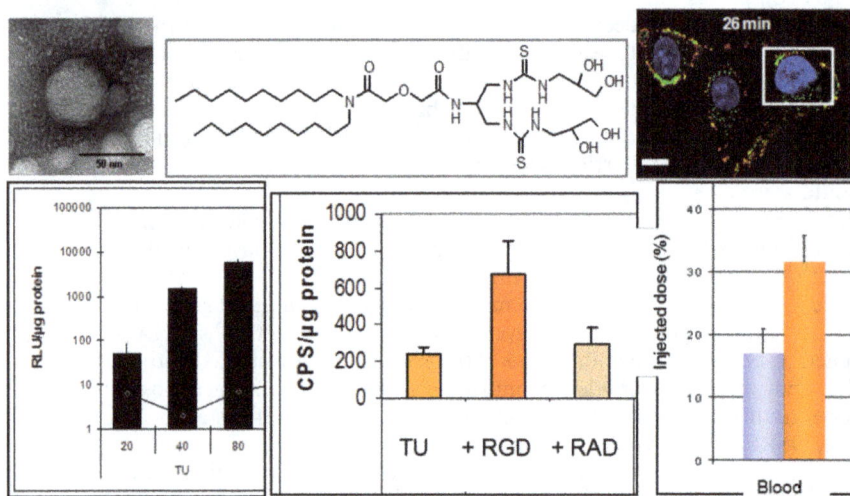

Figure 3. Selected thiourea lipid forming small vesicles as shown by cryoelectron microscopy. Thiourea lipids were shown to efficiently release DNA into the cells with a fast kinetic of DNA found in the nucleus, to transfect cells in a dose dependent manner. Targeting αvβ3 integrins was shown on EaHY cells by incorporation of a lipid-PEG-RGD or lipid-PEG-RAD in the formulation. Residence time of the rhodamine labelled liposomes in the blood showed a two fold increase as compared to pegylated cationic liposomes.

A screening of different lipid length, spacer chemical nature and lipid head hydrophilicity allowed obtaining amphiphilic molecules, easy to formulate and forming unilamellar vesicles of 60 to 80nm [11-13].

Comparing cationic and thiourea based lipids, we found that the last ones were internalised by the cells by different mechanisms less based on clathrin endocytosis but involving membrane destabilisation and caveolae endocytosis [14]. Six times less thiourea lipoplexes were shown to be internalised into the cells as compared to polyamine lipoplexes showing that non-specific interaction had been reduced. Targeting could then be achieved, as shown by incorporating RGD motives at the surface of the lipoplexes [15].

Following labelled DNA into the cells showed that DNA was more efficiently released by thiourea lipoplexes as compared to cationic lipoplexes, and that DNA reached the nucleus in a shorter time-scale [11].

In vivo evaluation indicated that pegylated thiourea lipoplexes showed an increase by a factor 3 in the mice blood, 30 minutes post intraveineous injection. Luciferase expression levels remained however too low as this stage to envision a therapeutic evaluation.

Targeting these vectors remains an excellent approach due to lower non specific interactions as compared to their cationic counterpart.

POLOXAMERS

Poloxamers are triblock copolymers of high interest. These polymers constituted of polyethylene oxide-polypropylene oxide do not bear chemical functions able to interact with DNA; however co-injection of polymer and DNA increases gene expression *in vivo*. The mechanism of this improvement is not fully understood but recent studies gave some insight into the way it works.

Poloxamers are composed of a hydrophobic polymer at the center flanked by two slightly more hydrophilic polymers. This structure gives them the property to self-assemble in an aqueous medium, according to the proportion of each polymer and to the temperature.

The hydrophobic part is prone to interact with lipid membranes [16] and to destabilise it as shown on lipid monolayers [17] and liposome models [18]. One can hypothesize then that poloxamers improve gene expression by a direct increase of gene transfer into the cell *via* cell membrane destabilisation. Unfortunately, it is not that simple. First, labelled poloxamers were not observed at the cell membrane *in vitro* but rather inside the cells, meaning that not only the unimers interact with the membrane but also that aggregates of poloxamers are internalised [19, 20]. Relation between membrane destabilisation and gene expression in the muscle *in vivo* has not been evidenced by paired MRI and optical imaging studies despite the fact that L64 was chosen for its membrane destabilising effect [21]. Several other poloxamers were shown to increase gene expression without exhibiting permeabilising properties. For instance P103, P105 and F127 increased gene expression in the muscle *in vivo* without inducing lactase deshydrogenase release *in vitro* [22].

Interestingly, other copolymers of different nature such as copolymers where the polyethylene oxide was replaced by a polymethyloxazoline also led to gene expression improvement in the muscle *in vivo* [23].

A similar mechanism could be expected for all these polymers. In particular, an indirect activation of transcription factors through a prior membrane interaction could explain gene expression improvement. Indeed, Sriadibhatla *et al.* showed that implementing the plasmid promoter by sequences recognised by the transcription factor NF-κB increased gene expression level [24]. This was since reproduced by other groups *in vitro* [20] and *in vivo* [22] confirming the involvement of this factor in gene expression mediated by triblock copolymers.

In vitro, gene expression improvement was obtained by addition of poloxamers to a cationic delivery agent such as polyethyleneimine, increasing both uptake of the polyplex and nuclear transport of DNA [25]. However *in vivo*, as the copolymers do not interact with DNA [18] and do not necessarily destabilise the cell membrane to induce a gene expression increase, this means that the membrane alteration due to the needle injection should be enough to deliver DNA inside the cells. This tend to show that activation of transcription factors helps the DNA already present into the cells to cross the nuclear membrane. However, this effect was not evidenced by addition of L64 copolymer to electrotransferred cells *in vitro* or in the muscles *in vivo*. Only a pre-treatment cell with the polymer prior electroporation could slightly improve the number of cell transfected and the gene expression level [20].

This means that the mechanism of transfection mediated by poloxamers, and physical methods, in general might not still be fully understood, but unequivocally involve multiple effects [26, 27] (*Figure 4*).

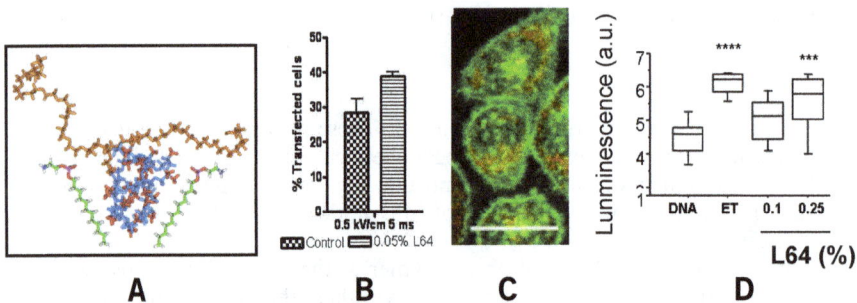

Figure 4. Representative scheme of pluronic interaction with membrane models (A), transfection increase by pre-treatment of CHO cells then electropermeabilisation application (B), cell internalisation of rhodamine labelled-L64 (C) and gene expression increase in mice muscle (D).

Poloxamer/DNA co-administration appeared to be a method of choice for gene transfer in the muscle due to its practical easiness: gene expression increase by simple co-injection of poloxamer and DNA, the fact that some poloxamers are already approved by the FDA. However, a closer look to these polymers reveals that some are quite toxic: the ratio between PEO and PPO is fundamental in this issue; the concentration range leading to gene expression improvement is relatively small. These polymers remain however extremely interesting tools for their physical properties of auto-assembly and temperature dependency and have undoubtly great potential in delivery which have not all been exploited yet.

CATIONIC AMPHIPATHIC HISTIDINE-RICH PEPTIDES FOR THE DELIVERY OF PLASMID DNA AND SIRNAS

Non-viral delivery of nucleic acids (plasmid DNA, antisense oligonucleotides, siRNAs, mRNA) into mammalian cells has been performed using a variety of compounds of unrelated structure including linear and branched polymers, cationic lipids and peptides. Notably, among all, the latter family is the least explored, although peptides have great biotechnological potential as key parameters such as product identification, large scale production and quality control are possible. In addition, peptides have a reduced size and they are biodegradable. Altogether, synthetic peptides possess interesting properties for future biomedical applications.

Gene delivery systems have to be multi-functional; in particular they should stabilise the nucleic acid and protect it from nucleases, promote cellular uptake and ensure that the nucleic acid reaches the desired intracellular compartment (nucleus for plasmid DNA while for siRNAs it is the cytoplasm). While most cationic compounds are able to complex DNA or siRNAs and favour cell uptake through non-specific endocytosis, it is the capacity of the transporter to induce the escape of the nucleic acid from the endosomes that mostly determines the efficiency of a system. A strategy that has proven particularly effective for endosome disruption consists in using compounds that are able to induce a "proton sponge" mechanism. Briefly, it consists in using compounds as for example polyethylenimines which can capture the protons entering the endosomes during the acidification process [28]. This in turn induces swelling of the endosomes that leads to membrane disruption. Interestingly, Midoux *et al.* showed that coupling histidine residues to polylysine strongly increases the transfection efficiency [29]. In fact, the imidazole group of histidine which has a pKa around 6 confers a proton sponge activity to the modified polylysines.

With this in mind, we focussed our efforts in the last years on the development of pH responsive, cationic amphipathic peptides. We started our study by evaluating the DNA transfection capabilities of LAH4 and derivatives thereof. LAH4 with the sequence **KKALLALALHHLAHLALHLALALKKA** was initially designed as a model peptide to study the membrane disturbing properties of α-helical amphipathic antibacterial peptides [30]. Our results demonstrated that the presence of histidine and lysine residues is not sufficient to obtain an efficient transfection agent. Of crucial importance are the number of histidine residues, their position in the sequence and the pH at which the peptides change from an in-plane to a transmembrane alignment [31]. Furthermore, evaluation of LAH4 isomers where the angle subtended by the positively charged histidine residues at pH 5 was varied (LAH4 has an angle of 100°), showed that an angle of 80° (peptide **KKALLAHALHLLALLALHLAHALKKA** called LAH4-L1) is optimal for DNA transfection [32].

More recently, we investigated whether: (1) peptides of the LAH4 family are able to deliver siRNAs into cells and (2) whether it is possible to find other residues than histidines which are able to activate the proton sponge mechanism.

1. We studied the potential of LAH4 and derivatives thereof to deliver siRNA into human retinoblasts. Our results showed that the LAH4 peptides are able to efficiently deliver siRNAs into the cells [33]. Indeed, when we compared the efficiency of our best peptide with three commercially available cationic compounds, namely Lipofectamine, DOTAP and PEI, we found peptides of the LAH4 family to be the most efficient agents. This high efficiency may be related to the great capacity of the peptides to favour association of the siRNA with the cells, as shown by experiments performed with a fluorescently labelled siRNA.

2. Although structurally related to its cationic analogues, such as lysine and ornithine, 2, 3-diaminopropionic acid (Dap) is characterized by distinctly lower proton ionization. We recently provided evidence that, when incorporated into a LAH4 peptide in place of histidines, Dap confers a high transfection activity to the peptide [34]. We thus showed that Dap residues represent an alternative to histidines to obtain pH responsive peptides.

In conclusion, we have developed a family of cationic amphipathic peptides that has proven to be remarkably effective with both DNA and siRNA delivery that often equals or outperforms commercially available cationic non-viral vectors.

DELIVERY OF DNA INTO MUSCLE BY ELECTROPORATION

Considering the limitations of viral based gene delivery (safety concerns, such as immune response, possible mutagenesis and carcinogenesis, and high production costs), the delivery of therapeutic genes to target cells upon direct *in vivo* administration of non-viral vectors, *i.e.*, plasmids, is of great value for the development of gene therapy. However, the use of plasmids is plagued by poor transfer efficiency, intracellular penetration and nuclear localization, low expression level and immunostimulatory properties of plasmid DNA. Therefore, technical improvements in gene delivery methods have definitely proven critical in the eventual success of gene transfer. Among the different non-viral strategies currently under study, the physical *in vivo* electroporation technique has proven to be one of the most efficient and simple methods, which could be applied in gene therapy and as a laboratory tool to study gene function. This technique is particularly efficient for gene transfer into the skeletal or smooth muscle, allowing their possible use as an endocrine organ for the secretion of therapeutic proteins.

Electrotransfer is based on a DNA solution injection into a targeted tissue, followed by the application onto the tissue of a defined set of electric pulses. The delivery of electric pulses enhances DNA uptake, resulting in a 100- to 1000-fold increase in gene expression (in comparison with naked DNA administration). This technique can be applied to any tissue, but the skeletal muscle is particularly suitable, mainly because it constitutes a large and easily accessible volume of tissue in which DNA electroporation is very efficient. Indeed the persistence of DNA in an episomal state for months and the ability of skeletal muscle to secrete proteins allow multiple therapeutic approaches such as direct gene transfer for muscle disorders, DNA vaccination or systemic delivery of therapeutic proteins to be considered.

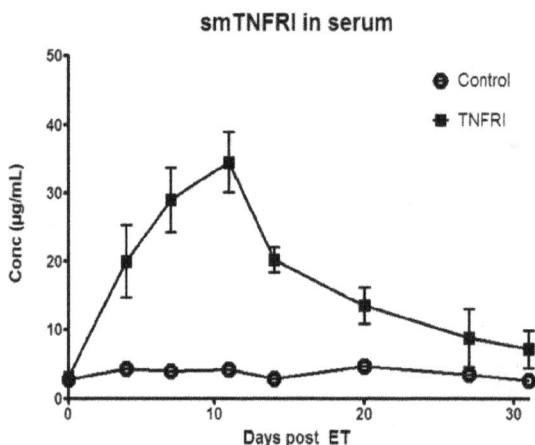

Figure 5. Expression of soluble TNF receptor in the mdx tibialis anterior muscle. 30µg of control plasmid (empty vector) and plasmid coding for the soluble mouse TNFα receptor I (TNFRI), were electroporated in the tibialis anterior muscle of 2 months old male mdx mice by electrotransfer. Serum levels of TNFRI were measured at day 0, 4, 7, 11, 14, 20, 27 and 31 by ELISA (DY425, R&D Systems).

We could apply *in vivo* electroporation to successfully reach therapeutic levels of a secreted TNFα soluble receptor I fused to a mutine IgG1 constant fraction in three different mouse models corresponding to a normal skeletal muscle, a smooth muscle, and a fragile dystrophic muscle:
- A single DNA electroporation in a normal skeletal muscle led to circulating levels of the secreted protein of about 5ng/ml for more than 6 months, that was able to inhibit the progression of a collagen induced arthritis disease in DBA1 mice [35].
- A single DNA electroporation into the ocular ciliary smooth muscle led to expression and secretion of the soluble receptor in the ocular fluids. This secreted protein was able to drastically inhibit the clinical and histological inflammation scores in rats with an endotoxin induced uveitis [36].
- A single DNA electroporation into a fragile dystrophic muscle of the *mdx* mouse strain led to circulating levels of the protein for at least one month, as illustrated in the shown figure below. Histological analysis of these muscles showed a biological effect on the fibrosis induced by the disease (unpublished data) (*Figure 5*).
Finally, these examples illustrate that DNA electroporation into skeletal or smooth muscle is able to induce secretion of therapeutic levels of a given protein, opening the door to further developments towards the clinics.

IMAGING PLASMID DELIVERY TO MUSCLE

There is presently no easy way for imaging plasmid delivery. However, associated phenomenon as gene expression resulting from DNA transfer into cell nuclei, or membrane modification accompanying the DNA transfer into cells can be imaged.

Fluorescent proteins

Recently the use of DNA coding fluorescent proteins opened avenue for non-invasive imaging of tissue transfection in the anaesthetized animal. In addition to allow observation on the living animal, non-invasive imaging techniques have the advantage of improving statistical analysis, the same animal being its own control for longitudinal studies.
DNA coding the green fluorescent protein GFP was used to evaluate different conditions of electrotransfer of the mouse tibial cranial muscle [37]. Nevertheless, fluorescence of GFP (λ ex 470nm λ em 515nm) is strongly attenuated by tissue absorption. However, for mouse muscle electrotransfer because of a high transfection level and a relative homogeneous distribution of transfected fibers, the partial amount of fluorescence detected can be considered representative of the fluorescence in the whole muscle. The minimum light absorption of biological tissues is occurring at wavelength close to 650-700nm (near infra-red). Different fluorescent proteins with excitation and emission wavelength approaching these values have been proposed, as, for example the "Katushka" protein with a high brightness in the far red (λ ex 588nm, λ em 635nm) [38], which has been used to study the transfection of the mouse tibial cranial muscle [39].

Bioluminescence

Another imaging method for evaluation of muscle transfection is based on *in situ* enzymatic bioluminescence production, by using plasmid DNA coding firefly luciferase. Luminescence centered at 560nm, resulting from the reaction between luciferase and luciferin, has the advantage of a high quantum yield associated to a very low background level of luminescence [40]. The Luciferin substrate can be injected *i.p.* or locally in the considered tissue. A particular advantage of the *i.p.* injection substrate is a wide-spread distribution at luciferase production sites. When possible, advantage of local luciferin injection is its higher sensitivity with reduced substrate consumption.

As shown in the (*Figure 6*), we observed a very good correlation between the luminescence level of the tibial cranial muscle of the mouse as measured *in vivo* by non-invasive optical imaging, and, *in vitro* on sample homogenate of the same muscle. In addition dose effect observed *in vitro* with increasing amount of DNA injected was similarly observed from *in vivo* measured luminescence. Thus, optical imaging can be considered as a sensitive and relevant technique to quantify variations of the luciferase activity *in vivo* in the tibial cranial muscle of the mouse. We have described and discussed in more details all these data in a previous publication [41].

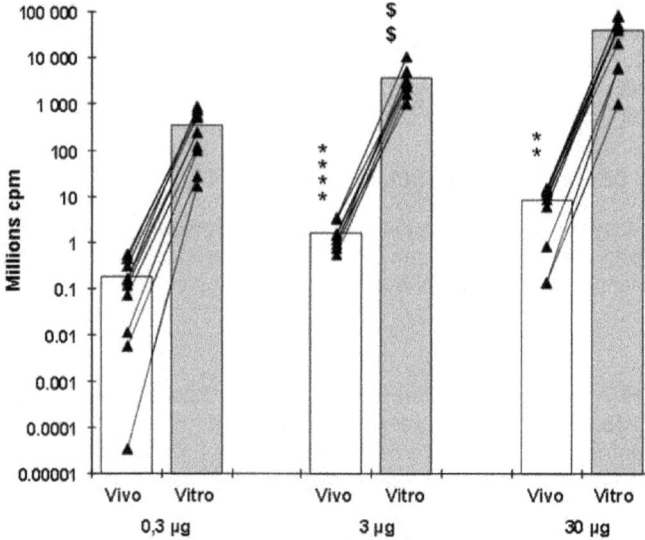

Figure 6. Comparison between the *in vivo* and *in vitro* measurements of luciferase activity of tibial cranial muscle after electrotransfer with a luciferase encoding plasmid. Values are mean ± SEM of the integrated values of luminescence in ROI of the tibial cranial muscle 8 days after electrotransfer of 0.3, 3 or 30µg of pCl luc plasmid as measured *in vivo* (white columns) and *in vitro* 3 hours later or more (grey columns) on the same muscles. Individual values are represented by black triangles and the lines links values measured *in vivo* and *in vitro* on the same muscles. *In vivo* background was substracted from the luminescence measured. *In vitro* background luminescence was negligeable. Dose effect: - *in vitro* ****p < 0.0001 between electrotransfer with 0.3 and 3µg of plasmid, **p< 0.01 between 3 and 30 µg of plasmid - *in vivo* $$p< 0.01 between electrotransfer with 0.3 and 3µg of plasmid. Correlation between *in vitro* and *in vivo* measurements: r2 = 0.796, p<0.0001, n=28 (C. Bloquel *et al.* [41]).

Magnetic resonance imaging (MRI)

The specific membrane events allowing gene transfer are difficult to study. But the occurrence of membrane modifications can be sometime evidenced from the cell permeabilization to small molecules. With MRI it is possible to visualize and evaluate the uptake of a contrast agent (Gadolinium-dotarem) by the permeabilized muscle fibers

[42]. Thus for mouse muscle electrotransfer, co-localisation between zones transfected and those permeabilized to the Gadolinium-Dotarem was shown [42]. We also observed a correlation between the volume permeabilized to the Gadolinium-Dotarem and transfection level [21]. Consequently use of MRI could be useful for visualising indirectly zone of therapeutic gene transfer in human by transfection methods inducing permeabilization to small molecules such as electrotransfer (*Figure 6*).

In conclusion, imaging techniques presently allow the non-invasive monitoring and evaluation of transfection of muscle and other tissues. Multimodality is possible, as for example for evaluation of muscle permeabilization and transfection using successively MRI and optical imaging [21]. Recent development of optical imaging system will allow 3D visualisation of fluorescence or luminescence *in vivo* emission. The possibility to combine optical imaging with X-scan gives bones reference points, which will allow to determine and accurately to compare the biodistribution of parameters obtained by different imaging modalities.

ACKNOWLEDGMENTS

This work has been performed with the support of the EC-DG research through the FP6-Network of Excellence, CLINIGENE: LSHB-CT-2006-018933

REFERENCES

1. Byk G, Scherman D, Schwartz B, Dubertret C. *Lipopolyamines as transfection agents and pharmaceutical uses thereof.* US Patent 2001, n°6171612.

2. Rhinn H, Largeau C, Bigey P, Lai Kuen R, Richard M, Scherman D, *et al.* How to make siRNA lipoplexes efficient? Add a DNA cargo. *Biochim Biophys Acta* 2009; 1790: 219-30.

3. Schlegel A, Largeau C, Bigey P, Bessodes M, Lebozec K, Scherman D, *et al.* Anionic polymers for decreased toxicity and enhanced *in vivo* delivery of siRNA complexed with cationic liposomes. *J Control Releas* 2011; 152: 393-401.

4. Khoury M, Louis-Plence P, Escriou V, Noël D, Largeau C, Cantos C, *et al.* Efficient new cationic liposome formulation for systemic delivery of small interfering RNA silencing tumor necrosis factor alpha in experimental arthritis. *Arthritis Rheum* 2006; 54: 1867-77.

5. Khoury M, Escriou V, Courties G, Galy A, Yao R, Largeau C, *et al.* Efficient suppression of murine arthritis by combined anticytokine small interfering RNA lipoplexes. *Arthritis Rheum* 2008; 58: 2356-67.

6. Courties G, Seiffart V, Presumey J, Escriou V, Scherman D, Zwerina J, *et al.* In vivo RNAi-mediated silencing of TAK1 decreases inflammatory Th-1 and Th-17 cells through targeting of myeloid cells. *Blood* 2010; 116: 3505-16.

7. Courties G, Baron M, Presumey J, Escriou V, VanLent P, Scherman D, *et al.* Cytosolic phospholipase A2a gene silencing in the myeloid lineage alters development of Th1 responses and reduces disease severity in collagen-induced arthritis. *Arthritis Rheum* 2011; 63: 681-90.

8. Rousseau J, Escriou V, Perrot P, Picarda G, Charrier C, Scherman D, *et al.* Advantages of bioluminescence imaging to follow siRNA or chemotherapeutic treatments in osteosarcoma preclinical models. *Cancer Gene Ther* 2010; 17: 387-97.

9. Rousseau J, Escriou V, Lamoureux F, Brion R, Chesneau J, Battaglia S, *et al.* Formulated siRNAs targeting Rankl prevent osteolysis and enhance chemotherapeutic response in osteosarcoma models. *J Bone Mineral Res* 2011; 26: 2452-62.

10. Nicolazzi C, Garinot M, Mignet N, Scherman D, Bessodes M. Cationic lipids for transfection. *Curr Med Chem* 2003; 10: 1263-77.

11. Tranchant I, Mignet N, Crozat E, Chain J, Girard C, Scherman D, *et al*. DNA complexing lipopolythiourea *Bioconjug Chem* 2004; 15: 1342-8.

12. Leblond J, Mignet N, Largeau C, Seguin J, Scherman D, Herscovici J. Lipopolythiourea transfecting agents: lysine thiourea derivatives. *Bioconjug Chem* 2008; 19: 306-14.

13. Leblond J, Mignet N, Largeau C, Spanedda MV, Seguin J, Scherman D, *et al*. Lipopolythiourea a new non cationic system for gene transfer. *Bioconjug Chem* 2007; 18: 484-93.

14. Breton M, Leblond J, Seguin J, Midoux P, Scherman D, Herscovici J, *et al*. Comparative gene transfer between cationic and thiourea lipoplexes. *J Gene Med* 2010; 12: 45-54.

15. Leblond J, Mignet N, Leseurre L, Largeau C, Bessodes M, Scherman D, *et al*. Design, synthesis and evaluation of enhanced DNA binding lipopolythiourea. *Bioconjug Chem* 2006; 17: 1200-8.

16. Firestone M, Wolf A, Seifert S. Small-angle X-ray scattering study of the interaction of poly(ethylene oxide)-b-poly(propylene oxide)-b-poly(ethylene oxide) triblock copolymers with lipid bilayers. *Biomacromolecules* 2003; 4: 1539-49.

17. Gau-Racine J, Lal J, Zeghal M, Auvray L. PEO-PPO block copolymer vectors do not interact directly with DNA but with lipid membranes. *J Phys Chem B* 2007; 111: 9900-7.

18. Pembouong G, Morellet N, Kral T, Hof M, Scherman D, Bureau MF, *et al*. Triblock copolymer L64 destabilizes lipidic membranes and does not interact with DNA. *J Control Release* 2011; 151: 57-64.

19. Sahay G, Batrakova E, Kabanov AV. Different internalization pathways of polymeric micelles and unimers and their effects on vesicular transport. *Bioconjug Chem* 2008; 19: 2023-9.

20. Wasungu L, Marty AL, Bureau MF, Kischler A, Bessodes M, Teissié J, *et al*. Pre-treatment of cells with pluronic L64 increases DNA transfection mediated by electrotransfer. *J Control Release* 2010; 149: 117-25.

21. Bureau MF, Jugé I, Seguin J, Scherman D, Rager MN, Mignet N. Muscle transfection and permeabilisation induced by electrotransfer or pluronic L64. *Biochim Biophys Acta* 2010; 1800: 537-43.

22. Alimi D, Leborgne C, Pembouong G, van Wittenberghe L, Mignet N, Scherman D, *et al*. Evaluation of the muscle gene transfer activity of a series of amphiphilic triblock copolymers. *J Gene Med* 2009; 11: 1114-24.

23. Brissault B, Kischler A, Leborgne C, Jarroux N, Cheradame H, Guis C. Amphiphilic poly[(propylene glycol)-block-(2-methyl-2-oxazoline)] copolymers for gene transfer in skeletal muscle. *Chem Med* 2007; 2: 1202-7.

24. Sriadibhatla S, Yang Z, Gebhart C, Alakhov VY, Kabanov A. Transcriptional activation of gene expression by pluronic block copolymers in stably and transiently transfected cells. *Mol Ther* 2006; 13: 804-13.

25. Astafieva I, Maksimova I, Lukanidin E, Alakhov V, Kabanov A. Enhancement of the polycation-mediated DNA uptake and cell transfection with Pluronic P85 block copolymer. *FEBS Lett* 1996; 389: 278-80.

26. Sahay Z, S. Sriadibhatla, Kabanov AV. Amphiphilic block copolymers enhance cellular uptake and nuclear entry of polyplex-delivered DNA. *Bioconjug Chem* 2008; 19: 1987-94.

27. Batrakova EV, Kabanov AV. Pluronic block copolymers: evolution of drug delivery concept from inert nanocarriers to biological response modifiers. *J Control Release* 2008; 130: 98-106.

28. Kichler A, Leborgne C, Coeytaux E, Danos O. Polyethylenimine-mediated gene delivery: a mechanistic study. *J Gene Med* 2001; 3: 135-44.

29. Midoux P, Monsigny M. Efficient gene transfer by histidylated polylysine/pDNA complexes. *Bioconjug Chem* 1999; 10: 406-11.

30. Bechinger B. Towards membrane protein design: pH-sensitive topology of histidine-containing polypeptides. *J Mol Biol* 1996; 263: 768-75.

31. Kichler A, Leborgne C, Marz J, Danos O, Bechinger, B. Histidine-rich amphipathic peptide antibiotics promote efficient delivery of DNA into mammalian cells. *Proc Natl Acad Sci USA* 2003; 100: 1564-8.

32. Mason AJ, Martinez A, Glaubitz C, Danos O, Kichler A, Bechinger B. The antibiotic and DNA-transfecting peptide LAH4 selectively associates with, and disorders, anionic lipids in mixed membranes. *FASEB J* 2006; 20: 320-2.

33. Langlet-Bertin B, Leborgne C, Scherman D, Bechinger B, Mason AJ, Kichler A. Design and evaluation of histidine-rich amphipathic peptides for siRNA delivery. *Pharm Res* 2010; 27: 1426-36.

34. Lan Y, Langlet-Bertin B, Abbate V, Vermeer LS, Kong X, Sullivan KE, *et al*. Incorporation of 2,3-diaminopropionic acid into linear cationic amphipathic peptides produces pH-sensitive vectors. *Chembiochem* 2010; 11: 1266-72.

35. Bloquel C, Bessis N, Boissier MC, Scherman D, Bigey P. Gene therapy of collagen-induced arthritis by electrotransfer of hTNF: a soluble receptor I variants. *Hum Gen Ther* 2004; 15: 189-201.

36. Bloquel C, Bejjani RA, Bigey P, Bedioui F, Doat M, Ben Ezra D, *et al*. Plasmid electrotransfer of eye ciliary muscle: principles and therapeutic efficacy using hTNF-alpha soluble receptor in uveitis. *FASEB J* 2006; 20: 389-91.

37. Andre FM, Gehl J, Sersa G, Preat V, Hojman P, Eriksen J, *et al*. Efficiency of high- and low-voltage pulse combinations for gene electrotransfer in muscle, liver, tumor, and skin. *Hum Gene Ther* 2008; 19: 1261-71.

38. Shcherbo D, Merzlyak EM, Chepurnykh TV, Fradkov AF, Ermakova GV, Solovieva EA, *et al*. Bright far-red fluorescent protein for whole-body imaging. *Nat Methods* 2007; 4: 741-6.

39. Hojman P, Eriksen J, Gehl J. *In vivo* imaging of far-red fluorescent proteins after DNA electrotransfer to muscle tissue. *Biol Proced Online* 2009; 11: 253-62.

40. Luker GD, Luker KE. Optical imaging: current applications and future directions. *J Nucl Med* 2008; 49: 1-4.

41. Bloquel C, Trollet C, Pradines E, Seguin J, Scherman D, Bureau MF. Optical imaging of luminescence for *in vivo* quantification of gene electrotransfer in mouse muscle and knee. *BMC Biotechnol* 2006; 6: 16.

42. Paturneau-Jouas M, Parzy E, Vidal G, Carlier PG, Wary C, Vilquin JT, *et al*. Electrotransfer at MR imaging: tool for optimization of gene transfer protocols. Feasibility study in mice. *Radiology* 2003; 228: 768-75.

A6-2
Overview of novel plasmid vectors and preclinical applications

CORINNE MARIE[1,2]*, DANIEL SCHERMAN[1,2]

[1]*CNRS, UMR8151, Paris, F-75006 France; Inserm, U1022, Paris, F-75006 France; Université Paris Descartes, Sorbonne Paris Cité, Faculté de Pharmacie, Chemical and Genetic Pharmacology and Imaging Laboratory, Paris, F-75270 France; École Nationale Supérieure de Chimie de Paris, Chimie ParisTech, Paris, F-75005 France.*
[2]*UPCGI, Inserm U1022 - CNRS UMR8151, Faculté des Sciences Pharmaceutiques et Biologiques, 4, avenue de l'Observatoire, 75270 Paris Cedex 06, France.*
daniel.scherman@parisdescartes.fr
corinne.marie@parisdescartes.fr
* Corresponding author

INTRODUCTION

The ultimate success of gene therapy relies on the administration of a safe delivery vehicle that mediates therapeutic levels of transgene expression in a targeted organ, which might have to be persistent in several instances. To deliver eukaryotic genes into living organisms, more than eight families of vectors have been described, which are mainly virus-related. Although non-viral gene vectors mostly comprise plasmid DNA derivatives, the number of studies involving this subclass has recently increased and now accounts for more than 18% of all gene therapy clinical trials, just behind those involving adenoviruses and retroviruses [1]. This recent evolution most probably results from the concomitant improvement of the non-viral vectors, eukaryotic expression cassettes and physical delivery techniques (*e.g.*: electroporation, sonoporation, hydrodynamics-based delivery, etc.).

The development of nonviral gene vectors has involved the optimization of both (1) the eukaryotic expression cassette, which comprises the identification of tissue-specific regulatory elements, such as promoters or micro RNAs to counteract host immune responses by preventing transgene expression in antigen-presenting cells, and/or the use of species-specific codon optimized therapeutic genes and (2) the plasmid backbones by removing the antibiotic resistance markers for an increased safety.

Indeed, regulatory agencies [2] have recommended the elimination, from plasmid backbones, of genes encoding proteins which catabolyse antibiotics used in human health, such as beta-lactam antibiotics or tetracyclin. The removal of antibiotic resistance markers from plasmid backbones will preclude their transfer to endogenous flora of treated patients and will decrease manufacturing costs by dismissing the necessity of evaluating putative residual antibiotics or derived products in plasmid

DNA-based medicines. In addition to an enhanced biosafety, the removal of antibiotic resistance genes also leads to a decrease in plasmid size and to a lightening of the metabolic burden imposed on the bacterial host for DNA plasmid replication as well as for transcription and translation of the antibiotic resistance markers during plasmid production [3]. The reduction in prokaryotic sequences and plasmid size also tends to increase gene expression levels [4], possibly resulting from a higher transfection efficacy and migration ability in the viscous cytosolic environment, but also seems to reduce heterochromatin formation favouring gene silencing in liver [5].

BIOSAFE NON-VIRAL VECTORS

To date, three main types of non-viral vectors devoid of antibiotic resistance markers have been described: (1) linearized double strand DNA molecules, (2) minicircles, and (3) biosafe miniplasmids. The two former ones do not contain any prokaryotic sequences.

Linearized cassettes can be generated *in vitro* by either polymerase chain reaction or specific endonuclease processing after plasmid propagation in bacteria. The endonuclease processing technique has been used by Mologen AG, a pharmaceutical company that developed MIDGE (Minimalistic Immunogenic Defined Gene Expression) vectors for DNA-based therapies and vaccines against colorectal carcinoma [6] or Leishmania infection [7].

Minicircles are circular molecules derived from a conventional plasmid that contains a eukaryotic expression cassette flanked by recombinase-recognized sequences. The recombination event is activated at the end of plasmid propagation in *Escherichia coli*, and results in the formation of two circularized molecules: a minicircle carrying the eukaryotic expression cassette and a smaller plasmid containing the rest of the vector backbone. Minicircles are thereafter purified by using various techniques (see chapters by Schleef *et al.*). Although minicircles present the obvious advantage of being totally free of prokaryotic-derived sequences, their large scale and cost effective production still requires some additional on-going adjustments.

We and others have therefore developed antibiotic-free systems to produce biosafe miniplasmids ([8] for a recent review). Their propagation and maintenance rely on the same basic principle: the growth of the bacterial host strain is conditioned by the presence of the plasmid to be produced.

Plasmidic expression vectors can harbor either: (1) *lac* operator sequences that titrate a repressor bound to an essential chromosomal gene promoter/operator region (*e.g.* pORT derivatives), (2) a suppressor t-RNA coding sequence enabling the complete translation of a protein playing a role in a biosynthetic pathway (pCOR and pFAR derivatives) and (3) a replication origin encoding an RNA molecule involved in the regulation of an essential or a lethal chromosomal *E. coli* gene *via* an RNA/RNA interference mechanism (pMINI and NTC derivatives).

The pCOR derivatives have been mostly used in gene therapy approaches and led, for examples, to an efficient treatment of β-thalassemic mouse anemia after intramuscular electotransfer of erythropoietin gene or of limb ischemia with fibroblast growth factor 1, which even reached phase III clinical studies (see Table 2 in [8] for a recent review; Tamaris phase III trial on NV1FGF). On the other hand, pORT and NTC derivatives have mainly been used as gene vectors in a DNA vaccination context. Strong immunogenic responses (cellular and humoral) were stimulated after injection of pORT derivatives encoding either the HIV-1 gag protein, human papillomavirus type 16 E7 or *Leishmania infantum* LACK antigens and of NTC derivatives encoding influenza H5 hemagglutinin (see Table 2 in [8] for a recent review and [9]).

pFAR4: A NOVEL ANTIBIOTIC-FREE PLASMID VECTOR

Recently, our group has developed a novel antibiotic-free selection system which is based on the suppression of a nonsense mutation introduced into an essential chromosomal *E. coli* gene by a plasmid-borne function [10]. The nonsense mutation was introduced into the *E. coli thyA* gene that encodes a thymidylate synthase. In parallel, a novel vector, which only contains a suppressor t-RNA coding sequence, an origin of replication and a multiple cloning site, was entirely synthesized to eliminate redundant sequences and to reduce plasmid size. The growth characteristics of pFAR4-containing optimized bacterial producer strain in selective medium were similar to those of a routinely used laboratory strain propagated in the presence of antibiotics.

The *in vivo* potency of pFAR4 expression vector has been demonstrated after plasmid injection into muscle, skin, tumour followed by electrotransfer, which consists of applying electric field-mediated intracellular delivery via a mechanism mostly composed of cell permeabilisation and electrophoretic DNA migration, thus promoting an efficient transit passage through cell membranes and the viscous cytoplasm [4].

In muscles, a pFAR4 derivative expressing the reporter luciferase gene from the ubiquitous cytomegalovirus promoter promoted elevated transgene expression. In a therapeutic context, the biosafe miniplasmid was also found to be a potent gene vector. Indeed, the injection and electrotransfer of a pFAR4 derivative carrying a gene encoding a species-specific codon optimized microdystrophin expressed from the minimal muscle-specific MCK (muscle creatine kinase) promoter into muscle of *mdx* mice led to a superior level of transfected muscle fibers than after injection of a microdystrophin-encoding AAV vector plasmid (in collaboration with H. Foster and G. Dickson, RHUL, London, UK).

For DNA-based vaccination, which aims at stimulating cellular and/or humoral immune responses, plasmid DNA can also be electroporated into either skin that presents the advantage of being easily accessible and containing a large of number of antigen-presenting cells, or into tumours for a recruitment of immune cells at the targeted site [11]. Interestingly, in B16F10 transplanted tumour cells transfected by the pFAR4 derivative, we detected a higher luciferase activity (by about a log) than in those transfected by the control vector [10]. Outstandingly, in skin, whereas luciferase activity decreased within 3 weeks after intradermal electrotransfer of a conventional expression vector, sustained luciferase expression was observed with the luciferase-encoding pFAR4 plasmid [10]. In addition, in a DNA vaccination assay, a strong immune response was obtained after the intradermal injection of a pFAR4 derivative encoding a HIV-1 antigenic determinant (in collaboration with A. Brave and B. Wharen; Karolinska Institutet, Stockholm, Sweden).

To target hepatocytes, plasmid DNA can be hydrodynamically injected *via* the tail vein. This technique, which consists of injecting a large volume (8-10% v/rodent body weight) of a plasmid solution over a short period (a few seconds), allows the transfection of ~40% of liver cells ([12], for a review). With either a ubiquitous (CAG) or a liver-specific (hAAT) promoter, the pFAR4 derivatives promoted a higher alkaline phosphatase activity in sera (> 20-fold, 7 days post injection), in comparison with similar plasmids carrying a kanamycin resistance marker gene. Interestingly, in a therapeutic context, injection of a pFAR4 derivative expressing the enzyme sulfamidase from the hAAT promoter into liver of mice suffering from the lysosomal storage mucopolysaccharidosis IIIA disease led to a high level of therapeutic protein in sera (~30 times the wild-type levels, 7 days post injection). Although the seric sulphamidase level appeared to slowly decrease with time, it was still more than 10 times superior to wild-type therapeutic level at least 6 months post plasmid delivery. The secreted and circulating therapeutic protein was then efficiently endocytosed by neighboring cells *via* a mechanism involving mannose 6-P receptors. This led to a phenotypic correction, measured by the reduction in glycosaminoglycan (GAGs) accumulation, in all organs (unpublished data). Thus, pFAR4 vector appears to efficiently deliver therapeutic gene into hepatocytes and could therefore be used to treat metabolic genetic diseases (such as lysosomal storage or hemophilia diseases) that require protein secretion from the liver. For a translation to clinics, the recent results obtained by D. Liu *et al.* [13], who used an image-guided hydrodynamic procedure coupled with a computer controlled injection device for gene delivery in large animals, appear extremely promising. We therefore expect that major developments in this field will continue emerging in the next few years.

In summary, either in a therapeutic or DNA-based vaccination context, the biosafe pFAR4 miniplasmid appears to be an efficient gene vector to transfect muscle, skin, tumour or liver cells. We are currently assessing the pFAR4 potency as a non-viral vector to deliver reprogramming genes to generate induced Pluripotent Stem cells (iPS cells). In addition, in order to obtain a sustained transgene expression in highly dividing cells, we are also merging the pFAR4 plasmid and the sleeping beauty transposon technology that allows random transgene integration into the host genome, unlike retroviruses that tend to mediate gene insertion in actively transcribed regions (see chapter by Z. Izsvak *et al.*, A6-5). Preliminary results indicate that the reduced size of pFAR4 appears to mediate higher transgene integration efficiency, most probably resulting from an increased gene transfection and/or transposition. Clearly, the ongoing research studies aiming at favoring site-specific gene integration into host genomes represent another major challenge for the future.

Finally, we believe that the ongoing development of plasmid vectors could also benefit to the field of gene therapy using viral vectors. Indeed during the production of viral particles, nonspecific nicking of the plasmid backbone sequence can occur, leading to unexpected packing of prokaryotic plasmid backbones and of antibiotic resistance markers that can represent up to 6% of the total vector genome of the recombinant adeno-associated virus (rAAV) [14]. Thus, the use of biosafe plasmids for the production of viral vectors could also be envisioned for an increased biosafety.

CONCLUDING REMARKS

Over the last 15 years, plasmid vectors were often seen as gene vectors that present the main following advantages: safe as non-integrating, cheaper to produce and store than viral vectors, and devoid of immunogenicity. Nevertheless, three major hurdles remained to be overcome: (1) transient expression in some tissues due to the loss of non-replicating vectors upon cell division, (2) epigenetic responses linked to the presence of sequences of prokaryotic origin on the plasmid, and (3) inefficient delivery of DNA molecules into cells of a specific organ. Major progresses have been made to overcome these limitations, which we expect, will be further pursued. In addition, the merging of newly developed technologies (biosafe miniplasmids, sleeping beauty transposon systems, improved localized plasmid delivery techniques,...) should lead to a safer and more efficient gene therapy, towards an increase in successful preclinical and clinical trials.

C. Marie, D. Scherman

Acknowledgments

This work was supported by the European Commission under the MOLEDA STREP (Number #512034) and the CliniGene Network of Excellence Grants (Number #LSHB-CT-2006-018933) of the Sixth Framework Programme.

We apologize to authors whose work could not be directly cited due to space limitations.

References

1. Gene Therapy Clinical Trials Worldwide (2010). http://wwwwileycom//legacy/wileychi/genmed/clinical/

2. World Health Organization. WHO Expert Committee on Biological Standardization, 56th meeting. *WHO Tech Rep Ser,* 2005.

3. Mairhofer J, Cserjan-Puschmann M, Striedner G, Nöbauer K, Razzazi-Fazeli E, Grabherr R. Marker-free plasmids for gene therapeutic applications: lack of antibiotic resistance gene substantially improves the manufacturing process. *J Biotechnol* 2010; 146: 130-7.

4. Bloquel C, Fabre E, Bureau MF, Scherman D. Plasmid DNA electrotransfer for intracellular and secreted proteins expression: new methodological developments and applications. *J Gene Med* 2004; 6: S11-3.

5. Riu E, Chen ZY, Xu H, He CY, Kay MA. Histone modifications are associated with the persistence or silencing of vector-mediated transgene expression *in vivo. Mol Ther* 2007; 15: 1348-55.

6. Wittig B, Märten A, Dorbic T, Weineck S, Min H, Niemitz S, *et al.* Therapeutic vaccination against metastatic carcinoma by expression-modulated and immunomodified autologous tumor cells: a first clinical phase I/II trial. *Hum Gene Ther* 2001; 12: 267-78.

7. Lopez-Fuertes L, Pérez-Jiménez E, Vila-Coro AJ, Sack F, Moreno S, Konig SA, *et al.* DNA vaccination with linear minimalistic (MIDGE) vectors confers protection against *Leishmania major* infection in mice. *Vaccine* 2002; 21: 247-57.

8. Vandermeulen G, Marie C, Scherman D, Préat V. New generation of plasmid backbones devoid of antibiotic resistance marker for gene therapy trials. *Mol Ther* 2011; 19: 1942-9.

9. Luke J, Carnes AE, Hodgson CP, Williams JA. Improved antibiotic-free DNA vaccine vectors utilizing a novel RNA based plasmid selection system. *Vaccine* 2009; 27: 6454-59.

10. Marie C, Vandermeulen G, Quiviger M, Richard M, Préat V, Scherman D. pFARs, Plasmids free of antibiotic resistance markers, display high-level transgene expression in muscle, skin and tumour cells. *J Gene Med* 2010; 12: 323-32.

11. van Drunen Littel-van den Hurk S, Hannaman D. Electroporation for DNA immunization: clinical application. *Expert Rev Vaccines* 2010; 9: 503-17.

12. Sawyer GJ, Rela M, Davenport M, Whitehorne M, Zhang X, Fabre JW. Hydrodynamic gene delivery to the liver: theoretical and practical issues for clinical application. *Curr Gene Ther* 2009; 9: 128-35.

13. Suda T, Suda K, Liu D. Computer-assisted hydrodynamic gene delivery. *Mol Ther* 2008; 16: 1098-104.

14. Chadeuf G, Ciron C, Moullier P, Salvetti A. Evidence for encapsidation of prokaryotic sequences during recombinant adeno-associated virus production and their *in vivo* persistence after vector delivery. *Mol Ther* 2005; 12: 744-53.

The CliniBook: Clinical gene transfer
Edited by Odile Cohen-Haguenauer – EDK, Paris © 2012, pp. 271-276

A6-3
Filling a gap: S/MAR-based replicating minicircles

Niels Heinz[1], Sandra Broll[2], Martin Schleef [3], Christopher Baum[1], Juergen Bode[1]*

[1]*Hannover Medical School (MHH), Institute of Experimental Haematology, OE 6960, D-30625 Hannover, Germany.*
[2]*Helmholtz Centre for Infection Research (HZI), Department Mol Biotech, Braunschweig, Germany.*
[3]*PlasmidFactory GmbH, D-33607 Bielefeld, Germany.*
bode.juergen@mh-hannover.de
* Corresponding author

Promising vectors for cell- and tissue modification do not depend on integration but rather behave as independent functional units replicating as an episome. Since most episomes persist in the nucleus in multiple copies, this status is a way to enhance the added genomic information in the absence of repeat-induced silencing phenomena.

WHAT VIRAL SYSTEMS CAN TELL

Until recently all episomes maintained in mammalian cells were of viral origin and required at least one viral protein (EBNA1 in case of EBV-derived plasmids) to enable replication, usually in a narrow host range. After lytic infection its 172 kb genome persists in B-lymphocytes as an extrachromosomal multicopy plasmid.

The mechanism according to which EBV replicates is well understood: the EBV latent origin has been identified and named OriP (origin of plasmid replication). It extends over 1.7-kb and contains two functional elements, the family of repeats (FR) and the dyad symmetry (DS) element, both binding sites for a trans-acting factor, EBV nuclear antigen-1 (EBNA-1). DS is a 120-bp region containing two EBNA-1-binding sites separated by 9-bp, serving as replication initiation region (IR). The second element, FR, comprises twenty EBNA-1 binding sites. EBNA1 complexes on DS and FR interact by a DNA looping mechanism in a way reminding of scaffold attachment factor A (SAF-A), which has been implicated in the retention of a new class of S/MAR-based episomes, upon which this contribution is centered [1, 2]. Such an attachment to the internal fibrogranular network within the nucleus (called "nuclear scaffold" or "-matrix") enables authentic segregation by non-covalent attachment to mitotic chromosomes according to the "hitchhiking principle" [3].

Since viral episomes may lead to transformation of recipient cells, the time had come for a new vector generation relying on Ori-associated factors intrinsic to the eukaryotic cellular replication machinery. Following the EBV paradigm a synthetic episome was expected to require three functions:

(i) chromosome association ("molecular glue"),
(ii) DNA strand-separation propensity,
(iii) functions of an replication initiation ("IR"-) region.

These prerequisites are naturally met by yeast, in which case an Ori is specified by ~125 base pair DNA-segments, so called autonomously replicating sequences (ARSs). As part of plasmids, ARS elements enable the existence as autonomous entities in the absence of sequence rearrangements or integration. While central properties of the ORC are evolutionarily conserved, replication promoting sequences are not. Thus, for decades the nature of replication origins has remained elusive for metazoa.

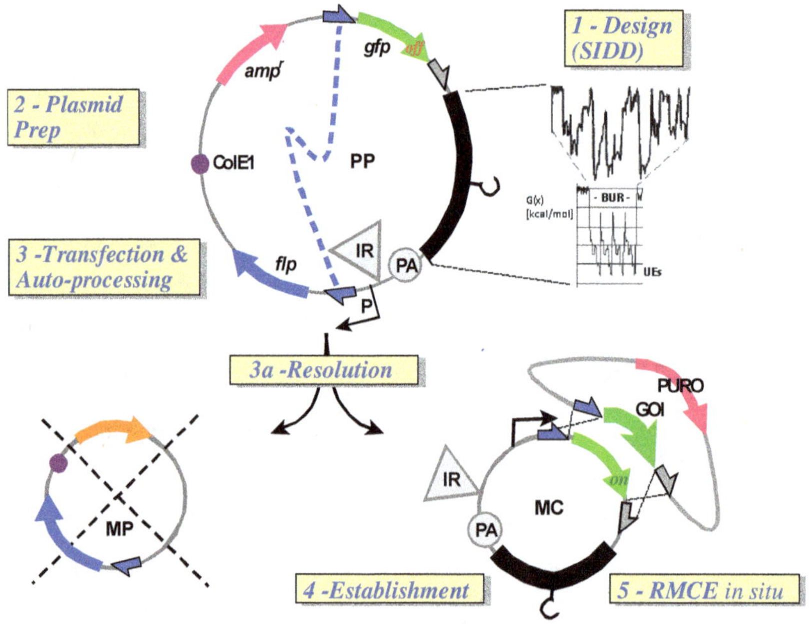

Figure 1. MCs are generated from parental plasmids *in situ* using a setup in which Flp recombinase is encoded on the vector backbone (blue arrow) together with the other auxiliary sequences. Central features of this MC-lifecycle are:

1. SIDD-driven design of the S/MAR in conjunction wit other regulatory elements.
2. Preparation of the "parental plasmid" (PP).
3. Transfection starts auto-conversion of the PP to Minicircle (MC) and Miniplasmid (MP), by Flp expression, which is driven by a strategically-positioned promoter (P).
3a. Resolution by Flp acting on two identical target sites (blue *FRT*s). Due to a promoter-switch, the process can be monitored by GFP expression and used for FACsorting.
4. MC establishment followed by *e.g.* the recovery of the respective fluorescent cells.
5. Replacement of the selection marker (eGFP or drug-selection marker) by the ultimate gene of interest via RMCE, *i.e.* a donor vector acting on the remaining set of "heterospecific" FRTs (blue and gray half-arrow).
Further options: • a second MC can be established subsequently or in parallel enabling elaborate expression protocols. • "Floxing" the S/MAR would enable withdrawal of the MC by the action of Cre.
• Constructs with proven performance will enter large-scale production (PlasmidFactory) after re-cloning the eukaryotic FRT-flanked section (*i.e.* the MC-equivalent) into a high-performance vector system.

FROM ARS TO S/MARS

There are definite relationships between ARSs and scaffold/matrix attachment regions (S/MARs; [3]). DNA segments with scaffold association (and thereby SIDD- [1, 3]) potential could be shown to include an ARS consensus sequence (ACS), suggesting a relation between S/MAR and ARS activities. The established strand-separation potential of S/MARs (SIDD diagrams in *Figure 1*) lends support to the idea that there is a regular association with origins of replication, which in turn motivated the generation of an S/MAR plasmid. This vector, pEPI, in fact, proved replication potential in a variety of eukaryotic cell systems. Available evidence indicates that it is the S/MAR element recruiting components of the cellular replication apparatus to support authentic replication and segregation by serving functions (i) and (ii) that were found to depend on its position at the downstream end of an active transcription unit [1, 2]. After its establishment in the nuclear architecture the replication apparatus of the host cell is utilized enabling S/MAR episomes to replicate once in early S phase in synchrony with the cellular genome.

FROM S/MAR-PLASMIDS TO MINICIRCLES: pFAR PRINCIPLES

Besides a limited cloning capacity remaining shortcomings of first-generation S/MAR-plasmid-episomes were silencing actions exerted by the bacterial vector parts. Moreover, plasmid-vectors do not comply with pFAR principles [4]. These restrictions could be overcome by removing all plasmid-derived and auxiliary sequences. Other than conventional minicircles (MCs) that persist only in non-dividing tissues, these efforts led to the first MC applicable for the modification of dividing cells due to its authentic replication and segregation behavior [2, 3].

The conversion of S/MAR-plasmids (so called "parental plasmids"/PPs) to minicircles mostly relies on site-specific recombinases (SSRs). In case two identical, equally oriented SSR-target-sites are parts of a given DNA segment, the PP will experience a recombinase-mediated crossover leading to resolution, *i.e.* the generation of two circular derivatives both maintaining the original supercoiled (ccc-) status [1]. These two daughter molecules are the miniplasmid (MP; containing the prokaryotic vector parts and accessory sequences) in addition to the MC composed from the eukaryotic sequences of choice. In principle, the MC mimics a functional chromatin domain in that a DNA loop ends in S/MAR element(s).

Since we have established a multi-purpose, mostly Flp-recombinase-based toolbox [5, 6] to enable the inversion, excision and (RMCE-mediated) integration of appropriately-flanked expression cassettes, we preferred the Flp/FRT over alternative SSRs that are otherwise applied to this end. We will further elaborate this toolbox below in a way that it will permit not only excision, but also the subsequent systematic elaboration of the minicircle by a principle called "flirting RMCE" [6]. *Figure 1* provides an overview regarding these actions.

Supported by bioinformatic (SIDD-) routines effective S/MAR modules (BURs, cf. *Figure 1*) can be predicted or designed. On this basis we derived a further minimized ~3 kb minicircle consisting of only one active transcription unit in addition to a still functional 730 bp sub-S/MAR [2]. Once established in the nuclear architecture, this entity proves an almost unlimited replication potential in dividing cells and its derivatives are currently investigated for their potential to modify tissues, stem cells and zygotes. In the latter case the authentic ccc-status enables facilitated passage of the nuclear membrane, effectively circumventing, for instance, the need of pronuclear injection of the vector [7]. Parallel efforts use a bovine fibroblast line to firmly establish the MC before these cells serve as a donor for somatic nuclear cell transfer (SCNT). Initial results support the value of these experiments for generating viable transgenic offspring.

NUCLEAR ESTABLISHMENT – A PREREQUISITE FOR LONG-TERM FUNCTION

Efficient maintenance of episomes requires their authentic replication. The process is initiated during an "establishment" phase, *i.e.* the interval between vector transduction and its functional association with the nuclear substructures providing replication potential. At this stage the vector acquires a chromatin structure to mediate long term maintenance, which is unprecedented by other types of episomes. This is reflected by the fact that stable matrix-association permits the recovery of clonal lines based upon one or several distinct minicircles that can be accommodated in parallel (opening numerous options for the expression of multiple-subunit proteins and the design of novel non-integrating inducible vector systems). Current work confirms that episomal establishment depends on the above conditions (i) – (ii) and emphasizes the auxiliary role of replicator functions (iii) that can be provided by IR minimal elements from either the β-globin or – preferentially – the lamin B gene (cooperation with A. Athanassiadou, University of Padras [8]). Nuclear establishment can be supported in case the host cell chromatin structure becomes relaxed histone hyperacetylation prior to transfection [2].

Various parameters are now available to safely confirm persistence of the episomal state. While full-length PCR may provide a preliminary hint, Southern-blot and Hirt-extraction protocols may strengthen the evidence in case they are combined with ATP-dependent nuclease treatment [2]. Though demanding, the most comprehensive information on copy number and -status is enabled by metaphase-FISH [1]. The approach generates multiple distinct fluorescent spots in association with the chromosomes when we have to deal with intact episomes. Alternatively, we find a single intense doublet of signals, one on each chromatid, indicating co-integration events that occurred during continued cultivation. While integration is noted for up to 40% of clones in case of S/MAR plasmids (PPs) this is rarely found for MCs [1].

CLONES RESULTING FROM MC TRANSFER, THEIR MODIFICATION AND WITHDRAWAL

It is of note that expression levels for both, established S/MAR-plasmids and minicircles vary by 2-3 orders of magnitude. Considering that this wide range refers to just a two-fold variation of copy numbers (typically 4-8) and that, for MCs, the variation is not due to silencing, these findings underline a widely different clonal behavior of cells. Proof of concept was obtained by the isolation of single clones and long- term stability of the respective, symmetrical expression profiles.

Our expanded SSR-toolbox permits several novel options, which are just listed as they are part of an extensive review [1]:

• The efficient establishment of MCs by FACsorting depends on the optimum time point of this step and varies depending on the respective clone and cell line. A more convenient strategy to this end is a time-delimited drug-selection procedure. This procedure involves the removal of the selection marker (SM), preferentially as part of a "flirting-RMCE" strategy (*Figure 1*). This setup covers both, deletion of the SM-cassette and its exchange for any GOI in one or a series of successive cassette exchanges steps.

• The removal of potentially transforming expression units is an essential part of, for instance, ongoing protocols for inducing a pluripotent status without entering the risks associated with a TIC (tumor-inducing cell-) status. Since clone establishment during reprogramming stringently depends on persistent S/MAR functions over a period of at least 2 weeks, it is an anticipated that "floxing" the S/MAR enables its SSR-induced removal. According to our experience, this step is not endangered by an aberrant genomic integration of remaining MC-sequences, as recombination occurs in tight association with the SSR until the products are released as ccc-circles to be lost during replication.

FROM BENCH TO THE PRODUCTION SITE: USE OF AVAILABLE ROUTINES

While the minicircle production process could continuously be refined in various cooperations, we have demonstrated that MC generation is also possible *in situ, i.e.* in the recipient mammalian cell itself. At present this "all-in-one" strategy (*Figure 1*) primarily serves exploratory purposes to optimize minicircle functions of the mentioned nature. In cases of success the presence of appropriate restriction sites adjacent to the FRTs will enable the rational transfer and insertion of the GOI - S/MAR - pA cassette to create a parental plasmid in the context of existing industrial-scale MC production routes (PlasmidFactory, Bielefeld). This technology will enable highly pure MC preparations with a defined superhelical status. Only these joint efforts will guarantee episomes meeting the requirements of cell- and gene therapy as well as genetic vaccination.

IN SUMMARY

Replicating S/MAR-minicircles combine the properties of efficient transient expression systems (facilitated membrane transfer and physical stability leading to an extended transcriptional burst) with those of stable expression systems. The transition between both phases is smooth such that comprehensive procedures for a variety of purposes can be envisaged. In the near future significant progress is anticipated from the incorporation of IR elements and the application of new concepts for initial selection by providing cells with a selection advantage. This may be done by the genuine form of a protein that compensates a mutant form causing a genetic disease or, alternatively, by expression of siRNA to suppress a mutated form.

ACKNOWLEDGMENTS

This work has been performed with the support of the EC-DG research through the FP6-Network of Excellence, CLINIGENE: LSHB-CT-2006-018933.

Abbreviations

ACS: ARS consensus sequence.

BUR: base-unpairing region.

Ccc: covalently closed circular.

DP: donor plasmid (an auxiliary vector providing the RMCE donor cassette).

Flirting: flanked by identical FRTs.

Floxing: flanked by loxP sites.

FRT: Flp-recognition target.

GOI: gene of interest.

MC: minicircle.

MP: miniplasmid (containing auxiliary sequences needed during production).

pFAR: plasmid free of antibiotic resistance genes.

PP: parental plasmid (*i.e.* the plasmid precursor of the MC).

RMCE: recombinase-mediated cassette exchange (here: Flp-RMCE).

SM: Selection marker.

S/MAR: scaffold/matrix attachment region.

SSR: site-specific recombination/recombinase.

REFERENCES

1. Nehlsen K, Broll SW, Kandimalla R, Heinz N, Heine M, Binius S, *et al. Replicating minicircles: overcoming the limitations of transient and of stable expression systems.* In: Schleef M, ed. New York: Wiley-VCH Verlag, 2012 (in press).

2. Broll S, Oumard A, Hahn K, Schambach A, Bode J. Minicircle performance depending on S/MAR-nuclear matrix interactions. *J Mol Biol* 2010; 395: 950-65.

3. Gluch A, Vidakovic M, Bode J. Scaffold/matrix attachment regions (S/MARs): relevance for disease and therapy, protein-protein interactions as new drug targets. In : Klussmann E, Scott JD, eds. *Handbook of experimental pharmacology*. Paris: Springer, 2008: 67-103.

4. Marie C, Vandermeulen G, Quiviger M, Richard M, Préat V, Scherman D. pFARs, Plasmids free of antibiotic resistancemarkers, display high-level transgene expression in muscle, skin and tumour cells. *J Gene Med* 2010; 12: 323-32.

5. Turan S, Galla M, Ernst E, Qiao J, Voelkel C, Schiedlmeier B, *et al.* Recombinase-mediated cassette exchange (RMCE): traditional concepts and current challenges. *J Mol Biol* 2011; 407: 193-221.

6. Turan S, Bode J. Site-specific recombinases: from "tag-and-target" to "tag-and-exchange": based genomic modifications. *FASEB J* 2012 (in press).

7. Iqbal K, Barg-Kues B, Broll S, Bode J, Niemann H, Kues WA. Cytoplasmic injection of circular plasmids allows targeted expression in mammalian embryos. *BioTechniques* 2009; 47: 959-68.

8. Giannakopoulos A, Stavrou EF, Zarkadis I, Zoumbos N, Thrasher AJ, Athanassiadou A. The functional role of S/MARs in episomal vectors as defined by the stress-induced destabilization profile of the vector sequences. *J Mol Biol* 2009; 387: 1239-49.

The CliniBook: Clinical gene transfer
Edited by Odile Cohen-Haguenauer – EDK, Paris © 2012, pp. 277-283

A6-4
Manufacturing and QC of plasmid based vectors

Marco Schmeer, Martin Schleef*

PlasmidFactory GmbH and Co. KG, Meisenstrasse 96, D-33607 Bielefeld, Germany.
martin.schleef@plasmidfactory.com
* Corresponding author

Plasmid-DNA is frequently used in non-viral gene therapy and gene vaccination but also for production of viral vectors. Hence, the requirements, especially for the pharmaceutical manufacturing of such vectors, have improved significantly. Here we summarize the main features of production and quality control of plasmid DNA.

Introduction

Recent promising results in the fields of gene therapy and genetic vaccination underline the need for the development of industrial scale processes for the production of plasmid DNA in an adequate quality, tailor-made for the intended applications. If the DNA will be used *e.g.* as an ancillary product for GMP viral vector production or an active pharmaceutical ingredient (API), such as *e.g.* antibodies, other functional proteins or RNA, this requires to fulfil the respective regulatory guidelines as well as a production process of a sufficient scale, *i.e.* milligram but even gram or kilogram scale productions have to be made possible [1, 2].

Plasmids have been successfully produced as a drug substance already years ago [1]. Frequently, process design can make use of a technology that is generic for at least plasmids of up to 10 kbp, but the requirement for producing plasmids with higher capacities led to the design of different process types – either for large vectors or those tending to be instable due to their size or sequence structure.

The plasmid DNA manufacturing process consists of two main process steps, cultivation of *E. coli* (preferably done by fermentation to ensure reproducible working conditions and quality profiles of the resulting plasmid DNA) and downstream processing. During and after the production process a variety of quality controls (QCs) is performed to ensure the adequate product purity and hence product quality.

Fermentation

The manufacturing of plasmid DNA starts with the transformation of the appropriate and characterised host cell, typically *E. coli* K-12 derivatives, with a fully characterised plasmid. The resulting bacteria stocks or cell banks have to be characterized to be of sufficient quality for a further manufacturing. Hence, already at this stage, certain QC assays have to be performed with this cell bank material as in-process controls or for lot release (*Table I*). The aspect of productivity and quality with respect to the content of plasmid forms very much depends on the host strain used and the proper cultivation parameters [3], *e.g.* temperature, culture media, etc.

Table I. QC assays performed with cell bank material for plasmid manufacturing.

Test	Analytical method
Plasmid	
Plasmid identity and integrity	Restriction digestion and agarose gel Sequencing (double strand)
Plasmid yield (µgDNA/gBiomass)	Quick plasmid DNA purification with subsequent spectrophotometric determination (260 nm)
Plasmid stability (segregative)	Replica plating on LB medium with and without antibiotic
***E. coli* host**	
Host identity	API-20E
	16S rRNA
	RADP fingerprinting
	Riboprinting
Purity	
Presence of bacterial and fungal contaminants (microbial purity)	Plating and streaking on selective media
Lytic and lysogenic bacteriophages	Plaque test on indicator host with and without prior UV-induction
Filling	
Test of containers	Visual inspection
Test of volume	Gravimetric analysis
Productivity and performance	
Pilot cultivation	Cultivation under final conditions ($\leq$ 5 L bioreactor)

Today´s technology for the generation of complex bacterial growth media uses soy bean peptones to avoid animal-derived protein sources due to problems occurred by BSE or TSE. Generally, in order to avoid BSE risk materials as recommended by regulatory guidelines, the use of synthetic growth media should be favoured [4]. By using a fully defined synthetic glycerol medium 45 mg dm^{-3} plasmid DNA could be produced. Recent developments allow even higher productivities.

The transformed of *E. coli* cells typically grow over night, sufficient to obtain large amounts of cell paste with a high amount of plasmid DNA. Cultivation is a "semi-generic" process: with some plasmids the same process type may be used, with others (typically those used for virus production with their repetitive elements such as ITR for AAV or LTR for lentiviral transfer plasmids but also other repetitive or homopolymeric sequences) for each new plasmid a cultivation process development is required.

The biomass resulting from the cultivation needs to be separated from the supernatant liquid of the culture. In lab scale this can be performed by batch centrifugation, in large scale by flow-through centrifugation or cell concentration with tangential flow filtration processes. The biomass is subject to QC tests for product content and absence of any contamination and will be further processed after release for manufacturing. For subsequent purification, the produced biomass is separated from the culture medium and can be stored at low temperatures (-20 °C).

DOWNSTREAM PROCESSING AND CHROMATOGRAPHY

Plasmid molecules are usually released from the *E. coli* host cells by alkaline lysis. This process step is critical because major contamination sources of plasmid DNA productions, *e.g.* the bacterial chromosomal DNA (chrDNA), RNA and bacterial endotoxins are released at this step, too [1]. Removal of these is a major task in plasmid manufacturing. Intact, *i.e.* high-molecular bacterial chromosomal DNA can be at least partially removed together with bacterial debris within the lysis separation and filtration. However, the resulting cleared lysate still contains a high amount of contaminating substances [5]. RNA has a short half life, but is still a substantial contamination in plasmid preparations and may block the binding capacity in *e.g.* anion exchange chromatography. Therefore, an enzymatic digestion of RNA prior to the chromatographic step is usually applied [6]. In pharmaceutical manufacturing processes, the use of RNase A, which is typically prepared from bovine pancreas, has to be avoided using recombinant RNase or, even better, manufacturing processes that completely avoid the use of RNase. In these cases, the RNA is removed, *e.g.* by specific purification techniques [3].

Downstream processing (DSP), starting from the cleared lysate, comprises the second phase of plasmid manufacturing, separating the plasmid DNA from soluble biomolecules (*e.g.* host chromosomal DNA, RNA, nucleotides, lipids, residual proteins, amino acids, saccharides), salts and buffer components. This is done by chromatography, typically anion exchange chromatography [1, 6, 7] plus additional cleaning steps. The applicable chromatographic process depends on the required purity of the plasmid product.

Alternative chromatographic technologies make use of size exclusion chromatography for small scales, reverse phase chromatography or hydrophobic interaction chromatography. Other approaches describe plasmid DNA purification systems for the selective removal of contaminants or improved binding capacity for the intended plasmid product (*e.g.* monolithic stationary phase) [8 ,9].

A very efficient chromatographic way to purify plasmids from contaminants is affinity chromatography binding a certain sequence stretch of the plasmid, as we could demonstrate for the specific purification of minicircle DNA (see chapter "Development of *minicircle* vectors" within this book).

Recent manufacturing technology makes use of removing the undesired open-circular (oc) and linear plasmid forms as well as of fragmented chrDNA deriving from the bacterial chromosome. The removal of damaged plasmid forms can be demonstrated by agarose gel electrophoresis (AGE) and capillary gel electrophoresis (CGE), the removal of chrDNA by qPCR ([3], PlasmidFactory, unpublished).

This second phase of plasmid manufacturing ends with bulk purified plasmid DNA being formulated within the appropriate buffer or solution for further processing or storage and application.

Plasmid **DNA** quality

Plasmid DNA quality mainly depends on the type of manufacturing as well as storage and application. Specifications for product release are well defined, but subject to ongoing improvements regarding the state-of-the-art on production processes and analytical techniques. *Table II* shows a selection of relevant quality control tests for in-process-control (IPC) and product release.
The most important contaminations and the respective QC tests are briefly described in the following sections.

Table II. Test assays and required quality controls for the quality assurance and product release of plasmid DNA.

Test	Analytical method
DNA concentration	UV-Absorption (260 nm)
Appearance	Visual inspection
DNA homogeneity (ccc content)	Densitometry after agarose gel electrophoresis (AGE)
DNA homogeneity (ccc content)	Capillary gel electrophoresis (CGE)
DNA purity	UV-Scan (220-320 nm)
RNA	Visual inspection after AGE
Endotoxin (LPS)	Limulus Amebocyte Lysate (LAL) test
Bacterial chromosomal DNA	Quantitative PCR
Total protein	Bicinchoninic acid (BCA) test
Host cell derived protein	ELISA
Bioburden	Presence of bacterial and fungal contaminants (bioburden: TAMC, TYMC)
Plasmid identity	Restriction digestion and agarose gel
Plasmid identity	Sequencing (double strand)

Bacterial chromosomal DNA

A major impurity in plasmid DNA preparations is the host chromosomal DNA (chrDNA). While with standard (*e.g.* kit-) procedures contaminations of plasmid DNA with chrDNA were in the range of 10% or more, novel purification technologies allow a reduction to <1%. One critical step is the alkaline lysis, where the chrDNA is a component of the flaky material which is generated by the alkaline lysis. Chromosomal DNA is extremely shear-sensitive, which can easily result in DNA fragmentation. Some chrDNA fragments migrate in one distinct band in agarose gel electrophoresis (AGE) or do not even enter the gel - being detected within the gel slot. Smaller fragments can be detected as an undefined smear by overloading the agarose gel. The most sensitive assay is a special real time PCR method to quantify chrDNA contaminations [10].

Other host cell impurities

Other host cell impurities have to be reduced to a minimum concentration during the purification process of plasmid DNA: proteins, RNA as well as lipopolysaccharides

(LPS endotoxins). The presence of proteins can be detected by colorimetric assays, like the BCA test (bicinchoninic acid).

Quantification of residual RNA is especially important if the plasmid is purified without using RNase, see above. It can be performed directly by fluorescence assays (Ribogreen) after digestion of the plasmid DNA with DNase or after AGE. A novel technique is the determination of RNA by quantitative RT-PCR.

Bacterial LPS endotoxins have a pyrogenic effect on mammalian cells, hence reduction in this impurity is necessary. LPS can be determined by kinetic measurement of *Limulus* polyphenus lysate (LAL) reaction with endotoxins.

Plasmid identity

A simple analytical method for determining plasmid identity is restriction digestion of the plasmid DNA followed by AGE. The length of the restriction fragments can be estimated by comparison with a linear DNA size marker (*e.g.* 1 kb ladder). The determined fragments have to conform to the calculated fragments or to a reference DNA with respect to identity. In our experience, four different enzymes each with a minimum two restriction sites should be used. Since the band pattern after digest is the same for monomer and multimer forms of a plasmid, it is strongly recommended to also check the undigested plasmid, at least on an agarose gel.

The exact nucleotide sequence has to be determined by sequencing the plasmid DNA.

Plasmid topology

Plasmids isolated from *E. coli* may exist in different topologies. The only really active form of plasmid DNA is the covalently closed circle (*ccc*). Single strand breaks lead to the open circular (*oc*), double strand breaks to the linear form. Such damages in the plasmid integrity may lead to inactivation, especially if the damage is within the therapeutically active part of the construct. Additionally, single and double strand breaks lead to certain changes in the effective size of the plasmid.

The structural homogeneity of plasmid DNA is usually determined by AGE. Different bands in AGE of a plasmid sample may be assigned to different plasmid forms. The assignment of bands to the different topologies, however, is not easy since the electrophoretic mobility of plasmids of different shape changes with the electrophoretic operating conditions [11]. In addition, the quantification of forms based on the signal intensity of stained bands in AGE may not be reliable. Up to now, the only reliable method to quantify the amount of the different active and inactice forms of the plasmid is capillary gel electrophoresis (CGE) [3, 12].

Storage stability of plasmid DNA

Recent studies ([12] and PlasmidFactory, unpublished results) show in detail potential alterations of plasmid DNA at different storage conditions. However, we have shown that highly purified plasmid DNA can be stored at -20 or -80°C for several years without alteration. A different situation is obvious for plasmid DNA stored at +4 °C and even more at room temperature. Here, during storage the amount of *ccc* forms decreased dramatically resulting in increasing amounts of the damaged *oc* and later even linear forms. This strongly indicates that such storage conditions promote plasmid DNA instability, which could have an impact at least on transfection efficiency.

An alternative approach to store plasmid DNA would be lyophilization of the plasmid DNA product. Here, a complete resuspension without significantly decreasing the quality of the plasmid DNA product is only possible with highly purified plasmid DNA (PlasmidFactory, unpublished data). However, at least the resulting plasmid DNA concentration and the relative amount of intact *ccc* forms have to be carefully checked after resuspending the DNA.

Plasmid stability during application

The physical and chemical stability of plasmid DNA is a requirement for development of DNA-based pharmaceuticals, which can be stored, shipped and applied even under critical environmental conditions.

The use of *e.g.* gene-gun, jet-injection or electroporation devices has been developed in recent years for the application of plasmid DNA drugs. However, it requires further evaluation with respect to plasmid stability. Monitoring the changes from *ccc* into damaged *oc* or linear topologies during the application, as well as optimizing the applied protocols with respect to different tissues, plasmid size, buffers and intended depth of injection, are essential. The analysis of the topology of plasmids used in gene therapy or DNA vaccination by CGE allows the determination of the integrity and distribution of the topology of the plasmid DNA. This issue is of importance not only with respect to pharmaceutical aspects of the homogeneity of the plasmid API, but also allows optimization of the application process with respect to the plasmid integrity.

To evaluate potentially destructive forces on plasmid DNA by jet-injection, CGE analysis of the pCMV-*lacZ* plasmid before and after jet-injection was performed and has been published in collaboration with Walther *et al.* [13].

ACKNOWLEDGMENTS

This work has been performed with the support of the EC-DG research through the FP6-Network of Excellence, CLINIGENE: LSHB-CT-2006-018933.

REFERENCES

1. Schleef M. Issues of large-scale plasmid manufacturing. In: Rehm HJ, Reed G, Pühler A, Stadler P, eds. *Biotechnology. Recombinant proteins, monoclonal antibodies and therapeutic genes*, vol. 5a. Weinheim: Wiley-VCH, 1999: 443-70.

2. Hoare M, Levy MS, Bracewell DG, Doig SD, Kong S, Titchener-Hooker N, *et al.* Bioprocess engineering issues that would be face in producing a DNA vaccine at up to 100m³ fermentation scale for an influenza pandemic. *Biotechnol Prog* 2005; 21: 1577-92.

3. Schleef M, Schmidt T. Animal-free production of *ccc*-supercoiled plasmids for research and clinical applications. *J Gene Med* 2004; 6 : 45-53.

4. EMEA. *Note for guidance on minimising the risk of transmitting animal spongiform encephalopathy agents via human and veterinary medicinal products*. CPMP/410/01, rev1, London, 2001.

5. Schorr J, Moritz P, Schleef M. Production of plasmid DNA in industrial quantities according to cGMP guidelines. In: Lowrie DB, Whalen RG, eds. *DNA vaccines: methods and protocols*. Totowa NJ: Humana Press 1999: 11-21.

6. Stadler J, Lemmens R, Nyhammar T. Plasmid DNA purification. *J Gene Med* 2004; 6 : 54-66.

7. Voß C, Schmidt T, Schleef M. From bulk to delivery: plasmid manufacturing and storage. In: Schleef M, ed. *DNA pharmaceuticals: formulation and delivery in gene therapy, DNA vaccination and immunotherapy.* Weinheim: Wiley-VCH, 2005: 23-42.

8. Lemmens R, Olsson U, Nyhammar T, Stadler J. Supercoiled plasmid DNA: selective purification by thiophilic/aromatic adsorption. *J Chromatogr B* 2003; 784: 291-300.

9. Strancar A, Podgornik A, Barut M, Necina R. Short monolithic columns as stationary phases for biochromatography. *Adv Biochem Eng Biotechnol* 2002; 76: 49-85.

10. Smith GJ, Helf M, Nesbet C, Betita HA, Mek J, Ferre F. Fast and accurate method for quantitating *E. coli* host cell DNA contamination in plasmid DNA preparations. *Electrophoresis* 1999; 26: 518-26.

11. Garner MM, Chrambach A. Resolution of circular, nicked and linear DNA, 4 kb in length, by electrophoresis in polyacrylamide solutions. *Electrophoresis* 1992; 13: 176-8.

12. Schleef M, Baier R, Walther W, Michel ML, Schmeer M. Long-term stability studa and topology analysis of plasmid DNA by capillary gel electrophoresis. *BioProcess Int* 2006; 4: 38-40.

13. Walther W, Stein U, Fichtner I, Voss C, Schmidt T, Schleef M, *et al.* Intratumoral low volume jet-injection for efficient non-viral gene transfer. *Mol Biotechnol* 2002; 21: 105-15.

The CliniBook: Clinical gene transfer
Edited by Odile Cohen-Haguenauer – EDK, Paris © 2012, pp. 284-289

A6-5
Sleeping Beauty transposon based gene therapy

ZSUZSANNA IZSVÁK*, ZOLTÁN IVICS

*Max Delbrück Centrum for Molecular Medicine, Robert Rossle Strasse 10,
Berlin D-13122, Germany*
zizsvak@mdc-berlin.de
* Corresponding author

NON-VIRAL VECTOR SYSTEMS

Non-viral vector systems generally suffer from inefficient cellular delivery and limited duration of transgene expression due to the lack of genomic insertion and resulting degradation and/or dilution of the vector in transfected cell populations. In post-mitotic tissues, non-viral vectors may provide long-lasting transgene expression; however, in the absence of long-term nuclear maintenance in dividing cell types such as stem cells, even efficient introduction of nucleic acids into cells does not guarantee long-term transgene expression. In principle, non-viral vector systems based on scaffold/matrix attachment region (S/MAR)-containing episomal vectors that can promote replication and maintenance in mammalian cells could potentially offer long-term expression in dividing cell types. Alternatively, *transposable elements* could ideally unite the advantages of integrating viral vectors with those of non-viral delivery systems.

DNA-BASED TRANSPOSONS

DNA-based transposons are natural gene delivery vehicles. Similarly to retroviruses, these elements integrate into the chromosomes of host cells, but their life-cycle does not involve reverse transcription, and they are not infectious. In nature, these elements exist as single units containing the transposase gene flanked by terminal inverted repeats (TIRs) that carry transposase binding sites (*Figure 1*). However, under laboratory conditions, it is possible to use transposons as bi-component systems, in which virtually any DNA sequence of interest can be placed between the transposon TIRs and mobilized by *trans*-supplementing the transposase in the form of an expression plasmid or mRNA synthesized *in vitro*. In the transposition process, the transposase enzyme mediates the excision of the element from its donor plasmid, followed by reintegration of the transposon into a chromosomal locus (*Figure 1*). This feature makes transposons natural and easily controllable non-viral DNA delivery vehicles. Furthermore, synthetically produced mRNA can serve as a source of the transposase, thereby limiting the duration of transposase expression and lowering the risk of "rehopping" of the already integrated transposon-based vector.

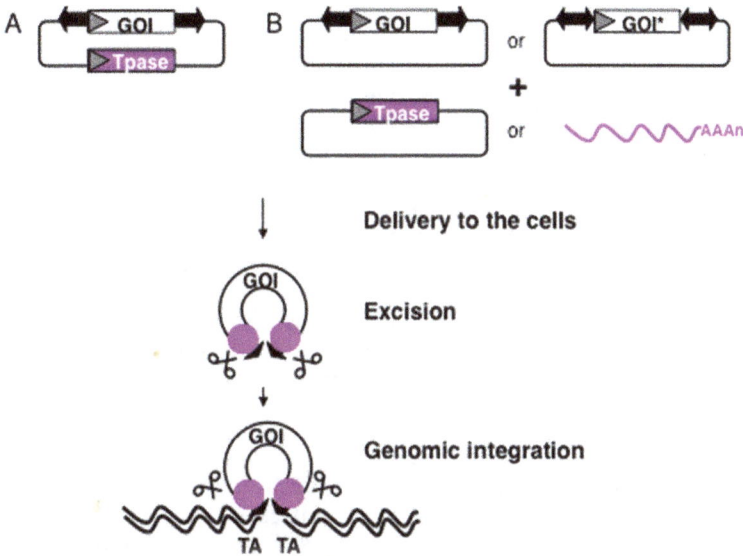

Figure 1. DNA-based transposons.

TRANSPOSON-BASED, NON-VIRAL INTEGRATING VECTOR SYSTEMS

Transposon-based, non-viral integrating vector systems represent a novel technology that opens up new possibilities for gene therapy. Due to stable chromosomal insertion, these systems can result in robust, long-term expression of the integrated transgene. The plasmid-based *Sleeping Beauty* (SB) transposon system [1] has become a popular tool for non-viral, therapeutic transgene delivery. The *SB* transposon has a favorable safety profile as compared to widely used retro/lentiviral approaches as it does not target transcriptionally active regions for integration (reviewed in [2]), and are less prone to reverse transcriptase-induced mutations/rearrangements. In contrast to viruses, transposons have low intrinsic activity, and are self-regulated. Interaction with cellular host factors appear to allow wild type transposons to persist in the host without producing serious levels of genetic damage. Notably, the plasmid-based transposon vectors have reduced immune complications, and have no strict limitation of the size of expression cassettes, and not require active cell division to integrate (reviewed in [2-4]). These features of SB are particularly favorable attributes for stable, long-term expression in various primary and stem cells [4-7]. As an important issue regarding the implementation of clinical trials, transposon vectors can be maintained and propagated as plasmid DNA, making them simple and inexpensive to manufacture (*i.e.* GMP vector production). In sum, the emerging technology of SB-mediated gene transfer shows clear advantages over other gene transfer methods, and might offer a safer alternative to viral approaches.

DELIVERY

Since transposons are not infectious, it is necessary to combine the plasmid-based transposon vectors with technologies capable of efficient delivery of these non-viral vectors into cells. Since the efficiency of transposition is dependent on the efficiency of uptake of the introduced plasmids into the cell nuclei, delivery is a rate-limiting factor in transposition, and is thus of paramount importance. In principle, any non-viral technology developed for transferring nucleic acids into cells can be combined with transposon vectors (reviewed in [3]). Alternatively, the development of hybrid vector systems combining the natural ability of viruses to traverse cell membranes with efficient genomic insertion mediated by the *SB* system is a promising strategy (reviewed in [2-4]).

Recently, a large-scale genetic screen to derive hyperactive transposases by *in vitro* evolution yielded a hyperactive transposase mutant, SB100X [5] (Molecule of the Year in 2009). This hyperactive SB system represents the first non-viral vector capable of stable gene transfer coupled with long-term therapeutic gene expression at a comparable efficiency to viral strategies, thereby addressing the bottle-neck problem of classical non-viral delivery. SB shows efficient transposition in human, including primary cells, and provides long-term transgene expression in preclinical animal models. The *SB* vector-based gene transfer was already tested in a clinical settings (reviewed in [2-4]).

In *ex vivo* applications, *easy-to-transfect* cell types conventional transfection technologies have been successfully adapted to deliver the transposon system in to cells [6]. In *hard-to-transfect* cells including primary stem cells, delivery of transposon-based vectors can be significantly facilitated by nucleofection, a procedure based on electroporation that transfers nucleic acids directly into the nucleus [6]. Indeed, nucleofection facilitated transposition in various stem cells including $CD34^+$ hematopoietic progenitors, primary T cells and human embryonic stem cells (reviewed in [2-4]). Importantly, in the context of the hematopoietic system, this *ex vivo* gene delivery procedure apparently did not compromise the potential of transposon-marked $CD34^+$ cells to differentiate normally into the erythroid, megakaryocytic, granulocyte/monocyte/macrophage [5] as well as into the $CD4^+CD8^+$ T, $CD19^+$ B, $CD56^+CD3$- NK, and $CD33^+$ myeloid lineages [8]. Similarly, the use of the SB100X system yielded robust gene transfer efficiencies into human mesenchymal stem cells, muscle stem/progenitor cells (myoblasts), iPSCs [7] and T cells [9]. These cells are relevant targets for stem cell biology and for regenerative medicine and gene- and cell-based therapies of complex genetic diseases. Importantly, expression of the SB100X hyperactive transposase did not adversely influence the differentiation or function of these adult stem/progenitor cells, nor was there any evidence of any cytogenetic abnormalities [7]. The robustness and feasibility of this non-viral, transposon-based procedure may significantly facilitate clinical realization of *ex vivo* stem cell therapy for the treatment of hematopoietic disorders and cancer, which has led to its application in humans [10].

In the context of *iPSC technology*, it was recently demonstrated that *SB* transposon-mediated delivery of the myogenic PAX3 transcription factor into iPSCs coaxed their differentiation into $MyoD^+$ myogenic progenitors and multinucleated myofibers [7], suggesting that PAX3 may serve as a myogenic "molecular switch" in iPSCs, a finding that has implications for cell therapy of congenital degenerative muscle diseases, including Duchenne muscular dystrophy.

Recent developments of non-viral delivery techniques, including liposomal formulations, nanoparticles, advanced electroporation methods such as nucleofection and cell penetrating peptides can significantly enhance transfer of nucleic acids into therapeutically relevant cell types, even *in vivo* (reviewed in [2, 3]).

Any expression vector system should ideally support long-term expression of the therapeutic genes. By using classical, plasmid-based, non-viral delivery approaches, expression from the extrachromosomal plasmid rapidly declines following delivery. Transgenes delivered by non-viral approaches often form long, repeated arrays (concatemers) that are targets for transcriptional silencing by heterochromatin formation. Notably, the cargo DNA itself may provoke transgene silencing, particularly the type of promoter used to drive expression of the gene of interest. In addition, long-term expression of transgenes delivered by retroviruses has been shown to be compromised by transcriptional silencing. The cut and paste mechanism of DNA transposition results in a clean individual integrating cassette at the insertion locus. Indeed, vector integrations delivered by the SB system only rarely (<2% of all insertions) undergo silencing in HeLa cells [11]. Furthermore, advantages of the SB system include its inert transcriptional activities [12, 13], therefore it is not expected to generate significant epigenetic turbulance at the site of integration. With careful promoter choice, several studies have established that SB-mediated transposition provides long-term expression *in vivo*. Notably, stable transgene expression from SB vectors was seen in mice after gene delivery in the liver, lung, brain and blood after hematopoietic reconstitution *in vivo* (reviewed in [3]). Thus, it appears that transposon vectors have the capacity to provide long-term expression of a therapeutic gene both *in vitro* and *in vivo*.

CHALLENGES AND STRATEGIES

Developing the SB transposon system further, for more efficient and safe gene delivery, applicable for clinical use would be extremely important. Our current research aims at directing transposon-based, non-viral gene delivery research towards clinical applications by developing clinically acceptable gene delivery modalities by optimizing its performance as a gene expression vector and improving its biosafety profile. The new, hyperactive SB100X-based vector system appears to be a potentially safer, but still efficient alternative of the integrating retro/lentiviral vectors. The SB100X system might have a special value in disease models, where the use of retro/lentiviral vectors was demonstrated to raise significant safety concerns.

In order to fill the gap between the vector development and clinical trials, the strategy could be the following: (1) try the SB system in disease models that were already on clinical trials, using retroviral vectors, but safety was a serious issue; (2) try the SB system in disease models that were already on clinical trials, using non-viral approaches, but efficacy was a limiting factor; (3) include certain *ex vivo* therapeutic approaches where the SB system was demonstrating safety and efficacy; (4) include models where the transposon/iPS-based regenerative technology has a potential; (5) combine the plasmid-based integration vectors with the cutting-edge DNA delivery strategies.

BIOSAFETY OF THE SB TRANSPOSON SYSTEM

Unlike the LTRs of retroviruses, the TIRs of *SB* vectors have low enhancer/promoter activity [12, 13] In order to improve the safety profile of the *SB* system further chromatin boundary elements (*insulators*) flanking the transposon-contained expression cassettes to prevent accidental *trans*activation of cellular promoters [12, 13].

Target site selection properties suggest that *SB* might be safer for therapeutic gene delivery than the integrating viral vectors that are currently used in clinical trials. In contrast to retro/lentiviral integration, *SB* integration can be considered fairly random on the genomic level, and the transcriptional status of targeted genes apparently does not influence the integration profile of *SB* (reviewed in [2]). Nevertheless, a systematic assessment of potential genotoxic effects associated with genomic integration of transposon vectors will need to be performed either in cell-based assays and/or in animal models to provide clinically relevant data. Indeed, the potential of genotoxic effects elicited by transcriptional upregulation of proto-oncogenes and other signaling genes upon random transposon insertion is a relatively unexplored area of research. Investigations into these questions will be required to document safety of the *SB* system for prospective clinical trials.

Furthermore, with any vector that integrates into chromosomes in a nearly random manner, the risk of genotoxicity is not zero. To learn how natural, target-selective transposons recognize a specific target DNA, and to apply this strategy to randomly integrating transposons is a real challenge. We have established a targeting strategy, and showed that *Sleeping Beauty* can be targeted into desired loci in the genome [14], demonstrating for the first time that it was possible to override the integration pathway of an otherwise randomly integrating vector. The proof of principle of target-selected *SB* insertion was assessed by employing a molecular strategy of targeting the *SB transposon* to a predetermined genomic locus within a 2.5-kb window at a frequency of >10% [14]. Ongoing work in the authors' laboratory is dedicated to translate the strategy to physiologically relevant, endogenous sites in the human genome. This direction of research could significantly enhance the safety feature of a therapeutic vector.

It was recently found that overexpression of the *SB* transposase can have cytotoxic effects [15]. The molecular mechanism of transposase cytotoxicity is currently not entirely understood, but it is unlikely due to uncontrolled cleavage of genomic DNA by the transposase [15]. At any rate, careful dosing of the transposase as well as the transposon donor plasmids in gene delivery experiments appears to be of fundamental importance; luckily, with plasmid-based vectors such as the *SB* transposon system, this can easily be achieved.

The transposon-based vector generated a considerable interest in developing new, safe, simple and efficient technologies for somatic gene transfer. The past few years have seen a steady growth in interest in applying the *SB* system for gene therapy. These strategies included haemophilia A and B, junctional epidermolysis bullosa, tyrosinemia I, Huntington disease sickle cell disease, mucopolysaccharidosis, cancer and type 1 diabetes. In addition, important steps have been made towards *SB*-mediated gene transfer in the lung for potential therapy of α-1-antitrypsin deficiency, cystic fibrosis and a variety of cardiovascular diseases (reviewed in [2-4]). The first clinical application of the *SB* system is currently ongoing using autologous T cells gene-modified with *SB* vectors [9] carrying a chimeric antigen receptor (CAR) to render the T cells cytotoxic specifically toward CD19-positive lymphoid tumors (reviewed in [3]). The ease and reduced cost associated with manufacturing of clinical-grade, plasmid-based SB vectors is an obvious advantage when compared with recombinant viral vectors.

The hyperactive SB100X system was a Highlight of the Year (ESGT, 2009), and the Molecule of the Year, 2009. Further reseach on the system is necessary to see if the vector could indeed fulfill these high expectations. The combination of the cutting-edge developments might help to meet the goal of establishing next-generation, clinically feasible, non-viral gene delivery paradigms for therapeutic purposes.

ACKNOWLEDGMENTS

This work has been performed with the support of the EC-DG research through the FP6-Network of Excellence, CLINIGENE: LSHB-CT-2006-018933.

REFERENCES

1. Ivics Z, Hackett PB, Plasterk RH, Izsvák Z. Molecular reconstruction of *Sleeping Beauty*, a Tc1-like transposon from fish, and its transposition in human cells. *Cell* 1997; 91: 501-10.

2. Ivics Z, Izsvák Z Non-viral gene delivery with the *Sleeping Beauty* transposon system. *Hum Gene Ther* 2011; 22: 1043-51.

3. Izsvak Z, Hackett PB, Cooper LJ, Ivics Z. Translating *Sleeping Beauty* transposition into cellular therapies: victories and challenges. *Bioessays* 2010; 32: 756-67.

4. Vandendriessche T, Ivics Z, Izsvak Z, Chuah MK. Emerging potential of transposons for gene therapy and generation of induced pluripotent stem cells. *Blood* 2009; 114: 1461-8.

5. Mates L, Chuah MK, Belay E, Jerchow B, Manoj N, Acosta-Sanchez A, *et al*. Molecular evolution of a novel hyperactive *Sleeping Beauty* transposase enables robust stable gene transfer in vertebrates. *Nat Genet* 2009; 41: 753-61.

6. Izsvák Z, Chuah MK, Vandendriessche T, Ivics Z. Efficient stable gene transfer into human cells by the Sleeping Beauty transposon vectors. *Methods* 2009; 49: 287-97.

7. Belay E, Matrai J, Acosta-Sanchez A, Ma L, Quattrocelli M, Mates L, *et al*. Novel hyperactive transposons for genetic modification of induced pluripotent and adult stem cells: a non-viral paradigm for coaxed differentiation. *Stem Cells* 2010; 28: 1760-71.

8. Xue X, Huang X, Nodland SE, Mátés L, Ma L, Izsvák Z, *et al*. Stable gene transfer and expression in cord blood-derived CD34+ hematopoietic stem and progenitor cells by a hyperactive *Sleeping Beauty* transposon system. *Blood* 2009; 114: 1319-30.

9. Jin Z, Maiti S, Huls H, Singh H, Olivares S, Mátés L, *et al*. The hyperactive *Sleeping Beauty* transposase SB100X improves the genetic modification of T cells to express a chimeric antigen receptor. *Gene Ther* 2011; 18: 849-56.

10. Williams DA. Sleeping beauty vector system moves toward human trials in the United States. *Mol Ther* 2008; 16: 1515-6.

11. Grabundzija I, Irgang M, Mátés L, Belay E, Matrai J, Gogol-Döring A, *et al*. Comparative analysis of transposable element vector systems in human cells. *Mol Ther* 2010; 18: 1200-9.

12. Walisko O, Schorn A, Rolfs F, Devaraj A, Miskey C, Izsvak Z, Ivics Z Transcriptional activities of the *Sleeping Beauty* transposon and shielding its genetic cargo with insulators. *Mol Ther* 2008; 16: 359-69.

13. Dalsgaard T, Moldt B, Sharma N, Wolf G, Schmitz A, Pedersen FS, Mikkelsen JG. Shielding of sleeping beauty DNA transposon-delivered transgene cassettes by heterologous insulators in early embryonal cells. *Mol Ther* 2009; 17: 121-30.

14. Ivics Z, Katzer A, Stuwe EE, Fiedler D, Knespel S, Izsvak Z. Targeted sleeping beauty transposition in human cells. *Mol Ther* 2007; 15: 1137-44.

15. Galla M, Schambach A, Falk CS, Maetzig T, Kuehle J, Lange K, *et al*. Avoiding cytotoxicity of transposases by dose-controlled mRNA delivery. *Nucleic Acids Res* 2011; 39: 7147-60.

The CliniBook: Clinical gene transfer
Edited by Odile Cohen-Haguenauer – EDK, Paris © 2012, pp. 290-294

A6-6
Development of *minicircle* vectors

MARCO SCHMEER, ANJA RISCHMÜLLER, MARTIN SCHLEEF*

PlasmidFactory GmbH and Co. KG, Meisenstrasse 96, D-33607 Bielefeld, Germany.
martin.schleef@plasmidfactory.com
* Corresponding author

Today, *minicircle* DNA is the system of choice in order to overcome the disadvantages of plasmids. This circular DNA molecule derives from plasmid DNA but lacks those elements of plasmids necessary for amplification in bacteria but not useful or even in doubt for clinical applications.

INTRODUCTION

Plasmids consist of a bacterial origin of replication (*ori*), a selection marker (typically antibiotic resistance element), and the gene cassette containing the gene of interest (GOI). But only the latter element is needed for the intended, *e.g.* therapeutic application. Hence, the optimal vector would contain only this gene cassette with the GOI and no other elements as especially the antibiotic resistance elements are considered redundant and a safety problem. The state-of-the-art approach meeting these (even regulatory) requirements is the *minicircle*. Several attempts to pruduce such biomolecules have been published over the last years but now, for the first time, it becomes possible to produce *minicircle* DNA in appropriate amounts and, most of all, an appropriate quality applicable for future therapeutic use.

MANUFACTURING OF *MINICIRCLE* DNA

Minicircles derive from parental plasmids, specially designed for *minicircle* production, containing at least antibiotic resistance markers, the *ori* and the gene cassette of interest (GOI) which is flanked by two special recombination sequences (*Figure 1*). By an intramolecular recombination the GOI plus one of the signal sequence elements is cut out of that parental plasmid, finally resulting in almost only the GOI in a circular molecule – the *minicircle*. The residual part, the so-called mini-plasmid, contains the *ori* and the selection marker. For an overview see *Figure 1*.
Several enzymes have been used so far to achieve this intramolecular recombination, *e.g.* tyrosine recombinases as the integrase of bacteriophage lambda, the Cre recombinase from bacteriophage P1, and the flp recombinase.
The recombination events of the Cre recombinase (lox sites) and of the flp recombinase (FRT sites) result in identical or highly similar sites and thus the recombination is bidi-

rectional and fully reversible, resulting in several multimer structures due to intramolecular as well as intermolecular recombination [1, 2]. Thus, Bigger and co-workers constructed a parental plasmid with one lox site being mutated to prefer unidirectional recombination. But, although the generation of monomeric *minicircle* molecules was improved, a high amount of concatamers was still observed [3].

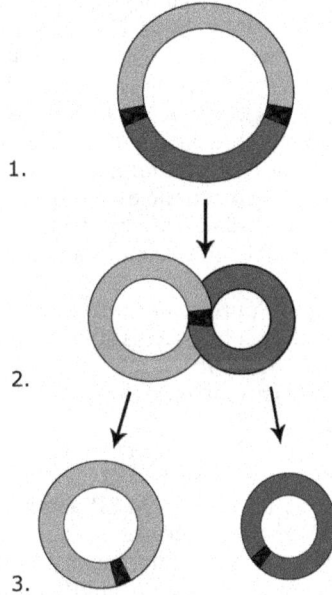

Figure 1. *Minicircle* recombination. A parental plasmid (1) is cis-recombined (2) resulting in two separate circles (3) one being a mini-plasmid and the other the *minicircle*. Dark gray: *minicircle* with gene of interest; light gray: miniplasmid containg *ori* and antibiotic resistance cassette; black: recombination sequences.

The integrase of bacteriophage PhiC31, a serine recombinase, has been shown to be unidirectional, *i.e. minicircle* production can be driven to a high percentage [4]. This enzyme mediates recombination events between an attP and an attB site, resulting in recombination products containing attL and attR sites [5, 6]. Unfortunately, the recombination efficacy is still too low, at least for a large scale process, and still several multimeric forms can be observed.

The ParA resolvase, a serine recombinase of the multimer resolution system of the broad host range plasmids RK2 and RP4, mediates only intra-molecular recombination between the corresponding resolution (res) sites [7-9]. Hence, the recombination reaction is catalyzed in only one direction to completion and no multimers or other concatamers occur during *minicircle* production [10].

Additionally, the integration of recombinase expression systems into the same plasmid that contains the corresponding recombination sites led to complete recombination when the ParA resolvase system was applied [10] as determined by quantitative real-time PCR [11].

However, after successful recombination, the *minicircle* has to be isolated from a mixture of three types of circular DNA molecules: *minicircles*, miniplasmids, and maybe residual amounts of parental plasmids. One approach is to linearize the miniplasmids and the parental plasmids by restriction digestion, and to isolate the still circular minicircle by ultracentrifugation in caesium chloride [3]. Unfortunately, this procedure causes high costs whereas the yield of resulting *minicircle* DNA is relatively low.

Bigger and coworkers [3] developed a method that degrades the remaining miniplasmid DNA and parental plasmid DNA (pDNA) by specific restriction digestion being later applied for PhiC31 [12] *via* the co-expression of a restriction enzyme. The homing endonuclease used in this procedure (I-Sce I) is expressed together with the PhiC31 recombinase as a bicistronic messenger RNA (mRNA). This endonuclease recognizes an 18-bp sequence incorporated into the backbone sequence of the parental plasmid DNA. Miniplasmids as well as parental plasmids are then degraded by linearization and the activity of *E. coli* exonucleases. However, it has been reported that, when using this system even 240 min after induction of the recombinase and the endonuclease, certain amounts of miniplasmids and parental plasmids are still detectable [12].

A very efficient chromatographic way to purify *minicircle* DNA from the remaining mini plasmid and any other contaminating substances is affinity chromatography. Here, a target sequence has to be present on the *minicircle*, able to reversibly attach to *e.g.* a recombinant protein linked to the solid chromatography material in order to allow its retention on the affinity chromatograghy.

Further improving non-viral plasmid or *minicircle* vectors, the combination of *minicircle* and S/MAR sequence elements was published in collaboration with Broll *et al.* [13], where a truncated small (733 bp long) S/MAR sequence in combination with eGFP under the control of a SV40-promoter was used to monitor the duration of expression in eukaryotic cells. The mg-scale affinity chromatography based production of the M18 minicircle was achieved by PlasmidFactory (Bielefeld, Germany) to allow larger scale experimental analysis published subsequently by Broll and coworkers [13].

As soon as the large scale production of *minicircle* vectors will be reproducibly possible, they will be the system of choice for direct application into human or animal or where the manufacturing of viral particles or antibodies requires the specific features of those. The European authority for the evaluation of medical products (EMA) already proposed in the guidelines for medical gene transfer products to avoid selection markers like resistances against antibiotics (CPMP/BWP/3088/99).

EXAMPLES OF SUCCESSFULLY PRODUCED *MINICIRCLE* DNA

The *minicircle* manufacturing system established by PlasmidFactory makes use of the highly efficient ParA resolvase. The recombination process results in a mixture of *minicircle* and miniplasmid, the parental plasmid is already efficiently removed due to the >99% recombination efficacy.

For purification of the *minicircle* DNA a proprietary affinity chromatography is used. Here, a distinct sequence motif on the *minicircle* binds to a protein structure bound to magnetic beads. After removal of the surrounding solvent and several washing steps the *minicircle* is eluated. Additional chromatography steps finally result in a highly purified product. Typical results of some of the comprehensive quality tests are shown in *Table I*. *Figure 2* shows examples of *minicircles* produced as described above.

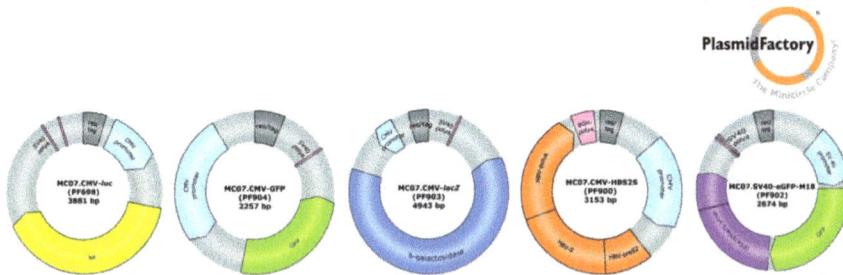

Figure 2. Examples of highly purified *minicircles* produced by PlasmidFactory (Bielefeld, Germany) as described.

Comparison of plasmid and *minicircle*-mediated gene expression shows improved performance of the *minicircle* in different cell lines, *i.e.*, *minicircle* vectors improve transfection efficiency and transgene expression, mainly due to size reduction, reduced CpG content, but also due to the high purity of such DNA product.

Table I. Typical results of some of the comprehensive quality tests.

Minicircle product	Size (bp)	ccc content (%)	Bact. Chrom. DNA
MC.CMV-luc	3881 bp	95%	0.081%
MC.CMV-GFP	2257 bp	98%	0.026%
MC.CMV-lacZ	4943 bp	96%	0.015%

ACKNOWLEDGMENTS

This work has been performed with the support of the EC-DG research through the FP6-Network of Excellence, CLINIGENE: LSHB-CT-2006-018933.

REFERENCES

1. Sadowski P. Site-specific recombinases: changing partners and doing the twist. *J Bacteriol* 1986; 165: 341-7.

2. Gilbertson L. Cre-lox recombination: creative tools for plant biotechnology. *Trends Biotechnol* 2003; 21: 550-5.

3. Bigger BW, Tolmachov O, Collomber JM, Fragkos M, Palaszewski I, Coutelle C. An araC-controlled bacterial cre expression system to produce DNA minicircle vectors for nuclear and mitochondrial gene therapy. *J Biol Chem* 2001; 276: 23018-27.

4. Chen ZY, He CY, Ehrhardt A, Kay MA. Minicircle DNA vectors devoid of bacterial DNA result in persistent and high-level transgene expression *in vivo*. *Mol Ther* 2003; 8: 495-500.

5. Thorpe HM, Smith MC. *In vitro* site-specific integration of bacteriophage DNA catalyzed by a recombinase of the resolvase/invertase family. *Proc Natl Acad Sci USA* 1998; 95: 5505-10.

6. Thorpe HM, Wilson SE, Smith MC. Control of directionality in the site-specific recombination system of the Streptomyces phage phiC31. *Mol Microbiol* 2000; 38: 232-41.

7. Eberl L, Kristensen CS, Givskov M, Grohmann E, Gerlitz M, Schwab H. Analysis of the multimer resolution system encoded by the *parCBA* operon of broad-host-range plasmid RP4. *Mol Microbiol* 1994; 12: 131-41.

8. Smith MC, Thorpe HM. Diversity in the serine recombinases. *Mol Microbiol* 2002; 44: 299-307.

9. Thomson JG, Ow DW. Site specific recombination systems for the genetic manipulation of eukaryotic genomes. *Genesis* 2006; 44: 465-76.

10. Jechlinger W, Azimpour Tabrizi T, Lubitz W, Mayrhofer P. Minicircle DNA immobilized in bacterial ghosts: *in vivo* production of safe non-viral DNA delivery vehicles. *J Mol Microbiol Biotechnol* 2004; 8: 222-31.

11. Mayrhofer P, Blaesen M, Schleef M, Jechlinger W. Minicircle-DNA production by site specific recombination and protein-DNA interaction chromatography. *J Gene Med* 2008; 10: 1253-69.

12. Chen ZY, He CY, Kay MA. Improved production and purification of minicircle DNA vector free of plasmid bacterial sequences and capable of persistent transgene expression *in vivo*. *Hum Gene Ther* 2005; 16: 126-31.

13. Broll S, Oumard A, Hahn K, Schambach A, Bode J. Minicircle performance depending on S/MAR-nuclear matrix interactions. *J Mol Biol* 2009; 395: 950-65.

The CliniBook: Clinical gene transfer
Edited by Odile Cohen-Haguenauer – EDK, Paris © 2012, pp. 295-303

A6-7
Exon skipping therapy for DMD using antisense oligomer technology

Linda Popplewell, Jagjeet Kang, Alberto Malerba, Keith Foster, George Dickson*

School of Biological Sciences, Royal Holloway, University of London, Egham Hill, Egham, Surrey, TW20 0EX, United Kingdom.
g.dickson@rhul.ac.uk
* Corresponding author

Introduction - Concepts and chemistries

Duchenne muscular dystrophy (DMD) is a severe genetic disease, characterized by progressive, and ultimately lethal, muscle-wasting caused by the lack of functional dystrophin protein in skeletal muscles. Expression of this fundamental protein is prevented by frame-disrupting deletions or duplications or, less commonly, nonsense or missense mutations in the *DMD* gene. Mutations that maintain the reading frame of the gene allow expression of truncated, but semi-functional, dystrophin protein; such deletions are characteristic of the less severe muscular disease, Becker muscular dystrophy (BMD).

As yet, there is no gene therapy available within the clinic for the treatment of DMD. However, exon skipping is the most advanced of the gene therapies currently being developed, and holds great promise as a treatment for certain DMD deletions [1]. The theory behind exon skipping is the use of antisense oligonucleotides (AOs) to sterically mask specific RNA sequence motifs on the pre-mRNA, so that assembly of the spliceosome on the target exon is prevented, and the target exon is subsequently spliced out of the mature gene transcript. Where the deletions allow, AOs could thus be used to transform a DMD phenotype into a BMD phenotype by skipping certain exons to restore the reading frame of the *DMD* gene. Indeed, AOs have been shown to restore truncated dystrophin expressed *in vitro* in DMD patient cells [2] and in animal models of the disease *in vivo* [3]. Interestingly, asymptomatic intragenic *DMD* deletions exist, suggesting that exon skipping may have the potential to revert a DMD phenotype to a normal phenotype.

The chemistry of AO backbone used has a profound effect on efficacy, toxicity and half-life. The available backbone chemistries confer high biostability and target specificity and include phosphorodiamidate morpholino oligomers (PMOs), peptide nucleic acids (PNAs), locked nucleic acids (LNAs), and 2'-O-methyl phosphorothioates (2OMePS), which also have the advantage of recruiting RNaseH for RNA target degradation. LNA AOs have been shown to have potential toxicity issues, while PNAs are expensive and have poor water solubility. While both 2OMePS and

PMO chemistries have excellent safety profiles, PMOs appear to produce more consistent and sustained exon skipping in the *mdx* mouse model of DMD [4], in human muscle explants [5], and dystrophic canine muscle cells *in vitro* [6]. PMOs also have the advantage of being easily conjugated to cell-penetrating peptides (CPPs), which improve delivery to mammalian cells, in particular to the heart, and enhance antisense activity [7].

PRECLINICAL DYSTROPHIN EXON SKIPPING STUDIES IN THE *MDX* MOUSE

The *mdx* mouse, the most used animal model for DMD, carries a nonsense point mutation (C→T) in exon 23. Only rare revertant dystrophin-positive fibres are produced in its skeletal and cardiac muscles due to skipping of one or more exons correctly reframing the transcript. The mature truncated mRNA lacking the exon 23 in the *mdx* mouse does not produce a functional protein, making this mouse the ideal animal model for preclinical studies of the exon skipping strategy for DMD. Additionally, the sarcolemmal integrity seen within the *mdx* mouse is an added bonus for AO exon skipping studies. This therapeutic approach has been achieved by using different AO chemistries, among which the most promising are the 2OMePS and the PMO. The latter is particularly resistant to endonucleases and possesses a high affinity to the sequence target which make it particularly suitable for *in vivo* applications. The sequence of the antisense oligonucleotide has been optimized during the years and it is very effective, inducing skipping up to 95%. The choice of an effective dosing regimen for PMO administration is also a pivotal parameter to reduce the amount of AO necessary for systemic delivery.

It has recently been demonstrated in *mdx* mouse that even a low dosage such as 4 weekly injections of 5 mg/kg PMO induces a significant increase in dystrophin expression [4]. However, due to the mechanism of the AO action, repeated chronic administration of AO is necessary to guarantee a continuous production of dystrophin. A recent report showed that systemic delivery of low, clinically applicable, doses of PMO for up to 1 year is safe in *mdx* mice and ameliorates the pathology of skeletal muscles [8]. Furthermore, the rescued dystrophin expression partially recovers limb strength and results in motor activity and movement behaviour of *mdx* that is indistinguishable from normal wild-type C57BL10 mice (*Figure 1*). However, naked AO are not able to enter the relatively undamaged cardiomyocytes and indeed no dystrophin expression is observed in cardiac muscles after systemic delivery of AO [8]. Analysis of the cardiac muscles of *mdx* mice treated for 1 year with PMO to induce exon 23 skipping in skeletal muscle showed evident signs of increased fibrotic histopathology and cardiomyocyte permeability in cardiac muscles of PMO treated mice [9]. Therefore, in the presence of sketetal muscle dystrophin restoration and the absence of cardiac muscle dystrophin restoration, the exercise-induced chronotrophic effects on the heart has the potential to accelerate the existing cardiac dysfunction and pathology noted in DMD patients. While the efficiency of some PMOs to induce exon skipping in human DMD RNAs, or the functionality of derived human truncated dystrophin protein may be relatively low, these data suggest that reduced dystrophin expression may be sufficient to allow improvement of the day-to-day activities in treated DMD patients.

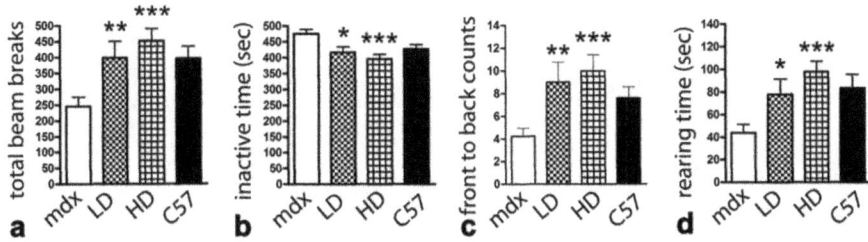

Figure 1. Physical activity is completely normalised in mdx mice following chronic PMO administration. *Mdx* mice were treated for a period of 50 weeks over which 5 cycles of repeated low dose (LD: 5mg/kg/week) and high dose (HD: 50mg/kg/week) PMO administered intravenously. Mice were analysed after 50 weeks of treatment with open field behavioural activity cages. Graphs show the detailed measurement related to the parameters "total activity" (a), "inactive time" (b), "front to back counts" (c), "rearing time" (d). (mean±S.E.M, Mann-Whitney test between treated and untreated *mdx* mice, ***:$p<0.001$, **:$p<0.01$, *:$p<0.05$) (Figure adapted from Malerba *et al.* [8]).

PRECLINICAL DYSTROPHIN EXON SKIPPING STUDIES IN DMD MUSCLE CULTURES

DMD is caused by a diverse array of mutations. According to the Leiden Duchenne muscular dystrophy database, deletions account for 72% of all mutations; those out-of-frame deletions for which exon skipping would restore the reading frame are summarised in *Table I*. As exon skipping is mutation-specific, personalized AO therapy is required. The continued development and analysis of AOs for the targeting of other *DMD* exons is therefore vital.

There have been many studies published describing the in-depth analyses of AO arrays, designed using a number of tools for the targeted skipping of certain *DMD* exons [10, 11]. Taken collectively, bioactive AOs are suggested to target certain serine/arginine (SR)-rich protein-binding motifs, bind to their target more strongly, either as a result of being longer or by being able to access their target site more easily, have their target sites within the exon, rather than intronically, and nearer to the splice acceptor site. However, an AO possessing all of these properties will not necessarily be bioactive; thus the empirical analysis of designed AOs for targeted exon skipping is still essential, and provides the foundation for any AO clinical trial. The methodological details of such analysis have recently been described in Popplewell *et al.*, 2011 [12]. Briefly, arrays of designed AOs are transfected (using lipofection or nucleofection) into either normal human skeletal muscle cells or DMD patient muscle cells, carrying appropriate deletions. Harvested RNA is subjected to nested RT-PCR analysis for the establishment of specific exon skipping at the genetic level in both cell types; detection of dystrophin protein on Western blot or immunocytochemistry in DMD patient cells confirms restoration of dystrophin protein expression as a result of exon skipping. To be cost-effective and safe, the choice of AO for each targeted exon would be expected to produce skipping at low doses and to have persistence of action. Therefore, timecourse and dose-response studies are routinely performed to ensure complete target optimization. Such detailed empirical analyses have been performed for a range of *DMD* exons, but in particular for exon 51 [2, 13], exon 53 [14] and exon 45 [15]; skipping of these exons would have the potential to treat 13%, 8% and 8% of DMD patients respectively (see *Table 1*).

Table I. DMD deletions for which exon skipping would be therapeutic.

Exon to skip	Therapeutic for DMD exonic deletions	Frequency (%)
2	3-7	2
8	3-7, 4-7, 5-7, 6-7	4
43	44, 44-47	5
44	35-43, 45, 45-54	8
45	18-44, 44, 46-47, 46-48, 46-49, 46-51, 46-53	13
46	45	7
50	51, 51-55	5
51	50, 45-50, 48-50, 49-50, 52, 52-63	15
52	51, 53, 53-55	3
53	45-52, 48-52, 49-52, 50-52, 52	9

Adapted from van Deutekom et al. [24]

CLINICAL TRIALS OF DYSTROPHIN EXON SKIPPING IN DMD PATIENTS

On the basis of *in vitro* and *in vivo* pre-clinical studies in DMD patient cells and in animal models, a number of patient trials, phase I and more recently phase 2, have been undertaken. In the first of these, four DMD patients carrying appropriate deletions received a single intramuscular injection of high dose of an AO with a 2OMePS backbone (PRO051), which targets exon 51. Each patient showed specific exon 51 skipping, myofibre expression of dystrophin protein, which was detectable at 3 to 12% of normal levels four weeks after injection. No clinically adverse events were detected [16]. In the second trial, the AO AVI-4658, which has PMO backbone and targets a slightly different intraexonic sequence (+68+95) of exon 51, has been injected intramuscularly in a dose-escalating trial into nine DMD boys. At the higher doses, this PMO AO produced good levels of local dystrophin protein production in treated muscles; the intensity of dystrophin staining was up to 42% of that seen in healthy muscle. The treatment had no adverse effects [17]. The clinical evaluation has been extended to 12 week systemic delivery of both exon 51 AOs and results have very recently been reported. Both chemistries showed no adverse effects and dose-dependent restoration of dystrophin production was clearly seen; functionality of this expressed dystrophin protein was established by the detection of other dystrophin-associated proteins at the sarcolemma (for AVI-4658), and by a modest, but not statistically significant, improvement in the patient six minute walk test after 12 weeks of extended treatment (for PRO051) [18, 19]. However, such studies highlight some other interesting findings; the best responders were patients with a deletion of exon 49 – 50, suggesting that sequence context of deletions may influence exon skipping frequencies or the resultant truncated dystrophin proteins have differential stabilities. On the basis of results seen in the *mdx* model using various dosing regimen over extended periods [4, 8, 9, 20], further phase II and phase III clinical studies are planned.

The drug company AVI BioPharma has performed preclinical studies with AVI-5038 in collaboration with the charity Charley's fund. AVI-5038 is a PMO conjugated to a cell-penetrating peptide (PPMO), designed to target skipping of exon 50 of the dystrophin gene. PPMOs have been used in the *mdx* animal model and shown to have improved deliverability to both skeletal and cardiac muscle, thus improving efficacy. Repeated weekly intravenous bolus injection over four weeks at a low dose of this PPMO was shown to be well-tolerated; however higher doses administered weekly for 12 weeks showed significant toxicological effects, particularly in relation to the kidney. As yet this problem has not been resolved, and an unconjugated version of the same PMO (AVI-4038) is currently being developed for clinical trial. There are a number of alternative peptide conjugates [21, 22] that show promise as enhancers of deliverability and are undergoing rapid pre-clinical development; however, toxicological and immunogenic profiles of these new conjugates are yet to be established. The next planned UK phase I trial by the MDEX consortium will involve conjugation of a PMO developed for the targeted skipping of exon 53 [14], and is supported by a Wellcome fellowship. Prosensa-GlaxoSmithKline are currently performing a phase I trial using a 2OMePS AO for the targeted skipping of exon 45.

DESTRUCTIVE EXON SKIPPING TO INHIBIT MYOSTATIN

Recent work in the field of skeletal muscle structure and function strongly suggests that this tissue controls its own mass through a regulatory mechanism that involves an endogenous negative muscle mass regulator called myostatin or GDF 8. As the natural mutations in myostatin gene have led to increase in muscle mass in cattle, mice, dogs, as well as humans, various approaches have been explored in order to develop a strategy that would help in recovering loss of muscle mass and function in various muscle wasting conditions. Also, myostatin-null mice have significantly lower fat accumulation and increased insulin sensitivity, thereby elevating the likelihood that inhibiting myostatin signalling could be a potential therapy for type II diabetes as well as obesity. Therefore, myostatin inhibition could have a very favourable impact on public health.

In case of myostatin, a destructive exon skipping is the aim rather than reading frame restoration as is the case in *DMD* skipping. Using safe and controlled exon skipping approach, 374 nucleotide long exon 2 of myostatin mRNA was skipped by antisense oligonucleotides (AOs) resulting in an out-of-frame fusion of exons 1 and 3 in a murine skeletal muscle cell line, as well as in animal models. A significant increase in treated muscles was observed following systemic as well as intramuscular injections of different chemistries of AOs targeted at myostatin exon 2 (see *Figure 2*). A number of conjugates have been reported to enhance the deliverability of the AOs and the ones used for myostatin so far (Kang *et al.*, unpublished data) are vivo-morpholino [4] and B-PMO [21]. These studies indicate that (1) antisense-mediated destructive exon skipping can be induced in the myostatin RNA, (2) antisense AO treatment reduces myostatin bioactivity and enhances muscle mass *in vivo*, and (3) AO-induced myostatin exon-skipping is a potential therapeutic strategy to counter muscular dystrophy, muscular atrophy, cachexia and sarcopenia [22]. Future work in this field needs to be done to assess the electrophysiological impact of the antisense-mediated myostatin exon skipping in animals. A combined study to induce dual exon skipping has been reported and holds a promise for a better strategy for muscular degeneration ([23], Kang *et al.*, unpublished data).

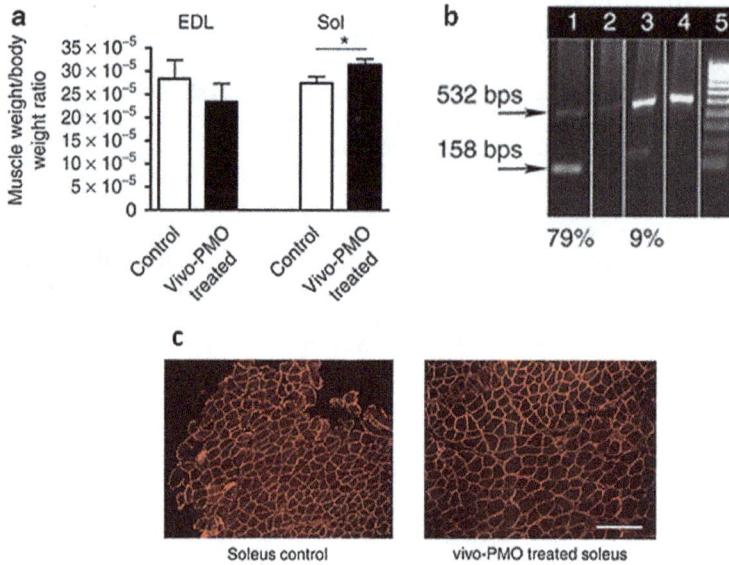

Figure 2. Systemic injection of PMO conjugated to octa-guanidine dendrimer (Vivo-PMO) results in a significant increase in muscle mass and myofibre size as a result of targeted myostatin exon skipping. Mice were treated with 6 mg/kg of Vivo-PMO-D3 by five weekly intravenous injections, and muscles harvested for RNA extraction and immunohistology 10 days later. (a) Weight of soleus and EDL muscle after treatment. Weights of soleus muscles were significantly increased (*t*-test, *P* < 0.034; *n* = 6), while weights of EDL muscles showed no significant change. (b) RT-PCR was carried out on 1 µg RNA from soleus and EDL muscles and products resolved on a 1.2% agarose gel. Track 1: Vivo-PMO treated soleus; Track 2: control soleus; Track 3: Vivo-PMO treated EDL; Track 4: control EDL. Much higher levels of skipping were observed in the soleus muscle relative to EDL muscle (79% *versus* 9%). (c) Representative dystrophin immunohistology indicating increased myofibre cross-sectional area (CSA) *in vivo*-PMO treated compared to control soleus muscle cryosections. Bar = 500 µm (Figure adapted from Kang *et al.* [22]).

CONCLUSIONS AND FUTURE PERSPECTIVES

AO-induced exon skipping has the potential to treat 77% of all patients with DMD, converting their disease phenotype to the less-severe BMD phenotype (see *Table 2*). The progress of clinical trials from phase I to phase II for AOs targeting exon 51 of the *DMD* gene and the results reported from these trails are extremely positive; repeated systemic injection of PMO and 2OMePS AO was well-tolerated and with no adverse effects. Higher doses of both chemistries were required to see exon skipping and consequent restoration of dystrophin expression. The scope of the DMD exon skipping trials is currently being extended to include targeting of exons 45 and 53. However, it should be noted that only 8%, 4%, 13% or 18% of DMD patient mutations should be convertible into a BMD phenotype by single AO exon 45, 50, 51 or 53 skipping, respectively. Personalized molecular medicine for each skippable DMD deletion is necessary and this would require the optimisation and clinical trial workup of many specific AOs. It has been suggested that multi-exon skipping, using cocktails of AOs or chemically linked AOs, around deletion hotspots (*e.g.* exons 45-55) may have the potential to treat approximately 65% of DMD patients. A multi-exon strategy has been shown to work in *mdx* mice, but this has not yet been achieved in DMD patient cells.

Table II. Applicability of exon skipping as a therapy for DMD.

Mutation type	% of all DMD patients	% within each mutation type with out-of-frame mutations	% of all patients with out-of-frame mutation type	% corrected by one exon skip	% corrected by two exon skip	Total % corrected by exon(s) skipping	% of patients treatable by exon skipping
Deletions	65	79	51	70	8	79[a]	51
Small mutations	27	40[b]	11	44	47	91[c]	25
Duplications	8	78	6	61	12	73[d]	6
% of all DMD patients	100	68	68	63	19	82	82[e]

Adapted from Aartsma-Rus et al. [25]

[a]Discrepancy in totals is due to rounding
[b]Remaining 60% due to introduction of translational truncation codons
[c]High percentage of correctable small mutations, relative to small percentage of out-of-frame mutations, is because small mutations within in-frame exons can be bypassed by skipping of the mutated exon
[d]Discrepancy in percentages of out-of-frame duplications and percentage correctable by exon skipping is due the over-representation of duplications in mutations that do not follow the reading frame rule
[e]Discounting rare mutations involving the cysteine-rich domain (3.7%) and very large deletions (>36 exons) or those that involve all actin-binding sites or C-terminal domain (1.3%), the theoretical applicability of exon skipping to DMD is close to 77%

There are further obstacles to be overcome for AO-induced exon skipping to be a viable gene therapy for DMD. The cost implications may end up being prohibitive for many patients; since AOs are rapidly cleared from the circulation, regular administrations of high doses of AO would be required for therapeutic effect. Secondly, although deliverability, particularly to the heart, is enhanced with the use of conjugated PMOs, their potential toxicological and immunogenic problems need to be addressed. Lastly, the need for personalized medicine will require the completion of many expensive, lengthy clinical trials of many AOs. Even so, the potential of combined AO-induced DMD and myostatin exon skipping being the first gene therapy for DMD available in the clinic is highly likely, and this certainly looks achievable within the very near future.

ACKNOWLEDGMENTS

This work has been performed with the support of the EC-DG research through the FP6-Network of Excellence, CLINIGENE: LSHB-CT-2006-018933.

REFERENCES

1. Trollet C, Athanasopoulos T, Popplewell L, Malerba A, Dickson G. Gene therapy for muscular dystrophy: current progress and future prospects. *Exp Opin Biol Ther* 2009; 9: 849-66.

2. Arechavala-Gomeza V, Graham IR, Popplewell LJ, Adams AM, Aartsma-Rus A, Kinali M, *et al.* Comparative analysis of antisense oligonucleotide sequences for targeted skipping of exon 51 during dystrophin pre-mRNA splicing in human muscle. *Hum Gene Ther* 2007; 18: 798-810.

3. Graham IR, Hill VJ, Manoharan M, Inamati GB, Dickson G. Towards a therapeutic inhibition of dystrophin exon 23 splicing in *mdx* mouse muscle induced by antisense oligoribonucleotides (splicomers): target sequence optimisation using oligonucleotide arrays. *J Gene Med* 2004; 6: 1149-58.

4. Malerba A, Thorogood FC, Dickson G, Graham IR. Dosing regimen has a significant impact on the efficiency of morpholino oligomer-induced exon skipping in *mdx* mice. *Hum Gene Ther* 2009; 20: 955-65.

5. McClorey G, Fall AM, Moulton HM, Iversen PL, Rasko JE, Ryan M, *et al.* Induced dystrophin exon skipping in human muscle explants. *Neuromuscul Disord* 2006; 16: 583-90.

6. McClorey G, Moulton HM, Iversen PL, Fletcher S, Wilton SD. Antisense oligonucleotide-induced exon skipping restores dystrophin expression *in vitro* in a canine model of DMD. *Gene Ther* 2006; 13: 1373-81.

7. Wu B, Li Y, Morcos PA, Doran TJ, Lu P, Lu QL. Octa-guanidine morpholino restores dystrophin expression in cardiac and skeletal muscles and ameliorates pathology in dystrophic *mdx* mice. *Mol Ther* 2009; 17: 864-71.

8. Malerba A, Sharp PS, Graham IR, Arechavala-Gomeza V, Foster K, Muntoni F, *et al.* Chronic systemic therapy with low-dose morpholino oligomers ameliorates the pathology and normalizes locomotor behavior in *mdx* mice. *Mol Ther* 2011; 19: 345-54.

9. Malerba A, Boldrin L, Dickson G. Long-term systemic administration of unconjugated morpholino oligomers for therapeutic expression of dystrophin by exon skipping in skeletal muscle: implications for cardiac muscle integrity. *Nucleic acid therapeutics* 2011; 21: 293-8.

10. Aartsma-Rus A, van Vliet L, Hirschi M, Janson AA, Heemskerk H, de Winter CL, *et al.* Guidelines for antisense oligonucleotide design and insight into splice-modulating mechanisms. *Mol Ther* 2009; 17: 548-53.

11. Popplewell LJ, Trollet C, Dickson G, Graham IR. Design of phosphorodiamidate morpholino oligomers (PMOs) for the induction of exon skipping of the human DMD gene. *Mol Ther* 2009; 17: 554-61.

12. Popplewell LJ, Graham IR, Malerba A, Dickson G. Bioinformatic and functional optimization of antisense phosphorodiamidate morpholino oligomers (PMOs) for therapeutic modulation of RNA splicing in muscle. *Methods Mol Biol* 2011; 709: 153-78.

13. Aartsma-Rus A, De Winter CL, Janson AAM, Kaman WE, van Ommen G-JB, Den Dunnen JT, *et al.* Functional analysis of 114 exon-internal AONs for targeted DMD exon skipping: indication for steric hindrance of SR protein binding sites. *Oligonucleotides* 2005; 15: 284-97.

14. Popplewell LJ, Adkin C, Arechavala-Gomeza V, Aartsma-Rus A, de Winter CL, Wilton SD, *et al.* Comparative analysis of antisense oligonucleotide sequences targeting exon 53 of the human DMD gene: implications for future clinical trials. *Neuromuscul Disord* 2010; 20: 102-10.

15. Aartsma-Rus A, Janson AA, Kaman WE, Bremmer-Bout M, Den Dennen JT, Baas F, *et al.* Therapeutic antisense-induced exon skipping in cultured muscle cells from six different DMD patients. *Hum Mol Genet* 2003; 12: 907-14.

16. van Deutekom JC, Janson AA, Ginjaar IB, Franzhuzen WS, Aartsma-Rus A, Bremmer-Bout M, *et al.* Local antisense dystrophin restoration with antisense oligonucleotide PRO051. *N Engl J Med* 2007; 357: 2677-87.

17. Kinali M, Arechavala-Gomeza V, Feng L, Cirak S, Hunt D, Adkin C, *et al*. Local restoration of dystrophin expression with the morpholino oligomer AVI-4658 in Duchenne muscular dystrophy: a single-blind, placebo-controlled, dose-escalation, proof-of-concept study. *Lancet Neurol* 2009; 8: 918-28.

18. Goemans NM, Tulinius M, van den Akker JT, Burm BE, Ekhart PF, Heuvelmans N, *et al*. Systemic administration of PRO051 in Duchenne's muscular dystrophy. *N Engl J Med* 2011; 364: 1513-22.

19. Cirak S, Arechavala-Gomeza V, Guglieri M, Feng L, Torelli S, Anthony K, *et al*. Exon skipping and dystrophin restoration in patients with Duchenne muscular dystrophy after systemic phosphorodiamidate morpholino oligomer treatment: an open-label, phase 2, dose-escalation study. *Lancet* 2011; 378: 595-605.

20. Wu B, Xiao B, Cloer C, Shaban M, Sali A, Lu P, *et al*. One-year treatment of morpholino antisense oligomer improves skeletal and cardiac muscle functions in dystrophic *mdx* mice. *Mol Ther* 2011; 19: 576-83.

21. Yin H, Moulton HM, Betts C, Seow Y, Boutilier J, Iverson PL, Wood MJ. A fusion peptide directs enhanced systemic dystrophin exon skipping and functional restoration in dystrophin-deficient *mdx* mice. *Hum Mol Genet* 2009; 18: 4405-14.

22. Kang JK, Malerba A, Popplewell L, Foster K, Dickson G. Antisense-induced myostatin exon skipping leads to muscle hypertrophy in mice following octa-guanidine morpholino oligomer treatment. *Mol Ther* 2011; 19: 159-64.

23. Kemaladewi DU, Hoogaars WM, van Heiningen SH, Terlouw S, de Gorter DJ, den Dunnen JT, *et al*. Dual exon skipping in myostatin and dystrophin for Duchenne muscular dystrophy. *BMC Med Genomics* 2011; 4 : 36.

24. van Deutekom JC, Bremmer-Bout M, Janson AA, Ginjaar IB, Baas F, den Dunnen JT, *et al*. Antisense-induced exon skipping restores dystrophin expression in DMD patient derived muscle cells. *Hum Mol Genet* 2001; 10: 1547-54.

25. Aartsma-Rus A, Fokkema I, Verschuuren J, Ginjaar I, van Deutekom J, van Ommen GJ, *et al*. Theoretic applicability of antisense-mediated exon skipping for Duchenne muscular dystrophy mutations. *Hum Mutat* 2009; 30: 292-9.

TECHNOLOGIES

Highlights on emerging technologies, iPS induction and genetic stability

COORDINATED BY
ODILE COHEN-HAGUENAUER

The CliniBook: Clinical gene transfer
Edited by Odile Cohen-Haguenauer – EDK, Paris © 2012, pp. 307-334

A7-1
Induction of pluripotency from adult somatic cells: a review

Émilie Bayart[1], Odile Cohen-Haguenauer[1,2] *

[1]CliniGene, École Normale Supérieure de Cachan, CNRS UMR 8113, 94235 Cachan, France; [2]Department of Medical Oncology, AP-HP, Hôpital Saint-Louis and Université Paris-Diderot, Sorbonne-Paris-Cité, 75475 Paris Cedex 10, France.
*Corresponding author
odile.cohen@lbpa.ens-cachan.fr

The lifespan of fully differentiated cells is short and they do not renew. Conversely, there is a pool of stem cells in tissues that holds extensive self-renewal capacity and is able to generate daughter cells which may further undergo differentiation into various lineages or terminally differentiate to reach a functional state. These adult stem cells (ASCs) can only generate a range of cell types specific to the tissue in which they reside and are thus called multipotent. In addition to ASCs, there are stem cells which hold an even broader differentiation potential, like the earliest possible, so-called embryonic stem cells (ESCs). ESCs can be isolated from the inner cell mass of the blastocyst before uterine implantation and maintained in culture without undergoing differentiation. They are able to generate all cell types of the embryo, but are not capable of initiating either the umbilical cord, trophoblasts or associated structures. These cells are described as being pluripotent. The successful derivation of human ESC lines extended their great potential to the study of human diseases and allowed to envisage the future prospect of regenerative medicine. However, this finding has also caused disquiet, as these cells were derived from *in vitro*-fertilized human embryos that in theory would have the potential to engineer a human being in full. However, besides significant ethical issues associated with the use of human embryos, this essentially is a limited source which, as such, also hinders broad therapeutic applications. A further disadvantage of ESCs is their unlimited proliferative capacity; this could cause tumour formation upon transplantation (so-called teratomas). Furthermore, ESCs would hardly be immune-compatible with a putative recipient patient, a feature which further restricts prospects for ESCs-based therapies. Several methods to generate patient-matched pluripotent cells have been developed, *e.g.* reprogramming through nuclear transfer to adult cells. Somatic cells could indeed be successfully reprogrammed to a pluripotent state by injecting the nucleus of an adult cell into an enucleated oocyte [1, 2] (reviewed in [3]). This leads to reprogramming of the somatic cell nucleus by the host cytoplasm. After several cell divisions, reprogrammed cells forms a blastocyst, which is at genetic match with the nuclear donor. Up to now, human somatic cell nuclear transfer, as it is called, is severely limited and is extremely demanding in terms of resources required. Also, the technique tends to cause some degree of cell damage and altogether is quite inefficient. As an alternative to oocytes, ESCs can be used for human somatic nuclei reprogramming [4]: this method also is rather inefficient and cannot be exploited for therapeutic applications given the resulting rate of tetraploid cells. Despite ethical and obvious technical limitations, somatic cell nuclear transfer clearly demonstrated that adult cells can be reprogrammed to a pluripotent state.

Recently, Takahashi and Yamanaka [5] achieved the conversion of mouse fibroblasts into ES-like cells, almost indistinguishable from mouse ES cells in terms of pluripotency, *via* the viral transduction of four transcription factors (Oct3/4, Sox2, Klf4 and c-Myc). The latter were already identified as being involved in early embryonic development as well as cell proliferation and supposed to play a crucial role in ES cell identity [6-10]. They demonstrated the characteristics of embryonic stem cells including the ability to form chimeric mice and contribute to the germ line. One year later, Yamanaka's team generated human iPS using the same strategy of forced expression based on four transcription factors [11]. These pioneer studies opened a new field for stem cell therapies and attracted public attention given the supposedly great potential of induced pluripotent cells (*Figure 1*).

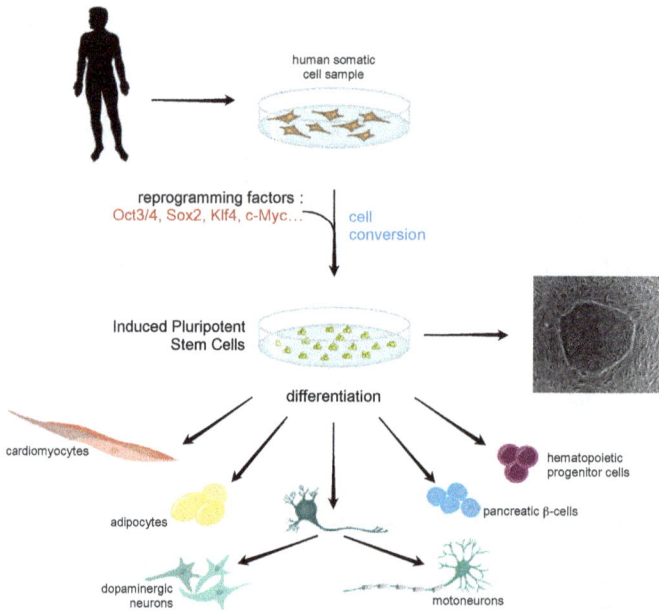

Figure 1. Schematic representation of adult somatic stem cells isolation and reprogramming into induced pluripotent stem cells (iPS) which in turn hold potential to re-differentiate into all three embryonic layers derived lineages (with the exception of germ-line cells).

Since these first demonstrations, many teams have successfully derived iPS cells from human somatic cells. Significant progress have been made and many methods have been reported which may combine transcription factors [12] and small chemicals [13, 14]. Up until now, the most currently used strategy for iPS generation aiming at basic research is gene-delivery *via* vectors systems. Retrovirus, lentivirus, adenovirus and plasmid are widely used. Human iPS cells are relevant to a wide range of applications such as test substrates for drugs, evaluation of toxicity, differentiation, disease modelling and therapeutics screens. Modelling both monogenic and multigenic diseases is currently being pursued in many laboratories, including big pharma, as well as the study of complex genetic traits and allelic variation. iPS cells can indeed be generated from cells sampled from affected-patients [15] once the phenotypic expression of the disease has been well-characterized in them: such information is unknown when considering ES cells. A summary of the current knowledge relating to both delivery systems and combinations of inducing factors as well as chemicals used to generate human iPS cells is presented below. This review also includes transgene-free reprogramming approaches which have been developed in order to circumvent vector integration-mediated risk for insertional mutagenesis.

DELIVERY METHODS

The reprogramming concept consists in the ectopic expression of a set of core pluripotency-related transcription factors in a somatic cell. In most case OCT4, SOX2, KLF4 and MYC are used and represent the commonly so-called OSKM cocktail. If successful, tightly compact colonies growing in ESC culture conditions appear on the culture dish. These colonies are morphologically, molecularly and phenotypically related to ES cells. Since 2007 and the first generation of human iPS cells by Yamanaka's team, more than 100 studies have been published which report on human iPS generation (For review see [16], http://intranet.cmrb.eu/reprogramming/home.html) which describes a number of studies published on mouse and human cells, among which some are pivotal.

Integrating vectors

Viral integrating vectors

In the original report of iPS induction, the delivery of pluripotency transcription factors was performed *via* gammaretroviral MLV (Moloney murine Leukemia Virus)-based vectors such as pMXs [11, 17] or pMSCV [15, 18, 19]. These vectors are replication-defective since regions encoding for the proteins necessary for additional rounds of virus replication and packaging are deleted from the viral genome. Defective gamma-retrovirus genomes have a cloning capacity up to 6-8kb, and are able to transduce target cells according to the envelope pseudotype under use. In actively dividing cells the efficiency of transgene delivery can reach up to 90%; a major limitation of this technology is that slowly- or non-dividing cells, such as neurons, are resistant to gamma-retrovirus-mediated transduction. It has been long identified that retrovirally-shuttled transgenes are silenced in ES cells [20, 21], as well as in iPS cells [15, 22] through mechanisms involving methylation and epigenetic modifications [23]. In fact, transgene silencing is important since iPS cells are being considered as duly and fully reprogrammed only upon both up-regulation of endogenous pluripotency genes and down-regulation of the transgene expression [24]. Despite practical advantages, gamma-retroviruses have been associated to major drawbacks in particular in clinical trials where insertional mutagenesis resulted in the development of malignancies. It thus became obvious that alternative approaches to retrovirus-mediated gene transfer should be considered especially when including a known oncogene like c-myc.

Unlike gamma-retrovectors, so far no malignancy resulting from insertional mutagenesis has been reported with Lentivectors. These distinct subclass of retrovirus vectors derive from either HIV-1, HIV-2 (human), SJV (simian) or EAIV (equine) and have been successfully used to generate iPS cells. A unique feature of lentiviruses is that they are able to transduce both non-dividing (slowly dividing or quiescent but metabolically active cells) and dividing cells, allowing the generation of iPS from most cell types. In addition, their cloning capacity is broader than that of gamma-retrovectors and they exhibit higher transduction efficiency, of human cells in particular. Like gamma-retrovectors, lentivectors are expected to be silenced during the reprogramming process. However, repression occurs to a lesser extent with lentivectors, a feature which in some instances may both prevent full reprogramming of cells [24] as well as indefinitely maintain unwanted expression of transcription factors and oncogenes used for reprogramming.

Non-viral integrating vectors

An alternative to viral vectors is the standard DNA transfection of plasmid DNA *via* liposomes or electroporation. However, compared to viruses, transduction efficiency is extremely low which makes it unlikely that a single cell will indeed capture all reprogramming factors at once. A major improvement was introduced with the development of polycistronic vectors expressing all induction factors driven by the same promoter. In these constructs, each cDNA is separated by a self-deleting 2A peptide sequence from picornaviruses [25, 26] which permits translation initiation from multiple sites or ribosomes re-entry once the protein encoded by the previous open reading frame has been released. Kaji *et al.* [27] were able to generate iPS from mouse cells and showed that a single copy of the polycistronic cassette was sufficient to achieve direct reprogramming. To date there is no evidence that human iPS could be obtained with this technology using "conventional" induction factors. However, one team was able to isolate human iPS cells when a mi-RNA involved in epigenetic modification was expressed and an antibiotics selection was applied for stable integration [28].

Integrating vectors and insertional mutagenesis

One major drawback of integrating delivery systems, whether viral or linear DNA vectors, towards induction of pluripotency is related to undesired transgene reactivation, a phenomenon which frequently occurs in differentiated cells derived from iPS, as this may lead to tumour formation resulting from *e.g.* over-expression of oncogene related factors such as c-*MYC*. Therefore, other transcription factors combinations have been investigated, which would exclude *c-MYC* and still allow full reprogramming [12, 22, 29, 30]. Another way to prevent re-expression of oncogene related factors is to control expression *via* a Tet-inducible system, which allows transgene repression in iPS like colony and further selection of fully reprogrammed cells [15, 31-35].
In addition, iPS cell lines generated with integrative vectors carry randomly distributed transgenes insertions [36] that harbour the risk for potential insertional mutagenesis and subsequent development of malignancies when inserted nearby sensitive sequences. In fact, Kane *et al.* [37] have shown that iPS cells could be generated without transcription factors, in merely transducing human fibroblasts with lentivectors only expressing the green fluorescent protein (GFP), though at very high multiplicity of infection (MOI). Primary fibroblasts transduced at MOI 200 gave rise to iPS cells which contain as many as 20 integration sites. This study comes as a striking illustration of the extent of deregulation into which insertional mutagenesis may result, reminiscent of helper retrovirus pathology induced in rodent.
In fact, the use of polycistronic vectors considerably reduces vector copy number integration per cell a feature which is expected to significantly decrease the risk for insertional mutagenesis. Based on the former observation that a single polycistronic cassette expres-

sing all transgenes under the same promoter from linear DNA is able to allow full re-programming of somatic cells, polycistronic gammaretroviral and lentiviral vectors have been developed which translate in the successful generation of human iPS cells [38, 39].

Excisable integrating vectors

Viral-derived excisable vectors and heterologous recombination system

As a next step towards safety improvement, excisable integrating vectors have been engineered in order to generate transgene-free iPS and help prevent above-mentioned drawbacks as well as the following. In addition to being placed under the control of viral promoters, the stable integration of transgenes encoding for transcription factors or oncogenes involved in cell proliferation such as *c-MYC*, harbours a substantial risk of malignant transformation should reprogramming factors not be fully silenced or incidentally be reactivated during differentiation. Moreover, viral promoter reactivation could lead to the deregulation of *cis*-neighbouring genes: the latter represents an additional mechanism which might compromise cell-cycle integrity. Excisable lentivirus vectors have been engineered which include both a *loxP* site in the 3'LTR and an inducible promoter driving transgene expression. During virus replication, the *loxP* site is duplicated in the 5'LTR so that the integrated transgenic cassette is flanked with a *loxP* site at both ends. The excision of the reprogramming factors follows the targeted and transient expression of Cre recombinase in transduced cells which induces a recombination event between *loxP* sites. Using this system, Jaenisch and his group [40] were able to generate transgene-free human iPS cells which are able to maintain their pluripotent state and display a global gene expression profile similar to human ES cells. These iPS cells could further differentiate into dopaminergic neurons [40]. The major limitation of this study is that reprogramming factors were primarily integrated at different independent sites which resulted in multiple transgenes excision upon Cre recombinase expression. In fact, multiple and simultaneous recombination reactions could lead to genome rearrangement and genomic instability. In order to overcome this drawback, Chang *et al.* [41] designed a polycistronic lentiviral vector encoding for defined reprogramming factors separated by 2A sequences resulting in the integration of a single reprogramming cassette floxed by two *loxP* sites. Following Cre recombinase mediated excision, the iPS cells lines generated harbour only three lentiviral LTR signatures which consist of a single *loxP* site that does not interrupt coding sequences, promoters or regulatory elements. Although conceptually elegant, this system holds a risk for non-specific recombination events and genomic instability should Cre recombinase expression not be tightly enough controlled .

Another commonly used heterologous recombination system is the Flp/FRT recombinase/targets system from *Saccharomyces cerevisiae* [42]. While it is supposedly less efficient than the *Cre/loxP* system [43] it conversely exhibits far less toxicity, a feature which is essential when working with primary cells [44]. To date, there has been no report of human iPS cells generation, while murine iPS cells have been generated using this system with a polycistronic lentivector in which the reprogramming cassette was flanked with two FRT sites. These mice iPS cells were further transduced with empty MLV retrovirus-like-particles which shuttle the Flp recombinase fused to the Gag-pol polyprotein. This process resulted in the complete removal of the reprogramming cassette [45]. Factor-free iPS resulting from heterologous recombination systems thus represent a more suitable source of cells towards human disease modelling. However, these iPS cells still harbour scars of insertion sites and are not "genetically clean" pluripotent stem cells, a feature which might still alleviate translation to cell-based therapies (*Figure 2*).

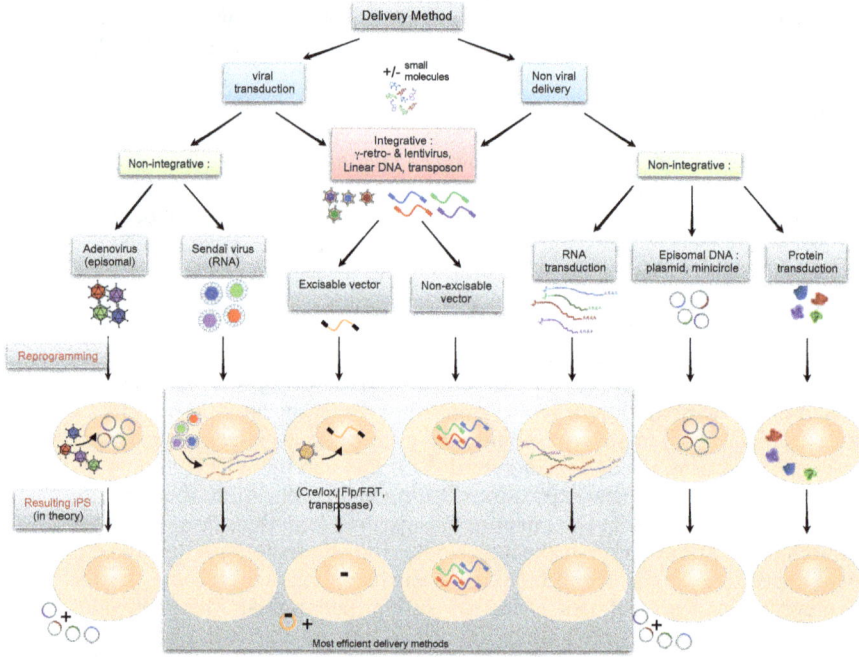

Figure 2. Schematic representation of technological options for iPS induction: viral, non-viral; integrative, non-integrative, transgene-free and resulting persistence or absence of genetic scars. The most efficient delivery methods are highlighted.

Transposon-derived excisable vectors

Besides viral derived systems, linear plasmids have also been tested for cell conversion which encode a polycistronic cassette floxed with two *loxP* sites [27]. While transgene-free mouse iPS were generated, so far there is no evidence that human iPSCs could. In order to address the reprogramming ability of their non-viral single-vector system in human cells, Kaji and co-workers enhanced stable transfection efficiencies using a *piggyBack* (*PB*) transposon-based delivery system which mediates genome integration at higher efficiency than would with linearized plasmids. Transposons are mobile genetic elements which can move from one position to another within the genome through an excision/insertion mechanism. As a vector system, *PB* transposon requires only 13 bp inverted terminal repeats (**ITRs**) and an active transposase, the enzyme which catalyses insertion and excision [46, 47]. The *PB* system is usually composed of a donor plasmid called transposon, which shuttles the transgenic sequence of interest flanked by the 5' and 3' ITRs. The latter is co-transfected with a transposase expressing helper plasmid that mediates integration [46-48]. Using these *PB*-based reprogramming vectors, both Kaji *et al.* [27] and Woltjen *et al.* [49], were able to generate human iPS cells from fibroblasts and subsequently delete the transgenes. In these studies, the authors demonstrated the traceless elimination of the reprogramming factors and scar-free excision of the inserted transposon without modifying the sequence of the integration site: this feature is unique to *PB*. Another transposon, the *Sleeping Beauty* (*SB*), was assembled in combining fragments of silent and defective Tc1/*mariner* elements from salmon fish [50]. The reconstructed *SB* showed the best transposition efficiency in vertebrate cells than any other transposon tested at that time. Most recently, a novel super-active transposase has been derived from *SB*: this SB100X mutant is a 100-fold more potent in HeLa cell lines compared to the originally resurrected *SB* [51]. Of note, it received the *molecule of the year* award in 2009. The efficiency of SB100X mediated transgene insertion is similar to viral transduction in generating both mouse and human iPS cells [52] but the integration/excision process is not entirely scar-free as with *PB*.

Both *piggyback* and *SB*-based system allow the removal of the reprogramming cassette and its site-specific exchange through a targeted recombination between the reprogramming cassette and a gene of interest, through the so-called Recombination-Mediated Cassette Exchange (RMCE) process. These features make the transposon/transposase system one of the best choices for delivering reprogramming factor into a broad range of somatic cells with view to generating "genetically clean" iPS cells [53]. However, transposon-based reprogramming is essentially depending on the delivery method which could represent a limitation when addressing some primary cells due to resistance or toxicity related to DNA transfection methods: lipofection, electroporation or nucleofection. In addition, it must be underlined that the transposition reaction in not always precise, as for instance Wang *et al.* [54] reported on alterations found in 5% of the transposition events. Moreover, the transposase promotes both deletion and integration at similar efficiencies, allowing the transposon to "jump" from site to site as long as the transposase is expressed: uncontrolled off-target repeated transposition could cause footprints and/or genetic rearrangement in the genome of human iPS cell generated. Therefore, the transposase expression window needs to be tightly controlled. Recently, Galla *et al.* [55] proposed an improved approach based on retrovirus particle-mediated mRNA transfer which allows transient and dose-controlled expression of SB100X. This was shown to both support efficient transposition and prevent related cytotoxicity. Although major improvements of both safety and quality of iPS cells are expected, the precise consequences of transposon-based system on the genomic stability of reprogrammed cells still need to be scrutinised and be it the case, ways of improvement sought.

Non-integrating vectors

Integration-free viral delivery

As persistent expression of reprogrammning factors should be avoided following iPSC generation, transient expression based on non-integrating vectors could help circumventing putative insertional mutagenesis. Along this line, integration-defective retrovectors have been engineered taking advantage of inactivating mutations introduced in the viral integrase. Integration-deficient gammaretroviral vectors have been described [56] which translate into very low titres. In addition to this bottleneck, their inability to transduce non-dividing cells makes it unlikely to fit the demands of most experiments. The so-called IDLV-platform (Integration Deficient Lentivirus Vectors) has attracted a lot of attention including with view to clinical translation in gene therapy settings. Therefore, like any episomal transgenic DNA IDLV may persist only transiently and be further diluted slowly with time and cell-divisions [57-59]. Surprisingly, so far, no iPS cells could be generated using integrase-defective lentivectors.

One of the first attempts to generate integration-free iPS cells was reported by Stadtfeld *et al.* [60], who used adenoviral vectors. These replication-defective vectors are in theory non-integrative in most cellular types. They are able to transduce a broad range of cell types in which they remain as episomes and mediate high transgene expression according to the promoter under use [61, 62]. Stadtfeld *et al.* [60], have generated mouse iPS cells from adult hepatocytes, which correspond to adenovirus vectors best tropism. However, this process only proved successful – although at very low efficiency – when using cells which were already genetically engineered with a stably integrated inducible *Oct4* expression cassette. More recently, with a payload of repeated infection cycles at MOI 250 with a series of adenovirus vectors expressing each a single reprogramming factor, human iPS cells could be generated from foetal fibroblasts although at much lower efficiency in reference to mouse cells [63]. When taking into account this very low efficiency, it is challenging to use adenoviral vectors with hope to generate fully reprogrammed iPS cells. Moreover, vector and transgene integration does happen, although at low frequency. Recombination occurred overall randomly at rates between 5.5 x 10(-3) and 1.1 x 10(-4) but with a preference for integration into genes [64]. Altogether, at this point, adenoviral vectors might need to combine with small molecules, before being considered routinely for the derivation of human iPS cells with full stemness characteristics.

The last but not least non-integrative viral strategy that has been developed towards iPS generation, takes advantage of F-deficient Sendai viral (SeV) vectors. The latter replicates under the form of a negative-sense single stranded RNA in the cytoplasm of infected cells, which neither involves DNA intermediates nor may be able to integrate into the host genome [65]. Since SeV vectors are: (i) very efficient at introducing foreign genes in a wide spectrum of host cells in many species and tissues; (ii) without identified pathogenicity for human and (iii) controllable for foreign gene expression [66], they have been considered as tools for gene transfer and therapy [67]. To date, human fibroblasts and terminally differentiated circulating T cells have been successfully reprogrammed: this is using SeV-based vectors which carry each of the reprogramming factors separately and a single infection cycle [68, 69]; and the system is commercially available. While it appears as a very appealing method, there might be limitations: for instance, the viral replicase is extremely sensitive to the nature of the transgenic sequences. In addition, because they constitutively replicate, SeV are difficult to eliminate from the host cells even at high number of passages. Nishimura *et al.* [70] have utmost recently reported promising results using improved SeV vectors. These new variant of replication defective Sendai vectors mediate persistent transgene expression (so called SeVdp), while first generation of recombinant vector are capable of strong but transient transgene expression [71]. These SeVdp allow to generate mouse iPS more efficiently. In adding interfering RNAs to the system, SeV virus genomes could be completely eliminated. This produces iPS cells devoid of exogenous nucleic acids which translates into interesting candidates for both disease modelling and cell therapy prospects, should safety be further demonstrated.

Transient episomal delivery

As an alternative to integration-defective virus, reprogramming approaches based on direct delivery of episomal vectors have been developed. These methods appear attractive since they are easy to carry out and do not require the production of viral particles. iPS cells could indeed be generated from mouse cells through both direct and transient delivery of plasmid DNA [72-74]. Si-Tayeb *et al.* [75] further addressed this option through direct delivery of plasmids otherwise used for lentivirus vectors production which encode for each reprogramming factors. Although these attempts met with some success providing two successive rounds of transfection were performed, this was at much lower rate than with lentivirus vectors. Of note, the iPS cell line generated was devoid of exogenous DNA. Along this line, Monserrat *et al.* [76] reported iPS generation from human cells in performing three consecutive cycles of transfections using the Poly(β-amino esters) polycation polymer to deliver a single polycistronic plasmid encoding for all reprogramming factors: the overall efficiency was still much lower than with virus-based systems. It may well be that fewer cells received the accurate dose of plasmids during the entire period required for reprogramming, with their premature dilution in actively dividing cells.

To circumvent the need for serial transfections and help solve the problem of episome dilution with cell divisions, Yu and colleagues [77] used oriP/Epstein-Barr nuclear antigen-1-based episomal vectors (oriP/EBNA1). The latter autonomously replicate as extra-chromosomal elements without integrating in the genome of cells whether dividing or not. These vectors can be maintained as stable episomes under drug selective pressure, which are progressively lost upon drug removal [78, 79]. In fact, human iPS cells were generated from human foreskin fibroblast in transfecting seven transcription factors which were expressed from three separate oriP/EBNA1 vectors. Vector- and transgene-free iPS cell lines were isolated using mere sub-cloning. However the reprogramming efficiency reported with this method proved as equally low as with other non-integrative systems [77]. More recently, two groups among which Yamanaka's reported the generation of iPS from human dermal fibroblast and dental pulp using a combination of three oriP/EBNA1 vectors encoding for six reprogramming factors [80]. In addition, Chou *et al.* [81] obtained iPS cells from adult peripheral blood mononuclear cells by performing a single transfection round with a single polycistronic oriP/EBNA1 vector which encodes for five reprogramming factors with a 10 to 100 fold increased efficiency compared to other transient episomal delivery systems [81]. The later study is promising considering that patients' peripheral blood samples are easily accessible.

Finally, in order to reduce the size of the reprogramming episomes and delete prokaryotic backbone sequences which may potentially be methylated, investigators have turned to minicircles. These entities represent an interesting option since they allow expression of reprogramming factors as both non-integrating and non-replicating episomes. Minicircle vectors are supercoiled DNA molecules that lack both a bacterial origin of replication and antibiotic resistance genes; therefore, they are primarily composed of an eukaryotic expression cassette. Compared to standard plasmid-DNA, minicircle vectors harbour higher transfection efficiencies and longer expression owing to decreased silencing mechanisms [82, 83] which can further be prevented by the addition of S/MARs derived sequences. A 2A-peptide-based polycistronic cassette including four reprogramming factors was used to perform several consecutive rounds of transfection which allowed Jia and colleagues [84] to generate iPS cells from human adipose stem cells with a ten-fold increase. These adipose iPS cells were devoid of vector integration. This group further published a standardized protocol for human iPS generation based on minicircle technology [85].

Significant improvements towards iPS generation have resulted from above described non-integrative strategies, but with the exception of Sendai-based vectors, all methods involve the expression of transgenes through an exogenous DNA intermediate. Although the resulting iPS cells were deemed to be transgene-free, the risk of exogenous DNA integration still persists, even at a very low rate. Therefore, careful analyses are required to scrutinize background integration and genetic stability in order to confirm that the resulting iPS cell lines are free from deleterious genetic modification.

Transgene free delivery methods

RNA delivery

Further down the road of preventing exogenous integration and suppress the risk of in-sertional mutagenesis, attempts have recently been made at the direct delivery of mRNAs encoding for the reprogramming factors. Plews *et al.* [86] first showed that *in vitro* trans-cribed capped mRNAs - which encompass 5' and 3' untranslated regions (UTRs) of the α-globin and encode for five reprogramming factors - resulted in increased expression of the endogenous genes responsible for cellular reprogramming. However this procedure proved insufficient to achieve full reprogramming. Few months later, Yakubov *et al.* [87] could successfully reprogram human foreskin fibroblasts by performing five consecutive transfections over several days using four *in vitro* transcribed capped mRNAs which com-prise IRES sequences in the 5'UTR and a polyA signal in the 3'UTR. The best results were obtained by Warren *et al.* [88] when synthetic capped mRNAs were produced with a strong translational initiation signal in the 5'UTR and the β-globin 3'UTR with a poly-A tail signal flanking the open reading frame. As a next step of sophistication, synthetic mRNAs were protected from innate antiviral response since *in vitro* transcription was per-formed with 5'methylcytidine substituting for cytidine and pseudo-uridine for uridin. Re-peated transfections of these synthetic mRNAs *via* cationic vehicles combined with an interferon inhibitor resulted in a conversion efficiency of about 2%; a figure which could be further increased in using chromatin structure modifiers in combination. The repro-gramming efficiency achieved with this strategy is higher than with any other system, when addressing a range of human somatic donor cells under test. However, the bottle-neck with this method stands in the need for repeated rounds of transfection that some fragile primary cells are not able to sustain. In addition, costs related to RNA-vectors production required for repeated cycles of delivery, currently are very high (*Figure 2*).

Protein delivery

A last strategy which is intended at avoiding the introduction of exogenous genetic ma-teriel into donor cells, is the delivery of reprogramming factors as proteins. A decade ago, Wilmut and colleagues showed that adult somatic cells could be reprogrammed back to an undifferentiated embryonic state using somatic cell nuclear transfer [89]. Along this line, Cho and co-workers [90] challenged cells with protein extracts derived from ES cells assuming that this could lead to similar results. Indeed, a single transfer of ES cells-derived proteins on primary cultures of mouse adult fibroblasts could fully convert iPS cells with a full differentiation potential. However, to date no human iPS cells could be generated using this approach, even when combined with chromatin re-modelling small chemicals [91]. This absence of efficacy on human cells has been attri-buted to insufficient concentration of factors from cell extracts. In order to improve these conditions, Zhou *et al.* [92], produced recombinant reprogramming factors in *E. coli* where a poly-arginine track was fused at the C-terminus in order to facilitate their pene-tration across the plasma membrane [93]. Following four cycles of exposure to the puri-fied recombinant proteins and the concomitant addition of a HDAC inhibitor, iPS cells were isolated from MEFs. However, again, so far attempts to establish human iPS cells using this method have been unsuccessful. In addition, substantially large amounts of purified recombinant proteins are required which make it unlikely to be tailored for rou-tine use. The same year, another group was luckier starting from the human HEK293 cell line engineered as a donor source to stably express one recombinant reprogramming factor also fused to a poly-arginine track. Human neonatal fibroblasts were exposed to protein extracts derived from the HEK293 cell line at regularly intervals, consisting of consecutive cycles of eight hours per week during six weeks, after which few iPS colonies could be isolated [94]. These protein-based strategies might be relevant when considering that iPS cell lines are completely devoid of exogenous DNA, thereby suppressing the risk for insertional mutagenesis which stems from integration of foreign DNA sequences into the genome. While poor efficiencies would require improvement the genuine prevention of genomic instability also needs to be demonstrated when considering in particular the extremely slow kinetics of the induction process based on proteins delivery.

REPROGRAMMING

Direct reprogramming is conceptually simple which involves ectopic introduction of defined factors that are capable of inducing cell conversion: the related induction technologies currently are widely used in many laboratories. However, this process still is extremely slow, inefficient, and depends on several parameters which affect efficiency, reproducibility in the process and the quality of the resulting iPS cells. As discussed in the previous section, one parameter is related to the method selected for reprogramming since virus-based systems are more efficient than the transfer of naked nucleic acids or the direct addition of proteins for example. However, the precise selection of those reprogramming factors that will be used in accordance with the donor cell types, also is a key element of success and/or safety which is discussed in the next section.

Reprogramming factors to facilitate stem cells induction

"Conventional" cocktails

Yamanaka's group was the first to report the generation of mouse and human iPS cells via overexpression of defined factors. Among 24 candidates known to be involved in embryonic development and maintenance, Yamanaka and co-workers shown that retroviral-mediated ectopic expression of *OCT4* (also known as *POU5F1*), *SOX2*, *KLF4* and *c-MYC* (so called OSKM cocktail) was sufficient to mediate full reprogramming of differentiated adult cells into stem cells [5, 95]. This canonical cocktail now has proved efficient on a wide range of human cell types with integrative delivery systems, in particular, as recently reviewed by Gonzalez *et al.* [16]. The OSKM cocktail was also shown to perform when introduced with non-integrative systems such as Sendai viruses [68-70] or mRNAs [88], and although at very low efficiency in particular with adenoviruses [92], episomal plasmids [76], and proteins [94].
As early as one month after the publication of Yamanaka's work on human cells, Thomson and colleagues reported the generation of human iPS using another reprogramming cocktail which also comprises *OCT4* and *SOX2*, and involves *NANOG* and *LIN28* (OSNL) instead of *KLF4* and *c-MYC* [12]. This reprogramming cocktail has also proved efficient in most cases when delivered by lentiviruses [16] or as mRNAs [87]. The stoichiometry of the reprogramming factors has been investigated: Papapetrou *et al.* [96] have shown that a high expression of *OCT4*, compared to others factors, is required with view to increasing conversion. When moving to polycistronic vectors, the main factor conditioning success is a high transduction efficacy. Cocktails including five factors such as OSKMN or OSKNL have further been tested in order to either improve the efficiency of iPS cells generation from common cell types such as keratinocytes and fibroblasts [31, 34] or facilitate the reprogramming of more difficult cells such as diseased patients' cell and vascular smooth muscle cells [15, 97]. The simultaneous use of six-reprogramming factors (OSKMNL) has further been attempted which met with ad-

ditional success with human new born foreskin and foetal dermis fibroblasts [98, 99]. A variety of other pluripotency-related factors have also been tested such as *UTF1* [100] with which more colonies where obtained when expressed along with **OSKM** in human primary fibroblasts. Similarly, a ten-fold increase could be observed when *SALL4* was co-expressed with **OSK** in human adult fibroblasts from dermis [101] (*Table I*).

Delivery Methods (group)	Delivery Methods	OCT4	SOX2	KLF4	c-MYC	L-MYC	LIN28	NANOG	TSV40	shRNAp53	Mir-302	ES cell	Butyrate	MEK inhibitor	poly(β-amino esters)	Valproic Acid	PMID
Integrating Vectors	Retrovirus	●	●	●	●												18035408
Integrating Vectors	Polycistronic retrovirus	●	●	●	●												19890879
Integrating Vectors	Lentivirus	●	●				●	●									18029452
Integrating Vectors	Inducible Lentivirus	●	●	●	●												18691744
Integrating Vectors	Inducible Lentivirus	●	●	●	●												20572011
Integrating Vectors	Inducible Lentivirus	●	●	●	●												18786420
Integrating Vectors	Inducible Lentivirus	●	●	●	●												20621045
Integrating Vectors	Inducible Lentivirus	●	●					●									20569691
Integrating Vectors	Polycistronic lentivirus	●	●	●	●												20682452
Integrating Vectors	Inducible polycistronic lentivirus	●	●	●	●												19109433
Integrating Vectors	Inducible Plasmid	●	●	●	●						●						20870751
Excisable integrating vector	Excisable (LoxP) lentivirus	●	●	●	●												19269371
Excisable integrating vector	Excisable (LoxP) polycistronic lentivirus	●	●	●	●												19415770
Excisable integrating vector	Excisable (FRT) polycistronic lentivirus	●	●	●	●												20385817
Excisable integrating vector	PiggyBack Transposon	●	●	●	●												19252477
Excisable integrating vector	PiggyBack Transposon	●	●	●	●										●		18511599
Excisable integrating vector	Inducible PiggyBack Transposon	●	●	●	●												19252478
Excisable integrating vector	Sleeping Beauty	●	●	●	●												Izsvak et al (2011)
Non-integrating vectors / pathways	Adenovirus	●	●	●	●												19697349
Non-integrating vectors / pathways	Sendaï virus	●	●	●	●												19838014
Non-integrating vectors / pathways	Sendaï virus	●	●	●	●												20621043
Non-integrating vectors / pathways	Lentivector (plasmid)	●	●				●	●						●			20682060
Non-integrating vectors / pathways	EBV based plasmid	●	●	●	●		●	●	●								19325077
Non-integrating vectors / pathways	EBV based plasmid	●	●	●	●		●	●	●								21243013
Non-integrating vectors / pathways	EBV based plasmid	●	●	●		●			●								21460823
Non-integrating vectors / pathways	Polycistronic plasmid	●	●	●	●										●		21285354
Non-integrating vectors / pathways	Minicircles	●	●				●	●									20139967/ 21212777
Non-integrating vectors / pathways	RNA	●	●	●	●												20188704
Non-integrating vectors / pathways	RNA	●	●	●	●												20888316
Non-integrating vectors / pathways	Proteins	●	●	●	●							●					20439621(Ro)
Non-integrating vectors / pathways	Proteins	●	●												●		19398399(Ro)
Non-integrating vectors / pathways	Proteins	●	●	●	●												19481515

Table I. This double entry table – with delivery methods in lines and induction factors or cocktails in columns – tentatively recapitulates the combination of technological options and factors used for induction of human iPS. The PMID of key papers describing the methods and its outcome are listed in the last column, in the matching line.

Reprogramming efficacy is tightly linked to cell proliferation

The efficiency with which cells can be converted is directly linked to cell cycle and division status. Indeed, a high proliferation rate appears to be required for efficient cell reprogramming [102]. As a consequence, when combined with OSKM both the SV40 large T antigen (SV40LT) and the Telomerase reverse transcriptase (h*TERT*) known to have positive effects on cell proliferation and prevention of cell senescence in protecting chromosome ends, increase the number of iPS colonies [15]. Along the same rationale, *REM2* or *CyclinD1* expression enhance reprogramming compared to the "conventional" cocktail alone and more importantly allow iPS generation without involving *c-MYC* [103]. As SV40LT is known to target p53, it has been hypothesized that p53 inhibition could also behave as a facilitator. Several studies have reported that the use of short hairpin RNAs (shRNAs) against p53 does indeed enhance cell conversion efficiency [100, 104, 105]. Further studies have defined p53 as a guardian against reprogramming [106] as i) p53-p21 pathway prevents iPS cells generation [107] and ii) during the reprogramming process, the levels of both p53 and p53 targets are increased and iii) p53 induces growth arrest and apoptosis [104, 105, 107]. Although Mah *et al.* [108] have postulated that these observations correspond to the innate immunity response induced by viral transduction, Hong *et al.* [107] reported that this response may indeed appear to be independent of viral integration. In further experiments, the introduction of shRNAs against p53 allowed iPS generation in the absence of *c-MYC* (OSK cocktail) as well as in the absence of *KLF4* (OS cocktail) on keratinocytes as shown by Kawamura *et al.* [104]. In postnatal neurons (although post-mitotic), the addition of a short hairpin RNAs (shRNA) against p53 to the OSKM cocktail is compulsory to successful reprogramming [109]. Another roadblock that is limiting reprogramming efficiency is the *Ink4a/ARF* locus which is linked to the p53 pathway. Indeed, shRNAs against *ARF* and/or *Ink4a* have been shown to greatly improve cell conversion efficiency in the absence of *c-MYC* in fetal lung fibroblasts [110].

• The obvious influence of cell-cycle regulators has also been evidenced using small chemical molecules. Indeed, the inhibition of either of or both the mitogen-activated protein kinase kinase (known as MEKK) signalling and Glycogene Synthase Kinase 3 (GSK3) pathways increases the number of fully reprogrammed colonies [75, 111]; in addition, this allows full reprogramming of neural precursors without a requirement for SOX2 and c-MYC [112]. Finally, MEK inhibitors promote the transformation of fibroblasts into stem cells with a 200-fold increase over the classical method in combination with an ALK5 (TGFβ receptor) inhibitor and thiazovivin [113]. While playing with identified key regulators of the cell-cycle clearly results in the facilitation of adults cell conversion into iPS, scrutiny is required on the potential associated payload when genetic stability and controlled proliferation might be at stake.

• Specific microRNAs (miRNA) have been shown to be involved in pluripotency and reprogramming [114] such as the miR-290 cluster which is believed to act downstream of *MYC* and is involved in features unique to EC cell-cycle [115]. The use of miR-291-3p, miR-294 or miR-295 combined with *OSK* cocktail increases the reprogramming efficiency in MEFs [116]. However, to date no human iPS generation has been reported using these miRNAs. Finally, recent studies have evidenced that both Oct4 and Sox2 play a pivotal role in miR-302 expression in human embryonic stem cells (hES) [117, 118]. MiR-302 indeed belongs to a class of miRNAs that functions as cytoplasmic gene silencers: this is in suppressing translation of targeted messenger RNAs (mRNA). A majority of miR-302-targeted genes are transcripts involved in development-related signals and oncogenes [119]. In human, miR-302 is predominantly expressed in hES and iPS cells, but not in differentiated cells [120, 121]. In using a vector which expresses a cDNA encoding for miR-302 and further selecting cells for its stable integration with antibiotics, Lin and co-workers [28] were able to achieve full reprogramming of cells from human hair follicles.

• Culture conditions can also modulate reprogramming efficiencies as a four-fold increase in human cell conversion efficiency is observed when MEFs are maintained under 5% O_2 hypoxic condition (like in stem-cell niches) during the reprogramming process which allows iPS generation with only two factors OCT4 and KLF4 [122]. This data is in keeping with well-identified observations of improved survival of hematopoietic stem cells [123] and the prevention of human ESCs differentiation [124] under low O_2 tension. In fact, pluripotency is regulated by the family of hypoxia inducible factors (HIFs) among which HIF-2α has been shown to act as an upstream regulator of OCT4 which in turn is also involved in both NANOG and SOX2 expression [125].

Overcoming epigenetic barriers

iPS reprogramming overall is a rather inefficient process. Somatic cell conversion obviously involves a massive reconfiguration of the chromatin structure, from DNA methylation to histone and nucleosome modifications. Chromatin remodelling, also known as the epigenetic barrier, is a rate-limiting step in somatic cell reprogramming since it holds the power to abrogate unwanted expression of lineage specific genes. The added value of chemical compounds which can modulate either DNA methylation status or chromatin modifications have emphasized the importance of epigenome in reprogramming. Subsequent improvement has been evidenced in various cell types. For example, the inhibition of DNA methylation during the conversion phase with the DNA methyltransferase (DNMT) inhibitor 5-azacytidine allows mouse iPSCs which exhibit an intermediate pattern to be fully reprogrammed [126]. Vitamin C also significantly improves reprogramming efficiency as it alleviates cell senescence [127] and induces DNA demethylation of gene sets specific to cell conversion [128]. Treatment with histone deacetylase (HDAC) inhibitors such as trichostatin A (TSA) or valproic acid (VPA), induces chromatin remodelling leading to up-regulation of ESC-specific genes [113], improvement of somatic cell reprogramming efficiency also allows cell conversion with only two factors: *OCT4* and *SOX2* [29]. Upon addition of VPA, cell conversion could be demonstrated *via* the direct delivery of recombinant proteins (OSKM cocktail) in mouse cells [92]. Recently, Picanço-Castro [129] and colleagues have generated iPS cells from human dermal fibroblasts in combining VPA with viral delivery of c-MYC, Sox2 and TCL1-A, a co-activator of the cell survival kinase AKT [130]. Butyrate also affects both histone H3 acetylation and promoter DNA methylation, thus altering the expression of endogenous pluripotency associated genes. As a consequence, it is expected to greatly enhance iPS cell derivation from human adult or fetal fibroblasts using 4 to 5 reprogramming genes; furthermore, its effect on reprogramming is more remarkable with an increase by over a 100- to 200-fold in the absence of either *KLF4* or MYC [131]. Along the same line, by inhibiting G9a histone methyltransferase, which mediates epigenetic repression of *OCT4* [132], iPS could be generated from MEFs using only two factors: *OCT4* and *KLF4* [30]. Other authors have also used Tranylcypromine (Parnate), an inhibitor of lysine-specific demethylase 1, which is responsible for K4 demethylation. They could successfully generate iPS cells from human keratinocytes again with *OCT4* and *KLF4* only [113]. However, chemical compounds could have deleterious side effects. For example, VPA has been shown to enhance recombination events [133, 134] and reduce the ability of cells to repair DNA double-strand breaks [135]. It might thus be wise to weigh out the use of these DNA-modifying molecules when considering the potential consequences of their use on the genetic stability of resulting iPS cells.

Bottlenecks towards clinical translation

Preventing the risk for induced oncogenesis

• Addressing the nature of reprogramming factors: In addition to the risk for insertional mutagenesis related to integration of foreign sequences into the cell genome, a forced expression of reprogramming factors may bring along an additional risk for the development of malignancy, when considering both the nature and the combination of inducing factors under use. In fact, among proposed procedures some are reminiscent of the generation of immortalized cell lines such as ectopic expression of telomerase reverse transcriptase (h*TERT*) and/or SV40 large T antigen (SV40LT) and their propensity for malignant transformation, *e.g.*: by adding a single oncogene such as H-ras [136-138]. Therefore, the potential added value to the reprogramming process related to the addition of these factors should be carefully weighed out in the eye of their potential incompatibility with clinical-relevant prospects. Similarly, the inclusion of the c-Myc proto-oncogene is also controversial as it is associated with tumour formation in iPSC-derived chimeric mice [5], despite a well-identified potent promoter of iPSC generation. This promotion capacity nevertheless is independent from its transformation property; indeed, other members of the Myc family such as L-Myc, or mutant c-Myc, share this ability to promote iPSC generation while showing more specific and efficient as compared to WT c-Myc [80, 139].
• Reducing the number of reprogramming factors: since the most efficient and commonly used methods to induce adult cell conversion involve the stable integration of transgenes with the concurrent risk for insertional mutagenesis, a critical path for improvement consists in the reduction of transduced reprogramming factors. So far, fibroblasts - which remain the most common donor cell type used in over 80% iPS experiments published so far [16] - were successfully reprogrammed using three-factors cocktails: whether including OSK [22, 39, 140-143], OSM [141] or OSN [144]; though at lower efficiency. Human keratinocytes, as well as mesenchymal cells from teeth and dental pulp have also been converted with OSK [18, 145, 146]. The endogenous expression of at least one of the reprogramming factors in some cell types obviously facilitates their full reprogramming. For instance, amniotic derived cells which spontaneously exhibit robust expression of *c-MYC*, could be converted with three-factors cocktails like either OSK [113, 147, 148] or OSN [149]. Along the same line, human melanocytes were found to express Sox2 and were reprogrammed with the OKM cocktail [35]. The challenge of cell conversion with the introduction of the two factors *OCT4* and *SOX2* only, met with success in human endothelial cells from umbilical cells that harbour endogenous expression of *KLF4* [150]. Similarly, foetal neural stem cells, which express high level of endogenous *SOX2,* could be converted using *OCT4* and *KLF4* [151] and further *via* ectopic expression of *OCT4* only [152]. However, these immature cells are relatively inaccessible and difficult to obtain and cannot be considered as straightforward sources for routine use. Such limitations might nevertheless be overcome: Giorgetti *et al.* reported promising results from studies involving CD133+ cells from cord blood which require expression of *OCT4* and *SOX2* only to convert into iPS cells [153]. As with other applications, including allogeneic blood stem cells transplantation, these cells which may be available from cell banks and are easy to isolate offer significant advantages over other adult somatic cell sources.

Donor cell type and differentiation efficiency

Embryonic tissues are the most easily prone to reprogramming, a process which results in this particular case in iPSCs which are nearly identical to fESCs. In contrast, reprogramming from commonly accessible adult tissues, which hold the utmost potential for disease modelling, is less efficient since it is limited by barriers related to donor's cells age and differentiation status [105, 110, 154]. Ageing cells harbour higher levels of Ink4/Arf, which limits the efficiency and fidelity of the reprogramming process [110]. Similarly, terminally differentiated blood cells can less efficiently be converted when compared to blood progenitors [154]. As mentioned above, various adult tissues show uneven susceptibility to reprogramming. For instance, keratinocytes reprogram more readily than fibroblasts [34]. Interestingly, iPSCs from stomach or liver cells harbour fewer integrated proviruses than fibroblasts, a feature which might indicate that lower expression levels of reprogramming factors may be required to achieve pluripotency [155]. Of note, cells can sit in intermediate states of reprogramming may so-called "interconvert" and achieve full conversion through sustained passages or treatment with chromatin-modifying agents [126, 156].

Fully reprogrammed generic iPSCs are highly similar to fESCs: like fESCs, iPSCs form teratomas *i.e.*: differentiated benign tumours which involve tissues from all three embryonic germ layers. Nevertheless both functional and molecular significant differences may be evidenced in iPSCs generated from various tissues. Human iPS cells have been suggested to be less prone to differentiation into either neural or blood tissue lineages [157, 158]. Since reversion of methylation is identified as a slow and inefficient process, it has been postulated that residual methylation remains within iPSCs. It was indeed recently shown that both mouse and human iPS cells exhibit noticeable variability in their epigenome. Genome-wide studies have revealed that although being close to ES cells [159-163], iPSC harbour differentially methylated regions (DMRs), which also vary from one line to another [160, 164, 165]. This particular feature also is associated with reprogramming variability [159, 166, 167]. In theory, the reprogramming process would likely erase all tissue specific marks; however, iPS cells do harbour DMRs which are hallmarks of the three-germ layers and of normal development status [160]. In most cases, different epigenetic features observed between iPS cells are characteristic of the tissue from which they originate which is defined as epigenetic memory [159-162]. In addition, it has been further shown that, at low passage, iPS cells retain persistent expression of somatic genes. This transcriptional memory is believed to result from both incomplete silencing of tissue specific genes and potentially incomplete reactivation of ES cell specific genes during the reprogramming process, a phenomenon which might partially be explained by promoters incomplete DNA methylation [163]. Residual epigenetic marks in fact antagonize differentiation into cell lineages distinct from the donor cell type and restrict the downstream process to the latter [160-162]. In studies performed with murine iPS cell lines, this epigenetic memory can be erased over time by extended culture [168]. Nevertheless this observation does not hold true in human iPS cells although cells show a gradual increase in their differentiation potential [162]. Interestingly, several rounds of reprogramming may expand iPS cell differentiation potential towards additional lineages as shown by Kim *et al.* [161].

Finally, the propensity to extended differentiation potential does not necessarily seem to correlate with the age of the donor. Along the same line of investigation, neither significant differences were identified between iPS cell lines originating from healthy *versus* diseased patients nor between lines reprogrammed with three *versus* four-factors [166]. Furthermore, the impact of reprogramming factors stable integration is controversial: Soldner *et al.* [40] claim that only viral excision can resolve the bottleneck of gene expression signature which is observed in differentiated progeny of iPS cells; on the other hand, Boulting *et al.* [166] were not able to detect any effect on differentiation in cell which display persistent transgene expression.

Is genetic instability a payload to reprogramming?

As previously mentioned, like ES cells, iPS cells exhibit variability in their epigenetic, transcriptional and differentiation potential, which in most case, represent a somatic memory originating from features specific to the donor cell. Bock and co-workers postulate that somatic cell memory provides a potential explanation to some iPS deviation although this phenomenon involves a small fraction of overall differences observed in the DNA methylation and gene expression profiles observed in iPS cell line [159].
Aberrant epigenetic profiles were reported in several studies [160, 167]. It thus appears that iPSC lines which were generated in various laboratories, using distinct technologies and derived from different germ layers, share numerous non-randomly distributed megabase-scale regions that are aberrantly methylated in a non-GC rich context. They are associated with alterations in CG methylation, histone modifications and gene expression. These differentially methylated regions observed in iPSCs are actually transmitted to their differentiated progeny at high rate [167].
When considering more subtle modifications, hiPS cell lines have been shown to contain an average of five protein-coding point mutations in the regions sampled (six protein-coding point mutations per exome estimate): this observation is concordant in cell-lines which had been derived by means of five different reprogramming methods. Most of these mutations were non-synonymous, nonsense or splice variants, and were enriched in genes mutated or having well-established causative effect in cancers. Of note, at least half of these reprogramming-associated mutations pre-existed in fact yet at low frequency in the fibroblast progenitors, the remaining half undoubtedly occurred during or after reprogramming [169]. When turning to copy number variations (CNVs) analysis through high-resolution nucleotide polymorphism array, significantly more CNVs are present in early-passage human iPS cells *versus* intermediate passage. Most CNVs are formed *de novo* and generate genetic mosaicism. Hussein and co-workers show evidence that the process of human iPS cells expansion in culture rapidly selects against affected mutated cells: this self-resolving dynamic subsequently drives the iPS line toward a genetic state resembling human ES cells [170]. Whereas experience gathered does validate the hypothesis that massive genetic alteration resolve in cell-catastrophe following death signals, more subtle genetic alterations can conversely accumulate and select in favour of mutated clones with selective growth advantage: in the X-SCiDs gene therapy clinical trials performed in both Paris and London, three years were required in patients *in vivo* for malignant clone outgrowth resulting in leukemia [171, 172].
These studies clearly indicate that both the reprogramming process and the subsequent expansion of iPSCs in culture may carry along the accumulation of genetic abnormalities at the chromosomal, sub-chromosomal and single-base levels. Hussein *et al.* [170] provide evidence that CNVs occurred more frequently at sites prone to replication stress. This observation suggests that the reprogramming process and the strong selection which is associated thereof, generate huge pressures on DNA replication and cell growth, which in turn result in genetic aberrations. Moreover, genetic amplification, deletion or point mutation lesions that arise in iPSCs mostly involve regions prone to cell-cycle regulation and cancer [169, 173, 174]. Although observed modifications during the amplification of iPSCs or their adaptation to culture conditions do not target a specific gene, the frequent association of genes affected with cancer gives cause for

concern. Ensuring cell safety and genome integrity of hiPS through extensive genetic screening should therefore become a standard procedure before any clinical use would be considered at all.

CONCLUSION

iPSCs represent a widely available, non-controversial and practically infinite source of pluripotent cells. Unlike human ESCs, their use is not restricted for ethical reasons, allowing most laboratories to develop research programmes involving this source of human pluripotent stem-cell lines. Since the first published demonstration from Yamanaka's laboratory that fibroblasts can be reprogrammed merely by retroviral delivery of four factors (OSKM), many alternative approaches have been developed in order to induce pluripotency starting from adult somatic cells. Integrative strategies based on retrovirus or transposons mediated gene transfer are most efficient and can be used for prominent current applications such as disease modelling and therapeutic screens, since the absence of persisting genetic modification is not an absolute prerequisite. In contrast, the generation of clinically relevant iPSCs intended for future cell therapy prospects requires technological approaches which do not leave genetic traces behind the cell conversion phase. Although methods based on proteins delivery [90, 92, 161] are relatively inefficient, strategies involving RNAs, directly or *via* Sendaï virus, and their potential improvement seem promising owing to the high efficiency of cell reprogramming [68, 69, 88].

However, 'safer' approaches without genetic scars, do not necessarily prevent variability in lineage-specific genes expression levels or the occurrence of aberrant epigenetic remodelling. Consequently, a pivotal challenge in the iPSC field is to determine how various methodologies affect the quality and the genomic integrity of iPSCs. Whole-genome sequencing and epigenome screening will probably play an important part in the validation of the iPS cell lines generated in terms of transcriptional signatures, epigenic status, genomic integrity, stability, differentiation and tumour potential. Prospects for human iPSCs-based cell therapies have been considered which raise enthusiasm toward regenerative medicine application and tissues replacement for treating injuries or diseases; iPSCs could in theory be generated in an autologous context. Beside a requirement for improved induction strategies and validation methodologies to ultimately warrant safety, iPSCs-based cell therapies will also require in many instances, the correction of genetic defects. Recently, the development of the "Zinc Finger Nuclease" (ZFN) technology enables efficient and precise genetic modifications *via* the induction of a double-strand break in a specific genomic target sequence, followed by the generation of desired modifications during subsequent DNA repair. This process is allowed as ZFN architecture links a DNA-binding domain of eukaryotic transcription factors customized to cleave a specific DNA target sequence and the nuclease domain of the FokI restriction enzyme. Li *et al.* [175] recently achieved *in vivo* genetic correction of haemophilia B *via* ZFN genome targeting and shown persistent correction. Although the relative efficiency of gene targeting still remains under the 1% range, clinical translation of ZFN gene targeting is currently underway in three Phase I clinical trial for the treatment of glioblastoma [176] and HIV [177, 178]. Recently, Yusa and co-workers [179] achieved biallelic correction of a point mutation in the gene *A1AT* responsible for α1-antitrypsin deficiency in diseased iPSCs, using a combination of ZFN and Piggy-Bac technologies, which restores both the structure and function of A1AT in liver cells derived *in vitro* and *in vivo*. Finally, new site-specific nucleases have been developed through engineering of Meganucleases and Transcription Activator-Like Effectors, so called TALENs. These nucleases mediate site-specific genome modifications in human pluripotent cells with similar efficiency and precision as do zinc-finger nucleases [180] (also see chapters A7-3 and A7-4, *ibid.*) and with far less toxicity, as reported. Once combining safe iPSCs induction and homologous recombination will become available, autologous cell-based therapies might be within reach providing clinically relevant cells can be established.

ACKNOWLEDGMENTS

This work has been performed with the support of the EC-DG research through the FP6-Network of Excellence, CLINIGENE: LSHB-CT-2006-018933. E.B. received a post-doctoral fellowship from DIM-Stem Pôle of Région Île-de-France.

REFERENCES

1. French AJ, Adams CA, Anderson LS, Kitchen JR, Hughes MR, Wood SH. Development of human cloned blastocysts following somatic cell nuclear transfer with adult fibroblasts. *Stem Cells* 2008; 26: 485-93.

2. Gurdon JB, Elsdale TR, Fischberg M. Sexually mature individuals of *Xenopus laevis* from the transplantation of single somatic nuclei. *Nature* 1958; 182: 64-5.

3. Gurdon JB, Melton DA. Nuclear reprogramming in cells. *Science* 2008; 322: 1811-5.

4. Cowan CA, Atienza J, Melton DA, Eggan K. Nuclear reprogramming of somatic cells after fusion with human embryonic stem cells. *Science* 2005; 309: 1369-73.

5. Takahashi K, Yamanaka S. Induction of pluripotent stem cells from mouse embryonic and adult fibroblast cultures by defined factors. *Cell* 2006; 126: 663-76.

6. Avilion AA, Nicolis SK, Pevny LH, Perez L, Vivian N, Lovell-Badge R. Multipotent cell lineages in early mouse development depend on SOX2 function. *Genes Dev* 2003; 17: 126-40.

7. Cartwright P, McLean C, Sheppard A, Rivett D, Jones K, Dalton S. LIF/STAT3 controls ES cell self-renewal and pluripotency by a Myc-dependent mechanism. *Development* 2005; 132: 885-96.

8. Li Y, McClintick J, Zhong L, Edenberg HJ, Yoder MC, Chan RJ. Murine embryonic stem cell differentiation is promoted by SOCS-3 and inhibited by the zinc finger transcription factor Klf4. *Blood* 2005; 105: 635-7.

9. Nichols J, Zevnik B, Anastassiadis K, Niwa H, Klewe-Nebenius D, Chambers I, Scholer H, Smith A. Formation of pluripotent stem cells in the mammalian embryo depends on the POU transcription factor Oct4. *Cell* 1998; 95: 379-91.

10. Niwa H, Miyazaki J, Smith AG. Quantitative expression of Oct-3/4 defines differentiation, dedifferentiation or self-renewal of ES cells. *Nat Genet* 2000; 24: 372-6.

11. Takahashi K, Tanabe K, Ohnuki M, Narita M, Ichisaka T, Tomoda K, Yamanaka S. Induction of pluripotent stem cells from adult human fibroblasts by defined factors. *Cell* 2007; 131: 861-72.

12. Yu J, Vodyanik MA, Smuga-Otto K, Antosiewicz-Bourget J, Frane JL, Tian S, *et al.* Induced pluripotent stem cell lines derived from human somatic cells. *Science* 2007; 318: 1917-20.

13. Huangfu D, Maehr R, Guo W, Eijkelenboom A, Snitow M, Chen AE, Melton DA. Induction of pluripotent stem cells by defined factors is greatly improved by small-molecule compounds. *Nat Biotechnol* 2008; 26: 795-7.

14. Shi Y, Do JT, Desponts C, Hahm HS, Scholer HR, Ding S. A combined chemical and genetic approach for the generation of induced pluripotent stem cells. *Cell Stem Cell* 2008; 2: 525-8.

15. Park IH, Lerou PH, Zhao R, Huo H, Daley GQ. Generation of human-induced pluripotent stem cells. *Nat Protoc* 2008; 3: 1180-6.

16. Gonzalez F, Boue S, Izpisua Belmonte JC. Methods for making induced pluripotent stem cells: reprogramming a la carte. *Nat Rev Genet* 2011; 12: 231-42.

17. Kitamura T, Koshino Y, Shibata F, Oki T, Nakajima H, Nosaka T, Kumagai H. Retrovirus-mediated gene transfer and expression cloning: powerful tools in functional genomics. *Exp Hematol* 2003; 31: 1007-14.

18. Aasen T, Raya A, Barrero MJ, Garreta E, Consiglio A, Gonzalez F, *et al*. Efficient and rapid generation of induced pluripotent stem cells from human keratinocytes. *Nat Biotechnol* 2008; 26: 1276-84.

19. Hawley RG, Lieu FH, Fong AZ, Hawley TS. Versatile retroviral vectors for potential use in gene therapy. *Gene Ther* 1994; 1: 136-8.

20. Jahner D, Stuhlmann H, Stewart CL, Harbers K, Lohler J, Simon I, Jaenisch R. *De novo* methylation and expression of retroviral genomes during mouse embryogenesis. *Nature* 1982; 298: 623-8.

21. Stewart CL, Stuhlmann H, Jahner D, Jaenisch R. *De novo* methylation, expression, and infectivity of retroviral genomes introduced into embryonal carcinoma cells. *Proc Natl Acad Sci USA* 1982; 79: 4098-102.

22. Nakagawa M, Koyanagi M, Tanabe K, Takahashi K, Ichisaka T, Aoi T, *et al*. Generation of induced pluripotent stem cells without Myc from mouse and human fibroblasts. *Nat Biotechnol* 2008; 26: 101-6.

23. Matsui T, Leung D, Miyashita H, Maksakova IA, Miyachi H, Kimura H, *et al*. Proviral silencing in embryonic stem cells requires the histone methyltransferase ESET. *Nature* 2010; 464: 927-31.

24. Hotta A, Ellis J. Retroviral vector silencing during iPS cell induction: an epigenetic beacon that signals distinct pluripotent states. *J Cell Biochem* 2008; 105: 940-8.

25. Ryan MD, Drew J. Foot-and-mouth disease virus 2A oligopeptide mediated cleavage of an artificial polyprotein. *Embo J* 1994; 13: 928-33.

26. Ryan MD, Flint M. Virus-encoded proteinases of the picornavirus super-group. *J Gen Virol* 1997; 78 : 699-723.

27. Kaji K, Norrby K, Paca A, Mileikovsky M, Mohseni P, Woltjen K. Virus-free induction of pluripotency and subsequent excision of reprogramming factors. *Nature* 2009; 458: 771-5.

28. Lin SL, Chang DC, Lin CH, Ying SY, Leu D, Wu DT. Regulation of somatic cell reprogramming through inducible mir-302 expression. *Nucleic Acids Res* 2011; 39: 1054-65.

29. Huangfu D, Osafune K, Maehr R, Guo W, Eijkelenboom A, Chen S, Muhlestein W, Melton DA. Induction of pluripotent stem cells from primary human fibroblasts with only Oct4 and Sox2. *Nat Biotechnol* 2008; 26: 1269-75.

30. Shi Y, Desponts C, Do JT, Hahm HS, Scholer HR, Ding S. Induction of pluripotent stem cells from mouse embryonic fibroblasts by Oct4 and Klf4 with small-molecule compounds. *Cell Stem Cell* 2008; 3: 568-74.

31. Buecker C, Chen HH, Polo JM, Daheron L, Bu L, Barakat TS, *et al*. A murine ESC-like state facilitates transgenesis and homologous recombination in human pluripotent stem cells. *Cell Stem Cell* 2010; 6: 535-46.

32. Hasegawa K, Zhang P, Wei Z, Pomeroy JE, Lu W, Pera MF. Comparison of reprogramming efficiency between transduction of reprogramming factors, cell-cell fusion, and cytoplast fusion. *Stem Cells* 2010; 28: 1338-48.

33. Loh YH, Hartung O, Li H, Guo C, Sahalie JM, Manos PD, *et al.* Reprogramming of T cells from human peripheral blood. *Cell Stem Cell* 2010; 7: 15-9.

34. Maherali N, Ahfeldt T, Rigamonti A, Utikal J, Cowan C, Hochedlinger K. A high-efficiency system for the generation and study of human induced pluripotent stem cells. *Cell Stem Cell* 2008; 3: 340-5.

35. Utikal J, Maherali N, Kulalert W, Hochedlinger K. Sox2 is dispensable for the reprogramming of melanocytes and melanoma cells into induced pluripotent stem cells. *J Cell Sci* 2009; 122: 3502-10.

36. Varas F, Stadtfeld M, de Andres-Aguayo L, Maherali N, di Tullio A, Pantano L, *et al.* Fibroblast-derived induced pluripotent stem cells show no common retroviral vector insertions. *Stem Cells* 2009; 27: 300-6.

37. Kane NM, Nowrouzi A, Mukherjee S, Blundell MP, Greig JA, Lee WK, *et al.* Lentivirus-mediated reprogramming of somatic cells in the absence of transgenic transcription factors. *Mol Ther* 2010; 18: 2139-45.

38. Carey BW, Markoulaki S, Hanna J, Saha K, Gao Q, Mitalipova M, Jaenisch R. Reprogramming of murine and human somatic cells using a single polycistronic vector. *Proc Natl Acad Sci USA* 2009; 106: 157-62.

39. Rodriguez-Piza I, Richaud-Patin Y, Vassena R, Gonzalez F, Barrero MJ, Veiga A, Raya A, Belmonte JC. Reprogramming of human fibroblasts to induced pluripotent stem cells under xeno-free conditions. *Stem Cells* 2010; 28: 36-44.

40. Soldner F, Hockemeyer D, Beard C, Gao Q, Bell GW, Cook EG, *et al.* Parkinson's disease patient-derived induced pluripotent stem cells free of viral reprogramming factors. *Cell* 2009; 136: 964-77.

41. Chang CW, Lai YS, Pawlik KM, Liu K, Sun CW, Li C, Schoeb TR, Townes TM. Polycistronic lentiviral vector for «hit and run» reprogramming of adult skin fibroblasts to induced pluripotent stem cells. *Stem Cells* 2009; 27: 1042-9.

42. O'Gorman S, Fox DT, Wahl GM. Recombinase-mediated gene activation and site-specific integration in mammalian cells. *Science* 1991; 251: 1351-5.

43. Nakano M, Ishimura M, Chiba J, Kanegae Y, Saito I. DNA substrates influence the recombination efficiency mediated by FLP recombinase expressed in mammalian cells. *Microbiol Immunol* 2001; 45: 657-65.

44. Schmidt-Supprian M, Rajewsky K. Vagaries of conditional gene targeting. *Nat Immunol* 2007; 8: 665-8.

45. Voelkel C, Galla M, Maetzig T, Warlich E, Kuehle J, Zychlinski D, *et al.* Protein transduction from retroviral Gag precursors. *Proc Natl Acad Sci USA* 2010; 107: 7805-10.

46. Cary LC, Goebel M, Corsaro BG, Wang HG, Rosen E, Fraser MJ. Transposon mutagenesis of baculoviruses: analysis of Trichoplusia ni transposon IFP2 insertions within the FP-locus of nuclear polyhedrosis viruses. *Virology* 1989; 172: 156-69.

47. Fraser MJ, Ciszczon T, Elick T, Bauser C. Precise excision of TTAA-specific lepidopteran transposons piggyBac (IFP2) and tagalong (TFP3) from the baculovirus genome in cell lines from two species of Lepidoptera. *Insect Mol Biol* 1996; 5: 141-51.

48. Fraser MJ, Cary L, Boonvisudhi K, Wang HG. Assay for movement of Lepidopteran transposon IFP2 in insect cells using a baculovirus genome as a target DNA. *Virology* 1995; 211: 397-407.

49. Woltjen K, Michael IP, Mohseni P, Desai R, Mileikovsky M, Hamalainen R, *et al.* piggyBac transposition reprograms fibroblasts to induced pluripotent stem cells. *Nature* 2009; 458: 766-70.

50. Ivics Z, Hackett PB, Plasterk RH, Izsvak Z. Molecular reconstruction of Sleeping Beauty, a Tc1-like transposon from fish, and its transposition in human cells. *Cell* 1997; 91: 501-10.

51. Mates L, Chuah MK, Belay E, Jerchow B, Manoj N, Acosta-Sanchez A, *et al.* Molecular evolution of a novel hyperactive Sleeping Beauty transposase enables robust stable gene transfer in vertebrates. *Nat Genet* 2009; 41: 753-61.

52. Iszvak Z, Escobar H, Johen S, Ivics Z, Kusk P, Thumann G. *The Sleeping Beauty-based non viral, integrating vector system, the next challenge.* Paris: e-chips, 2011: 73.

53. Belay E, Dastidar S, Vandendriessche T, Chuah MK. Transposon-mediated gene transfer into adult and induced pluripotent stem cells. *Curr Gene Ther* 2011; 11: 406-13.

54. Wang W, Lin C, Lu D, Ning Z, Cox T, Melvin D, *et al.* Chromosomal transposition of PiggyBac in mouse embryonic stem cells. *Proc Natl Acad Sci USA* 2008; 105: 9290-5.

55. Galla M, Schambach A, Falk CS, Maetzig T, Kuehle J, Lange K, *et al.* Avoiding cytotoxicity of transposases by dose-controlled mRNA delivery. *Nucleic Acids Res* 2011; 39: 7147-60.

56. Yu SS, Dan K, Chono H, Chatani E, Mineno J, Kato I. Transient gene expression mediated by integrase-defective retroviral vectors. *Biochem Biophys Res Commun* 2008; 368: 942-7.

57. Philippe S, Sarkis C, Barkats M, Mammeri H, Ladroue C, Petit C, Mallet J, Serguera C. Lentiviral vectors with a defective integrase allow efficient and sustained transgene expression *in vitro* and *in vivo. Proc Natl Acad Sci USA* 2006; 103: 17684-9.

58. Saenz DT, Loewen N, Peretz M, Whitwam T, Barraza R, Howell KG, *et al.* Unintegrated lentivirus DNA persistence and accessibility to expression in nondividing cells: analysis with class I integrase mutants. *J Virol* 2004; 78: 2906-20.

59. Yanez-Munoz RJ, Balaggan KS, MacNeil A, Howe SJ, Schmidt M, Smith AJ, *et al.* Effective gene therapy with nonintegrating lentiviral vectors. *Nat Med* 2006; 12: 348-53.

60. Stadtfeld M, Nagaya M, Utikal J, Weir G, Hochedlinger K. Induced pluripotent stem cells generated without viral integration. *Science* 2008; 322: 945-9.

61. Graham FL, Prevec L. Adenovirus-based expression vectors and recombinant vaccines. *Biotechnology* 1992; 20: 363-90.

62. He TC, Zhou S, da Costa LT, Yu J, Kinzler KW, Vogelstein B. A simplified system for generating recombinant adenoviruses. *Proc Natl Acad Sci USA* 1998; 95: 2509-14.

63. Zhou W, Freed CR. Adenoviral gene delivery can reprogram human fibroblasts to induced pluripotent stem cells. *Stem Cells* 2009; 27: 2667-74.

64. Stephen SL, Sivanandam VG, Kochanek S. Homologous and heterologous recombination between adenovirus vector DNA and chromosomal DNA. *J Gene Med* 2008; 10: 1176-89.

65. Lamb R, Kolakofsky D. *Paramyxoviridae: the viruses and their replication.* New York: Lippincott-Williams and Wilkins, 2001: 1177-204.

66. Tokusumi T, Iida A, Hirata T, Kato A, Nagai Y, Hasegawa M. Recombinant Sendai viruses expressing different levels of a foreign reporter gene. *Virus Res* 2002; 86: 33-8.

67. Li HO, Zhu YF, Asakawa M, Kuma H, Hirata T, Ueda Y, *et al.* A cytoplasmic RNA vector derived from nontransmissible Sendai virus with efficient gene transfer and expression. *J Virol* 2000; 74: 6564-9.

68. Fusaki N, Ban H, Nishiyama A, Saeki K, Hasegawa M. Efficient induction of transgene-free human pluripotent stem cells using a vector based on Sendai virus, an RNA virus that does not integrate into the host genome. *Proc Jpn Acad Ser B Phys Biol Sci* 2009; 85: 348-62.

69. Seki T, Yuasa S, Oda M, Egashira T, Yae K, Kusumoto D, *et al.* Generation of induced pluripotent stem cells from human terminally differentiated circulating T cells. *Cell Stem Cell* 2010; 7: 11-4.

70. Nishimura K, Sano M, Ohtaka M, Furuta B, Umemura Y, Nakajima Y, *et al.* Development of defective and persistent Sendai virus vector: a unique gene delivery/expression system ideal for cell reprogramming. *J Biol Chem* 2011; 286: 4760-71.

71. Griesenbach U, Inoue M, Hasegawa M, Alton EW. Sendai virus for gene therapy and vaccination. *Curr Opin Mol Ther* 2005; 7: 346-52.

72. Gonzalez F, Barragan Monasterio M, Tiscornia G, Montserrat Pulido N, Vassena R, Batlle Morera L, Rodriguez Piza I, Izpisua Belmonte JC. Generation of mouse-induced pluripotent stem cells by transient expression of a single nonviral polycistronic vector. *Proc Natl Acad Sci USA* 2009; 106: 8918-22.

73. Okita K, Hong H, Takahashi K, Yamanaka S. Generation of mouse-induced pluripotent stem cells with plasmid vectors. *Nat Protoc* 2010; 5: 418-28.

74. Okita K, Nakagawa M, Hyenjong H, Ichisaka T, Yamanaka S. Generation of mouse induced pluripotent stem cells without viral vectors. *Science* 2008; 322: 949-53.

75. Si-Tayeb K, Noto FK, Sepac A, Sedlic F, Bosnjak ZJ, Lough JW, Duncan SA. Generation of human induced pluripotent stem cells by simple transient transfection of plasmid DNA encoding reprogramming factors. *BMC Dev Biol* 2010; 10: 81.

76. Montserrat N, Garreta E, Gonzalez F, Gutierrez J, Eguizabal C, Ramos V, Borros S, Izpisua Belmonte JC. Simple generation of human induced pluripotent stem cells using poly-(beta)-amino esters as the non-viral gene delivery system. *J Biol Chem* 2011; 286: 12417-28.

77. Yu J, Hu K, Smuga-Otto K, Tian S, Stewart R, Slukvin, II, Thomson JA. Human induced pluripotent stem cells free of vector and transgene sequences. *Science* 2009; 324: 797-801.

78. Yates J, Warren N, Reisman D, Sugden B. A cis-acting element from the Epstein-Barr viral genome that permits stable replication of recombinant plasmids in latently infected cells. *Proc Natl Acad Sci USA* 1984; 81: 3806-10.

79. Yates JL, Warren N, Sugden B. Stable replication of plasmids derived from Epstein-Barr virus in various mammalian cells. *Nature* 1985; 313: 812-5.

80. Okita K, Matsumura Y, Sato Y, Okada A, Morizane A, Okamoto S, *et al*. A more efficient method to generate integration-free human iPS cells. *Nat Methods* 2011; 8: 409-12.

81. Chou BK, Mali P, Huang X, Ye Z, Dowey SN, Resar LM, *et al*. Efficient human iPS cell derivation by a non-integrating plasmid from blood cells with unique epigenetic and gene expression signatures. *Cell Res* 2011; 21: 518-29.

82. Chen ZY, He CY, Ehrhardt A, Kay MA. Minicircle DNA vectors devoid of bacterial DNA result in persistent and high-level transgene expression *in vivo*. *Mol Ther* 2003; 8: 495-500.

83. Chen ZY, He CY, Kay MA. Improved production and purification of minicircle DNA vector free of plasmid bacterial sequences and capable of persistent transgene expression *in vivo*. *Hum Gene Ther* 2005; 16: 126-31.

84. Jia F, Wilson KD, Sun N, Gupta DM, Huang M, Li Z, *et al*. A nonviral minicircle vector for deriving human iPS cells. *Nat Methods* 2010; 7: 197-9.

85. Narsinh KH, Jia F, Robbins RC, Kay MA, Longaker MT, Wu JC. Generation of adult human induced pluripotent stem cells using nonviral minicircle DNA vectors. *Nat Protoc* 2011; 6: 78-88.

86. Plews JR, Li J, Jones M, Moore HD, Mason C, Andrews PW, Na J. Activation of pluripotency genes in human fibroblast cells by a novel mRNA based approach. *PLoS One* 2010; 5: e14397.

87. Yakubov E, Rechavi G, Rozenblatt S, Givol D. Reprogramming of human fibroblasts to pluripotent stem cells using mRNA of four transcription factors. *Biochem Biophys Res Commun* 2010; 394: 189-93.

88. Warren L, Manos PD, Ahfeldt T, Loh YH, Li H, Lau F, *et al*. Highly efficient reprogramming to pluripotency and directed differentiation of human cells with synthetic modified mRNA. *Cell Stem Cell* 2010; 7: 618-30.

89. Wilmut I, Schnieke AE, McWhir J, Kind AJ, Campbell KH. Viable offspring derived from fetal and adult mammalian cells. *Nature* 1997; 385: 810-3.

90. Cho HJ, Lee CS, Kwon YW, Paek JS, Lee SH, Hur J, *et al.* Induction of pluripotent stem cells from adult somatic cells by protein-based reprogramming without genetic manipulation. *Blood* 2010; 116: 386-95.

91. Han J, Sachdev PS, Sidhu KS. A combined epigenetic and non-genetic approach for reprogramming human somatic cells. *PLoS One* 2010; 5: e12297.

92. Zhou H, Wu S, Joo JY, Zhu S, Han DW, Lin T, *et al.* Generation of induced pluripotent stem cells using recombinant proteins. *Cell Stem Cell* 2009; 4: 381-4.

93. Wadia JS, Dowdy SF. Protein transduction technology. *Curr Opin Biotechnol* 2002; 13: 52-6.

94. Kim D, Kim CH, Moon JI, Chung YG, Chang MY, Han BS, *et al.* Generation of human induced pluripotent stem cells by direct delivery of reprogramming proteins. *Cell Stem Cell* 2009; 4: 472-6.

95. Takahashi K, Okita K, Nakagawa M, Yamanaka S. Induction of pluripotent stem cells from fibroblast cultures. *Nat Protoc* 2007; 2: 3081-9.

96. Papapetrou EP, Tomishima MJ, Chambers SM, Mica Y, Reed E, Menon J, *et al.* Stoichiometric and temporal requirements of Oct4, Sox2, Klf4, and c-Myc expression for efficient human iPSC induction and differentiation. *Proc Natl Acad Sci USA* 2009; 106: 12759-64.

97. Lee TH, Song SH, Kim KL, Yi JY, Shin GH, Kim JY, *et al.* Functional recapitulation of smooth muscle cells via induced pluripotent stem cells from human aortic smooth muscle cells. *Circ Res* 2010; 106: 120-8.

98. Kamata M, Liu S, Liang M, Nagaoka Y, Chen IS. Generation of human induced pluripotent stem cells bearing an anti-HIV transgene by a lentiviral vector carrying an internal murine leukemia virus promoter. *Hum Gene Ther* 2010; 21: 1555-67.

99. Liao J, Wu Z, Wang Y, Cheng L, Cui C, Gao Y, *et al.* Enhanced efficiency of generating induced pluripotent stem (iPS) cells from human somatic cells by a combination of six transcription factors. *Cell Res* 2008; 18: 600-3.

100. Zhao R, Daley GQ. From fibroblasts to iPS cells: induced pluripotency by defined factors. *J Cell Biochem* 2008; 105: 949-55.

101. Tsubooka N, Ichisaka T, Okita K, Takahashi K, Nakagawa M, Yamanaka S. Roles of Sall4 in the generation of pluripotent stem cells from blastocysts and fibroblasts. *Genes Cells* 2009; 14: 683-94.

102. Ruiz S, Panopoulos AD, Herrerias A, Bissig KD, Lutz M, Berggren WT, Verma IM, Izpisua Belmonte JC. A high proliferation rate is required for cell reprogramming and maintenance of human embryonic stem cell identity. *Curr Biol* 2011; 21: 45-52.

103. Edel MJ, Menchon C, Menendez S, Consiglio A, Raya A, Izpisua Belmonte JC. Rem2 GTPase maintains survival of human embryonic stem cells as well as enhancing reprogramming by regulating p53 and cyclin D1. *Genes Dev* 2010; 24: 561-73.

104. Kawamura T, Suzuki J, Wang YV, Menendez S, Morera LB, Raya A, Wahl GM, Belmonte JC. Linking the p53 tumour suppressor pathway to somatic cell reprogramming. *Nature* 2009; 460: 1140-4.

105. Marion RM, Strati K, Li H, Murga M, Blanco R, Ortega S, *et al.* A p53-mediated DNA damage response limits reprogramming to ensure iPS cell genomic integrity. *Nature* 2009; 460: 1149-53.

106. Menendez S, Camus S, Izpisua Belmonte JC. p53: guardian of reprogramming. *Cell Cycle* 2010; 9: 3887-91.

107. Hong H, Takahashi K, Ichisaka T, Aoi T, Kanagawa O, Nakagawa M, Okita K, Yamanaka S. Suppression of induced pluripotent stem cell generation by the p53-p21 pathway. *Nature* 2009; 460: 1132-5.

108. Mah N, Wang Y, Liao MC, Prigione A, Jozefczuk J, Lichtner B, et al. Molecular insights into reprogramming-initiation events mediated by the OSKM gene regulatory network. *PLoS One* 2011; 6: e24351.

109. Kim J, Lengner CJ, Kirak O, Hanna J, Cassady JP, Lodato MA, *et al.* Reprogramming of post-natal neurons into induced pluripotent stem cells by defined factors. *Stem Cells* 2011; 29: 992-1000.

110. Li H, Collado M, Villasante A, Strati K, Ortega S, Canamero M, Blasco MA, Serrano M. The Ink4/Arf locus is a barrier for iPS cell reprogramming. *Nature* 2009; 460: 1136-9.

111. Raya A, Rodriguez-Piza I, Guenechea G, Vassena R, Navarro S, Barrero MJ, *et al.* Disease-corrected haematopoietic progenitors from Fanconi anaemia induced pluripotent stem cells. *Nature* 2009; 460: 53-9.

112. Silva J, Barrandon O, Nichols J, Kawaguchi J, Theunissen TW, Smith A. Promotion of repro-gramming to ground state pluripotency by signal inhibition. *PLoS Biol* 2008; 6: e253.

113. Li W, Zhou H, Abujarour R, Zhu S, Young Joo J, Lin T, *et al.* Generation of human-induced pluripotent stem cells in the absence of exogenous Sox2. *Stem Cells* 2009; 27: 2992-3000.

114. Mallanna SK, Rizzino A. Emerging roles of microRNAs in the control of embryonic stem cells and the generation of induced pluripotent stem cells. *Dev Biol* 2010; 344: 16-25.

115. Wang Y, Baskerville S, Shenoy A, Babiarz JE, Baehner L, Blelloch R. Embryonic stem cell-specific microRNAs regulate the G1-S transition and promote rapid proliferation. *Nat Genet* 2008; 40: 1478-83.

116. Judson RL, Babiarz JE, Venere M, Blelloch R. Embryonic stem cell-specific microRNAs promote induced pluripotency. *Nat Biotechnol* 2009; 27: 459-61.

117. Card DA, Hebbar PB, Li L, Trotter KW, Komatsu Y, Mishina Y, Archer TK. Oct4/Sox2-regulated miR-302 targets cyclin D1 in human embryonic stem cells. *Mol Cell Biol* 2008; 28: 6426-38.

118. Marson A, Levine SS, Cole MF, Frampton GM, Brambrink T, Johnstone S, *et al.* Connecting microRNA genes to the core transcriptional regulatory circuitry of embryonic stem cells. *Cell* 2008; 134: 521-33.

119. Lin SL, Chang DC, Chang-Lin S, Lin CH, Wu DT, Chen DT, Ying SY. Mir-302 reprograms human skin cancer cells into a pluripotent ES-cell-like state. *RNA* 2008; 14: 2115-24.

120. Suh MR, Lee Y, Kim JY, Kim SK, Moon SH, Lee JY, *et al.* Human embryonic stem cells express a unique set of microRNAs. *Dev Biol* 2004; 270: 488-98.

121. Wilson KD, Venkatasubrahmanyam S, Jia F, Sun N, Butte AJ, Wu JC. MicroRNA profiling of human-induced pluripotent stem cells. *Stem Cells Dev* 2009; 18: 749-58.

122. Yoshida Y, Takahashi K, Okita K, Ichisaka T, Yamanaka S. Hypoxia enhances the generation of induced pluripotent stem cells. *Cell Stem Cell* 2009; 5: 237-41.

123. Ezashi T, Das P, Roberts RM. Low O2 tensions and the prevention of differentiation of hES cells. *Proc Natl Acad Sci USA* 2005; 102: 4783-8.

124. Morrison SJ, Csete M, Groves AK, Melega W, Wold B, Anderson DJ. Culture in reduced levels of oxygen promotes clonogenic sympathoadrenal differentiation by isolated neural crest stem cells. *J Neurosci* 2000; 20: 7370-6.

125. Forristal CE, Wright KL, Hanley NA, Oreffo RO, Houghton FD. Hypoxia inducible factors reg-ulate pluripotency and proliferation in human embryonic stem cells cultured at reduced oxygen tensions. *Reproduction* 2010; 139: 85-97.

126. Mikkelsen TS, Hanna J, Zhang X, Ku M, Wernig M, Schorderet P, *et al.* Dissecting direct re-programming through integrative genomic analysis. *Nature* 2008; 454: 49-55.

127. Esteban MA, Wang T, Qin B, Yang J, Qin D, Cai J, *et al.* Vitamin C enhances the generation of mouse and human induced pluripotent stem cells. *Cell Stem Cell* 2010; 6: 71-9.

128. Chung TL, Brena RM, Kolle G, Grimmond SM, Berman BP, Laird PW, Pera MF, Wolvetang EJ. Vitamin C promotes widespread yet specific DNA demethylation of the epigenome in human em-bryonic stem cells. *Stem Cells* 2010; 28: 1848-55.

129. Picanco-Castro V, Russo-Carbolante E, Reis LC, Fraga AM, de Magalhaes DA, Orellana MD, *et al.* Pluripotent reprogramming of fibroblasts by lentiviral mediated insertion of SOX2, C-MYC, and TCL-1A. *Stem Cells Dev* 2011; 20: 169-80.

130. Laine J, Kunstle G, Obata T, Sha M, Noguchi M. The protooncogene TCL1 is an Akt kinase coactivator. *Mol Cell* 2000; 6: 395-407.

131. Mali P, Ye Z, Hommond HH, Yu X, Lin J, Chen G, Zou J, Cheng L. Improved efficiency and pace of generating induced pluripotent stem cells from human adult and fetal fibroblasts. *Stem Cells* 2008; 26: 1998-2005.

132. Feldman N, Gerson A, Fang J, Li E, Zhang Y, Shinkai Y, Cedar H, Bergman Y. G9a-mediated irreversible epigenetic inactivation of Oct-3/4 during early embryogenesis. *Nat Cell Biol* 2006; 8: 188-94.

133. Defoort EN, Kim PM, Winn LM. Valproic acid increases conservative homologous recombination frequency and reactive oxygen species formation: a potential mechanism for valproic acid-induced neural tube defects. *Mol Pharmacol* 2006; 69: 1304-10.

134. Sha K, Winn LM. Characterization of valproic acid-initiated homologous recombination. *Birth Defects Res B Dev Reprod Toxicol* 2010; 89: 124-32.

135. Purrucker JC, Fricke A, Ong MF, Rube C, Rube CE, Mahlknecht U. HDAC inhibition radiosensitizes human normal tissue cells and reduces DNA double-strand break repair capacity. *Oncol Rep* 2010; 23: 263-9.

136. Elenbaas B, Spirio L, Koerner F, Fleming MD, Zimonjic DB, Donaher JL, *et al.* Human breast cancer cells generated by oncogenic transformation of primary mammary epithelial cells. *Genes Dev* 2001; 15: 50-65.

137. Hahn WC, Counter CM, Lundberg AS, Beijersbergen RL, Brooks MW, Weinberg RA. Creation of human tumour cells with defined genetic elements. *Nature* 1999; 400: 464-8.

138. Lundberg AS, Randell SH, Stewart SA, Elenbaas B, Hartwell KA, Brooks MW, *et al.* Immortalization and transformation of primary human airway epithelial cells by gene transfer. *Oncogene* 2002; 21: 4577-86.

139. Nakagawa M, Takizawa N, Narita M, Ichisaka T, Yamanaka S. Promotion of direct reprogramming by transformation-deficient Myc. *Proc Natl Acad Sci USA* 2010; 107: 14152-7.

140. Hockemeyer D, Soldner F, Cook EG, Gao Q, Mitalipova M, Jaenisch R. A drug-inducible system for direct reprogramming of human somatic cells to pluripotency. *Cell Stem Cell* 2008; 3: 346-53.

141. Lowry WE, Richter L, Yachechko R, Pyle AD, Tchieu J, Sridharan R, Clark AT, Plath K. Generation of human induced pluripotent stem cells from dermal fibroblasts. *Proc Natl Acad Sci USA* 2008; 105: 2883-8.

142. Vallier L, Touboul T, Brown S, Cho C, Bilican B, Alexander M, *et al.* Signaling pathways controlling pluripotency and early cell fate decisions of human induced pluripotent stem cells. *Stem Cells* 2009; 27: 2655-66.

143. Yehezkel S, Rebibo-Sabbah A, Segev Y, Tzukerman M, Shaked R, Huber I, *et al.* Reprogramming of telomeric regions during the generation of human induced pluripotent stem cells and subsequent differentiation into fibroblast-like derivatives. *Epigenetics* 2011; 6: 63-75.

144. Choi KD, Yu J, Smuga-Otto K, Salvagiotto G, Rehrauer W, Vodyanik M, Thomson J, Slukvin I. Hematopoietic and endothelial differentiation of human induced pluripotent stem cells. *Stem Cells* 2009; 27: 559-67.

145. Oda Y, Yoshimura Y, Ohnishi H, Tadokoro M, Katsube Y, Sasao M, *et al.* Induction of pluripotent stem cells from human third molar mesenchymal stromal cells. *J Biol Chem* 2010; 285: 29270-8.

146. Tamaoki N, Takahashi K, Tanaka T, Ichisaka T, Aoki H, Takeda-Kawaguchi T, *et al*. Dental pulp cells for induced pluripotent stem cell banking. *J Dent Res* 2010; 89: 773-8.

147. Nagata S, Toyoda M, Yamaguchi S, Hirano K, Makino H, Nishino K, *et al*. Efficient reprogramming of human and mouse primary extra-embryonic cells to pluripotent stem cells. *Genes Cells* 2009; 14: 1395-404.

148. Ye L, Chang JC, Lin C, Sun X, Yu J, Kan YW. Induced pluripotent stem cells offer new approach to therapy in thalassemia and sickle cell anemia and option in prenatal diagnosis in genetic diseases. *Proc Natl Acad Sci USA* 2009; 106: 9826-30.

149. Zhao HX, Li Y, Jin HF, Xie L, Liu C, Jiang F, *et al*. Rapid and efficient reprogramming of human amnion-derived cells into pluripotency by three factors OCT4/SOX2/NANOG. *Differentiation* 2010; 80: 123-9.

150. Ho PJ, Yen ML, Lin JD, Chen LS, Hu HI, Yeh CK, *et al*. Endogenous KLF4 expression in human fetal endothelial cells allows for reprogramming to pluripotency with just OCT3/4 and SOX2: brief report. *Arterioscler Thromb Vasc Biol* 2010; 30: 1905-7.

151. Hester ME, Song S, Miranda CJ, Eagle A, Schwartz PH, Kaspar BK. Two factor reprogramming of human neural stem cells into pluripotency. *PLoS One* 2009; 4: e7044.

152. Kim JB, Greber B, Arauzo-Bravo MJ, Meyer J, Park KI, Zaehres H, Scholer HR. Direct reprogramming of human neural stem cells by OCT4. *Nature* 2009; 461: 649-3.

153. Giorgetti A, Montserrat N, Aasen T, Gonzalez F, Rodriguez-Piza I, Vassena R, *et al*. Generation of induced pluripotent stem cells from human cord blood using OCT4 and SOX2. *Cell Stem Cell* 2009; 5: 353-7.

154. Eminli S, Foudi A, Stadtfeld M, Maherali N, Ahfeldt T, Mostoslavsky G, Hock H, Hochedlinger K. Differentiation stage determines potential of hematopoietic cells for reprogramming into induced pluripotent stem cells. *Nat Genet* 2009; 41: 968-76.

155. Aoi T, Yae K, Nakagawa M, Ichisaka T, Okita K, Takahashi K, Chiba T, Yamanaka S. Generation of pluripotent stem cells from adult mouse liver and stomach cells. *Science* 2008; 321: 699-702.

156. Chan EM, Ratanasirintrawoot S, Park IH, Manos PD, Loh YH, Huo H, *et al*. Live cell imaging distinguishes bona fide human iPS cells from partially reprogrammed cells. *Nat Biotechnol* 2009; 27: 1033-7.

157. Feng Q, Lu SJ, Klimanskaya I, Gomes I, Kim D, Chung Y, *et al*. Hemangioblastic derivatives from human induced pluripotent stem cells exhibit limited expansion and early senescence. *Stem Cells* 2010; 28: 704-12.

158. Hu BY, Weick JP, Yu J, Ma LX, Zhang XQ, Thomson JA, Zhang SC. Neural differentiation of human induced pluripotent stem cells follows developmental principles but with variable potency. *Proc Natl Acad Sci USA* 2010; 107: 4335-40.

159. Bock C, Kiskinis E, Verstappen G, Gu H, Boulting G, Smith ZD, *et al*. Reference maps of human ES and iPS cell variation enable high-throughput characterization of pluripotent cell lines. *Cell* 2011; 144: 439-52.

160. Doi A, Park IH, Wen B, Murakami P, Aryee MJ, Irizarry R, *et al*. Differential methylation of tissue- and cancer-specific CpG island shores distinguishes human induced pluripotent stem cells, embryonic stem cells and fibroblasts. *Nat Genet* 2009; 41: 1350-3.

161. Kim K, Doi A, Wen B, Ng K, Zhao R, Cahan P, *et al*. Epigenetic memory in induced pluripotent stem cells. *Nature* 2010; 467: 285-90.

162. Kim K, Zhao R, Doi A, Ng K, Unternaehrer J, Cahan P, *et al*. Donor cell type can influence the epigenome and differentiation potential of human induced pluripotent stem cells. *Nat Biotechnol* 2011; 29, 1117-9

163. Ohi Y, Qin H, Hong C, Blouin L, Polo JM, Guo T, *et al*. Incomplete DNA methylation underlies a transcriptional memory of somatic cells in human iPS cells. *Nat Cell Biol* 2011; 13: 541-9.

164. Ball MP, Li JB, Gao Y, Lee JH, LeProust EM, Park IH, *et al.* Targeted and genome-scale strategies reveal gene-body methylation signatures in human cells. *Nat Biotechnol* 2009; 27: 361-8.

165. Stadtfeld M, Apostolou E, Akutsu H, Fukuda A, Follett P, Natesan S, *et al.* Aberrant silencing of imprinted genes on chromosome 12qF1 in mouse induced pluripotent stem cells. *Nature* 2010; 465: 175-81.

166. Boulting GL, Kiskinis E, Croft GF, Amoroso MW, Oakley DH, Wainger BJ, *et al.* A functionally characterized test set of human induced pluripotent stem cells. *Nat Biotechnol* 2011; 29: 279-86.

167. Lister R, Pelizzola M, Kida YS, Hawkins RD, Nery JR, Hon G, *et al.* Hotspots of aberrant epigenomic reprogramming in human induced pluripotent stem cells. *Nature* 2011; 471: 68-73.

168. Polo JM, Liu S, Figueroa ME, Kulalert W, Eminli S, Tan KY, *et al.* Cell type of origin influences the molecular and functional properties of mouse induced pluripotent stem cells. *Nat Biotechnol* 2010; 28: 848-55.

169. Gore A, Li Z, Fung HL, Young JE, Agarwal S, Antosiewicz-Bourget J, *et al.* Somatic coding mutations in human induced pluripotent stem cells. *Nature* 2011; 471: 63-7.

170. Hussein SM, Batada NN, Vuoristo S, Ching RW, Autio R, Narva E, *et al.* Copy number variation and selection during reprogramming to pluripotency. *Nature* 2011; 471: 58-62.

171. Hacein-Bey-Abina S, Garrigue A, Wang GP, Soulier J, Lim A, Morillon E, *et al.* Insertional oncogenesis in 4 patients after retrovirus-mediated gene therapy of SCID-X1. *J Clin Invest* 2008; 118: 3132-42.

172. Howe SJ, Mansour MR, Schwarzwaelder K, Bartholomae C, Hubank M, Kempski H, *et al.* Insertional mutagenesis combined with acquired somatic mutations causes leukemogenesis following gene therapy of SCID-X1 patients. *J Clin Invest* 2008; 118: 3143-50.

173. Laurent LC, Ulitsky I, Slavin I, Tran H, Schork A, Morey R, *et al.* Dynamic changes in the copy number of pluripotency and cell proliferation genes in human ESCs and iPSCs during reprogramming and time in culture. *Cell Stem Cell* 2011; 8 : 106-18.

174. Mayshar Y, Ben-David U, Lavon N, Biancotti JC, Yakir B, Clark AT, *et al.* Identification and classification of chromosomal aberrations in human induced pluripotent stem cells. *Cell Stem Cell* 2010; 7: 521-31.

175. Li H, Haurigot V, Doyon Y, Li T, Wong SY, Bhagwat AS, *et al.* In vivo genome editing restores haemostasis in a mouse model of haemophilia. *Nature* 2011; 475: 217-21.

176. Reik A, Zhou Y, Hamlett A, Wagner J, Mendel MC, Flinders CW, *et al.* Zinc finger nucleases targeting the glucocorticoid receptor allow IL-13 zetakine transgenic CTLs to kill glioblastoma cells *in vivo* in the presence of immunosuppressing glucocorticoids. *Mol Ther* 2008; 16 (1s): S13-4.

177. Holt N, Wang J, Kim K, Friedman G, Wang X, Taupin V, *et al.* Human hematopoietic stem/progenitor cells modified by zinc-finger nucleases targeted to CCR5 control HIV-1 *in vivo*. *Nat Biotechnol* 2010; 28: 839-47.

178. Perez EE, Wang J, Miller JC, Jouvenot Y, Kim KA, Liu O, *et al.* Establishment of HIV-1 resistance in CD4+ T cells by genome editing using zinc-finger nucleases. *Nat Biotechnol* 2008; 26: 808-16.

179. Yusa K, Rashid ST, Strick-Marchand H, Varela I, Liu PQ, Paschon DE, *et al.* Targeted gene correction of alpha1-antitrypsin deficiency in induced pluripotent stem cells. *Nature* 2011; 478: 391-4.

180. Hockemeyer D, Wang H, Kiani S, Lai CS, Gao Q, Cassady JP, *et al.* Genetic engineering of human pluripotent cells using TALE nucleases. *Nat Biotechnol* 2011; 29: 731-4.

The CliniBook: Clinical gene transfer
Edited by Odile Cohen-Haguenauer – EDK, Paris © 2012, pp. 335-340

A7-2
Genetic modification of adult stem cells and induced pluripotent stem cells with emerging transposon technologies

THIERRY VANDENDRIESSCHE[1,2]*, MARINEE K.L. CHUAH[1,2]*

[1]Department of Gene Therapy and Regenerative Medicine, Free University of Brussels
(VUB), Faculty of Medicine and Pharmacy, University Medical Center - Jette,
Laarbeeklaan 103, B-1090 Brussels, Belgium.
[2]Department of Molecular Cardiovascular Medicine, University of Leuven, University
Hospital Campus Gasthuisberg, Belgium.
thierry.vandendriessche@vub.ac.be
marinee.chuah@vub.ac.be
* Corresponding authors

INTRODUCTION

The use of autologous adult stem cells for gene and cell therapy applications may warrant the introduction of a therapeutic gene into these cells to first correct the underlying gene defect. Similarly, there is a need to efficiently and safely introduce genes into induced pluripotent stem (iPS) cells to express therapeutic proteins in their differentiated progeny. Gene transfer into stem cells can be accomplished either by non-viral transfection or following transduction using viral vectors. Unfortunately, non-viral plasmids integrate inefficiently into stem cells and are rapidly diluted and/or degraded in a dividing stem cell population and its progeny. Consequently, in the absence of stable gene integration, expression from plasmid-based vectors typically declines in the days after transfection, especially in dividing cells. To ensure continuous expression, the gene of interest would need to be stably integrated into the target cell genome. The use of non-viral gene delivery approaches in conjunction with the latest generation transposon technology may potentially overcome some of these limitations and pave the way towards novel and improved gene therapy applications [1, 2]. Transposon and transposase constructs can be delivered to the target cells by transfection with carrier molecules that facilitate their entry into the target cells. Some of the transfection methods such as electroporation, nucleofection, magnetofection had all been used for *ex vivo* gene delivery of transposon/transposase constructs, resulting in long-term and efficient transgene expression. The use of transposons may overcome some of the manufacturing and regulatory hurdles associated with viral vectors, and allow for stable expression of the therapeutic gene in stem cells and their progeny. To turn DNA transposons into a gene delivery tool, a binary system has been developed that comprises (1) an expression plasmid that encodes the transposase and (2) a donor plasmid containing the DNA to be integrated, which is flanked in *cis* by the transposon terminal repeat sequences required for transposition (see Izsvak Z. and Ivics Z., *ibid*. chapter A6-5). The transposase binds these terminal repeat sequences and catalyzes the excision of the gene of interest from the donor plasmid as well as its insertion into the genome of the host cell. The DNA transposons *Sleeping Beauty* (*SB*), *piggyBac* (*PB*) and *Tol2* hold promise for gene transfer into stem/progenitor cells. Only *SB* and *PB* have been used for gene transfer into adult stem cells or iPS cells, which will be highlighted here.

Sleeping Beauty and PiggyBac

The vast majority of DNA transposons in vertebrate genomes had become silent by accumulating inactivating mutations [3]. To convert transposons into a robust gene transfer vector it was necessary to first overcome the effects of these inactivating mutations. Active transposons could be reconstituted by "reverse evolution" from silent ancestral transposons of vertebrates. This had been accomplished by the reconstruction of the *SB* transposon system from its evolutionary inactivated form in fish genomes [4]. Subsequently, by using a high-throughput, polymerase chain reaction-based, DNA-shuffling strategy, a library of mutant transposase genes was established to identify pairwise, synergistic combinations of these hyperactive mutations [5]. The most hyperactive version, here after referred to as SB100X, was 100-fold more potent in HeLa cell lines compared with the originally resurrected SB, based on the efficiency of mobilizing a transposon that is integrated into the chromosome. The generation of this novel and robust SB100X paved the way towards its use in stem cell gene transfer studies. The *PB* transposon was derived from the cabbage looper moth *Trichoplusia ni* and was initially discovered in baculovirus [6]. For gene delivery experiments, the PB system is also reconfigured as a binary system with a donor plasmid that contains the transposon with the gene of interest and a helper plasmid that expresses the transposase. Several strategies have recently been devised to further boost the efficiency of PB transposition based on codon-optimization or mutating the transposase or by mutating the inverted repeats [7-9].

Adult stem cells

One of the early hyperactive versions of SB led to modest stable *in vitro* transfection efficiencies in human CD34+ HSCs [10]. However, efficient *in vivo* gene marking could not be demonstrated after transplantation of transposon-modified CD34+ HSC into immunodeficient mice. In contrast, we showed that efficient and stable nonviral gene transfer into *bona fide* HSCs could be achieved with the hyperactive SB100X [5]. To achieve this, CD34+ HSCs obtained from cord blood were transfected by electroporation with a transposon encoding a marker (neomycin resistance gene, Neo^R) or a reporter gene (green fluorescent protein, GFP) and a plasmid expressing SB100X. Up to 40% of the hematopoietic colonies expressed GFP encoded by the *SB* transposon. In contrast, fewer GFP+ colonies could be obtained with any of the early-generation SB transposases. The transfected CD34+ cells retained their ability to differentiate *in vitro* along distinct lympho-hematopoietic lineages, though the transfection methods itself triggered some cytotoxic effects. Most importantly, CD34+ HSCs that had been transfected with the transposon/SB100X constructs were able to functionally reconstitute irradiated immunodeficient NOD-SCID IL2R$\gamma_c$$^{-/-}$ mice. Interestingly, common transposon integration sites were found in both the myeloid and lymphoid lineages, indicating that transposition had likely occurred in *bona fide* HSCs (or an early progenitor) capable of hematopoietic reconstitution. To our knowledge, our results demonstrated for the first time that transposons could be used for efficient gene marking *in vivo* after hematopoietic reconstitution with transfected HSCs. Since over the past 20 years it has been particularly challenging to develop an efficient, non-viral gene delivery system to genetically modify HSCs, this study overcomes this bottleneck. Subsequent studies independently confirmed these earlier findings, using similar approaches [11, 12]. By further optimizing the promoters used to drive expression of the transposase and the reporter gene in the transposon, long-term *in vivo* expression of the reporter gene could be demonstrated in lymphoid and myeloid lineages [11, 12].

We also demonstrated the superior stable gene transfer efficiency of SB100X in other stem cell popultaions, including mesenchymal stem cells (MSCs) and muscle stem/progenitor cells (*i.e.* myoblasts), which are important targets for regenerative medicine and gene therapy [13]. We showed that both MSCs and myoblasts could be engineered with a transposon encoding coagulation factor IX (FIX) along with SB100X, resulting in sustained production of biologically active FIX. This could pave the way towards a potential gene therapy approach for hemophilia.

SB100X showed no biased integration within genes, as opposed to γ-retroviral or lentiviral vectors [5], which may diminish the risk of insertional oncogenesis. Moreover, in contrast to the g-retroviral *long terminal repeat (LTR)*, the terminal repeat sequences of *SB* have low intrinsic promoter/enhancer activity and consequently cannot readily activate endogenous genes that flank the transposon integration sites [14].

As an alternative, *PB* was used to stably deliver genes into cord blood derived CD34+ HSC. Stem cells were transfected by electroporation using a *PB* transposon encoding GFP and human or mouse codon-optimized *PB* vectors, yielding up to 15% GFP-positive hematopoietic colonies (CFU-E) [5] and unpublished). The *PB*-transfected CD34+ cells retained their ability to differentiate *in vitro* along distinct lympho-hematopoietic lineages using conventional clonogenic assays, consistent with the results obtained with the SB system. It would appear however, that SB100X was still more efficient than PB to achieve stable gene expression in HSCs and its progeny.

INDUCED PLURIPOTENT STEM CELLS

iPS cells have been generated by transient transfection of the reprogramming genes with non-viral vectors. However, the efficiency of iPS cell induction with non-viral vectors is rather modest and was unsuccessful in many primary human cell types [15]. Several recent studies provide an alternative, more efficient, and safer strategy that involves non-viral integration of reprogramming genes, followed by their removal [16, 17]. This was achieved by incorporating all four reprogramming genes into a single *PB* vector. The most important and unique feature of this approach is that reintroduction of the PB transposase by transient transfection resulted in the excision of the reprogramming cassette from the iPS cell [16, 17]. This "traceless excision" paradigm using PB technology prevent re-expression of the reprogramming factors in the iPS cell induction and diminishes the risk of insertional oncogenesis, while maintaining a relatively robust reprogramming efficiency. Alternatively, the reprogramming cassette could be flanked with lox P sites allowing for its subsequent excision in iPS cells by CRE recombinase if transgene-free iPS cells are needed. However, transposons could also be used to genetically correct iPS cells by conferring stable expression of a gene of interest following its stable genomic integration. Obviously, in this case, removal of the transposon encoding the therapeutic gene is not desirable. Interestingly, if the reprogramming cassette encoded by the transposon is flanked by lox P sites it could potentially be replaced by the (therapeutic) gene of interest by CRE recombinase-mediated cassette exchange (RMCE). In addition to the *PB* transposon system, different strategies are being explored to generate iPS cells devoid of the reprogramming cassette using episomal plasmid vectors, Sendai RNA virus based vectors, mRNA and protein delivery. A comprehensive side-by-side comparative study may be required to assess the relative efficiency of human iPS generation using these different methods.

Directed differentiation of iPS cells into the desired, clinically relevant, transplantable cell types is mandatory for therapeutic or other applications. We have shown that transposon-mediated gene delivery into iPS cells can be used to control their differentiation. In particular, using the SB100X transposon system, we have demonstrated that *de novo* expression of the myogenic PAX3 transcription factor in mouse iPS cells resulted in their coaxed differentiation into myogenic cells [13]. This suggested that transposon-based PAX3 delivery could serve as a myogenic "molecular switch" that may replicate the normal myogenic developmental program, consistent with the induction of MYOD expression leading to multinucleated myotube formation.

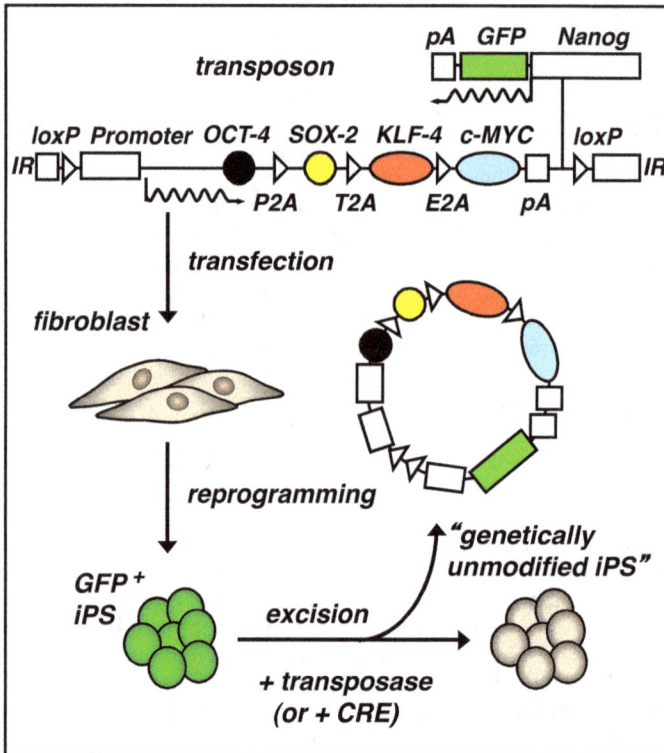

Figure 1. Transposon-based reprogramming as a non-viral paradigm for iPS generation. The transposon contains a single, polycistronic transcript that encodes Oct-4, Sox-2, Klf-4 and c-Myc respectively and flanked between the two IRs. Each of this factors is separated by a viral 2A peptide. These 4 reprogramming factors are driven from an internal promoter. A nanog promoter-driven GFP expression cassette is incorporated downstream of the 4 factors. This entire reprogramming cassette is flanked with loxP sites allowing for its subsequent excision in iPS cells by either *de novo* expression of the transposases or the CRE recombinase.

FUTURE PERSPECTIVES

Although these different independent studies confirmed the potential of *SB* or *PB* transposons for genetic modification of stem/progenitor cells, there are still some outstanding issues that need to be addressed before transposons can be used for stem cell gene transfer in patients. First, due to the intrinsic cytotoxicity of electroporation it is necessary to develop alternative gene transfer approaches and/or to further optimize the nucleofection conditions to reduce acute cell mortality. Second, genomic integration is not site-specific and the risk of insertional oncogenesis cannot formally be excluded. Additional studies are therefore needed to rigorously assess the genotoxic risk of *SB* and *PB* transposons in tumor-prone mouse models or sensitive *in vitro* genotoxicity assays. To further reduce the risk of insertional oncogenesis in HSCs, insulators could be used [18] or the transposase could be engineered with designer proteins to allow for site-specific interactions with specific DNA sequences and facilitate targeted genomic integration into chromosomal "safe harbors". Third, another concern relates to the potential inadvertent genomic integration of the SB or PB transposase-encoding expression plasmid, which may contribute to an increased genotoxic risk. This concern could be overcome by providing the SB or PB transposase as mRNA or protein. Fourth, expression of the gene of interest may be prone to transcriptional silencing but this could be overcome using insulators [18]. Finally, it is important to demonstrate that *SB* or *PB* transposons can correct a genetic disorder by HSC gene transfer in clinically relevant animals that model the corresponding human disease.

ACKNOWLEDGEMENTS

This work was supported by the 6th and 7th EU framework program (grant agreement n°222878, PERSIST; INTHER & CLINIGENE), FWO, GOA EPIGEN (VUB) and AFM. We wish to thank the members of our laboratories and our collaborators for their contributions to some of the work described herein.

This work has been performed with the support of the EC-DG research through the FP6-Network of Excellence, CLINIGENE: LSHB-CT-2006-018933.

REFERENCES

1. VandenDriessche T, Ivics Z, Izsvak Z, Chuah MK. Emerging potential of transposons for gene therapy and generation of induced pluripotent stem cells. *Blood* 2009; 114: 1461-8.

2. Ivics Z, Izsvak Z. Transposons for gene therapy! *Curr Gene Ther* 2006; 6: 593-607.

3. Ivics Z, Kaufman CD, Zayed H, Miskey C, Walisko O, Izsvak Z. The Sleeping Beauty transposable element: evolution, regulation and genetic applications. *Curr Iss Mol Biol* 2004; 6 : 43-55.

4. Ivics Z, Hackett PB, Plasterk RH, Izsvak Z. Molecular reconstruction of Sleeping Beauty, a Tc1-like transposon from fish, and its transposition in human cells. *Cell* 1997; 91: 501-10.

5. Mates L, Chuah MK, Belay E, Jerchow B, Manoj N, Acosta-Sanchez A, *et al.* Molecular evolution of a novel hyperactive Sleeping Beauty transposase enables robust stable gene transfer in vertebrates. *Nat Genet* 2009; 41: 753-61.

6. Cary LC, Goebel M, Corsaro BG, Wang HG, Rosen E, Fraser MJ. Transposon mutagenesis of baculoviruses: analysis of Trichoplusia ni transposon IFP2 insertions within the FP-locus of nuclear polyhedrosis viruses. *Virology* 1989; 172: 156-69.

7. Wu SC, Meir YJ, Coates CJ, Handler AM, Pelczar P, Moisyadi S, *et al.* piggyBac is a flexible and highly active transposon as compared to sleeping beauty, Tol2, and Mos1 in mammalian cells. *Proc Natl Acad Sci USA* 2006; 103: 15008-13.

8. Lacoste A, Berenshteyn F, Brivanlou AH. An efficient and reversible transposable system for gene delivery and lineage-specific differentiation in human embryonic stem cells. *Cell Stem Cell* 2009; 5: 332-42.

9. Yusa K, Zhou L, Li MA, Bradley A, Craig NL. A hyperactive piggyBac transposase for mammalian applications. *Proc Natl Acad Sci USA* 2011; 108: 1531-6.

10. Hollis RP, Nightingale SJ, Wang X, Pepper KA, Yu XJ, Barsky L, *et al.* Stable gene transfer to human CD34+ hematopoietic cells using the Sleeping Beauty transposon. *Exp Hematol* 2006; 34: 1333-43.

11. Xue X, Huang X, Nodland SE, Mates L, Ma L, Izsvak Z, *et al.* Stable gene transfer and expression in cord blood-derived CD34+ hematopoietic stem and progenitor cells by a hyperactive Sleeping Beauty transposon system. *Blood* 2009; 114: 1319-30.

12. Sumiyoshi T, Holt NG, Hollis RP, Ge S, Cannon PM, Crooks GM, *et al.* Stable transgene expression in primitive human CD34+ hematopoietic stem/progenitor cells, using the Sleeping Beauty transposon system. *Hum Gene Ther* 2009; 20: 1607-26.

13. Belay E, Matrai J, Acosta-Sanchez A, Ma L, Quattrocelli M, Mates L, *et al.* Novel hyperactive transposons for genetic modification of induced pluripotent and adult stem cells: a nonviral paradigm for coaxed differentiation. *Stem Cells* 2010; 28: 1760-71.

14. Walisko O, Schorn A, Rolfs F, Devaraj A, Miskey C, Izsvak Z, *et al.* Transcriptional activities of the Sleeping Beauty transposon and shielding its genetic cargo with insulators. *Mol Ther* 2008; 16: 359-69.

15. Okita K, Hong H, Takahashi K, Yamanaka S. Generation of mouse-induced pluripotent stem cells with plasmid vectors. *Nat Protoc* 2010; 5: 418-28.

16. Woltjen K, Michael IP, Mohseni P, Desai R, Mileikovsky M, Hamalainen R, *et al.* piggyBac transposition reprograms fibroblasts to induced pluripotent stem cells. *Nature* 2009; 458: 766-70.

17. Yusa K, Rad R, Takeda J, Bradley A. Generation of transgene-free induced pluripotent mouse stem cells by the piggyBac transposon. *Nat Methods* 2009; 6: 363-9.

18. Dalsgaard T, Moldt B, Sharma N, Wolf G, Schmitz A, Pedersen FS, *et al.* Shielding of sleeping beauty DNA transposon-delivered transgene cassettes by heterologous insulators in early embryonal cells. *Mol Ther* 2009; 17: 121-30.

The CliniBook: Clinical gene transfer
Edited by Odile Cohen-Haguenauer – EDK, Paris © 2012, pp. 341-353

A7-3
Targeted genome engineering approaches based on rare-cutting endonucleases: a tentative summary

FRÉDÉRIC PÂQUES[1], JULIANNE SMITH[2*]

[1]Cellectis S. A. and [2]Cellectis Therapeutics, 8, rue de la Croix Jarry, 75013 Paris, France.
smith@cellectis.com
*Corresponding author

The successful treatment of several X-SCID patients [1], followed by similar results with ADA-SCID [2], WAS [3], ALD [4], and β-thalassaemia patients [5], has shown that gene therapy is an effective way to address genetic diseases. All of these clinical trials were based on the delivery of a therapeutic transgene, using a viral vector that stably integrates into the genome of patient derived cells. The use of integrative vectors is required in dividing cells in order to avoid transgene loss and ensure long-term correction of the genetic defect. However, this requirement has resulted in severe adverse events (SAEs) associated with the insertion of the viral vector in the vicinity of a proto-oncogene, resulting in its transcriptional activation. Several cases of malignant cell proliferation have been detected in X-SCID [6-8], Chronic Granulomatous Disease (CGD) [9, 10], and more recently, WAS patients, illustrating one of the inherent drawbacks of the use of integrative vectors. Thus, in spite of the large amount of alleged "non coding" DNA in the human genome, gain of function by insertional mutagenesis represents a major risk.

However, this picture has to be put into perspective. First, similar integrative viral vectors have been used in cancer immunotherapy [11], and no malignant transformation has been observed. Since these approaches rely on the modification and transfer of T lymphocytes (instead of hematopoetic stem cells [HSCs] in the case of X-SCID,CGD and WAS), the absence of lymphoproliferation might reflect a reduced proficiency of T cells for malignant transformation, or a different pattern of vector integration [12]. Second, extensive efforts have been made towards the development of safer vectors, devoid of strong *cis*-activating elements in their LTRs [13-15]. These self-inactivating (SIN) gamma-retrovirus and lentivirus-based vectors are now in clinic [4, 16-20] and the coming years should tell us whether they have the expected safety properties. However, one should keep in mind that in spite of the occurrence of SAEs, gene therapy by gene transfer has already saved many lives, and for patients who do not have an HLA-identical donor remains a viable option.

Nevertheless, SAEs as well as other complications associated with the semi-random integration of viral vectors have fostered a growing interest for more precise approaches that aim at controlling the integration of therapeutic transgenes [21]. This interest has been further supported by the development of a large and diverse toolbox for targeted genome modification. The development of several technological platforms has generated new possibilities for the creation of animal models, improved crop plants, and cell lines for screening and protein production. However, no potential application has created as much excitement as the use of targeted genome modifications for therapeutic purposes.

At least three types of gene targeting (GT) approaches, described in *Figure 1*, have been envisioned: targeted gene insertion, gene correction and gene inactivation [21]. Targeted gene insertion strategies involve the insertion of a DNA sequence into a chosen chromosomal locus. This approach could alleviate not only the safety concerns associated with insertional mutagenesis, but also transgene extinction or inadequate expression, two other major issues. This type of approach is dependent on the identification of a "safe harbor" allowing for stable expression of the transgene without any impact on other genes, including neighboring ones [22]. Gene correction is the ultimate form of targeted modification: instead of pasting, somewhere into the genome, an exogenous functional copy, one erases the genetic defect at the endogenous gene. In contrast, gene inactivation consists in introducing a mutation into a functional gene. This inactivation can be achieved in association with targeted gene insertion or by the generation of small insertions and deletions within the gene, often referred to as targeted mutagenesis (TM). Homologous gene targeting (HGT) was one of the first methods for targeted genome engineering [23-26]. HGT is based on homologous recombination, a natural mechanism for DNA repair, and can be used to generate the three types of events described in *Figure 1*. Its major drawback remains its low efficiency, in the range of 10^{-6} to 10^{-9} of treated mammalian cells. The correction of the HBBs alleles by gene targeting in ES or iPS from humanized mouse models by different groups remains a milestone in the field [27-29]. However, these studies also accurately highlight the limits of the system, with the use of intensive selection protocols (and as a consequence high levels of cell expansion) to alleviate the low rates of homologous recombination. It seems difficult today to translate these experiments into a clinical approach for human patients.

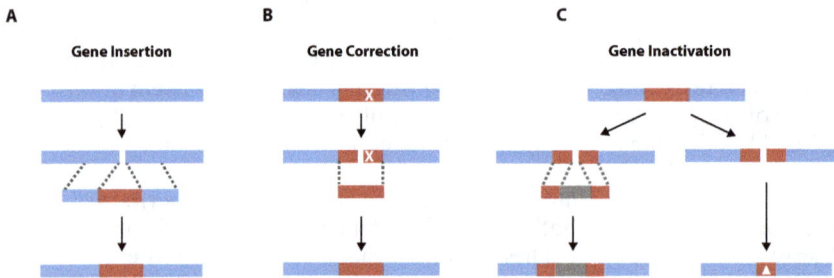

Figure 1. Gene targeting approaches. All of the following events can be stimulated by the generation of site-specific double-strand breaks using rare-cutting endonucleases. A. Gene insertion consists in the addition of a DNA sequence at a chosen chromosomal site. For gene therapy purposes, a therapeutic expression cassette is targeted to a safe harbor locus *via* flanking sequences that are homologous to the genomic locus. B. Gene correction. A genetic defect in the genome is repaired with donor DNA that contains wild-type sequences homologous to the mutated gene. C. Gene inactivation can be achieved by homologous recombination *via* gene insertion, where an insertion into the coding sequence of a gene results in its inactivation. Alternatively the misrepair of DNA ends by error-prone non-homologous end joining can result in insertions or deletions of various sizes, leading to gene inactivation.

Thus, several groups have developed an extensive assortment of tools allowing for precise AND efficient genome surgery. These approaches have been reviewed extensively elsewhere [21], and we will in this short review focus on the use of rare cutting endonucleases, the most successful approach so far.

THE WORLD OF RARE-CUTTING ENDONUCLEASES

There are today four families of rare cutting endonucleases used in genome engineering; Meganucleases (or Homing Endonucleases), Zinc Finger Nucleases, Transcription-Activator-Like Nucleases and Chemical Nucleases (*Figure 2*).

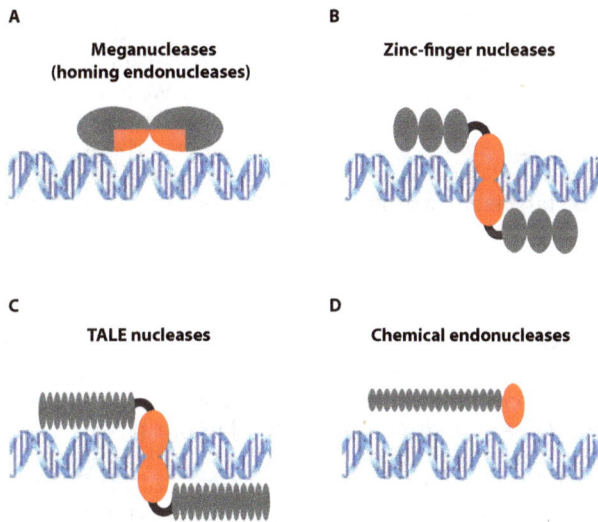

Figure 2. Sequence-specific endonucleases used for gene targeting. A. Engineered meganucleases are derived from natural meganucleases (or homing endonucleases) from the LAGLIDAG family. These proteins contain two distinct DNA binding domains with a catalytic center (red) embedded in the DNA binding interface. B. Zinc-finger nucleases are chimeric endonucleases resulting from the fusion of polydactyl DNA binding domains (*i.e.* strings of zinc fingers) with the catalytic domain of the bacterial FokI restriction enzyme. C. TALE nucleases are chimeric endonucleases that consist of a DNA binding domain derived from TAL effectors fused to the catalytic domain of the Fok1 nuclease. TAL effectors have a unique type of DNA binding domain, containing a series of 33-35 amino acids repeats, where each base pair from the DNA target is contacted by a single repeat. D. Chemical endonucleases consist of a DNA binding polymer (TFO, polyamine, etc.) conjugated with a distinct chemical or peptidic catalytic moiety.

Meganucleases

The meganuclease story starts with the identification, in the 80's, of the HO [30] and I-SceI [31] yeast nucleases, found to recognize unusually long target sites and to trigger gene transfer by a process that mimics targeted insertion (or to be more exact, that the researcher mimics when they use targeted insertion). These proteins are called meganucleases (alluding to the size of their target) or homing endonucleases [32], referring to the "homing process" triggered by I-SceI and many other endonucleases. I-SceI has been used since the 90's in genome engineering experiments in mammalian cells [33, 34], and plants [35, 36], and a large body of experiments in a wide variety of cell types and organisms has demonstrated the robustness of the technology [21].

The meganuclease family has several hundred members today, and at least five different sub-families have been identified [37], the best characterized one being the "LAGLI-DADG" family, named after a conserved peptide sequence, that includes the yeast nuclease I-SceI. The substantial size of this meganuclease family (> 200 members) suggests that many proteins could be used in the same way as I-SceI. It is also possible to use the degeneracy displayed at certain positions of the cleavage site to add new degrees of freedom, and thereby cleave more targets [38]. Furthermore, the dimeric or pseudo-dimeric structure of LAGLIDADG proteins permits the design of chimeric molecules [39, 40], a process that further enlarges the sequence space attainable by natural meganucleases and their derivatives. Nevertheless, it is the redesign of the DNA binding interface, permitting the targeting of a sequence every few hundred bps, that will allow the complexity of the genome to be fully addressed. We have described in detail the methods used to produce engineered meganucleases derived from I-CreI, combining semi-rational design, and high-throughput screening [41-44]. Other scaffolds than I-CreI can be used [45, 46], and one can expect that this diversification will both increase the space of targetable sequences, and allow for further refinements in terms of activity and specificity.

Zinc finger nucleases

Zinc Finger Proteins (ZFPs) are among the most abundant DNA binding proteins in humans, including many transcription factors. They include at least one zinc Finger (ZF) motif, consisting of a $\beta\beta\alpha$ fold organized around a zinc atom [47]. Polydactyl ZFPs can include several ZFs, with each ZF contacting a DNA triplet. This modular organization was discovered with the tridimensional structure of Zif268, which includes three contiguous ZFs wrapped around the major groove of the DNA double helix [48, 49]. Thus, the design of artificial ZFPs binding chosen targets can be achieved by simple combinatorial assembly of individual ZFs with known recognition patterns [50-52]. In order to target the largest possible sequence space, several groups launched a real hunt for new building blocks, and ZFs recognizing most GNN, ANN and CNN triplets were available relatively early [53, 54]. Today, a large number of triplets, including TNNs are available [55, 56].

However, the refined structure of Zif268 [49] also suggests cross-talk between adjacent ZFs, with certain ZFs having the possibility to establish hydrogen bonds with adjacent triplets. Thus, in a polydactyl, the ability of individual ZFs to bind their cognate triplets proved to be context dependent [57], which strongly impacted the success rate of modular assembly [58]. Several groups developed strategies to cope with these unexpected attrition rates, and clever experimental designs have been described, including sequential assembly [59], and the use of overlapping building blocks including more than one ZF [56, 60].

Engineered polydactyls are only DNA binders, and to be used as tools, they need an effector. ZFPs have been tethered to various protein domains, including nucleases. Shortly after the Klug and Pabo groups reported the basis for ZFP engineering [50-52], the Chandrasegaran group described the first Zinc Finger Nucleases (ZFNs) resulting from the fusion of Zif268 with the catalytic domain of the bacterial FokI restriction enzyme [61]. Due to the intrinsic properties of FokI, these fusions need to dimerize to cleave DNA [62], and most ZFNs today consist of heterodimers, each monomer comprising 3 or 4 ZFs and a FokI domain [63].

Transcription-activator-like nucleases

Recently, a third class of protein endonucleases has emerged, based on Transcription Activator-Like Effectors (TALE), a family of proteins from plant pathogens from the *Xanthomonas* genus [64]. TALEs have a unique type of DNA binding domain, containing a series of 33-35 amino acid repeats, differing essentially at two positions [65, 66]. Each base pair from the DNA target is contacted by a single repeat, with the specificity resulting from the two variant amino acids of the repeat. So far, individual repeats have been shown to bind their cognate target independently. This absence or near absence of observed context dependence contrasts with what is observed with meganucleases and ZFPs. TALEs appear today to be the only peptidic DNA binding domains that can be assembled rationally by modular assembly, using a simple recognition code [67-72].
As for ZFPs, TALEs could be fused to transcription factors [73], and to the well characterized FokI cleavage domain. The first TALENs (Transcription Activator-Like Effector Nucleases) proved to be both efficient and very specific [67, 69-71], which probably accounts for the rapid diffusion of the technology.

Chemical nucleases

Chemical endonucleases include a variety of artificial rare cutters comprising a DNA-binding polymer and a DNA-reactive agent [74, 75]. At least one of the two moieties is not peptidic, and such reagents have to be synthesized *in vitro* and introduced into the target cell.
The DNA binding polymer can be a triplex-forming oligonucleotides (TFO) [76, 77], or a Peptidic Nucleic Acid (PNA) [78], but other types of polymers, such as polyamides could be envisioned (for review see [75]). Various active domains have been described including psoralen [79], topoisomerase inhibitor (camptothecin) [77], bypiridine [80], or a restriction enzyme [76]. While in principle promising [78], this approach has not been validated by a large body of results.

WHERE DO WE STAND TODAY

Today, the efficiency of rare cutting endonucleases is largely validated, but the strength and limits of each technology, as well as their potential for therapeutic applications, is still under discussion. It should be noted that the first rare cutting endonucleases in clinic today are not for the correction of a deficient gene using homologous recombination (HR) but for the inactivation of a functional gene, by Non Homologous End-Joining (NHEJ), a non-templated repair mechanism.
Double-strand breaks (DSBs) generated by Meganucleases, ZFNs and MNs can all be repaired by two types of DNA repair pathways: HR or NHEJ [21]. HR is the natural pathway underlying HGT whereas NHEJ is an error prone DSB repair pathway, that can result in the introduction of indels (small insertions and deletions) into the targeted sequence, and can be used to inactivate the open reading frames of chosen genes by targeted mutagenesis (TM) [81, 82].
Several groups have shown that rare cutting endonucleases can significantly stimulate HGT in immortalized cell lines [21]. Some of these studies describe the efficient engineering of genes involved in genetic diseases, such as IL2RG [83, 84], Rag1 [44] and F9 [85], as well as the insertion of transgenes into potential "safe harbors" [84, 86]. However, achieving the same results in primary cells, in particular stem cells, has proven to be more difficult. Using a ZFN targeting the human IL2RG gene, Lombardo *et al.*

reported an unusually high efficacy of about 40% of HGT in Jurkat and K562 cells [84]. However, this efficacy dropped to 5% in human ES cells and 0.1% in HSCs [84]. Since the publication of these results in 2007, they have remained by far the highest published figures, and in the case of HSCs, nearly the only ones. Similarly, in induced pluripotent stem (iPS) cells, several studies have already demonstrated the possibility of using ZFNs for HGT [87-89]. However, as observed with ES cells and HSCs, absolute frequencies, although higher than spontaneous events, remain low ($\geq 10^{-4}$). Thus, it is commonly accepted today that in contrast with mouse ES cells, human stem cells are difficult to engineer by HGT.

During the same period of time, very conclusive results were achieved for nuclease-induced gene disruption through NHEJ. Several studies have shown that nuclease-mediated TM was efficient in Drosophila, immortalized mammalian cells, fertilized fish eggs, rat oocytes, and plants. In addition, up to 50% and 17% of TM could be achieved in T cells and HSCs, respectively [82, 90]. Several studies suggest that whereas HR is associated with the S and G2 phase of dividing cells, NHEJ occurs throughout the cell cycle [91]. Thus, it is tempting to speculate that NHEJ-based approaches are simply more robust, in a much broader spectrum of cell types. Additionally, in contrast with HGT, nuclease-mediated TM does not require the presence of a homologous molecule for templated repair of the DSB, which alleviates issues related to co-delivery of the repair matrix. However, the diversity of experimental designs (notably regarding vectorization) makes it difficult to directly compare the results achieved for TM and for HGT. No systematic analysis has been conducted to evaluate the efficacy of nuclease-mediated TM and HGT in several cell types in a single study (what would be the equivalent of Lombardo *et al.* for nuclease-mediated HGT). Interestingly, Zou *et al.* observed 4.6×10^{-6} of ZFN-induced TM in the PIG-A gene of ES cells, whereas the same ZFN could induce 100 times more HGT [88], a result that contrasts with idea that NHEJ is more prevalent in primary cells.

The high rate of gene disruptions in therapeutically relevant cells, applied to an unmet medical need, fostered the first clinical trials involving a rare cutting endonuclease. Disruption of CCR5, the major HIV-1 co-receptor, in T cells in order to introduce HIV resistance. This approach is based, in part, on the finding that the CCR5delta32 allele, which produces a truncated form of the molecule, is associated with a strong resistance to HIV-1 infection in homozygous individuals [92]. In order to provide an autologous source of *CCR5$^{-/-}$* cells, Perez *et al.* used a ZFN to cleave the human CCR5 gene in human T cells [82]. Under nonselective conditions, 23% of T cell clones carried a disrupted CCR5 allele, and about one-third of these cells harbored a bi-allelic disruption. This study was rapidly followed by clinical trials based on the ZFN-inactivation of CCR5 in T cells from HIV patients (NCT00842634, NCT01044654, NCT01252641). Initial results from these studies indicate that patients display improved immune cell counts and reduced viral loads (to an undetectable level in one patient) after temporary suppression of classic antiretroviral treatment [93]. Today, several other clinical trials based on nuclease-mediated gene disruptions are being planned, including disruption of CCR5 in HSCs and the nuclease-mediated inactivation of the glucocorticoïd receptor in T cells (for the treatment of malignant gliomas in the presence of high doses of steroids).

The successful use of targeted modifications (HGT or TM) for gene therapy requires a minimal efficacy, which remains to be determined for each application. The efficacy required depends in part on the dominant or recessive nature of the mutated allele, on whether the phenotype is cell autonomous, but also on disease-specific parameters. It is generally admitted that for most diseases, a significant therapeutic effect requires at least 1% of the treated cells to be modified (although in several cases, such as Sickle Cell Anemia, much higher figures are usually considered). Another factor that may be important in determining success is a selective growth advantage of the modified cells. Positive selection for corrected cells, was observed in the treatment of SCID animal models [94-99] and was key to the success of SCID clinical trials (as illustrated by the results with and without ADAPEG for ADA SCID patients [2, 100, 101]). Similarly, a selective advantage for transplanted *CCR5⁻ᐟ⁻* T cells in the context of an HIV infection has been described [82]. Thus, selection may play a decisive role in the ongoing HIV trials using the CCR5 disruption.

However, the initiation of a clinical trial does not depend only on technical results, but also on the demonstration of an acceptable risk/benefit ratio that results from many other parameters, including the existence of an efficient (even if not perfect) alternative treatment. After different ups and downs, the global outcome of the X-SCID clinical trials has proven to be rather positive, with 17 out of the 20 treated patients having today a restored immune system [102]. Moreover, new γ-retroviral and lentiviral vectors with potentially better safety properties are already in clinic [4, 16-20]. In these conditions, one can understand that the development of HGT-based strategies remains important, but was not a priority for diseases such as X-SCID, WAS, ALD and SCA, for which classical gene transfer with γ-retroviral vectors, SIN γ retroviral vectors and lentiviral vectors were already providing potential solutions.

Nevertheless, the use of nuclease-mediated HGT still represents an attractive way to address many orphan diseases, and several strategies have been envisioned to increase recovery of targeted cells. The use of *ex vivo* selection in several studies with iPS cells have shown that drug selection can strongly enhance yield [87-89]. However, for therapeutic applications it will be important to be able to subsequently eliminate the selectable marker. Optimized vectorization protocols may also play a key role, in particular for HGT approaches, which require the introduction of the nuclease and a repair substrate. Finally, it is important to remember that the toolbox of enzymes that can be used for HGT is constantly increasing. The recent emergence of TALENs, which display surprisingly high levels of specificity, might result in a more complex landscape. Initial success in immortalized mammalian cells [70, 71], as well as human iPS and ES cells [103] has already been described. Given the strong interest in targeted genome engineering for therapeutic applications, one can expect that nuclease-mediated approaches based on HR have not had their last word.

REFERENCES

1. Cavazzana-Calvo M, Hacein-Bey S, de Saint Basile G, Gross F, Yvon E, Nusbaum P, *et al.* Gene therapy of human severe combined immunodeficiency (SCID)-X1 disease. *Science* 2000; 288: 669-72.

2. Aiuti A, Slavin S, Aker M, Ficara F, Deola S, Mortellaro A, *et al.* Correction of ADA-SCID by stem cell gene therapy combined with nonmyeloablative conditioning. *Science* 2002; 296: 2410-3.

3. Boztug K, Schmidt M, Schwarzer A, Banerjee PP, Diez IA, Dewey RA, *et al.* Stem-cell gene therapy for the Wiskott-Aldrich syndrome. *N Engl J Med* 2010; 363: 1918-27.

4. Cartier N, Hacein-Bey-Abina S, Bartholomae CC, Veres G, Schmidt M, Kutschera I, *et al.* Hematopoietic stem cell gene therapy with a lentiviral vector in X-linked adrenoleukodystrophy. *Science* 2009; 326: 818-23.

5. Cavazzana-Calvo M, Payen E, Negre O, Wang G, Hehir K, Fusil F, *et al*. Transfusion independence and HMGA2 activation after gene therapy of human beta-thalassaemia. *Nature* 2010; 467: 318-22.

6. Howe SJ, Mansour MR, Schwarzwaelder K, Bartholomae C, Hubank M, Kempski H, *et al*. Insertional mutagenesis combined with acquired somatic mutations causes leukemogenesis following gene therapy of SCID-X1 patients. *J Clin Invest* 2008; 118: 3143-50.

7. Hacein-Bey-Abina S, Garrigue A, Wang GP, Soulier J, Lim A, Morillon E, *et al*. Insertional oncogenesis in 4 patients after retrovirus-mediated gene therapy of SCID-X1. *J Clin Invest* 2008; 118: 3132-42.

8. Hacein-Bey-Abina S, Von Kalle C, Schmidt M, McCormack MP, Wulffraat N, Leboulch P, *et al*. LMO2-associated clonal T cell proliferation in two patients after gene therapy for SCID-X1. *Science* 2003; 302: 415-9.

9. Ott MG, Schmidt M, Schwarzwaelder K, Stein S, Siler U, Koehl U, *et al*. Correction of X-linked chronic granulomatous disease by gene therapy, augmented by insertional activation of MDS1-EVI1, PRDM16 or SETBP1. *Nat Med* 2006; 12: 401-9.

10. Stein S, Ott MG, Schultze-Strasser S, Jauch A, Burwinkel B, Kinner A, *et al*. Genomic instability and myelodysplasia with monosomy 7 consequent to EVI1 activation after gene therapy for chronic granulomatous disease. *Nat Med* 2010; 16: 198-204.

11. Kohn DB, Dotti G, Brentjens R, Savoldo B, Jensen M, Cooper LJ, *et al*. CARs on track in the clinic. *Mol Ther* 2011; 19: 432-8.

12. Recchia A, Bonini C, Magnani Z, Urbinati F, Sartori D, Muraro S, *et al*. Retroviral vector integration deregulates gene expression but has no consequence on the biology and function of transplanted T cells. *Proc Natl Acad Sci USA* 2006; 103: 1457-62.

13. Nienhuis AW, Dunbar CE,Sorrentino BP. Genotoxicity of retroviral integration in hematopoietic cells. *Mol Ther* 2006; 13: 1031-49.

14. Montini E, Cesana D, Schmidt M, Sanvito F, Bartholomae CC, Ranzani M, *et al*. The genotoxic potential of retroviral vectors is strongly modulated by vector design and integration site selection in a mouse model of HSC gene therapy. *J Clin Invest* 2009; 119: 964-75.

15. Modlich U, Navarro S, Zychlinski D, Maetzig T, Knoess S, Brugman MH, *et al*. Insertional transformation of hematopoietic cells by self-inactivating lentiviral and gammaretroviral vectors. *Mol Ther* 2009; 17: 1919-28.

16. D'Costa J, Mansfield SG,Humeau LM. Lentiviral vectors in clinical trials: current status. *Curr Opin Mol Ther* 2009; 11: 554-64.

17. Humeau LM, Binder GK, Lu X, Slepushkin V, Merling R, Echeagaray P, *et al*. Efficient lentiviral vector-mediated control of HIV-1 replication in CD4 lymphocytes from diverse HIV+ infected patients grouped according to CD4 count and viral load. *Mol Ther* 2004; 9: 902-13.

18. Galy A, Roncarolo MG,Thrasher AJ. Development of lentiviral gene therapy for Wiskott Aldrich syndrome. *Expert Opin Biol Ther* 2008; 8: 181-90.

19. Galy A,Thrasher AJ. Gene therapy for the Wiskott-Aldrich syndrome. *Curr Opin Allergy Clin Immunol* 2011; 11: 545-50.

20. Fischer A, Hacein-Bey-Abina S,Cavazzana-Calvo M. Gene therapy for primary adaptive immune deficiencies. *J Allergy Clin Immunol* 2011; 127: 1356-9.

21. Silva G, Poirot L, Galetto R, Smith J, Montoya G, Duchateau P, Paques F. Meganucleases and other tools for targeted genome engineering: perspectives and challenges for gene therapy. *Curr Gene Ther* 2011; 11: 11-27.

22. Sadelain M, Papapetrou EP,Bushman FD. Safe harbours for the integration of new DNA in the human genome. *Nat Rev Cancer* 2011; 12: 51-8.

23. Thomas KR, Capecchi MR. Site-directed mutagenesis by gene targeting in mouse embryo-derived stem cells. *Cell* 1987; 51: 503-12.

24. Doetschman T, Maeda N, Smithies O. Targeted mutation of the Hprt gene in mouse embryonic stem cells. *Proc Natl Acad Sci USA* 1988; 85: 8583-7.

25. Smithies O, Gregg RG, Boggs SS, Koralewski MA, Kucherlapati RS. Insertion of DNA sequences into the human chromosomal beta-globin locus by homologous recombination. *Nature* 1985; 317: 230-4.

26. Rothstein RJ. One-step gene disruption in yeast. *Methods Enzymol* 1983; 101: 202-11.

27. Chang JC, Ye L, Kan YW. Correction of the sickle cell mutation in embryonic stem cells. *Proc Natl Acad Sci USA* 2006; 103: 1036-40.

28. Hanna J, Wernig M, Markoulaki S, Sun CW, Meissner A, Cassady JP, *et al.* Treatment of sickle cell anemia mouse model with iPS cells generated from autologous skin. *Science* 2007; 318: 1920-3.

29. Wu LC, Sun CW, Ryan TM, Pawlik KM, Ren J, Townes TM. Correction of sickle cell disease by homologous recombination in embryonic stem cells. *Blood* 2006; 108: 1183-8.

30. Kostriken R,Heffron F. The product of the HO gene is a nuclease: purification and characterization of the enzyme. *Cold Spring Harb Symp Quant Biol* 1984; 49: 89-96.

31. Colleaux L, d'Auriol L, Betermier M, Cottarel G, Jacquier A, Galibert F, Dujon B. Universal code equivalent of a yeast mitochondrial intron reading frame is expressed into *E. coli* as a specific double strand endonuclease. *Cell* 1986; 44: 521-33.

32. Chevalier BS, Stoddard BL. Homing endonucleases: structural and functional insight into the catalysts of intron/intein mobility. *Nucleic Acids Res* 2001; 29: 3757-74.

33. Choulika A, Perrin A, Dujon B, Nicolas JF. Induction of homologous recombination in mammalian chromosomes by using the I-SceI system of *Saccharomyces cerevisiae. Mol Cell Biol* 1995; 15: 1968-73.

34. Rouet P, Smih F,Jasin M. Expression of a site-specific endonuclease stimulates homologous recombination in mammalian cells. *Proc Natl Acad Sci USA* 1994; 91: 6064-8.

35. Puchta H, Dujon B, Hohn B. Homologous recombination in plant cells is enhanced by *in vivo* induction of double strand breaks into DNA by a site-specific endonuclease. *Nucleic Acids Res* 1993; 21: 5034-40.

36. Puchta H, Dujon B,Hohn B. Two different but related mechanisms are used in plants for the repair of genomic double-strand breaks by homologous recombination. *Proc Natl Acad Sci USA* 1996; 93: 5055-60.

37. Stoddard BL. Homing endonucleases: from microbial genetic invaders to reagents for targeted DNA modification. *Structure* 2011; 19: 7-15.

38. Barzel A, Privman E, Peeri M, Naor A, Shachar E, Burstein D, et al. Native homing endonucleases can target conserved genes in humans and in animal models. *Nucleic Acids Res* 2011; 39: 6646-59.

39. Chevalier BS, Kortemme T, Chadsey MS, Baker D, Monnat RJ, Stoddard BL. Design, activity, and structure of a highly specific artificial endonuclease. *Mol Cell* 2002; 10: 895-905.

40. Epinat JC, Arnould S, Chames P, Rochaix P, Desfontaines D, Puzin C, *et al.* A novel engineered meganuclease induces homologous recombination in yeast and mammalian cells. *Nucleic Acids Res* 2003; 31: 2952-62.

41. Arnould S, Chames P, Perez C, Lacroix E, Duclert A, Epinat JC, *et al.* Engineering of large numbers of highly specific homing endonucleases that induce recombination on novel DNA targets. *J Mol Biol* 2006; 355: 443-58.

42. Smith J, Grizot S, Arnould S, Duclert A, Epinat JC, Chames P, *et al.* A combinatorial approach to create artificial homing endonucleases cleaving chosen sequences. *Nucleic Acids Res* 2006; 34: e149.

43. Arnould S, Perez C, Cabaniols JP, Smith J, Gouble A, Grizot S, et al. Engineered I-CreI derivatives cleaving sequences from the human XPC gene can induce highly efficient gene correction in mammalian cells. *J Mol Biol* 2007; 371: 49-65.

44. Grizot S, Smith J, Daboussi F, Prieto J, Redondo P, Merino N, et al. Efficient targeting of a SCID gene by an engineered single-chain homing endonuclease. *Nucleic Acids Res* 2009; 37: 5405-19.

45. Takeuchi R, Certo M, Caprara MG, Scharenberg AM, Stoddard BL. Optimization of *in vivo* activity of a bifunctional homing endonuclease and maturase reverses evolutionary degradation. *Nucleic Acids Res* 2009; 37: 877-90.

46. Takeuchi R, Lambert AR, Mak AN, Jacoby K, Dickson RJ, Gloor GB, et al. Tapping natural reservoirs of homing endonucleases for targeted gene modification. *Proc Natl Acad Sci USA* 2011; 108: 13077-82.

47. Pabo CO, Peisach E, Grant RA. Design and selection of novel Cys2His2 zinc finger proteins. *Annu Rev Biochem* 2001; 70: 313-40.

48. Pavletich NP, Pabo CO. Zinc finger-DNA recognition: crystal structure of a Zif268-DNA complex at 2.1 A. *Science* 1991; 252: 809-17.

49. Elrod-Erickson M, Rould MA, Nekludova L, Pabo CO. Zif268 protein-DNA complex refined at 1.6 A: a model system for understanding zinc finger-DNA interactions. *Structure* 1996; 4: 1171-80.

50. Rebar EJ, Pabo CO. Zinc finger phage: affinity selection of fingers with new DNA-binding specificities. *Science* 1994; 263: 671-3.

51. Choo Y, Sanchez-Garcia I, Klug A. *In vivo* repression by a site-specific DNA-binding protein designed against an oncogenic sequence. *Nature* 1994; 372: 642-5.

52. Choo Y, Klug A. Selection of DNA binding sites for zinc fingers using rationally randomized DNA reveals coded interactions. *Proc Natl Acad Sci USA* 1994; 91: 11168-72.

53. Dreier B, Fuller RP, Segal DJ, Lund CV, Blancafort P, Huber A, Koksch B, Barbas CF 3rd. Development of zinc finger domains for recognition of the 5'-CNN-3' family DNA sequences and their use in the construction of artificial transcription factors. *J Biol Chem* 2005; 280: 35588-97.

54. Beerli RR, Barbas CF 3rd. Engineering polydactyl zinc-finger transcription factors. *Nat Biotechnol* 2002; 20: 135-41.

55. Maeder ML, Thibodeau-Beganny S, Osiak A, Wright DA, Anthony RM, Eichtinger M, et al. Rapid open-source engineering of customized zinc-finger nucleases for highly efficient gene modification. *Mol Cell* 2008; 31: 294-301.

56. Sander JD, Dahlborg EJ, Goodwin MJ, Cade L, Zhang F, Cifuentes D, et al. Selection-free zinc-finger-nuclease engineering by context-dependent assembly (CoDA). *Nat Methods* 2011; 8: 67-9.

57. Isalan M, Choo Y, Klug A. Synergy between adjacent zinc fingers in sequence-specific DNA recognition. *Proc Natl Acad Sci USA* 1997; 94: 5617-21.

58. Ramirez CL, Foley JE, Wright DA, Muller-Lerch F, Rahman SH, Cornu TI, et al. Unexpected failure rates for modular assembly of engineered zinc fingers. *Nat Methods* 2008; 5: 374-5.

59. Greisman HA, Pabo CO. A general strategy for selecting high-affinity zinc finger proteins for diverse DNA target sites. *Science* 1997; 275: 657-61.

60. Isalan M, Klug A, Choo Y. A rapid, generally applicable method to engineer zinc fingers illustrated by targeting the HIV-1 promoter. *Nat Biotechnol* 2001; 19: 656-60.

61. Kim YG, Cha J, Chandrasegaran S. Hybrid restriction enzymes: zinc finger fusions to Fok I cleavage domain. *Proc Natl Acad Sci USA* 1996; 93: 1156-60.

62. Smith J, Bibikova M, Whitby FG, Reddy AR, Chandrasegaran S, Carroll D. Requirements for double-strand cleavage by chimeric restriction enzymes with zinc finger DNA-recognition domains. *Nucleic Acids Res* 2000; 28: 3361-9.

63. Carroll D. Progress and prospects: zinc-finger nucleases as gene therapy agents. *Gene Ther* 2008; 15: 1463-8.

64. Bogdanove AJ, Schornack S, Lahaye T. TAL effectors: finding plant genes for disease and defense. *Curr Opin Plant Biol* 2010; 13: 394-401.

65. Moscou MJ, Bogdanove AJ. A simple cipher governs DNA recognition by TAL effectors. *Science* 2009; 326: 1501.

66. Boch J, Scholze H, Schornack S, Landgraf A, Hahn S, Kay S, *et al*. Breaking the code of DNA binding specificity of TAL-type III effectors. *Science* 2009; 326: 1509-12.

67. Christian M, Cermak T, Doyle EL, Schmidt C, Zhang F, Hummel A, Bogdanove AJ, Voytas DF. Targeting DNA double-strand breaks with TAL effector nucleases. *Genetics* 2010; 186: 757-61.

68. Cermak T, Doyle EL, Christian M, Wang L, Zhang Y, Schmidt C, *et al*. Efficient design and assembly of custom TALEN and other TAL effector-based constructs for DNA targeting. *Nucleic Acids Res* 2011; 39: e82.

69. Mahfouz MM, Li L, Shamimuzzaman M, Wibowo A, Fang X, Zhu JK. *De novo*-engineered transcription activator-like effector (TALE) hybrid nuclease with novel DNA binding specificity creates double-strand breaks. *Proc Natl Acad Sci USA* 2011; 108: 2623-8.

70. Miller JC, Tan S, Qiao G, Barlow KA, Wang J, Xia DF, *et al*. A TALE nuclease architecture for efficient genome editing. *Nat Biotechnol* 2011; 29: 143-8.

71. Mussolino C, Morbitzer R, Lutge F, Dannemann N, Lahaye T, Cathomen T. A novel TALE nuclease scaffold enables high genome editing activity in combination with low toxicity. *Nucleic Acids Res* 2011; 39: 9283-93.

72. Li T, Huang S, Zhao X, Wright DA, Carpenter S, Spalding MH, Weeks DP, Yang B. Modularly assembled designer TAL effector nucleases for targeted gene knockout and gene replacement in eukaryotes. *Nucleic Acids Res* 2011; 39: 6315-25.

73. Zhang F, Cong L, Lodato S, Kosuri S, Church GM, Arlotta P. Efficient construction of sequence-specific TAL effectors for modulating mammalian transcription. *Nat Biotechnol* 2011; 29: 149-53.

74. Pingoud A, Silva GH. Precision genome surgery. *Nat Biotechnol* 2007; 25: 743-4.

75. Schleifman EB, Chin JY, Glazer PM. Triplex-mediated gene modification. *Methods Mol Biol* 2008; 435: 175-90.

76. Eisenschmidt K, Lanio T, Simoncsits A, Jeltsch A, Pingoud V, Wende W, Pingoud A. Developing a programmed restriction endonuclease for highly specific DNA cleavage. *Nucleic Acids Res* 2005; 33: 7039-47.

77. Arimondo PB, Thomas CJ, Oussedik K, Baldeyrou B, Mahieu C, Halby L, *et al*. Exploring the cellular activity of camptothecin-triple-helix-forming oligonucleotide conjugates. *Mol Cell Biol* 2006; 26: 324-33.

78. McNeer NA, Chin JY, Schleifman EB, Fields RJ, Glazer PM, Saltzman WM. Nanoparticles deliver triplex-forming PNAs for site-specific genomic recombination in CD34+ human hematopoietic progenitors. *Mol Ther* 2010; 19: 172-80.

79. Majumdar A, Muniandy PA, Liu J, Liu JL, Liu ST, Cuenoud B, Seidman MM. Targeted gene knock in and sequence modulation mediated by a psoralen-linked triplex-forming oligonucleotide. *J Biol Chem* 2008; 283: 11244-52.

80. Simon P, Cannata F, Perrouault L, Halby L, Concordet JP, Boutorine A, *et al*. Sequence-specific DNA cleavage mediated by bipyridine polyamide conjugates. *Nucleic Acids Res* 2008; 36: 3531-8.

81. Liang F, Han M, Romanienko PJ, Jasin M. Homology-directed repair is a major double-strand break repair pathway in mammalian cells. *Proc Natl Acad Sci USA* 1998; 95: 5172-7.

82. Perez EE, Wang J, Miller JC, Jouvenot Y, Kim KA, Liu O, *et al.* Establishment of HIV-1 resistance in CD4+ T cells by genome editing using zinc-finger nucleases. *Nat Biotechnol* 2008; 26: 808-16.

83. Urnov FD, Miller JC, Lee YL, Beausejour CM, Rock JM, Augustus S, *et al.* Highly efficient endogenous human gene correction using designed zinc-finger nucleases. *Nature* 2005; 435: 646-51.

84. Lombardo A, Genovese P, Beausejour CM, Colleoni S, Lee YL, Kim KA, *et al.* Gene editing in human stem cells using zinc finger nucleases and integrase-defective lentiviral vector delivery. *Nat Biotechnol* 2007; 5: 1298-306.

85. Li H, Haurigot V, Doyon Y, Li T, Wong SY, Bhagwat AS, *et al. In vivo* genome editing restores haemostasis in a mouse model of haemophilia. *Nature* 2011; 475: 217-21.

86. Lombardo A, Cesana D, Genovese P, Di Stefano B, Provasi E, Colombo DF, *et al.* Site-specific integration and tailoring of cassette design for sustainable gene transfer. *Nat Methods* 2011; 8: 861-9.

87. Yusa K, Rashid ST, Strick-Marchand H, Varela I, Liu PQ, Paschon DE, *et al.*Targeted gene correction of alpha1-antitrypsin deficiency in induced pluripotent stem cells. *Nature* 2011; 478: 391-4.

88. Zou J, Maeder ML, Mali P, Pruett-Miller SM, Thibodeau-Beganny S, Chou BK, *et al.* Gene targeting of a disease-related gene in human induced pluripotent stem and embryonic stem cells. *Cell Stem Cell* 2009; 5: 97-110.

89. Hockemeyer D, Soldner F, Beard C, Gao Q, Mitalipova M, DeKelver RC, *et al.* Efficient targeting of expressed and silent genes in human ESCs and iPSCs using zinc-finger nucleases. *Nat Biotechnol* 2009; 27: 851-7.

90. Holt N, Wang J, Kim K, Friedman G, Wang X, Taupin V, *et al.* Human hematopoietic stem/progenitor cells modified by zinc-finger nucleases targeted to CCR5 control HIV-1 *in vivo. Nat Biotechnol* 2010; 28: 839-47.

91. Delacote F, Lopez BS. Importance of the cell cycle phase for the choice of the appropriate DSB repair pathway, for genome stability maintenance: the trans-S double-strand break repair model. *Cell Cycle* 2008; 7: 33-8.

92. Samson M, Libert F, Doranz BJ, Rucker J, Liesnard C, Farber CM, *et al.* Resistance to HIV-1 infection in caucasian individuals bearing mutant alleles of the CCR-5 chemokine receptor gene. *Nature* 1996; 382: 722-5.

93. Ledford H. Targeted gene editing enters clinic. *Nature* 2011; 471: 16.

94. Tsai EJ, Malech HL, Kirby MR, Hsu AP, Seidel NE, Porada CD, *et al.* Retroviral transduction of IL2RG into CD34+ cells from X-linked severe combined immunodeficiency patients permits human T- and B-cell development in sheep chimeras. *Blood* 2002; 100: 72-9.

95. Yates F, Malassis-Seris M, Stockholm D, Bouneaud C, Larousserie F, Noguiez-Hellin P, *et al.* Gene therapy of RAG-2-/- mice: sustained correction of the immunodeficiency. *Blood* 2002; 100: 3942-9.

96. Bunting KD, Sangster MY, Ihle JN, Sorrentino BP. Restoration of lymphocyte function in Janus kinase 3-deficient mice by retroviral-mediated gene transfer. *Nat Med* 1998; 4: 58-64.

97. Candotti F, Johnston JA, Puck JM, Sugamura K, O'Shea JJ, Blaese RM. Retroviral-mediated gene correction for X-linked severe combined immunodeficiency. *Blood* 1996; 87: 3097-102.

98. Hacein-Bey S, Basile GD, Lemerle J, Fischer A, Cavazzana-Calvo M. gammac gene transfer in the presence of stem cell factor, FLT-3L, interleukin-7 (IL-7), IL-1, and IL-15 cytokines restores T-cell differentiation from gammac(-) X-linked severe combined immunodeficiency hematopoietic progenitor cells in murine fetal thymic organ cultures. *Blood* 1998; 92: 4090-7.

99. Soudais C, Shiho T, Sharara LI, Guy-Grand D, Taniguchi T, Fischer A, Di Santo JP. Stable and functional lymphoid reconstitution of common cytokine receptor gamma chain deficient mice by retroviral-mediated gene transfer. *Blood* 2000; 95: 3071-7.

100. Kohn DB, Hershfield MS, Carbonaro D, Shigeoka A, Brooks J, Smogorzewska EM, *et al*. T lymphocytes with a normal ADA gene accumulate after transplantation of transduced autologous umbilical cord blood CD34+ cells in ADA-deficient SCID neonates. *Nat Med* 1998; 4: 775-80.

101. Bordignon C, Notarangelo LD, Nobili N, Ferrari G, Casorati G, Panina P, *et al*. Gene therapy in peripheral blood lymphocytes and bone marrow for ADA- immunodeficient patients. *Science* 1995; 270: 470-5.

102. Fischer A, Hacein-Bey-Abina S, Cavazzana-Calvo M. 20 years of gene therapy for SCID. *Nat Immunol* 2010; 11: 457-60.

103. Hockemeyer D, Wang H, Kiani S, Lai CS, Gao Q, Cassady JP, *et al*. Genetic engineering of human pluripotent cells using TALE nucleases. *Nat Biotechnol* 2011; 29: 731-4.

The CliniBook: Clinical gene transfer
Edited by Odile Cohen-Haguenauer – EDK, Paris © 2012, pp. 354-367

A7-4
Targeted genome modifications with designer nucleases

CHRISTIEN BEDNARSKI[1,2], EVA-MARIA HÄNDEL[2], TONI CATHOMEN[1,2]*

[1]Laboratory of Cell and Gene Therapy, Center for Chronic Immunodeficiency, University Medical Center Freiburg, Engesserstr. 4, D-79108 Freiburg, Germany; [2]Institute of Experimental Hematology, Hannover Medical School, Carl-Neuberg-Strasse 1, D-30625 Hannover, Germany.
toni.cathomen@uniklinik-freiburg.de
*Corresponding author

BACKGROUND

Everyday cells are exposed to DNA damaging agents, either endogenous or environmental factors. With the help of different DNA repair pathways the cell maintains the integrity of the genome and prevents transformation. However, what happens if a defect is present from birth on, *e.g.* a mutation that impedes a specific function? Base substitutions, deletions and insertions in a locus can lead to frame-shift mutations within the coding sequence of a gene and result in loss of function of the gene product. For example, the most frequent mutation responsible for the congenital disorder cystic fibrosis is a deletion of a base triplet in the *CFTR* gene. The *CFTR* gene encodes for a chloride channel located in epithelial cell membranes of many exocrine tissues. The mutated CFTR protein lacks the amino acid phenylalanine at position 508. As a consequence, the protein is incorrectly folded and degraded rapidly. The absence of the CFTR chloride channel at the cell surface results in defective ion conductance, leading to bacterial infection in the lung, to pancreatic fibrosis and intestinal malabsorption and obstruction [1, 2]. The disorder X-linked severe combined immunodeficiency (X-SCID) is caused by mutations in the *IL2RG* gene, including stop codons that terminate translation of the IL-2Rγ protein prematurely. IL-2Rγ is an essential subunit of many receptors that are essential for differentiation of hematopoietic stem cells to mature T and NK cells. In affected patients the loss severely limits the cellular and humoral immune response [3, 4].

Patients with inherited disorders have to deal with the lifelong symptoms because available medication achieves only a transient improvement and does not eliminate the basic defect. Gene therapy, on the other hand, could provide a permanent cure for these patients. Currently, the practical implementation of this therapy is based on gene addition, through which the loss of function of the affected protein is compensated. Vectors for gene addition carry the coding sequence and all control elements to successfully express the transgene of interest. The transferred expression cassette can be integrated into the genomic DNA or remain extra-chromosomally, respectively. The up and downsides of some successfully conducted gene therapy trials are described in more details in other chapters of this book. One of the shortcomings of the use of retroviral vectors for gene transfer involves the risk of inducing leukemia or myelodysplasia, as shown in some clinical trials [5-7]. The transforming characteristics were mostly based on the enhancer function residing in the long terminal repeats (LTR) of the retroviral vectors [8]. If integration occurred close to cellular proto-oncogenes, such as the *LIM domain Only 2* (*LMO-2*) gene, the LTR increased transcription of these endogenous genes, which in turn led to uncontrolled proliferation and final transformation of the cells [9]. The generation of optimized retro- and lentiviral vectors, in which the transgene is under the control of an internal promoter, proved to be safer but even those vectors can induce elevated proliferation through integration in the proximity of proto-oncogenes, such as *EviI* [10]. Hence, even though gene therapy has shown great potential to overcome basic defects for several diseases, the randomly integrating nature of retro- and lentiviral vector systems rendered transgene expression unreliable and unpredictable.

TARGETED GENOME ENGINEERING

To preserve genome integrity, targeted genome editing is favored over random integration approaches. Homologous recombination (HR) is a cellular mechanism that has been harnessed to integrate transgenes in a targeted fashion or to facilitate the exchange of homologous DNA sequences in order to replace a mutated DNA sequence with a correct copy. The frequency of HR under normal conditions is rather low (1 event per 10^6 cells) and has to be stimulated to be utilized for therapeutic approaches. It has been shown that the HR frequency can be significantly increased (up to 10,000-fold) by introducing a targeted DNA double-strand break (DSB) in the locus of interest with designer nucleases [11-15]. Different types of artificial nucleases have been used for homology directed targeting studies: zinc-finger nucleases (ZFNs) [16-18], recombinant homing endonucleases (rHEs) [19-23] and transcription activator-like effector nucleases (TALENs) [24, 25]. All of these engineered nucleases consist of a DNA binding domain for targeted DNA recognition and a catalytical cleavage domain to introduce the DSB. Thus, the use of chimeric nucleases makes it possible to perform precise genome surgery at a desired locus and to exploit this for gene therapy.

The targeted introduction of a DSB via engineered nucleases activates one of two DNA repair pathways of the cell, non-homologous end joining (NHEJ) or homology directed repair (HDR) (*Figure 1*). NHEJ is the predominant DSB repair pathway that is mainly active in the G1-phase of the cell cycle. It is a fast but error-prone pathway because processed ends are directly ligated, which often results in imprecise repair with small insertions and deletions at the break site. Consequently, NHEJ has been proven to be extremely efficient to create knockout mutations in animal or plant model organisms [26-31]. The HDR pathway is based on HR and takes place preferentially in S/G2-phase of the cell cycle when, under natural conditions, homologous sequences are available for repairing a DSB. HDR is a process that is activated in somatic cells mainly as a response of DSB induced by collapsing replication forks. Furthermore, HDR is activated in germ cells in which the crossing over events contribute to the recombination of genetic material. Since the HDR pathway also accepts exogenous DNA as a template for HR, it can be harnessed for introducing precise modifications in complex genomes and is therefore an attractive and promising technique for gene therapy.

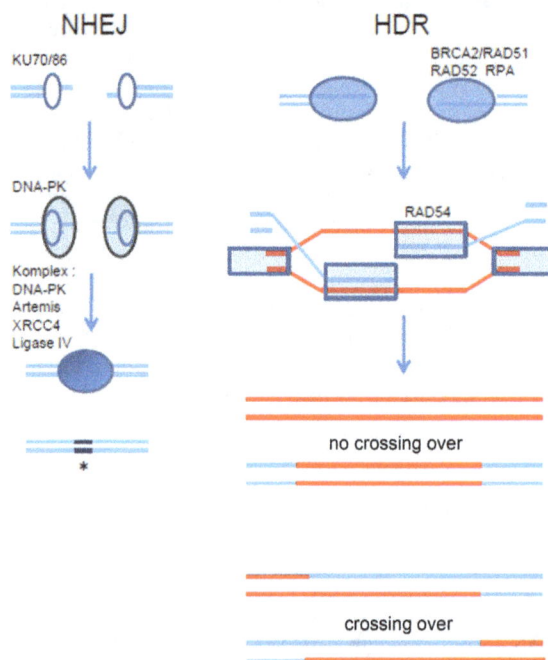

Figure 1. Major repair pathways of DNA double strand breaks (DSBs) in mammalian cells. In the non-homologous end joining pathway KU70 and KU86 bind initially as heterodimers to the DSB and recruit the catalytic subunit DNA-PKcs. DNA-PKcs phosphorylates itself and, in turn, facilitates Artemis activity that processes the DNA ends at the DSB. Subsequently, the XRCC4/DNA ligaseIV-complex is responsible for the ligation of the blunted ends. In the homology directed repair (HDR) pathway replication protein A (RPA) makes the single stranded DNA strands accessible *via* strand resection and recruits RAD52. This complex is then replaced by BRCA2/RAD51, which allows the single-stranded DNA to invade the homologous sequences and so to form a template for the polymerase. RAD54's helicase activity unwinds the DNA surrounding the DSB whereas RAD51 promotes stand inversion and homologous paring of the single strands during branch migration. The structure is resolved either via gene conversion (no crossing over) or by DNA strand exchange (crossing over) *via* resolvases (Figure modified from Vasileva *et al.* [32]).

Depending on which major DSB repair pathway is utilized, the genome engineering approach can have different outcomes (*Figure 2*). By employing a designer nuclease with an appropriately designed DNA donor, a mutated sequence can be corrected directly *in situ*. A second application of HDR is targeted gene addition, which is based on the targeted insertion of a whole gene expression cassette at a site of interest, *e.g.* the integration of a therapeutic gene cassette into a "safe harbor" site of the genome, such as the *PPP1R12C locus* (also known as *AAVS1*). As opposed to retro-/lentiviral or transposon based random integration approaches, respectively, the expression of a transgene in *AAVS1* has been shown to be long-lasting, even if the cells are differentiated. Furthermore, integration seems without physiological consequence to the cell, *i.e.* without impairing cellular function or inducing transformation [33-38].
Targeted gene disruption or targeted deletion are genome modification approaches

based on NHEJ with the purpose of knocking out a gene function (*Figure 2*). As mentioned above, ZFN and/or TALEN-mediated gene knockout was applied successfully in many model organisms, including *Drosophila*, *C. elegans*, zebrafish and rats, in order to investigate gene function *in vivo*. For many of these organisms, designer nuclease mediated gene knockout was the first efficient possibility to perform reverse genetics, as opposed to classical forward genetics that relied on random mutatagenesis, and hence represents a major breakthrough for basic research in the respective fields [26-30, 39, 40]. An additional application is targeted deletion of a DNA sequence using two autonomously operating designer nucleases to delete *e.g.* entire loci [41-44].

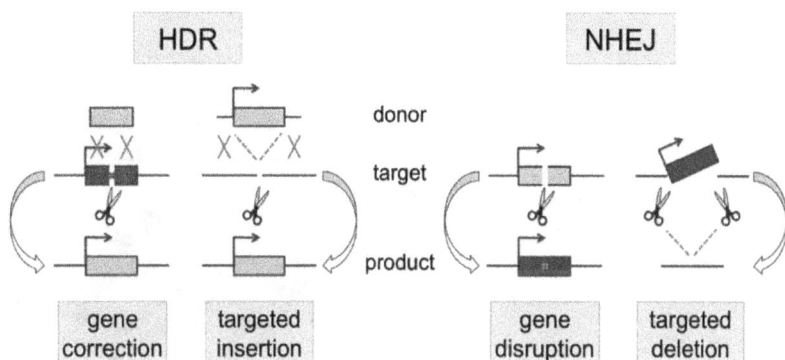

Figure 2. Targeted genome modification with engineered nucleases. Nuclease-based genome engineering relies on either of the two major repair pathways, HDR and NHEJ. HDR is preferred if a sufficiently high intranuclear concentration of donor DNA is available to be harnessed either for direct gene correction or for targeted integration, *e.g.* into a safe harbor (depending on donor DNA design). Error-prone NHEJ can be used to insert mutations in a targeted fashion, which in turn can lead to gene disruption. Simultaneous expression of two autonomous designer nucleases is used to insert a targeted chromosomal deletion (Figure from Händel *et al.* [18]).

In order to perform gene therapy *ex vivo*, stem cells are isolated from an organism to facilitate genome editing with designer nucleases, followed by reimplantation of the genetically modified cells. Another promising strategy is based on genetic engineering of patient derived induced pluripotent stem cells (iPSCs). Successfully corrected iPSCs could then be re-differentiated into the desired cell types before transplantation as demonstrated with some cell lineages.

A third approach involves direct *in vivo* gene targeting, which requires administration of both the therapeutic donor DNA and the modifying enzymes into the target organs. Successful *in vivo* genome editing was achieved in combining ZFN-mediated repair with adeno-associated virus based gene transfer to restore haemostasis in a mouse model of haemophilia [45].

ZINC-FINGER NUCLEASES

The most successfully used protein based nucleases are ZFNs, rHEs and TALENs. ZFNs are chimeric enzymes that consist of two major functional domains, the DNA binding domain and the catalytic domain of FokI endonuclease. Zinc-finger (ZF)-based DNA binding domains are frequently found in nature, especially in transcription factors [46-48]. The prototype is the murine transcription factor Zif268, which com-

prises a well-described DNA binding domain that carries three ZF modules. One single
ZF module consists of ~30 amino acids that fold into a DNA-recognizing α-helix and
two β-sheets (*Figure 3A*). The secondary structure is formed by complex formation of
the zinc ion with two cysteins und two histidines. The essential amino acids for DNA
binding are located in positions -1, 2, 3 and 6 relative to the start of the α-helix. Overall
three to six residues in the α-helix contribute to the specificity of DNA recognition
[49-52]. An arginine, frequently present in helix position -1 in eukaryotic transcription
factors, recognizes guanine in triplet position 1, and aspartic acid located in helix position 2 specifies binding to either an adenine or cytosine on the opposite strand of
the preceding triplet, leading to cross-strand interactions (*Figure 3B*) [46-48].

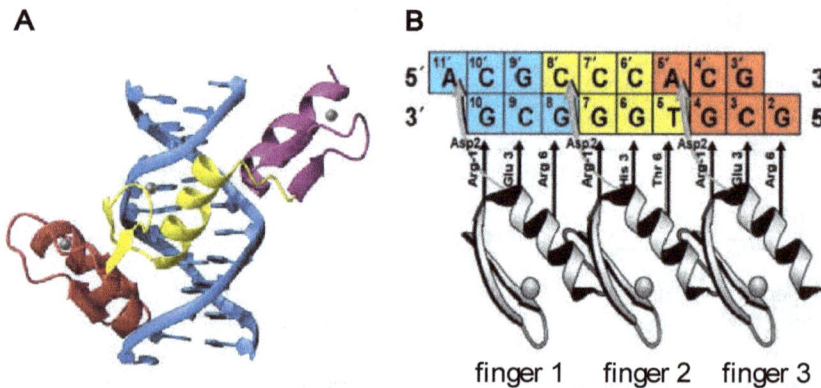

Figure 3. DNA recognition of zinc-finger motifs. (A) The DNA binding domain of Zif268 consists of
three ZF modules (depicted in red, yellow and purple). A module forms the typical zinc-finger
structure with a DNA recognizing α-helix and two β-sheets surrounding the zinc ion (grey). (B) Protein–DNA interaction model. Residues at positions -1, 2, 3 and 6 of the α-helix mediate DNA
recognition. Some ZF modules show additional cross-strand interactions with the neighboring
strand emanating from position 2 of the recognition helix [50, 52, 53] (Figure 3A from Pabo *et al.*
[46], Figure 3B modified from Klug [54]).

ZFNs currently used in gene therapy approaches consist of three to six ZF modules
per subunit [55-57]. Consequently, a heterodimeric ZFN pair recognizes a DNA stretch
of 18-36 bp, which should be long enough to define a statistically unique target site in
the human genome.
The catalytic domain of a ZFN originates from the type II restriction enzyme FokI
that has been isolated from *Flavobacerium okeanokoites* [58]. The natural enzyme has
to dimerize before passing through a conformational change that activates the enzyme
[59], leading to a staggered cut 9-13 bp distant from its recognition sequence.
As the natural FokI enzyme, ZFNs have to dimerize to cleave the target site. The dependency on dimerization contributes considerably to the specificity of ZFNs. For instance, the target sequence of a three-finger ZFN subunit comprises 9 bp, which occurs
statistically more than 11,000 times in the human genome. Indeed, the dimer interface
between the two ZFN monomers has been shown to play a crucial role in ZFN associated toxicity [60-63]. At least in theory, a ZFN subunit bound to its DNA target half-
site can dimerize through protein–protein interactions with a second ZFN monomer
that is not properly bound to DNA and would induce cleavage at target half-sites (*Figure 4A*). Furthermore, homodimerization of two identical ZFN monomers (*Figure 4B*)
could lead to unspecific cleavage in the genome. In both cases, this unspecific DNA

cleavage activity can induce significant cytotoxicity. An additional crucial parameter for ZFN specificity includes a highly specific DNA binding domain (*Figure 4C*). As previously mentioned, due to cross-strand interactions, context-based selection methods in general allows for the generation of more specific ZFNs and should therefore be favored for the production of highly specific DNA binding domains [16, 64-66]. An ideal ZFN would therefore encompass the following parameters: (i) highly specific DNA binding, (ii) obligate heterodimer, and (iii) weak dimer interface to prevent cleavage at target half-sites (*Figure 4D*). Miller *et al.* and Szczepek *et al.* optimized the interacting residues in the protein–protein interface of the FokI nuclease domain to allow more specific applications of ZFNs [60, 61]. Some charged amino acids in the dimerization interface of FokI were exchanged in order to create asymmetric FokI variants to prevent homodimerization and to destabilize the dimer interface.

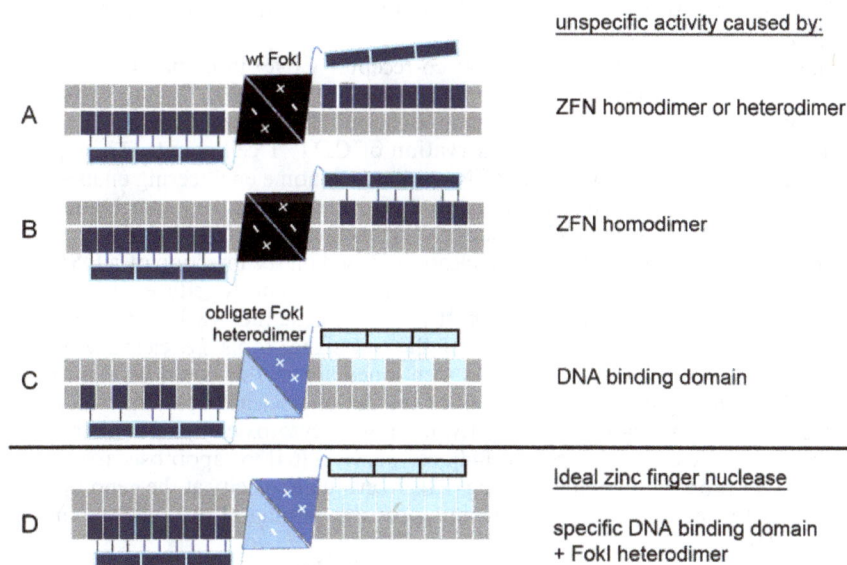

Figure 4. Unspecific ZFN activity caused by (A) cleavage at target half-sites, (B) homodimerization of identical monomers, and (C) unspecific DNA binding. (D) The ideal ZFN architecture contains a destabilized and asymmetric FokI dimer interface and an optimized DNA binding domain. Charged residues in the dimer interface are indicated by + and – (Figure modified from Cathomen and Joung [67]).

The third important feature besides the DNA binding and catalytic domain is the protein linker that connects these two domains. Investigations regarding different linker lengths and composition revealed highest ZFN activity at 6 bp long DNA spacers [14, 68]. This fact is due to the helicality of the DNA, i.e. with a 6 bp spacer the catalytic domains are located on the same side of the helix, thus in an optimal constellation for creating the DSB. Händel *et al.* showed that both length and sequence of the inter-domain linker determine ZFN activity and target-site specificity, and are therefore important parameters to be considered when designing ZFNs for genome editing [69]. In summary, the ideal ZFN system comprises a highly specific DNA-binding domain, an appropriate linker and an obligate heterodimieric FokI variant that prevents homodimerization.

APPLICATIONS

Some recent studies of ZFN-based gene targeting in mouse models, iPSCs and embryonic stem cells (ESCs) highlight their great potential and promising prospect in clinical settings. For example, Hockemeyer *et al.* showed efficient targeting of intron 1 of the *AAVS1* locus in human ESCs and iPSCs [38]. At the same time Zou *et al.* created a model for paroxysmal nocturnal hemoglobinuria by targeted insertion of a drug resistance gene into *PIG-A* in iPSCs [70]. Furthermore, ZFN-mediated gene targeting was used to correct the E6V mutation in the β-globin locus in iPSCs generated from patients suffering from sickle cell anemia [71]. A recent study in a haemophilia B mouse model demonstrated efficient *in vivo* ZFN-based targeting of the mutated *F9* gene in the liver using a hepatotropic AAV vector [45]. Recently, biallelic correction of a point mutation in the α-1 antitrypsin gene was achieved in human iPSCs using a ZFN-based targeting strategy [72].

The specific bi-allelic disruption of the HIV-1 co-receptor *CCR5* in human CD4+ T cells or CD34+ hematopoietic stem and progenitor cells (HSPCs) and the successful engraftment of those modified cells in an immunodeficient HIV mouse model resulted in significantly lower HIV-1 levels and preservation of CD4+ T cell counts [17, 57]. These two studies strikingly showed that ZFN-mediated genome engineering enables a novel genetic anti-HIV approach, which led to a clinical trial involving autologous T cells genetically modified at the *CCR5* locus (NCT00842634; NCT01044654).

Therapeutic gene targeting using designer nucleases is based on the insertion of a DSB into the human genome and therefore requires safety measurements to reduce nuclease associated cytotoxicity and genotoxicity. A bottleneck for gene therapy based on engineered nucleases can be unspecific activity of those designer tools, *i.e.* cleavage of the genome at so-called "off-target sites". As mentioned above, this could be due to suboptimal DNA binding parameters [55, 64] or the use of nuclease domains which do not prevent homodimerization [60, 61]. Evaluation of cytotoxicity can be determined quantitatively by cell cycle analysis [44], cell survival [64] or apoptosis assays using annexin-V or propidium iodide staining [73]. To evaluate toxicity at the genomic level DSB repair foci can be counted by staining for the gamma-H2AX histone or 53BP1 [60, 61, 74-76].

To determine the binding specificity *in vitro*, systematic evolution of ligands by exponential enrichment (SELEX) has been used. The *in vitro* binding profile can then be used to predict off-target sites in the human genome. Recently, two different genome wide approaches to determine the specificity of ZFNs in cells have been published [77, 78]. Using two different methodologies both groups evaluated the activity profile of the same *CCR5*-specific ZFNs. Deep-sequencing analysis revealed measurable off-target activities of these nucleases, with a major hot spot in the *CCR2* gene. However, other identified off-target loci did not overlap between the two studies, suggesting that both approaches were not comprehensive. This bias in the experimental outcome shows the need to develop more sensitive methods to identify possible off-target sites and to evaluate the associated genotoxic risks, especially with respect to potential upcoming clinical applications. However, both studies show that low ZFN concentrations, ameliorating ZFN architecture and prevention of homodimerization contributes to improve the ZFN cleavage specificity [79].

Besides above-mentioned ZFN features, the delivery system plays a crucial role in genome engineering. Of pivotal importance for gene therapy approaches are both tissue specific delivery of the ZFNs and prevention of random integration of the shuttle vector. A wide range of viral delivery vectors have been used towards targeted genome modification, including vectors based on adenovirus [17], integrase-deficient lentivirus [80, 81] and AAV [44, 45]. Although non-integrating in nature, those vehicles can passively integrate into natural or induced DSBs: however it is difficult and expensive to routinely sequence the whole genome for such events [44, 78, 82, 83]. Control elements, such as tissue specific promoters or micro RNAs, can be combined as part of the delivery vector design to achieve expression specific either to the cell type or to the differentiation state [84, 85]. An ideal way to achieve high level transient expression without unwanted integration might be delivery in form of ZFN-encoding mRNA [28, 29, 56, 86]. In particular, microinjection of mRNA into one-cell-embryos has proven to be very efficient for inducing gene disruption in zebrafish and rat [26, 28].

TRANSCRIPTION ACTIVATOR-LIKE EFFECTOR NUCLEASES (TALENs) AND OUTLOOK

ZFNs have been the most frequently used platform for genome modifications [87] but two major factors limit their widespread application: the time consuming generation of those highly specific nucleases and the limited targeting range of about one potential target site every 500 bp [16, 87, 88]. TALENs are a novel and alternative class of engineered nucleases based on the DNA binding properties of transcription activator-like effectors (TALEs) [89, 90]. Natural TALEs are transcription factors found in plant pathogenic bacteria of the genus *Xanthomonas*. During the infection cycle, TALEs are injected into plant cells by the pathogen and bind promoter sequences of the host cells in order to activate genes that contribute to bacterial growth and pathogen distribution [91, 92]. TALEs consist of an N-terminal translocation signal, a C-terminal transcriptional activation domain and a central DNA binding domain composed of highly conserved 34 residue long repeat units arranged as tandem arrays [93]. The simple 'one TALE repeat to one base' code was unraveled in 2009 by two independent groups [89, 90].

One advantage over ZFNs is that TALENs can be designed to target longer sites in the genome, which could contribute to higher specificity [24, 25]. When comparing ZFNs and TALENs at two human loci (*CCR5* and *IL2RG*), TALENs were as active as ZFNs but associated with less cytotoxicity [25]. Another superiority was demonstrated by showing that *CCR5* specific TALENs were capable of discriminating between the *CCR5* and the highly similar *CCR2* locus, which is distinct from the *CCR5* specific ZFNs [25]. However, whether TALENs show higher specificity and less nuclease-associated toxicity in general has to be investigated in more detail in future studies. In any case, first encouraging gene editing studies in iPSCs, zebrafish and rat zygotes have revealed that TALENs contain the same cleavage potential as ZFNs [24, 94, 95]. Furthermore, there has not been a single study reporting context-specific DNA binding by TALEs. This underscores both the true modular 'one TALE repeat unit to 1 nucleotide' recognition mode of DNA binding and the simplicity of generating TALENs as compared to ZFNs [79].

16 years have passed since the development of artificial ZFNs [13]. Ever since, designer nucleases have evolved into a successful and rapid tool to perform reverse genetics at a wide range of loci in many different cell types and organisms [14-17, 26-31, 38, 40, 70, 96]. Many efforts have been undertaken to make gene editing with designer nucleases more efficient and safer by optimizing the nuclease architectures [16, 24, 25, 60, 61, 65, 69], finding the right delivery tools, such as DNA-based vectors with optimized control elements or mRNA [17, 26, 27, 80-82, 84, 85, 97], and identifying "neutral harbor" sites, such as *AAVS1* and *ROSA26* [33, 34, 98, 99], for the safe integration of therapeutic transgene cassettes.

C. Bednarski et al.

Acknowledgments

This work was supported by the German Research Foundation (SPP1230-Ca311/2 and SFB738-C9), the Federal Ministry of Education and Research (InTherGD-01GU0834 and ReGene-01GN1003B), the European Commission's 7th Framework Programme (PERSIST-222878 and HeMiBio-266777), the FP6-NoE CliniGene, LSHB-CT-2006-018933, and the Mukoviszidose Institut gGmbH (S03/11).

References

1. Hoelen H, Kleizen B, Schmidt A, Richardson J, Charitou P, Thomas PJ, Braakman I. The primary folding defect and rescue of delta F508 CFTR emerge during translation of the mutant domain. *PLoS One* 2010; 5: e15458.

2. Boucher RC. An overview of the pathogenesis of cystic fibrosis lung disease. *Adv Drug Deliver Rev* 2002; 54: 1359-71.

3. Noguchi M, Yi HF, Rosenblatt HM, Filipovich AH, Adelstein S, Modi WS, Mcbride OW, Leonard WJ. Interleukin-2 receptor gamma chain mutation results in X-linked severe combined immunodeficiency in humans. *Cell* 1993; 73: 147-57.

4. Qasim W, Gaspar HB, Thrasher AJ. Progress and prospects: gene therapy for inherited immunodeficiencies. *Gene Ther* 2009; 16: 1285-91.

5. Howe SJ, Mansour MR, Schwarzwaelder K, Bartholomae C, Hubank M, Kempski H, *et al*. Insertional mutagenesis combined with acquired somatic mutations causes leukemogenesis following gene therapy of SCID-X1 patients. *J Clin Invest* 2008; 118: 3143-50.

6. Ott MG, Schmidt M, Schwarzwaelder K, Stein S, Siler U, Koehl U, *et al*. Correction of X-linked chronic granulomatous disease by gene therapy, augmented by insertional activation of MDS1-EVI1, PRDM16 or SETBP1. *Nat Med* 2006; 12: 401-9.

7. Hacein-Bey-Abina S, Garrigue A, Wang GP, Soulier J, Lim A, Morillon E, *et al*. Insertional oncogenesis in 4 patients after retrovirus-mediated gene therapy of SCID-X1. *J Clin Invest* 2008; 118: 3132-42.

8. Modlich U, Schambach A, Brugman MH, Wicke DC, Knoess S, Li Z, *et al*. Leukemia induction after a single retroviral vector insertion in Evi1 or Prdm16. *Leukemia* 2008; 22: 1519-28.

9. Hacein-Bey-Abina S, Von Kalle C, Schmidt M, McCcormack MP, Wulffraat N, Leboulch P, *et al*. LMO2-associated clonal T cell proliferation in two patients after gene therapy for SCID-X1. *Science* 2003; 302: 415-9.

10. Modlich U, Navarro S, Zychlinski D, Maetzig T, Knoess S, Brugman MH, *et al*. Insertional transformation of hematopoietic cells by self-inactivating lentiviral and gammaretroviral vectors. *Mol Ther* 2009; 17: 1919-28.

11. Rouet P, Smih F, Jasin M. Introduction of double-strand breaks into the genome of mouse cells by expression of a rare-cutting endonuclease. *Mol Cell Biol* 1994; 14: 8096-106.

12. Choulika A, Perrin A, Dujon B, Nicolas JF. Induction of homologous recombination in mammalian chromosomes by using the I-Scei system of *Saccharomyces cerevisiae*. *Mol Cell Biol* 1995; 15: 1968-73.

13. Kim YG, Cha J, Chandrasegaran S. Hybrid restriction enzymes: zinc finger fusions to Fok I cleavage domain. *Proc Natl Acad Sci USA* 1996; 93: 1156-60.

14. Bibikova M, Carroll D, Segal DJ, Trautman JK, Smith J, Kim YG, Chandrasegaran S. Stimulation of homologous recombination through targeted cleavage by chimeric nucleases. *Mol Cell Biol* 2001; 21: 289-97.

15. Urnov FD, Miller JC, Lee YL, Beausejour CM, Rock JM, Augustus S, *et al*. Highly efficient endogenous human gene correction using designed zinc-finger nucleases. *Nature* 2005; 435: 646-51.

16. Maeder ML, Thibodeau-Beganny S, Osiak A, Wright DA, Anthony RM, Eichtinger M, *et al*. Rapid open-source engineering of customized zinc-finger nucleases for highly efficient gene modification. *Mol Cell* 2008; 31: 294-301.

17. Perez EE, Wang JB, Miller JC, Jouvenot Y, Kim KA, Liu O, *et al*. Establishment of HIV-1 resistance in CD4+ T cells by genome editing using zinc-finger nucleases. *Nat Biotechnol* 2008; 26: 808-16.

18. Händel EM, Cathomen T. Zinc-finger nuclease based genome surgery: it's all about specificity. *Curr Gene Ther* 2011; 11: 28-37.

19. Smith J, Grizot S, Arnould S, Duclert A, Epinat JC, Chames P, *et al*. A combinatorial approach to create artificial homing endonucleases cleaving chosen sequences. *Nucleic Acids Res* 2006; 34: e149.

20. Redondo P, Prieto J, Munoz IG, Alibes A, Stricher F, Serrano L, *et al*. Molecular basis of xeroderma pigmentosum group C DNA recognition by engineered meganucleases. *Nature* 2008; 456: 107-11.

21. Grizot S, Smith J, Daboussi F, Prieto J, Redondo P, Merino N, *et al*. Efficient targeting of a SCID gene by an engineered single-chain homing endonuclease. *Nucleic Acids Res* 2009; 37: 5405-19.

22. Grosse S, Huot N, Mahiet C, Arnould S, Barradeau S, Le Clerre D, *et al*. Meganuclease-mediated inhibition of HSV1 infection in cultured cells. *Mol Ther* 2011; 19: 694-702.

23. Stoddard BL. Homing endonucleases: from microbial genetic invaders to reagents for targeted DNA modification. *Structure* 2011; 19: 7-15.

24. Miller JC, Tan SY, Qiao GJ, Barlow KA, Wang JB, Xia DF, *et al*. A Tale nuclease architecture for efficient genome editing. *Nat Biotechnol* 2011; 29: 143-8.

25. Mussolino C, Morbitzer R, Lütge F, Dannemann N, Lahaye T, Cathomen T. A novel Tale nuclease scaffold enables high genome editing activity in combination with low toxicity. *Nucleic Acids Res* 2011; 39: 9283-93.

26. Geurts AM, Cost GJ, Freyvert Y, Zeitler B, Miller JC, Choi VM, *et al*. Knockout rats via embryo microinjection of zinc-finger nucleases. *Science* 2009; 325: 433.

27. Beumer KJ, Trautman JK, Bozas A, Liu JL, Rutter J, Gall JG, Carroll D. Efficient gene targeting in Drosophila by direct embryo injection with zinc-finger nucleases. *Proc Natl Acad Sci USA* 2008; 105: 19821-6.

28. Doyon Y, McCammon JM, Miller JC, Faraji F, Ngo C, Katibah GE, *et al*. Heritable targeted gene disruption in zebrafish using designed zinc-finger nucleases. *Nat Biotechnol* 2008; 26: 702-8.

29. Meng XD, Noyes MB, Zhu LHJ, Lawson ND, Wolfe SA. Targeted gene inactivation in zebrafish using engineered zinc-finger nucleases. *Nat Biotechnol* 2008; 26: 695-701.

30. Morton J, Davis MW, Jorgensen EM, Carroll D. Induction and repair of zinc-finger nuclease-targeted double-strand breaks in *Caenorhabditis elegans* somatic cells. *Proc Natl Acad Sci USA* 2006; 103: 16370-5.

31. Townsend JA, Wright DA, Winfrey RJ, Fu FL, Maeder ML, Joung JK, Voytas DF. High-frequency modification of plant genes using engineered zinc-finger nucleases. *Nature* 2009; 459: 442-5.

32. Vasileva A, Jessberger R. Precise hit: adeno-associated virus in gene targeting. *Nat Rev Microbiol* 2005; 3: 837-47.

33. Sadelain M, Papapetrou EP, Bushman FD. Safe harbours for the integration of new DNA in the human genome. *Nat Rev Cancer* 2012; 12: 51-8.

34. Lombardo A, Cesana D, Genovese P, Di Stefano B, Provasi E, Colombo DF, *et al*. Site-specific integration and tailoring of cassette design for sustainable gene transfer. *Nat Methods* 2011; 8: 861-9.

35. Zou JZ, Sweeney CL, Chou BK, Choi U, Pan J, Wang HM, *et al*. Oxidase-deficient neutrophils from X-linked chronic granulomatous disease iPS cells: functional correction by zinc finger nuc-lease-mediated safe harbor targeting. *Blood* 2011; 117: 5561-72.

36. DeKelver RC, Choi VM, Moehle EA, Paschon DE, Hockemeyer D, Meijsing SH, *et al*. Functional genomics, proteomics, and regulatory DNA analysis in isogenic settings using zinc finger nuclease-driven transgenesis into a safe harbor locus in the human genome. *Genome Res* 2010; 20: 1133-42.

37. Smith JR, Maguire S, Davis LA, Alexander M, Yang FT, Chandran S, Ffrench-Constant C, Pe-dersen RA. Robust, persistent transgene expression in human embryonic stem cells is achieved with AAVS1-targeted integration. *Stem Cells* 2008, 26: 496-504.

38. Hockemeyer D, Soldner F, Beard C, Gao Q, Mitalipova M, DeKelver RC, *et al*. Efficient targeting of expressed and silent genes in human ESCs and iPSCs using zinc-finger nucleases. *Nat Biotechnol* 2009; 27: 851-7.

39. Foley JE, Maeder ML, Pearlberg J, Joung JK, Peterson RT, Yeh JRJ. Targeted mutagenesis in zebrafish using customized zinc-finger nucleases. *Nat Protoc* 2009; 4: 1855-68.

40. Mashimo T, Takizawa A, Voigt B, Yoshimi K, Hiai H, Kuramoto T, Serikawa T. Generation of knockout rats with X-linked severe combined immunodeficiency (X-Scid) using zinc-finger nucleases. *PLoS One* 2010; 5: e8870.

41. Sollu C, Pars K, Cornu TI, Thibodeau-Beganny S, Maeder ML, Joung JK, Heilbronn R, Cathomen T. Autonomous zinc-finger nuclease pairs for targeted chromosomal deletion. *Nucleic Acids Res* 2010; 38: 8269-76.

42. Lee HJ, Kim E, Kim JS. Targeted chromosomal deletions in human cells using zinc finger nuc-leases. *Genome Res* 2010; 20: 81-9.

43. Lee HJ, Kweon J, Kim E, Kim S, Kim JS. Targeted chromosomal duplications and inversions in the human genome using zinc finger nucleases. *Genome Res* 2012; 22: 539-48.

44. Händel EM, Gellhaus K, Khan K, Bednarski C, Cornu TI, Muller-Lerch F, Heilbronn R, Cathomen T. Versatile and efficient genome editing in human cells by combining zinc-finger nucleases with AAV vectors. *Hum Gene Ther* 2012; 23: 321-9.

45. Li HJ, Haurigot V, Doyon Y, Li TJ, Wong SNY, Bhagwat AS, *et al*. *In vivo* genome editing restores haemostasis in a mouse model of haemophilia. *Nature* 2011; 475: 217-21.

46. Pabo CO, Peisach E, Grant RA. Design and selection of novel Cys(2)His(2) zinc finger proteins. *Annu Rev Biochem* 2001; 70: 313-40.

47. Pavletich NP, Pabo CO. Zinc finger DNA recognition: crystal-structure of a Zif268-DNA complex at 2.1-A. *Science* 1991; 252: 809-17.

48. Klug A. The discovery of zinc fingers and their applications in gene regulation and genome ma-nipulation. *Annu Rev Biochem* 2010; 79: 213-31.

49. Hurt JA, Thibodeau SA, Hirsh AS, Pabo CO, Joung JK. Highly specific zinc finger proteins ob-tained by directed domain shuffling and cell-based selection. *Proc Natl Acad Sci USA* 2003; 100: 12271-6.

50. Isalan M, Choo Y, Klug A. Synergy between adjacent zinc fingers in sequence-specific DNA re-cognition. *Proc Natl Acad Sci USA* 1997; 94: 5617-21.

51. Imanishi M, Nakamura A, Morisaki T, Futaki S. Positive and negative cooperativity of modularly assembled zinc fingers. *Biochem Biophys Res Commun* 2009; 387: 440-3.

52. Isalan M, Klug A, Choo Y. Comprehensive DNA recognition through concerted interactions from adjacent zinc fingers. *Biochemistry* 1998; 37: 12026-33.

53. Fairall L, Schwabe JWR, Chapman L, Finch JT, Rhodes D. The crystal-structure of a 2 zinc-finger peptide reveals an extension to the rules for zinc-finger DNA recognition. *Nature* 1993; 366: 483-7.

54. Klug A. The discovery of zinc fingers and their development for practical applications in gene regulation and genome manipulation. *Q Rev Biophys* 2010; 43: 1-21.

55. Pruett-Miller SM, Connelly JP, Maeder ML, Joung JK, Porteus MH. Comparison of zinc finger nucleases for use in gene targeting in mammalian cells. *Mol Ther* 2008; 16: 707-17.

56. Meyer M, de Angelis MH, Wurst W, Kuhn R. Gene targeting by homologous recombination in mouse zygotes mediated by zinc-finger nucleases. *Proc Natl Acad Sci USA* 2010; 107: 15022-6.

57. Holt N, Wang JB, Kim K, Friedman G, Wang XC, Taupin V, *et al*. Human hematopoietic stem/progenitor cells modified by zinc-finger nucleases targeted to CCR5 control HIV-1 *in vivo*. *Nat Biotechnol* 2010; 28: 839-47.

58. Wah DA, Hirsch JA, Dorner LF, Schildkraut I, Aggarwal AK. Structure of the multimodular endonuclease FokI bound to DNA. *Nature* 1997; 388: 97-100.

59. Bitinaite J, Wah DA, Aggarwal AK, Schildkraut I. FokI dimerization is required for DNA cleavage. *Proc Natl Acad Sci USA* 1998; 95: 10570-5.

60. Szczepek M, Brondani V, Buchel J, Serrano L, Segal DJ, Cathomen T. Structure-based redesign of the dimerization interface reduces the toxicity of zinc-finger nucleases. *Nat Biotechnol* 2007; 25: 786-93.

61. Miller JC, Holmes MC, Wang JB, Guschin DY, Lee YL, Rupniewski, I, *et al*. An improved zinc-finger nuclease architecture for highly specific genome editing. *Nat Biotechnol* 2007; 25: 778-85.

62. Ramalingam S, Kandavelou K, Rajenderan R, Chandrasegaran S. Creating designed zinc-finger nucleases with minimal cytotoxicity. *J Mol Biol* 2011; 405: 630-41.

63. Doyon Y, Vo TD, Mendel MC, Greenberg SG, Wang JB, Xia DF, *et al*. Enhancing zinc-finger-nuclease activity with improved obligate heterodimeric architectures. *Nat Methods* 2011; 8: 74-9.

64. Cornu TI, Thibodeau-Beganny S, Guhl E, Alwin S, Eichtinger M, Joung J, Cathomen T. DNA-binding specificity is a major determinant of the activity and toxicity of zinc-finger nucleases. *Mol Ther* 2008; 16: 352-8.

65. Maeder ML, Thibodeau-Beganny S, Sander JD, Voytas DF, Joung JK. Oligomerized pool engineering (OPEN): an open-source protocol for making customized zinc-finger arrays. *Nat Protoc* 2009; 4: 1471-501.

66. Maeder ML, Yeh JRJ, Foley JE, Zou JH, Thibodeau-Beganny S, Cheng LH, Peterson RT, Joung JK. Further improvements and applications of Open (oligomerized pool engineering): a rapid, robust, and publicly available method for engineering customized zinc finger nucleases. *Mol Ther* 2009; 17: S162-3.

67. Cathomen T, Joung JK. Zinc-finger nucleases: the next generation emerges. *Mol Ther* 2008; 16: 1200-7.

68. Porteus MH, Baltimore D. Chimeric nucleases stimulate gene targeting in human cells. *Science* 2003; 300: 763.

69. Händel EM, Alwin S, Cathomen T. Expanding or restricting the target site repertoire of zinc-finger nucleases: the inter-domain linker as a major determinant of target site selectivity. *Mol Ther* 2009; 17: 104-11.

70. Zou JZ, Maeder ML, Mali P, Pruett-Miller SM, Thibodeau-Beganny S, Chou BK, *et al*. Gene targeting of a disease-related gene in human induced pluripotent stem and embryonic stem cells. *Cell Stem Cell* 2009; 5: 97-110.

71. Sebastiano V, Maeder ML, Angstman JF, Haddad B, Khayter C, Yeo DT, *et al*. *In situ* genetic correction of the sickle cell anemia mutation in human induced pluripotent stem cells using engineered zinc finger nucleases. *Stem Cells* 2011; 29: 1717-26.

72. Yusa K, Rashid ST, Strick-Marchand H, Varela I, Liu PQ, Paschon DE, *et al*. Targeted gene correction of alpha(1)-antitrypsin deficiency in induced pluripotent stem cells. *Nature* 2011; 478: 391-4.

73. Alwin S, Gere MB, Guhl E, Effertz K, Barbas CF, Sega DJ, Weitzman MD, Cathomen T. Custom zinc-finger nucleases for use in human cells. *Mol Ther* 2005; 1: 610-17.

74. Rogakou EP, Boon C, Redon C, Bonner WM. Megabase chromatin domains involved in DNA double-strand breaks *in vivo*. *J Cell Biol* 1999; 146: 905-15.

75. Schultz LB, Chehab NH, Malikzay A, Halazonetis TD. p53 binding protein 1 (53BP1) is an early participant in the cellular response to DNA double-strand breaks. *J Cell Biol* 2000; 151: 1381-90.

76. Wang B, Matsuoka S, Carpenter PB, Elledge SJ. 53BP1, a mediator of the DNA damage checkpoint. *Science* 2002; 298: 1435-8.

77. Pattanayak V, Ramirez CL, Joung JK, Liu DR. Revealing off-target cleavage specificities of zinc-finger nucleases by *in vitro* selection. *Nat Methods* 2011; 8: 765-70.

78. Gabriel R, Lombardo A, Arens A, Miller JC, Genovese P, Kaeppel C, *et al*. An unbiased genome-wide analysis of zinc-finger nuclease specificity. *Nat Biotechnol* 2011; 29: 816-23.

79. Mussolino C, Cathomen T. On target? Tracing zinc-finger-nuclease specificity. *Nat Methods* 2011; 8: 725-6.

80. Cornu TI, Cathomen T. Targeted genome modifications using integrase-deficient lentiviral vectors. *Mol Ther* 2007; 15: 2107-13.

81. Lombardo A, Genovese P, Beausejour CM, Colleoni S, Lee YL, Kim KA, *et al*. Gene editing in human stem cells using zinc finger nucleases and integrase-defective lentiviral vector delivery. *Nat Biotechnol* 2007; 25: 1298-306.

82. Gellhaus K, Cornu TI, Heilbronn R, Cathomen T. Fate of recombinant adeno-associated viral vector genomes during DNA double-strand break-induced gene targeting in human cells. *Hum Gene Ther* 2010; 21: 543-53.

83. Miller DG, Trobridge GD, Petek LM, Jacobs MA, Kaul R, Russell DW. Large-scale analysis of adeno-associated virus vector integration sites in normal human cells. *J Virol* 2005; 79: 11434-42.

84. Brown BD, Gentner B, Cantore A, Colleoni S, Amendola M, Zingale A, *et al*. Endogenous microRNA can be broadly exploited to regulate transgene expression according to tissue, lineage and differentiation state. *Nat Biotechnol* 2007, 25: 1457-67.

85. Brown BD, Venneri MA, Zingale A, Sergi LS, Naldini L. Endogenous microRNA regulation suppresses transgene expression in hematopoietic lineages and enables stable gene transfer. *Nat Med* 2006; 12: 585-91.

86. Foley JE, Yeh JRJ, Maeder ML, Reyon D, Sander JD, Peterson RT, Joung JK. Rapid mutation of endogenous zebrafish genes using zinc finger nucleases made by oligomerized pool engineering (Open). *PLoS One* 2009; 4: e4348.

87. Carroll D. Zinc-finger nucleases: a panoramic view. *Curr Gene Ther* 2011; 11: 2-10.

88. Mussolino C, Cathomen T. Tale nucleases: tailored genome engineering made easy. *Curr Opin Biotechnol* 2012; 23: 1-7.

89. Moscou MJ, Bogdanove AJ. A simple cipher governs DNA recognition by TAL effectors. *Science* 2009; 326: 1501.

90. Boch J, Scholze H, Schornack S, Landgraf A, Hahn S, Kay S, *et al*. Breaking the code of DNA binding specificity of TAL-type III effectors. *Science* 2009; 326: 1509-12.

91. Bogdanove AJ, Schornack S, Lahaye T. TAL effectors: finding plant genes for disease and defense. *Curr Opin Plant Biol* 2010; 13: 394-401.

92. Scholze H, Boch J. TAL effectors are remote controls for gene activation. *Curr Opin Microbiol* 2011; 14: 47-53.

93. Boch J, Bonas U. Xanthomonas AvrBs3 family-type III effectors: discovery and function. *Annu Rev Phytopathol* 2010; 48: 419-36.

94. Wood AJ, Lo TW, Zeitler B, Pickle CS, Ralston EJ, Lee AH, *et al*. Targeted genome editing across species using ZFNs and TALENs. *Science* 2011; 333: 307.

95. Hockemeyer D, Wang HY, Kiani S, Lai CS, Gao Q, Cassady JP, *et al*. Genetic engineering of human pluripotent cells using TALE nucleases. *Nat Biotechnol* 2011; 29: 731-4.

96. Mcnulty J, Noyes M, Smith T, Rayla A, Chu S, Meng XD, *et al*. Creating targeted genomic lesions in zebrafish using zinc finger nucleases. *Transgenic Res* 2010; 19: 139-40.

97. Porteus MH, Cathomen T, Weitzman MD, Baltimore D. Efficient gene targeting mediated by adeno-associated virus and DNA double-strand breaks. *Mol Cell Biol* 2003; 23: 3558-65.

98. Perez-Pinera P, Ousterout DG, Brown MT, Gersbach CA. Gene targeting to the ROSA26 locus directed by engineered zinc finger nucleases. *Nucleic Acids Res* 2011; december 14, online.

99. Irion S, Luche H, Gadue P, Fehling HJ, Kennedy M, Keller G. Identification and targeting of the ROSA26 locus in human embryonic stem cells. *Nat Biotechnol* 2007, 25: 1477-82.

PRE-CLINICAL STUDIES,
BIOSAFETY AND ANIMAL MODELS

Preclinical
assessment tools

COORDINATED BY
AMOS PANET,
NICOLE DÉGLON
AND
ANDREAS H. JACOBS

The CliniBook: Clinical gene transfer
Edited by Odile Cohen-Haguenauer – EDK, Paris © 2012, pp. 371-385

B1-1
Preclinical assessment tools: imaging gene transfer to the brain

Yannic Waerzeggers[1,2], Thomas Viel[1,2], Sonja Schäfers[2], Parisa Monfared[1,2],
Alexandra Winkeler[1,3], Andreas H. Jacobs[1,2,4]*

[1]*Laboratory for Gene Therapy and Molecular Imaging at the Max Planck Institute for
Neurological Research with Klaus-Joachim-Zülch-Laboratories of the Max Planck Society
and the Faculty of Medicine of the University of Cologne, Cologne, Germany.*
[2]*European Institute for Molecular Imaging (EIMI), University of Münster (WWU),
Münster, Germany.*
[3]*Laboratory for Experimental Molecular Imaging, Inserm U1023, University Paris Sud,
Paris, France.*
[4]*Department of Geriatric Medicine, Johanniter Hospital, Bonn, Germany.*
ahjacobs@uni-muenster.de
* Corresponding author

Introduction

In gene therapy specific genes are introduced, altered or eliminated with the aim to
restore hereditary diseases linked to a genetic defect or to impact cancer and infectious
diseases (*e.g.* HIV). Today, most gene therapy studies for brain disorders introduce
transgenes, that have the ability to restore the level of depleted neurotransmitters
(restorative gene therapy; *e.g.* dopamine replacement therapy in Parkinson's disease
(PD [1]) or that influence brain tumour growth (suicide or gene-directed enzyme prodrug therapy [2]). Transgene delivery can be carried out by synthetic vectors (liposomes, nanoparticles) or by vectors derived from viruses, bacteria or mammalian stem
cells [3]. Numerous targeted or oncolytic viral vectors, such as retroviruses, adenoviruses or lentiviruses [4-6], have been investigated over the past years and vector
tropism to specific cell types ameliorated [7-12]. Moreover, *in vivo* homing of neural
or mesenchymal stem and progenitor cells to sites of pathology has been exploited
for transgene delivery [13].

The efficacy of a certain gene therapy approach does not only depend on the delivered
transgene and gene-carrying vector, but also on the way the vector is delivered. Due
to the privileged localisation of most brain pathologies behind the blood-brain barrier,
systemic vector application is not the delivery route of choice. In most preclinical studies the vector is directly applied within the brain parenchyma or the ventricles by means
of simple needle injections [14]. By this approach vector distribution within the target
volume is often inhomogeneous and better results have been achieved by the use of
hollow fibres [15] or convection-enhanced delivery [16, 17]. Due to the relatively good

prediction of vector spread in the latter approach, this technique is mostly deployed in clinical trials [18]. In the past decade also the exceptional homing capabilities of stem cells to sites of brain pathology have been exploited for the use of stem cells as carrying vectors for therapeutic transgenes [19, 20], often combined with specific contrast agents [21, 22].

Table I. Comparative overview of molecular imaging systems.

technique (and used energy window)	spatial resolution	depth penetration	temporal resolution	sensitivity for detection of molecular probes	main advantages	main disadvantages	clinical use	operational costs
PET (high-energy γ-rays)	1-2 mm	no limit	minutes-hours	nanomolar	high sensitivity, quantitative, variety of available probes	cyclotron needed, short-lived radioisotopes, low resolution, single-to-noise ratio	yes	€€€
SPECT (low-energy γ-rays)	1-2 mm	no limit	minutes-hours	nanomolar	radioisotopes have longer half-lives than those used in PET, multiple probes can be detected simultaneously	sensitivity 10-100 times lower than PET, semiquantitative	yes	€€
MRI (radio-waves)	10-100 μm	no limit	minutes-hours	millimolar-micromolar	high spatial resolution and soft tissue contrast, functional information, versatile	low sensitivity, long acquisition and image processing times	yes	€€€
BLI (visible light)	several mm	centimeters	minutes	picomolar	high sensitivity, high through-put, transgene-based approach confers versatility	light emission prone to attenuation and scatter with increased tissue depth	no	€
FI (visible and NIR light)	1 mm	<10cm	seconds-minutes	picomolar	potential for multiplex imaging, high through-put, transgene-based approach confers versatility	excitation and emission light < 600nm prone to attenuation with increased tissue depth, autofluorescence	in development	€

MOLECULAR IMAGING (MI)

Over the last decade the development of efficient gene therapy protocols largely benefited from the development of molecular imaging strategies enabling the non-invasive assessment of gene transfer, gene function and therapy response [23]. Molecular imaging (MI) is a term that was developed in the late 1990s. MI seeks to shed new light on both structure and function by creating images that directly or indirectly reflect specific cellular and molecular events (*e.g.* gene expression), which can reveal pathways and mechanisms responsible for disease within the context of physiologically authentic and intact living subject environments [24]. MI may play a crucial role in the non-invasive assessment of all steps of a gene therapy protocol: (i) non-invasive determination of viable target tissue which may benefit from a biologic treatment paradigm, (ii) guidance of transgene delivery, (iii) assessment of the location, magnitude, and duration of transgene expression (the actual gene transfer), and (iv) monitoring of therapy response or of the downstream readouts of transgene expression during and after gene therapy [23, 25].

Molecular imaging involves nuclear, magnetic resonance (MRI) and *in vivo* optical imaging (OI) systems. These imaging techniques differ in a number of aspects like spatial and temporal resolution, depth penetration and tomographic ability, detection threshold (sensitivity), signal quantification, cost and ease of operation and clinical translatability, among others (*Table I*). As no single modality addresses all aspects related with gene transfer and gene therapy, the use of multi-modality platforms has gained much attention in order to take the best advantage of each technique. Multi-modality imaging with positron emission tomography (PET)/computed tomography (CT) or single photon emission computed tomography (SPECT)/CT have become everyday techniques in clinical practice and in preclinical and basic medical research. The development of hybrid PET/MRI systems is an active area of research at the present time and even other, less obvious combinations, including CT/MRI and PET/optical are being investigated [26]. In addition to the integration of instrumentation, there are parallel developments in synthesizing imaging agents that can be viewed by multiple imaging modalities, such as the combination of PET-optical [27, 28] and MR-optical [29-31] or PET-MR [32] compatible contrast agents.

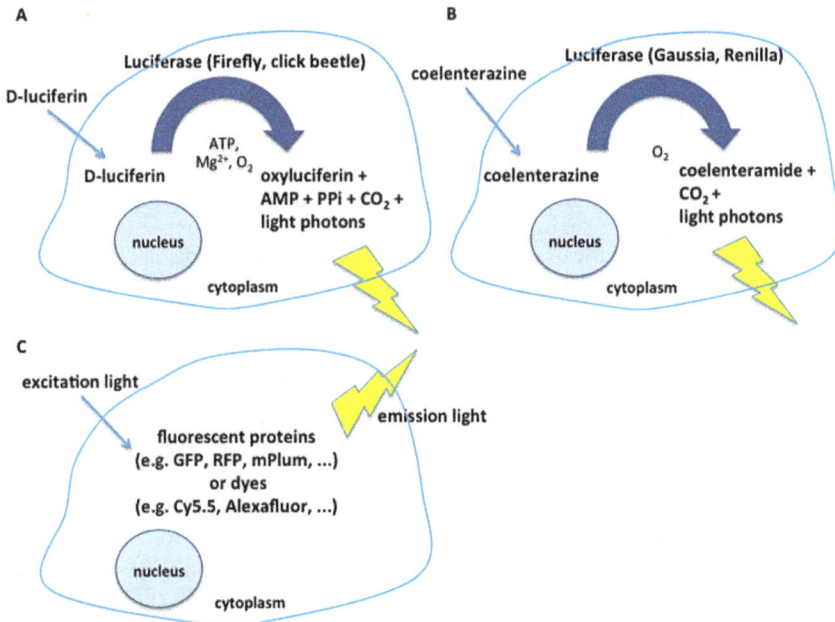

Figure 1. Schematic representation of bioluminescence and fluorescence imaging reporters. (A) Beetle luciferase enzymes (firefly, click beetle) expressed in cytoplasm of engineered cells catalyze production of light photons from the substrate luciferin in the presence of oxygen and ATP. (B) Gaussia and Renilla luciferases use coelenterazine as substrate and are independent of ATP. (C) Fluorescence imaging requires light of appropriate wavelength to excite a fluorescent reporter molecule (fluorescent protein or dye molecule), resulting in emission of light with a defined emission spectrum for each reporter protein or dye.

Optical imaging techniques

Optical techniques, including bioluminescence and fluorescence, are key technologies in preclinical research. Bioluminescence refers to the production of light of a specific wavelength by an energy-dependent enzymatic reaction of a luciferase enzyme with its substrate in the presence of oxygen and for some luciferases also other cofactors such as adenosine triphosphate (ATP) or Mg^{2+} (*Figure 1A,B*). Luciferase proteins with unique spectral characteristics and substrate requirements have been isolated from a variety of organisms, such as Photinus pyralis (Firefly luciferase; substrate: luciferin), Pyrophorus plagiophthalamus (click beetle luciferase; substrate luciferin), sea pansy (Renilla luciferase, substrate: coelenterazine) or marine copepod (Gaussia luciferase; substrate coelenterazine).

Due to the substrate specificity of different luciferase enzymes, such luciferases can be combined as dual reporters for bioluminescence imaging (BLI) of 2 different processes sequentially in the same living subject [33]. In the past decade, BLI has become indispensable for non-invasive monitoring of biological phenomena *in vivo*, such as gene expression and gene regulation, protein-protein interaction, cell (immune, stem or cancer cells) trafficking and tumourigenesis [34].

In fluorescence imaging an external light of appropriate wavelength excites a target fluorophore (fluorescent protein or dye) and the transferred light energy is emitted as a longer-wavelength, lower-energy light for imaging when the fluorophore returns back to its ground state (*Figure 1C*).

The key challenges for optical imaging are related to light scattering and attenuation by tissues compromising sensitivity and spatial resolution and to the use of planar imaging complicating quantification and the ability to resolve depth [35]. These hurdles can in part be overcome by the use of tomographic principles and by imaging in the near-infrared (NIR) spectrum, which decreases light absorption by hemoglobine and other tissue macromolecules and increases tissue penetration. Furthermore, at these wavelenghts nonspecific tissue autofluorescence is greatly reduced [36, 37]. Although optical molecular imaging techniques essentially have been used for studying small animal models, fluorescence applications for superficially accessible locations in clinical care are expected to expand, such as endoscopy, intraoperative scanning and breast or skin imaging [36].

Nuclear imaging techniques

Nuclear imaging techniques include PET and SPECT and are clinically the most used techniques to monitor biological function, including gene expression. In these techniques positron-emitting or gamma-emitting radionuclide imaging probes are used to detect biologically active molecules, as a result of the target-dependent sequestration of the systemically administered imaging probes.

After reaching the target organ, the radionuclide tracers are specifically retained as a result of transport, binding to receptors or antigens or reaction with enzymes. The tagged enzymes, receptors or transporters may be expressed endogenously and this methodology is used in conventional PET images, *e.g.* imaging of cell metabolism with radiolabelled glucose (2-[18F]fluoro-2-deoxy-D-glucose; [18F]FDG) targeted to the Glut-1 transporter and to the enzyme hexokinase, or these molecules can be expressed by exogenously introduced genes (called marker genes, imaging or reporter genes, see also below) a strategy mostly used for the evaluation of gene therapy protocols (*Table II*). Despite their unequalled sensitivity for clinical applications, the most important drawback of nuclear imaging techniques, besides radiation exposure and dependence on radiopharmaceutical production, is their moderate spatial resolution and lack to provide structural information.

Table II. Reporter genes for nuclear imaging.

reporter gene	working mechanism	reporter probe	imaging modality	references
herpes simplex virus type 1 thymidine kinase (HSV-1-*tk*)	HSV-1-TK phosphorylizes thymidine, pyrimidine nucleosides and acycloguanosine derivates which are then trapped within transduced cells (enzyme)	(i) pyrimidine nucleosides: [[123, 125, 131]I], [[124]I], [^{18}F] 5-iodo-2'-[^{18}F]fluoro-2'deoxy-1-β-D-arabino-furanosyluracil (FIAU); 5-ethyl-2'-[^{18}F]fluoro-2'deoxy-1-β-D-arabinosyl-furanosyl-uracil (FEAU); 1-(2'-deoxy-2'-[^{18}F]fluoro-5-iodo-1-β-D-ribofuranosyl)-uracil (FIRU); 29-[^{18}F]fluoro-5-methyl-1-beta-D-arabinofuranosyluracil (FMAU); 2-[^{18}F]fluoro-2-deoxy-5-iodovinyl-1--D-ribofuranosyl-uracil (IVFRU) (ii) acycloguanosine derivates: [^{18}F]ganciclovir (GCV); 8-[^{18}F]fluoro-9-[4-hydroxy-3-(hydroxymethyl)butyl]guanine (FPCV); 9-[4-[^{18}F]fluoro-3-(hydoxymethyl)butyl]guanine (FHBG); 9-[(3-[^{18}F]fluoro-1-hydroxy-2-propoxy)methyl]guanine (FHPG)	PET, SPECT	(50, 74, 75)
dopamine D2 receptor (D2R)	Receptor	[^{11}C]raclopride; N-[^{11}C]methylspiperone; 3-(2-[^{18}F]fluoroethyl)spiperone (FESP)	PET	(59, 76, 77)
human somatostatin receptor subtype 2 (hSSTR2)	somatostatin receptors mediate the various actions of somatostatin, a peptide that inhibits the release of growth hormone (receptor)	[[188]Re], [^{99m}Tc]somatostatin analogues; [^{111}In]DTPA-D-Phe1-octreotide; [^{68}Ga]DOTATOC; [^{111}In]DTPA-octreotide	PET; SPECT	(78-80)
sodium/iodide symporter (NIS)	NIS is an intrinsic transmembrane glycoprotein from the sodium/solute symporter family (transporter)	[[124]I]NaI and [[123, 125, 131]I]NaI; [^{99m}Tc]pertechnetate; [[186, 188]Re]perrhenate [^{18}F]tetrafluoroborate (TFB)	PET, SPECT	(60, 81-84)
norepinephrine transporter (NET)	NET mediates the transport of norepinephrine, dopamine and epinephrine across the cell membrane (transporter)	[[124]I] meta-iodobenzylguanidine (MIBG); [^{11}C]epinedrine (EPI); [^{11}C]hydroxyephedrine (HED)	PET	(85, 86)
human mitochondrial thymidine kinase (hTK2)	hTK2 phosphorylates deoxythymidine, deoxycytidine and deoxyuridine, as well as several antiviral and anticancer nucleoside analogs	[[124]I]FIAU; [^{18}F]FIAU; [^{18}F]FEAU	PET	(87)
human deoxycytidine kinase (dCK)	dCK has a high phosphorylation activity for thymidine analogs such as deoxycytidine, deoxyadenosine, deoxyguanosine, and several pyrimidine-based cytotoxic drugs (Ara-C, gemcitabine) (enzyme)	[^{18}F]FEAU; 1-(2'-deoxy-2'-[^{18}F]fluoro-beta-D-arabinofuranosyl)cytosine ([^{18}F]FAC)	PET	(88, 89)
type 2 cannabinoid receptor	G-protein coupled receptor	[^{11}C]GW405833	PET	(90)

Table III. Reporter genes for magnetic resonance imaging.

reporter gene	working mechanism	MR contrast/imaging modality	references
creatine kinase (CK), arginine kinase (AK)	CK or AK catalyzes ATP conversion to ADP, hereby producing phosphocreatine (PCr) or phosphoarginine, respectively	^{31}P MRS	(45, 91, 92)
cytosine deaminase (CD)	CD converts the pro-drug 5-fluorocytosine into the chemotherapeutic 5-fluorouracil which results in a chemical shift in the ^{19}F peak	^{19}F MRS	(93)
LacZ	β-galactosidase, the LacZ gene product, (i) catalyzes the hydrolysis of β-D-galactopyranosides, resulting in a chemical shift in the ^{19}F peak;	^{19}F MRS	(94, 95)
	(ii) catalyzes the hydrolysis of β-D-galactosides such as EgadMe, a chelated gadolinium caged by a galactopyranose molecule, thereby exposing the free coordination sites of the Gd;	T1	(44)
	(iii) induces the precipitation of ferric ions in the presence of S-Gal	T2/T2*	(65, 96)
tyrosinase	tyrosinase overexpression leads to the production of melanin followed by higher metal binding (endogenous or exogenous Fe)	T2/T2*	(41)
ferritin	intracellular iron (endogenous or exogenous Fe) storing protein	T2/T2*	(38, 39)
transferrin receptor (TfR)	TfR imports bloodstream iron or exogenous transferrin-MION/SPIO by internalising the iron-transferrin complex	T2/T2*	(40)
Mag A	Mag A is an iron transporter protein from the magnetotactic bacteria family	T2/T2*	(42, 43)
Lysin Rich Protein (LRP)	The LRP amino acid sequence is similar to the polypeptide poly-L-lysine (PLL) and provides MR contrast at the amide proton frequency	CEST	(48)
polyphosphate kinase (PPK)	PPK catalyzes the synthesis of inorganic polyphosphate (polyP) from ATP	^{31}P MRS	(47)
green fluorescent protein (GFP)	GFP expression results in a detectable change in macromolecule concentration	MTC	(49)

Magnetic resonance imaging (MRI)

Recent advances in magnetic resonance imaging (MRI), especially the advent of so-phisticated acquisition protocols as well as MR reporter genes, allow the concomitant registration of structural, functional and biochemical tissue information with high spatial resolution. Most important drawbacks of MRI include limited temporal resolution and low sensitivity. MRI relies on measuring magnetization of magnetic nuclei subjected to radiofrequency irradiation inside a magnetic field. A variety of nuclei can be studied: most commonly studied are properties of the hydrogen nucleus (proton: ^1H) within tissue water and organic compounds (proton or spin density; time constant, T1 and relaxation times T2 and T2*; CEST) but also individual proton signals within metabolites as well as a number of other nuclei such as ^{31}P, ^{13}C, ^{23}Na and ^{19}F can be detected with MR spectroscopy. The endogenous tissue contrast, which is mainly dependent on the different properties of tissue water, can be tailored using different pulse sequences and, if necessary, be further modified with exogenous contrast agents. These exogenous contrast agents alter the relaxation properties of tissue water and are usually based on either paramagnetic gadolinium (Gd^{3+}) chelates, that produce hyperintense "positive" contrast in T1-weighted MRI, or super-paramagnetic iron-oxide particles that produce 'negative' contrast in T2-weighted MRI. As a consequence, genes that increase the amount of intracellular iron ions (by either trapping or increasing their transport; ferritin [38, 39], transferrin [40], tyrosinase [41], MagA [42, 43]) or activate a modified Gd^{3+} chelate (β-galactosidase [44]) have been developed and studied as potential candidates for MR reporter genes that can be detected by T1- or T2-weigthed imaging. Moreover, the feasibility of other MR imaging methodologies, such as spectroscopy (MRS) or MRI with magnetization transfer contrast (MTC) or chemical exchange saturation transfer (CEST) to study the expression of creatine kinase (CK) [45], arginine kinase [45, 46], polyphosphate kinase (PPK) [47], Lysine Rich Proteins (LRP) [48] or green fluorescent protein (GFP) [49] have been demonstrated (*Table III*).

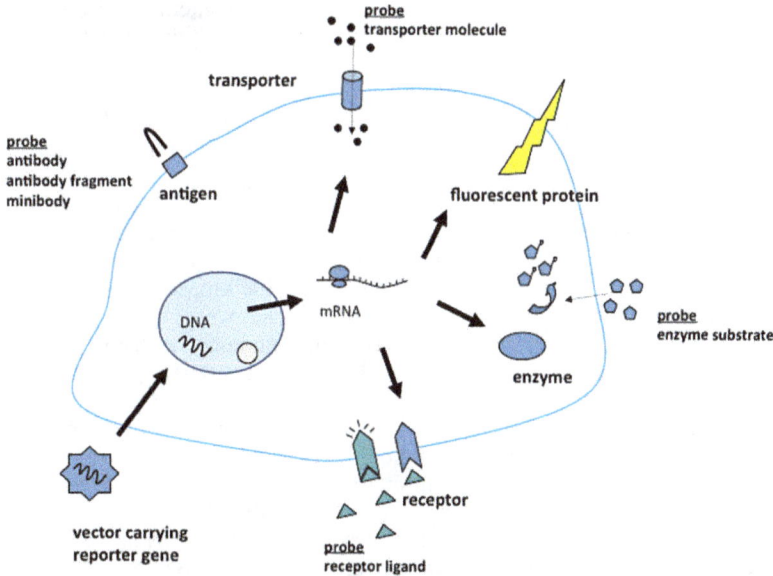

Figure 2. General paradigm for reporter gene imaging. In reporter gene imaging first, the reporter gene complex is transduced into target cells by a vector (viral or non-viral). Inside the transduced cell the reporter gene may integrate into the host genome or remain episomal. After initiation of reporter gene transcription the reporter gene product is expressed. The reporter gene product can be an enzyme, a membrane transporter, a membrane receptor, an artificial cell-surface antigen or a fluorescent protein. Usually a complementary reporter probe (a radiolabelled, paramagnetic or bioluminescent molecule) has to be administered and concentrates or emits light at the site of reporter gene expression. In fluorescence imaging no supplementary reporter probe is necessary, just external illumination. The level of reporter probe concentration or the intensity of emitted light is usually proportional to the level of reporter gene expression.

REPORTER GENES AND OTHER LABELLING STRATEGIES FOR MOLECULAR IMAGING

A reporter gene (also called marker or imaging gene) is a transgene, whose product can be readily detected and ideally quantified by a non-invasive imaging technique and which can be used to interrogate the spatio-temporal profile of a given *in vivo* biological process of interest. Key steps involved in reporter gene imaging and gene transfer in general are (i) transfer of the reporter construct to the target tissue followed by (ii) DNA transcription (the initiation of which can be controlled by specific promoter/enhancer elements) and subsequent (iii) mRNA translation into the gene product, all of which can be specifically visualized *in vivo* by utilizing reporter gene imaging. Moreover, reporter constructs can be tailored to the specific needs of a certain research issue, for instance of a gene therapy protocol [23]. Reporter gene constructs driven by constitutively active promoters can be used to identify the site, extent and duration of vector delivery and to monitor the efficiency of tissue and cell transduction [50], whereas the use of tissue-specific or inducible promoter-enhancer elements can be used to specifically direct gene expression to the target tissue (*e.g.* prostate [51], cancer [52] or brain cells [53]) diminishing side-effect to non-target tissue or to control transgene expression within the target tissue (*e.g.* by hormones or drugs [54]) allowing to control the ideal time-window for transgene expression, respectively. Once the marker gene is transcribed, the gene product can emit light, trap radiolabeled probes or modulate magnetic resonance contrast depending on the exact nature of the reporter product in combination with a complementary reporter probe or excitation light (*Figure 2*).

Furthermore, multimodality reporter constructs can be created containing two or more different (reporter) transgenes with a proportional and constant relationship in their co-expression over a wide range of expression levels allowing to maximally take advantage of the complementary information that can be provided by different MI techniques. Many reports on the construction and validation of several multimodality bifusion and triple fusion reporter genes in living animals exist. The first attempts to combine reporter genes involved two genes with the aim of dual modality imaging. Initially, the reporter gene for herpes simplex virus type 1 thymidine kinase (HSV-1-*tk*) was fused with the gene for GFP [55, 56], later similar approaches were used for a fluorescence/bioluminescence fusion gene [57], a HSV-1-tk/bioluminescence fusion gene [58] or for fusion of a fluorescence gene with other PET or MR reporter genes [59, 60]. Lately triple fusion genes have been validated, combining two optical reporter genes and one radionuclide reporter gene [61, 62]. Moreover, some commonly used reporter genes can be tracked by distinct imaging techniques. For instance the most commonly used PET reporter gene/reporter probe combination for preclinical imaging HSV-1-*tk*/9-(4-[^{18}F]-fluoro-3-[hydroxymethyl]butyl)guanine ([^{18}F]FHBG) not only can be non-invasively assessed with PET imaging but also with OI [63], whereas GFP or β-galactosidase expression can be imaged with fluorescence microscopy as well as with MRI [44, 49, 64, 65].

The use of double or triple transgene constructs can be particularly useful in gene therapy protocols by linking a therapeutic gene to a reporter gene, as most reporter genes don't have therapeutic functions. In such gene therapeutic paradigms direct measure of the expression and activity of the reporter gene gives indirect evaluation of the expression and activity of the therapeutic gene of interest due to the proportional co-expression of both genes. Such co-expression of 2 or more transgenes can be achieved by the use of dual promoters, by gene fusion into a single translational cassette or by certain translational linkers, such as the internal ribosomal entry site (IRES) [23]. The use of such combined vector constructs allows the non-invasive determination of the tissue dose of vector-mediated gene expression and, hence, the gene therapeutic capacity of the delivery system [25, 56, 66, 67] (*Figure 3*).

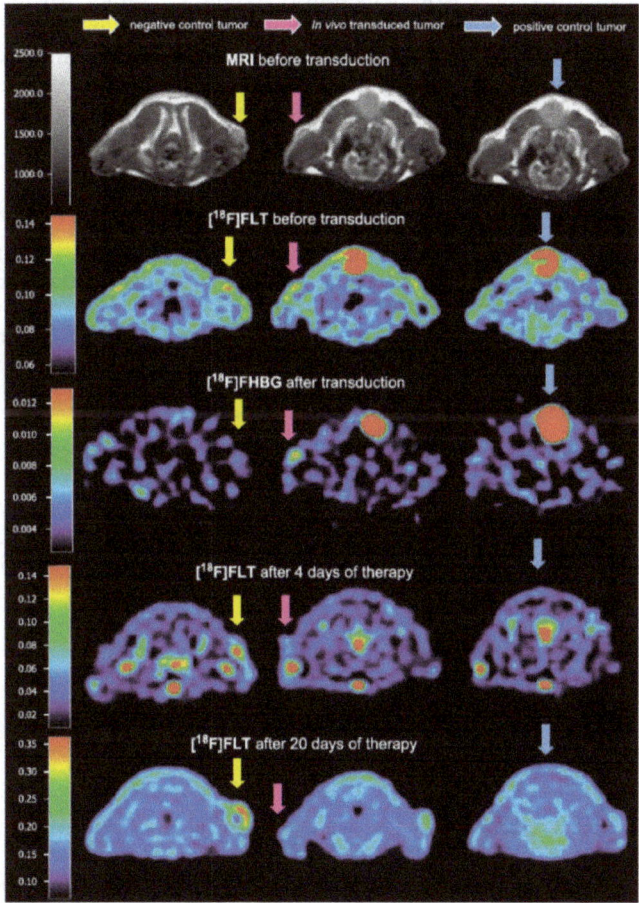

Figure 3. Non-invasive monitoring of gene therapy in experimental glioma. Multimodality imaging protocol of a mouse during treatment of s.c. gliomas after *in vivo* transduction with a vector containing the gene construct CITG and expressing the genes for cytosine deaminase (CD), a mutated form of HSV-1-thymidine kinase (tk39) and green fluorescent protein (GFP). A wild-type glioma served as negative control and a glioma stably expressing the gene construct CITG served as positive control. Row 1 (MRI) and row 2 ([18F]FLT-PET) display tumour morphology and proliferative activity and this information is used to guide vector application. Row 3 ([18F]FHBG-PET) illustrates the intensity of exogenous gene expression after *in vivo* transduction. Rows 4 and 5 ([18F]FLT-PET) show proliferative activity during early and late follow-up under therapy with the prodrugs 5-fluorocytosine and ganciclovir. The negative control tumour shows no expression of HSV-1-tk and an increase in size and proliferative activity in the course of therapy; the *in vivo* transduced tumor with a distinct tk expression in [18F]FHBG-PET, as well as the positive control tumor, disappear under therapy. Figure reprinted with permission from Jacobs *et al.* [25].

Most current *in vivo* MI strategies used to monitor gene transfer involve the use of reporter genes. However, also direct labelling of gene vectors or cells carrying vectors with contrast agents can be used for non-invasive imaging of gene transfer. The most commonly used cell/vector labels are based on Gd-chelates [68], manganese oxide [69] or iron oxide particles [70-72] for MR detection or contain a radiolabel, mostly [^{18}F]FDG or [^{64}Cu]PTSM for PET detection [73]. Although such labelling procedures are straightforward the main disadvantages are (i) label release or washout diminishing signal intensity, (ii) possible label reuptake by neighbouring cells impeding exact vector localisation and most of all (iii) independence of the image signal from the function of the transgene.

CONCLUSION

Gene transfer and cell replacement strategies have considerable potential to become a valuable treatment option for several inherited and acquired brain disorders. By introducing MI methods within the gene therapeutic protocol significant information on the functionality and efficacy of this promising therapy can be provided non-invasively which will ultimately result in the development and selection of safe, efficient and case-selective gene therapy protocols.

ACKNOWLEDGMENTS

Our work has been supported in part by the Deutsche Forschungsgemeinschaft (DFG-Ja98/1-2), the BMBF grant MoBiMed, the DAAD-INCa Joint Transnational Research Programme on Cancer and by the 6th FW EU grants EMIL (LSHC-CT-2004-503569), DiMI (LSHB-CT-2005-512146) and CliniGene NoE (LSHB-CT-2006-018933).

REFERENCES

1. Carlsson T, Bjorklund T, Kirik D. Restoration of the striatal dopamine synthesis for Parkinson's disease: viral vector-mediated enzyme replacement strategy. *Curr Gene Ther* 2007; 7: 109-20.

2. Jacobs A, Voges J, Reszka R, *et al.* Positron-emission tomography of vector-mediated gene expression in gene therapy for gliomas. *Lancet* 2001; 358: 727-9.

3. Briat A, Vassaux G. Preclinical applications of imaging for cancer gene therapy. *Expert Rev Mol Med* 2006;8: 1-19.

4. Sinn PL, Sauter SL, McCray PB Jr. Gene therapy progress and prospects: development of improved lentiviral and retroviral vectors: design, biosafety, and production. *Gene Ther* 2005; 12: 1089-98.

5. Frampton AR Jr, Goins WF, Nakano K, Burton EA, Glorioso JC. HSV trafficking and development of gene therapy vectors with applications in the nervous system. *Gene Ther* 2005; 12: 891-901.

6. Pedersini R, Vattemi E, Claudio PP. Adenoviral gene therapy in high-grade malignant glioma. *Drug News Perspect* 2010; 23: 368-79.

7. Belousova N, Mikheeva G, Gelovani J, Krasnykh V. Modification of adenovirus capsid with a designed protein ligand yields a gene vector targeted to a major molecular marker of cancer. *J Virol* 2008; 82: 630-7.

8. Hoffmann D, Wildner O. Comparison of herpes simplex virus- and conditionally replicative adenovirus-based vectors for glioblastoma treatment. *Cancer Gene Ther* 2007; 14: 627-39.

9. Magnusson MK, Henning P, Myhre S, *et al.* Adenovirus 5 vector genetically re-targeted by an Affibody molecule with specificity for tumor antigen HER2/neu. *Cancer Gene Ther* 2007; 14: 468-79.

10. Van der Perren A, Toelen J, Carlon M, *et al.* Efficient and stable transduction of dopaminergic neurons in rat substantia nigra by rAAV 2/1, 2/2, 2/5, 2/6.2, 2/7, 2/8 and 2/9. *Gene Ther* 2011; 18: 517-27.

11. Gonzalez AM, Leadbeater W, Podvin S, *et al.* Epidermal growth factor targeting of bacteriophage to the choroid plexus for gene delivery to the central nervous system via cerebrospinal fluid. *Brain Res* 2010; 1359: 1-13.

12. Cannon JR, Sew T, Montero L, Burton EA, Greenamyre JT. Pseudotype-dependent lentiviral transduction of astrocytes or neurons in the rat substantia nigra. *Exp Neurol* 2011; 228: 41-52.

13. Barresi V, Belluardo N, Sipione S, Mudo G, Cattaneo E, Condorelli DF. Transplantation of pro-drug-converting neural progenitor cells for brain tumor therapy. *Cancer Gene Ther* 2003; 10: 396-402.

14. Hellums EK, Markert JM, Parker JN, *et al.* Increased efficacy of an interleukin-12-secreting herpes simplex virus in a syngeneic intracranial murine glioma model. *Neuro-Oncology* 2005; 7: 213-24.

15. Oh S, Odland R, Wilson SR, *et al.* Improved distribution of small molecules and viral vectors in the murine brain using a hollow fiber catheter. *J Neurosurg* 2007; 107: 568-77.

16. Voges J, Reszka R, Gossmann A, *et al.* Imaging-guided convection-enhanced delivery and gene therapy of glioblastoma. *Ann Neurol* 2003; 54: 479-87.

17. Salegio EA, Kells AP, Richardson RM, *et al.* Magnetic resonance imaging-guided delivery of adeno-associated virus type 2 to the primate brain for the treatment of lysosomal storage disorders. *Hum Gene Ther* 2010; 21: 1093-103.

18. Debinski W, Tatter SB. Convection-enhanced delivery to achieve widespread distribution of viral vectors: predicting clinical implementation. *Curr Opin Mol Ther* 2010; 12: 647-53.

19. Aboody KS, Najbauer J, Danks MK. Stem and progenitor cell-mediated tumor selective gene therapy. *Gene Ther* 2008; 15: 739-52.

20. Miletic H, Fischer Y, Litwak S, *et al.* Bystander killing of malignant glioma by bone marrow-derived tumor-infiltrating progenitor cells expressing a suicide gene. *Mol Ther* 2007; 15: 1373-81.

21. Waerzeggers Y, Klein M, Miletic H, *et al.* Multimodal imaging of neural progenitor cell fate in rodents. *Mol Imaging* 2008; 7: 77-91.

22. Sun N, Lee A, Wu JC. Long term non-invasive imaging of embryonic stem cells using reporter genes. *Nat Protocols* 2009; 4: 1192-201.

23. Waerzeggers Y, Monfared P, Viel T, Winkeler A, Voges J, Jacobs AH. Methods to monitor gene therapy with molecular imaging. *Methods* 2009; 48: 146-60.

24. Massoud TF, Singh A, Gambhir SS. Noninvasive molecular neuroimaging using reporter genes: part I, principles revisited. *AJNR Am J Neuroradiol* 2008; 29: 229-34.

25. Jacobs AH, Rueger MA, Winkeler A, *et al.* Imaging-guided gene therapy of experimental gliomas. *Cancer Res* 2007; 67: 1706-15.

26. Cherry SR. Multimodality imaging: beyond PET/CT and SPECT/CT. *Semin Nucl Med* 2009; 39: 348-53.

27. Li C, Wang W, Wu Q, *et al.* Dual optical and nuclear imaging in human melanoma xenografts using a single targeted imaging probe. *Nucl Med Biol* 2006; 33: 349-58.

28. Xu H, Baidoo K, Gunn AJ, *et al.* Design, synthesis, and characterization of a dual modality positron emission tomography and fluorescence imaging agent for monoclonal antibody tumor-targeted imaging. *J Med Chem* 2007; 50: 4759-65.

29. Paproski RJ, Forbrich AE, Wachowicz K, Hitt MM, Zemp RJ. Tyrosinase as a dual reporter gene for both photoacoustic and magnetic resonance imaging. *Biomed Optics Express* 2011; 2: 771-80.

30. Nam T, Park S, Lee SY, *et al.* Tumor targeting chitosan nanoparticles for dual-modality optical/MR cancer imaging. *Bioconjug Chem* 2010; 21: 578-82.

31. Kamaly N, Kalber T, Ahmad A, *et al.* Bimodal paramagnetic and fluorescent liposomes for cellular and tumor magnetic resonance imaging. *Bioconjug Chem* 2008; 19: 118-29.

32. Jarrett BR, Gustafsson B, Kukis DL, Louie AY. Synthesis of 64Cu-labeled magnetic nanoparticles for multimodal imaging. *Bioconjug Chem* 2008; 19: 1496-504.

33. Shah K, Tang Y, Breakefield X, Weissleder R. Real-time imaging of TRAIL-induced apoptosis of glioma tumors *in vivo*. *Oncogene* 2003; 22: 6865-72.

34. Badr CE, Tannous BA. Bioluminescence imaging: progress and applications. *Trends Biotechnol* 2011; 29: 624-33.

35. Ntziachristos V, Ripoll J, Wang LV, Weissleder R. Looking and listening to light: the evolution of whole-body photonic imaging. *Nat Biotechnol* 2005; 23: 313-20.

36. Luker GD, Luker KE. Optical imaging: current applications and future directions. *J Nucl Med* 2008; 49: 1-4.

37. Hilderbrand SA, Weissleder R. Near-infrared fluorescence: application to *in vivo* molecular imaging. *Curr Opin Chem Biol* 2010; 14: 71-9.

38. Cohen B, Dafni H, Meir G, Harmelin A, Neeman M. Ferritin as an endogenous MRI reporter for noninvasive imaging of gene expression in C6 glioma tumors. *Neoplasia* 2005; 7: 109-17.

39. Genove G, DeMarco U, Xu H, Goins WF, Ahrens ET. A new transgene reporter for in vivo magnetic resonance imaging. *Nat Med* 2005; 11: 450-4.

40. Ichikawa T, Hogemann D, Saeki Y, *et al.* MRI of transgene expression: correlation to therapeutic gene expression. *Neoplasia* 2002; 4: 523-30.

41. Weissleder R, Simonova M, Bogdanova A, Bredow S, Enochs WS, Bogdanov A Jr. MR imaging and scintigraphy of gene expression through melanin induction. *Radiology* 1997; 204: 425-9.

42. Zurkiya O, Chan AW, Hu X. MagA is sufficient for producing magnetic nanoparticles in mammalian cells, making it an MRI reporter. *Magn Reson Med* 2008; 59: 1225-31.

43. Goldhawk DE, Lemaire C, McCreary CR, *et al.* Magnetic resonance imaging of cells overexpressing MagA, an endogenous contrast agent for live cell imaging. *Mol Imaging* 2009; 8: 129-39.

44. Louie AY, Huber MM, Ahrens ET, *et al.* In vivo visualization of gene expression using magnetic resonance imaging. *Nat Biotechnol* 2000; 18: 321-5.

45. Li Z, Qiao H, Lebherz C, *et al.* Creatine kinase, a magnetic resonance-detectable marker gene for quantification of liver-directed gene transfer. *Hum Gene Ther* 2005; 16: 1429-38.

46. Walter G, Barton ER, Sweeney HL. Noninvasive measurement of gene expression in skeletal muscle. *Proc Natl Acad Sci USA* 2000; 97: 5151-5.

47. Ki S, Sugihara F, Kasahara K, Tochio H, Shirakawa M, Kokubo T. Magnetic resonance-based visualization of gene expression in mammalian cells using a bacterial polyphosphate kinase reporter gene. *BioTechniques* 2007; 42: 209-15.

48. Gilad AA, McMahon MT, Walczak P, *et al.* Artificial reporter gene providing MRI contrast based on proton exchange. *Nat Biotechnol* 2007; 25: 217-9.

49. Perez-Torres CJ, Massaad CA, Hilsenbeck SG, Serrano F, Pautler RG. *In vitro* and *in vivo* magnetic resonance imaging (MRI) detection of GFP through magnetization transfer contrast (MTC). *NeuroImage* 2010; 50: 375-82.

50. Jacobs A, Tjuvajev JG, Dubrovin M, *et al*. Positron emission tomography-based imaging of transgene expression mediated by replication-conditional, oncolytic herpes simplex virus type 1 mutant vectors *in vivo*. *Cancer Res* 2001; 61: 2983-95.

51. Iyer M, Salazar FB, Wu L, Carey M, Gambhir SS. Bioluminescence imaging of systemic tumor targeting using a prostate-specific lentiviral vector. *Hum Gene Ther* 2006; 17: 125-32.

52. Badr CE, Niers JM, Morse D, *et al*. Suicidal gene therapy in an NF-kappaB-controlled tumor environment as monitored by a secreted blood reporter. *Gene Ther* 2011; 18: 445-51.

53. Vandier D, Rixe O, Besnard F, *et al*. Inhibition of glioma cells *in vitro* and *in vivo* using a recombinant adenoviral vector containing an astrocyte-specific promoter. *Cancer Gene Ther* 2000; 7: 1120-6.

54. Winkeler A, Sena-Esteves M, Paulis LE, *et al*. Switching on the lights for gene therapy. *PLoS One* 2007; 2: e528.

55. Jacobs A, Dubrovin M, Hewett J, *et al*. Functional coexpression of HSV-1 thymidine kinase and green fluorescent protein: implications for noninvasive imaging of transgene expression. *Neoplasia* 1999; 1: 154-61.

56. Jacobs AH, Winkeler A, Hartung M, *et al*. Improved herpes simplex virus type 1 amplicon vectors for proportional coexpression of positron emission tomography marker and therapeutic genes. *Hum Gene Ther* 2003; 14: 277-97.

57. Wang Y, Yu YA, Shabahang S, Wang G, Szalay AA. Renilla luciferase- Aequorea GFP (Ruc-GFP) fusion protein, a novel dual reporter for real-time imaging of gene expression in cell cultures and in live animals. *Mol Genet Genomics* 2002; 268: 160-8.

58. Ray P, Wu AM, Gambhir SS. Optical bioluminescence and positron emission tomography imaging of a novel fusion reporter gene in tumor xenografts of living mice. *Cancer Res* 2003; 63: 1160-5.

59. Kummer C, Winkeler A, Dittmar C, *et al*. Multitracer positron emission tomographic imaging of exogenous gene expression mediated by a universal herpes simplex virus 1 amplicon vector. *Mol Imaging* 2007; 6: 181-92.

60. Che J, Doubrovin M, Serganova I, Ageyeva L, Zanzonico P, Blasberg R. hNIS-IRES-eGFP dual reporter gene imaging. *Mol Imaging* 2005; 4: 128-36.

61. Ray P, De A, Min JJ, Tsien RY, Gambhir SS. Imaging tri-fusion multimodality reporter gene expression in living subjects. *Cancer Res* 2004; 64: 1323-30.

62. Ponomarev V, Doubrovin M, Serganova I, *et al*. A novel triple-modality reporter gene for whole-body fluorescent, bioluminescent, and nuclear noninvasive imaging. *Eur J Nucl Med Mol Imaging* 2004; 31: 740-51.

63. Liu H, Ren G, Liu S, *et al*. Optical imaging of reporter gene expression using a positron-emission-tomography probe. *J Biomed Opt* 2010; 15: 060505.

64. Kodibagkar VD, Yu J, Liu L, Hetherington HP, Mason RP. Imaging beta-galactosidase activity using 19F chemical shift imaging of LacZ gene-reporter molecule 2-fluoro-4-nitrophenol-beta-D-galactopyranoside. *Magn Reson Imaging* 2006; 24: 959-62.

65. Cui W, Liu L, Kodibagkar VD, Mason RP. S-Gal, a novel 1H MRI reporter for beta-galactosidase. *Magn Reson Med* 2010; 64: 65-71.

66. Klose A, Waerzeggers Y, Monfared P, *et al*. Imaging bone morphogenetic protein 7 induced cell cycle arrest in experimental gliomas. *Neoplasia* 2011; 13: 276-85.

67. Rueger MA, Ameli M, Li H, *et al*. [18F]FLT PET for non-invasive monitoring of early response to gene therapy in experimental gliomas. *Mol Imaging Biol* 2011; 13: 547-57.

68. Fiandaca MS, Varenika V, Eberling J, *et al*. Real-time MR imaging of adeno-associated viral vector delivery to the primate brain. *NeuroImage* 2009; 47 (suppl 2): T27-35.

69. Gilad AA, Walczak P, McMahon MT, *et al*. MR tracking of transplanted cells with positive contrast using manganese oxide nanoparticles. *Magn Reson Med* 2008; 60: 1-7.

70. Raty JK, Liimatainen T, Wirth T, *et al*. Magnetic resonance imaging of viral particle biodistribution *in vivo*. *Gene Ther* 2006; 13: 1440-6.

71. Valable S, Barbier EL, Bernaudin M, *et al*. *In vivo* MRI tracking of exogenous monocytes/macrophages targeting brain tumors in a rat model of glioma. *NeuroImage* 2008; 40: 973-83.

72. Kievit FM, Veiseh O, Fang C, *et al*. Chlorotoxin labeled magnetic nanovectors for targeted gene delivery to glioma. *ACS Nano* 2010; 4: 4587-94.

73. Fromes Y, Modo M, Herynek V, Hoehn, M, Waerzeggers Y, Jacobs AH. Cellular therapies and cell tracking. In: Ntziachristos V, Leroy-Willig A, Tavitian B, eds. *Textbook of in vivo imaging in vertebrates*. Chichester UK: John Wiley and Sons Ltd, 2007.

74. Tjuvajev JG, Doubrovin M, Akhurst T, *et al*. Comparison of radiolabeled nucleoside probes (FIAU, FHBG, and FHPG) for PET imaging of HSV1-tk gene expression. *J Nucl Med* 2002; 43: 1072-83.

75. Alauddin MM, Gelovani JG. Radiolabeled nucleoside analogues for PET imaging of HSV1-tk gene expression. *Curr Top Med Chem* 2010; 10: 1617-32.

76. MacLaren DC, Gambhir SS, Satyamurthy N, *et al*. Repetitive, non-invasive imaging of the dopamine D2 receptor as a reporter gene in living animals. *Gene Ther* 1999; 6: 785-91.

77. Umegaki H, Ishiwata K, Ogawa O, *et al*. Longitudinal follow-up study of adenoviral vector-mediated gene transfer of dopamine D2 receptors in the striatum in young, middle-aged, and aged rats: a positron emission tomography study. *Neuroscience* 2003; 121: 479-86.

78. Win Z, Al-Nahhas A, Rubello D, Gross MD. Somatostatin receptor PET imaging with Gallium-68 labeled peptides. *QJ Nucl Med Mol Imaging* 2007; 51: 244-50.

79. Cotugno G, Aurilio M, Annunziata P, *et al*. Noninvasive repetitive imaging of somatostatin receptor 2 gene transfer with positron emission tomography. *Hum Gene Ther* 2011; 22: 189-96.

80. Zhang H, Moroz MA, Serganova I, *et al*. Imaging expression of the human somatostatin receptor subtype-2 reporter gene with 68Ga-DOTATOC. *J Nucl Med* 2011; 52: 123-31.

81. Haberkorn U. Gene therapy with sodium/iodide symporter in hepatocarcinoma. *Exp Clin Endocrinol Diabetes* 2001; 109: 60-2.

82. Haberkorn U, Henze M, Altmann A, *et al*. Transfer of the human NaI symporter gene enhances iodide uptake in hepatoma cells. *J Nucl Med* 2001; 42: 317-25.

83. Niu G, Gaut AW, Ponto LL, *et al*. Multimodality noninvasive imaging of gene transfer using the human sodium iodide symporter. *J Nucl Med* 2004; 45: 445-9.

84. Jauregui-Osoro M, Sunassee K, Weeks AJ, *et al*. Synthesis and biological evaluation of [(18)F]tetrafluoroborate: a PET imaging agent for thyroid disease and reporter gene imaging of the sodium/iodide symporter. *Eur J Nucl Med Mol Imaging* 2010; 37: 2108-16.

85. Altmann A, Kissel M, Zitzmann S, *et al*. Increased MIBG uptake after transfer of the human norepinephrine transporter gene in rat hepatoma. Journal of nuclear medicine : official publication, Society of Nuclear Medicine 2003;44: 973-80.

86. Moroz MA, Serganova I, Zanzonico P, *et al*. Imaging hNET reporter gene expression with 124I-MIBG. *J Nucl Med* 2007; 48: 827-36.

87. Ponomarev V, Doubrovin M, Shavrin A, *et al*. A human-derived reporter gene for noninvasive imaging in humans: mitochondrial thymidine kinase type 2. *J Nucl Med* 2007; 48: 819-26.

88. Radu CG, Shu CJ, Nair-Gill E, *et al*. Molecular imaging of lymphoid organs and immune activation by positron emission tomography with a new [18F]-labeled 2'-deoxycytidine analog. *Nat Med* 2008; 14: 783-8.

89. Likar Y, Zurita J, Dobrenkov K, *et al.* A new pyrimidine-specific reporter gene: a mutated human deoxycytidine kinase suitable for PET during treatment with acycloguanosine-based cytotoxic drugs. *J Nucl Med* 2010; 51: 1395-403.

90. Vandeputte C, Evens N, Toelen J, *et al.* A PET brain reporter gene system based on type 2 cannabinoid receptors. *J Nucl Med* 2011; 52: 1102-9.

91. Koretsky AP, Brosnan MJ, Chen LH, Chen JD, Van Dyke T. NMR detection of creatine kinase expressed in liver of transgenic mice: determination of free ADP levels. *Proc Natl Acad Sci USA* 1990; 87: 3112-6.

92. Walter G, Barton ER, Sweeney HL. Noninvasive measurement of gene expression in skeletal muscle. *Proc Natl Acad Sci USA* 2000; 97: 5151-5.

93. Stegman LD, Rehemtulla A, Beattie B, *et al.* Noninvasive quantitation of cytosine deaminase transgene expression in human tumor xenografts with *in vivo* magnetic resonance spectroscopy. *Proc Natl Acad Sci USA* 1999;96: 9821-6.

94. Kodibagkar VD, Yu J, Liu L, Hetherington HP, Mason RP. Imaging beta-galactosidase activity using 19F chemical shift imaging of LacZ gene-reporter molecule 2-fluoro-4-nitrophenol-beta-D-galactopyranoside. *Magn Reson Imaging* 2006; 24: 959-62.

95. Yu JX, Kodibagkar VD, Liu L, Mason RP. A 19F-NMR approach using reporter molecule pairs to assess beta-galactosidase in human xenograft tumors *in vivo*. *NMR Biomed* 2008; 21: 704-12.

96. Bengtsson NE, Brown G, Scott EW, Walter GA. lacZ as a genetic reporter for real-time MRI. *Magn Reson Med* 2010; 63: 745-53.

The CliniBook: Clinical gene transfer
Edited by Odile Cohen-Haguenauer – EDK, Paris © 2012, pp. 386-393

B1-2
Persistent luminescence nanoparticles for *in vivo* imaging: characteristics and targeting

Thomas Maldiney*, Daniel Scherman, Cyrille Richard*

Unité de Pharmacologie Chimique et Génétique et d'Imagerie; CNRS, UMR 8151, Paris, F-75270 cedex France; Inserm, U 1022, Paris, F-75270 cedex France; Université Paris Descartes, Sorbonne Paris Cité, Faculté des Sciences Pharmaceutiques et Biologiques, Paris, F-75270 cedex France; ENSCP, Paris, F-75231 cedex France.
thomas.maldiney@parisdescartes.fr
cyrille.richard@parisdescartes.fr
* Corresponding authors

INTRODUCTION

In the last decade, optical imaging, exploiting photons as primary information, has witnessed major improvements for the grasping of physiological mechanisms or new diagnosis and therapeutic applications [1]. This growing interest is mainly associated to the practicalness offered by photonic probes and devices, but also to the relatively low cost of these techniques, compared to other common imaging modalities already used in medicine like MRI, PET or OCT. Among a wide panel of different optical probes used within the scientific community, light usually spread on inorganic semi-conductor quantum-dots (QD) [2], known to display one of the highest quantum yields or noteworthy photostability, as well as near-infrared fluorescent molecules, like Alexa Fluor®, that show better stability than the first organic dyes and some ability to evade autofluorescence from tissues. Nonetheless, these probes, based on fluorescence phenomenon, both require constant illumination which systematically induces autofluorescence from irradiated tissues and consequently a significant loss of sensitivity [3].
In order to avoid the need for permanent illumination, and suppress the disturbing background signal, we developed an alternative bioimaging technique based on crystalline materials bearing special optical property called persistent luminescence.

THE PRINCIPLE OF PERSISTENT LUMINESCENCE MATERIALS

Most of the time, long-lasting phosphors find applications in emergency lightings, safety indications, or road signs. Mimicking a capacitor, these materials can be excited under relatively high-energy photons (generally UV light or X-rays) a few minutes before use and subsequently emit in the visible region for several hours (without the need for further illumination). Recently, silicate phosphors have been paid considerable attention because of their ability to emit long-lasting afterglow in a large region of the visible spectrum. In 2003, Wang et al. reported the synthesis of enstatite ($MgSiO_3$) doped with several cations: Eu^{2+}, Mn^{2+}, and Dy^{3+}, responsible for bright red long-lasting phosphorescence [4]. This publication triggered our team's interest in the development of near-infrared persistent luminescence nanoparticles (referred to as PLNP) with formula $Ca_{0.2}Mg_{0.9}Zn_{0.9}Si_2O_6$, doped with Eu^{2+}, Mn^{2+}, and Dy^{3+}, intended for optical imaging in living animals [5].

SOL-GEL SYNTHESIS OF PERSISTENT LUMINESCENCE NANOPARTICLES FOR *IN VIVO* IMAGING

Inorganic phosphors are generally obtained through solid-state reaction, leading to micrometer-sized nanoparticles, hardly suitable for *in vivo* experiments. We gave our preference to the sol-gel synthesis under acidic condition that allows a lower calcination temperature and limits crystal growth (*Figure 1*) [6].

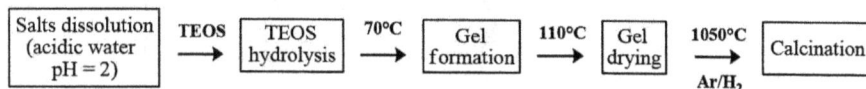

Figure 1. Sol-gel synthesis of persistent luminescence crystals.

Persistent luminescence nanoparticles (PLNP) were extracted by selective sedimentation after several centrifugation steps following wet grinding of the calcined product in diluted sodium hydroxide (*Figure 2*) [7].

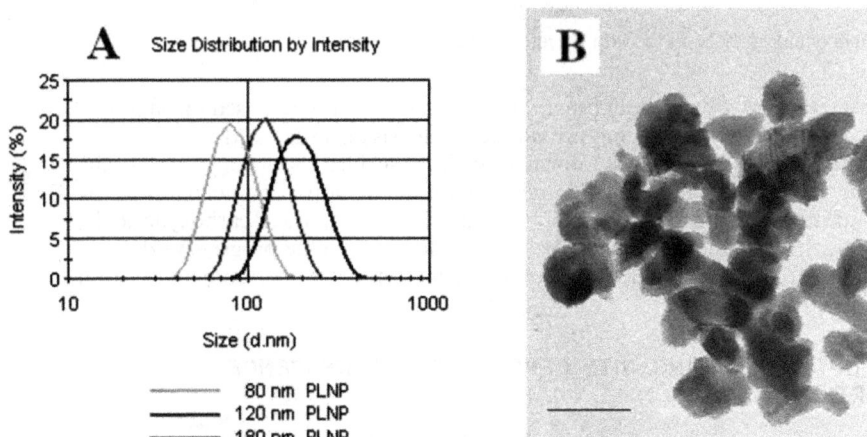

Figure 2. A. Dynamic light scattering measurements for different size populations. B. Transmission electron micrograph of 80nm PLNP (scale bar represents 100nm).

FUNCTIONALIZATION AND CHARACTERIZATION OF PERSISTENT LUMINESCENCE NANOPARTICLES

Surface properties such as charge, functional groups, and potential grafted molecules, are commonly known to have a major impact on the circulation of any colloidal system. In particular, several years of work with synthetic vectors revealed what is now established as the classical biodistribution patterns for negatively charged nanoparticles, rapidly opsonised and collected by reticulo-endothelial system (RES), mostly liver and spleen. Alternatively, its PEGylated neutral counterpart, is known to delay RES uptake by limiting charge recognition from circulating opsonins. For this reason, successful PLNP functionalization was thought critical towards relevant distribution of PLNP after intravenous injection (*Figure 3*) [7].

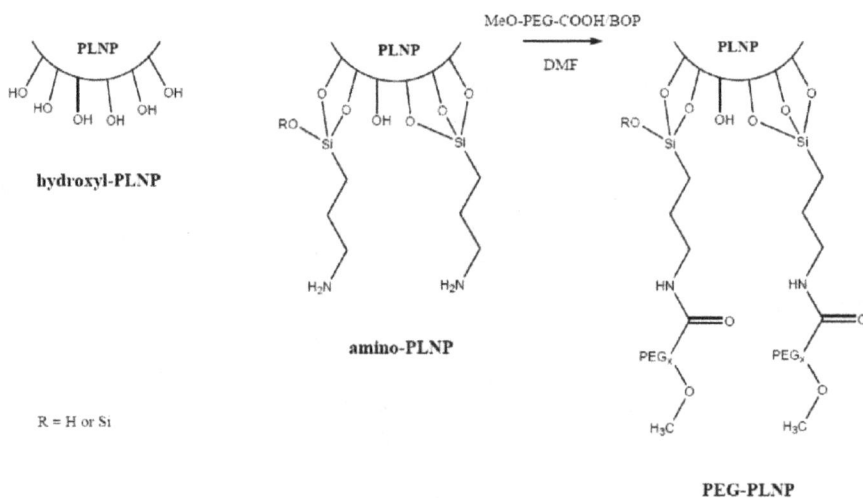

Figure 3. Functionalization of PLNP with polyethylene glycol.

Complete characterization of each functionalization step can be assessed through several chemical, physico-chemical, or even physical analysis techniques. Most often, zeta potential measurement brings first information about surface charge of the nanoparticle. Then, this result is generally completed with quantitative characterization by chemical titration (specific to certain functional groups like amines or carboxylic acids) or thermogravimetric analysis that records weight loss due to the progressive decomposition of organic material under thermal treatment (typical temperature range: from 20°C to 780°C).

IN VIVO OPTICAL IMAGING WITH PERSISTENT LUMINESCENCE NANOPARTICLES

As mentioned above, the main characteristic of these PLNP, compared to other optical probes based on fluorescence phenomenon, relies on their ability to be excited before the injection to small animals, and followed under the appropriate photon-counting system (cooled GaAs intensified charge-coupled device camera, Biospace Lab) without the need for constant illumination. The principle of bioimaging with PLNP is summarized in *Figure 4*.

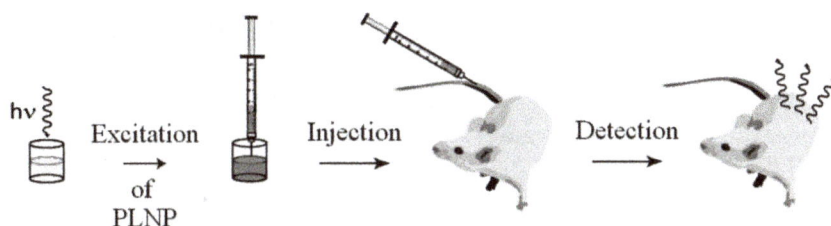

Figure 4. Bioimaging with PLNP.

We previously reported the influence of hydrodynamic diameter and surface coating, notably PEGylation, on the biodistribution of persistent luminescence nanoparticles in healthy and tumour-bearing mice [7]. This study confirmed classical biodistribution patterns observed with synthetic vectors, in particular the rapid capture of hydroxyl-PLNP (*Figure 5, left*), with global negative surface charge, within major RES organs, and liver in particular. Conversely, PEG-grafting was shown to greatly improve PLNP distribution after systemic injection in the tail vain of BALC/c mice (*Figure 5, right*).

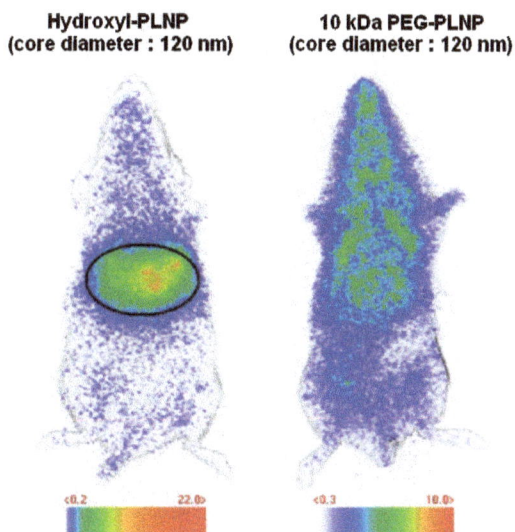

Figure 5. Comparative biodistribution of hydroxyl-PLNP and PEG-PLNP (15 minutes after the injection of 100µg materials in normal saline).

The ability of such persistent luminescence nanoparticles to freely circulate in the bloodstream was also shown to be highly dependent on the hydrodynamic diameter of the core particle. Indeed the smaller the particle, the smaller the amount of PLNP retrieved in RES organs and the longer sustained circulation.

These results on the biodistribution of PLNP *in vivo* prompted us to initiate further work on the development of PLNP as innovative optical tool intended for diagnosis applications, with special consideration for targeted PLNP, directed against specific diseases like cancer or rheumatoid arthritis.

IN VITRO TARGETING WITH PERSISTENT LUMINESCENCE NANOPARTICLES

Along with the need to evade RES uptake in order to notably improve PLNP distribution within the animal, comes the fundamental issue of reaching a given region of interest *in vivo*: how can the probe be specifically addressed to the designated malignancy? This difficult task is generally achieved by taking advantage of the specific and privileged interaction between a ligand (small molecules, antibody) and its dedicated target (receptor) [8]. In order to investigate this strategy, we designed two different strategies intended for the specific targeting of PLNP against cancer cells *in vitro* (*Figure 6*).

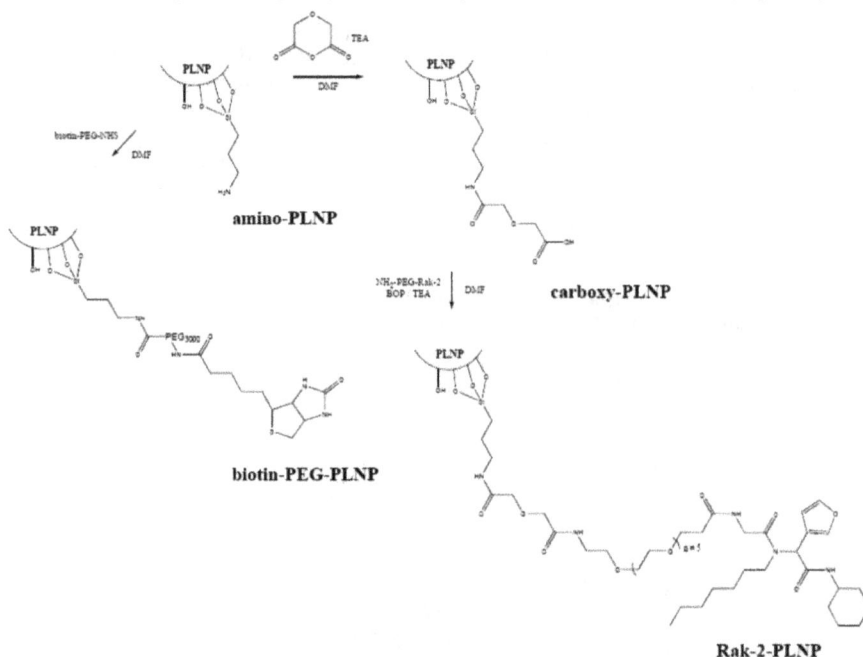

Figure 6. Functionalization of PLNP with biotin and Rak-2.

The first example relies on the recent discovery of a small molecule (Rak-2), reported for its high affinity toward PC-3 cells [9]. We have shown that functionalization of PLNP with a Rak-2 molecule by means of a small 250 daltons PEG spacer (*Figure 6*) allows preferential binding on PC-3 cells (*Figure 7*), compared to the control PLNP on which N-propyl amide was grafted instead of the targeting ligand [10].

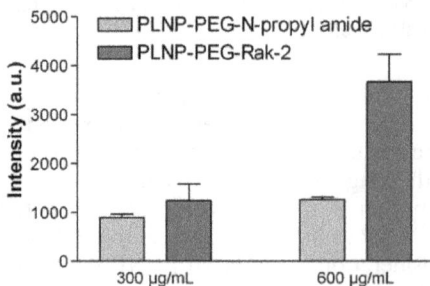

Figure 7. *In vitro* binding (30 minutes) of 180nm Rak-2-PLNP on PC-3 cells.

These preliminary *in vitro* results validate the first targeting strategy through specific ligand-target interaction.

By taking advantage of avidin-biotin technology, the second approach exploits biotinylated PLNP to target malignant cells transduced with a fusion protein called lodavin (composed of both avidin and the endocytotic low-density lipoprotein (LDL) receptor). Indeed, Lesch *et al.* recently produced a lentiviral vector expressing lodavin that could induce long-term expression of avidin on the surface of transduced glioma cells (referred to as BT4C+) [11]. We evaluated the ability of biotin-functionalized PLNP (*Figure 6*) to preferentially target transduced BT4C cells, which display avidin on the outer membrane, as compared to wild type BT4C (referred to as BT4C-). Additional control PLNP was obtained after biotin coverage with neutravidin.

Our data show that biotinylated PLNP were preferentially retained on glioma cells expressing the avidin fusion protein in reference to control cells (*Figure 8*). The significant decrease in PLNP binding on both BT4C- and BT4C+ cells after biotin saturation with neutravidin comes as a confirmation that the binding of biotin-PEG-PLNP on BT4C cells expressing the fusion protein occurred through a specific interaction between biotin and the avidin moiety of lodavin [12].

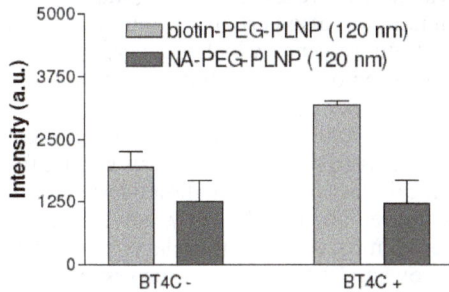

Figure 8. *In vitro* binding (15 minutes) of PLNP (150µg/mL) on BT4C cells.

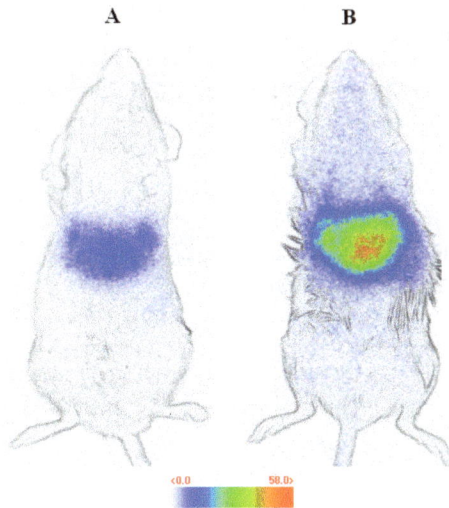

Figure 9. *In vivo* comparison of different PLNP compositions (injection of 100µg of PLNP) (A - $Ca_{0.2}Mg_{0.9}Zn_{0.9}Si_2O_6:Eu^{2+},Mn^{2+},Dy^{3+}$; B - $CaMgSi_2O_6:Eu^{2+},Mn^{2+},Pr^{3+}$).

PAVING THE WAY FOR NEW COMPOSITIONS AND IMPROVED OPTICAL PROPERTIES

Persistent luminescence provides a powerful tool for sensitive optical detection that allows complete suppression of autofluorescence from living tissues. However, when injected to small animals with view to follow real-time biodistribution *in vivo*, the luminescence signal does not show intense enough to provide long-term monitoring (several hours). This observation unveils the requirement to further develop new compounds with improved optical characteristics (*Figure 9*).

By focusing on the fundamental properties associated with persistent luminescence mechanism, we recently identified a novel composition ($CaMgSi_2O_6$, doped with Eu^{2+}, Mn^{2+}, and Pr^{3+}), somewhat related to the previous silicate, which displays a stronger near-infrared afterglow [13].

Upon intravenous injection of this new material, a significant benefit revealed *in vivo* both in the signal intensity and the duration of probe's monitoring.

CONCLUSION

Persistent luminescence offers an innovative tool for optical imaging. It allows not only real-time imaging in living animals, but also permits to completely suppress the troublesome background signal, autofluorescence, which is generally associated to the requirement for permanent illumination of fluorescent probes. Taking advantage of the sol-gel process, we were able to synthesize persistent luminescence nanoparticles, which harbour narrow distribution profiles and acceptable sizes for a broad spectrum of *in vivo* applications. Moreover, we successfully achieved accurate surface functionalization through relatively simple chemical reactions, which allows designing the surface coverage at will, according to the desired purpose. Notably, polyethylene glycol grafting, as well as smaller core diameter (80nm), significantly delayed nanoparticles uptake by reticulo-endothelial system, favouring PLNP access to the systemic circulation.

In addition to these first *in vivo* data, we report that such nanoparticles harbouring persistent luminescence could successfully be targeted to malignant cancer cells *in vitro* using different approaches, based on either specific ligand-protein recognition, or biotin-avidin technology. Conjugated to the discovery of a novel compound with improved optical characteristics, that increase both sensitivity and visualization time of the probe, our findings open great avenues for the future development of efficient nanoprobes able to target malignant tumours *in vivo*.

ACKNOWLEDGMENTS

This work has been performed with the support of the EC-DG research through the FP6-Network of Excellence, CLINIGENE: LSHB-CT-2006-018933.

REFERENCES

1. Weissleder R, Pittet MJ. Imaging in the era of molecular oncology. *Nature* 2008; 452: 580-9.

2. Medintz IL, Uyeda HT, Goldman ER, Mattoussi H. Quantum dot bioconjugates for imaging, labelling and sensing. *Nat Mater* 2005; 4: 435-46.

3. Frangioni JV. *In vivo* near-infrared fluorescence imaging. *Curr Opin Chem Biol* 2003; 7: 626-34.

4. Wang XJ, Jia D, Yen WM. Mn^{2+} activated green, yellow, and red long persistent phosphors. *J Lumin* 2003; 102-103: 34-7.

5. Le Masne de Chermont Q, Chanéac C, Seguin J, Pellé F, Maîtrejean S, Jolivet P, *et al*. Nanoprobes with near-infrared persistent luminescence for *in vivo* imaging. *Proc Natl Acad Sci USA* 2007; 104: 9266-71.

6. Le Masne de Chermont Q, Richard C, Seguin J, Chanéac C, Bessodes M, Scherman D. Silicates doped with luminescent ions: useful tools for optical imaging applications. *Proc SPIE* 2009; 7189: 71890B/1-9.

7. Maldiney T, Richard C, Seguin J, Wattier N, Bessodes M, Scherman D. Effect of core diameter, surface coating, and PEG chain length on the biodistribution of persistent luminescence nanoparticles in mice. *ACS Nano* 2011; 5: 854-62.

8. Byrne JD, Betancourt T, Brannon-Peppas L. Active targeting schemes for nanoparticle systems in cancer therapeutics. *Adv Drug Deliv Rev* 2008; 60: 1615-26.

9. Byk G, Partouche S, Weiss A, Margel S, Khandadash S. Fully synthetic phage-like system for screening mixtures of small molecules in live cells. *J Comb Chem* 2010; 12: 332-45.

10. Maldiney T, Byk G, Wattier N, Seguin J, Khandadash R, Bessodes M, *et al*. Synthesis and functionalization of persistent luminescence nanoparticles with small molecules and evaluation of their targeting ability. *Int J Pharm* 2012; 423: 102-7.

11. Lesch HP, Pikkarainen JT, Kaikkonen MU, Taavitsainen M, Samaranayake H, Lehtolainen-Dalkilic P, *et al*. Avidin fusion protein-expressing lentiviral vector for targeted drug delivery. *Hum Gene Ther* 2009; 20: 871-82.

12. Maldiney T, Kaikkonen MU, Seguin J, le Masne de Chermont Q, Bessodes M, Ylä-Herttuala S, *et al*. *In vitro* targeting of avidin-expressing glioma cells with biotinylated persistent luminescence nanoparticles. *Bioconjugate Chem* 2012. DOI: 10.1021/bc200510z.

13. Maldiney T, Lecointre A, Viana B, Bessière A, Bessodes M, Gourier D, *et al*. Controlling electron trap depth to enhance optical properties of persistent luminescence nanoparticles for *in vivo* imaging. *J Am Chem Soc* 2011; 133: 11810-5.

The CliniBook: Clinical gene transfer
Edited by Odile Cohen-Haguenauer – EDK, Paris © 2012, pp. 394-401

B1-3
Ex-vivo evaluation of gene-transfer vectors: efficacy, tropism and safety

Dror Kolodkin-Gal, Shay Tayeb, Abed Khalaileh, Gidi Zamir, Nikolai Kunicher, Amos Panet*

Departments of Biochemistry and Surgery, the Hebrew University-Hadassah Medical School, IMRIC, Jerusalem, Israel.
paneta@cc.huji.ac.il
* Corresponding author

INTRODUCTION

Viral vectors considered for therapeutic purposes, are usually evaluated, first onto cultured cells and subsequently in animal models, which are relevant for the target disease. As most gene therapy vectors are based on human viruses (*i.e.* AAV-2, adeno-5 and -2, HIV-1, and HSV-1), evaluation of these vectors in animal models is problematic as tissue and cell tropism may be different in various species. Thus, there is always a need to validate the animal model and to develop alternative assay systems for the evaluation of viral vectors designed for gene therapy. To meet this objective, we have developed a model based on an *ex vivo* organ culture system derived from human solid tissues with view to evaluating viral tropism and potential toxicity [1]. Organ cultures have been extensively applied in several fields of research, especially in physiological studies of the brain, in tissue metabolism and in drug toxicity assays. As little information is available regarding virus infection and spreading in a three dimensional solid tissue, we have applied the *ex vivo* system to the analysis of several viruses and viral vectors in order both to determine viral tropism within the different cell types constituting a tissue and to evaluate barriers within the solid tissue that restrict the spread of the virus. In addition, we compared viral tropism *ex vivo* in the same tissues being derived either from human or from mouse together with an *in vivo* mouse system. These comparative experiments were performed with view to determining to which extent our mouse experimental system would be relevant to certain viral vectors. Potential toxicity of viral vectors is currently tested before clinical trials by mean of animal models, in particular the mice. Since infection of mice by human viruses may not reflect the human condition, we have also applied the organ culture model with the relevant human and mouse tissues to validate currently available toxicology tests that involve mouse models. In this review, we summarize data from our studies, mostly related to the tropism of gene therapy vectors, in particular Adeno, HSV1 and Lenti, taking from our published work [1-8].

RESULTS

Preparation and maintenance of solid tissues in organ culture

Fresh tissues of normal skin, lung and colon and the corresponding malignant tumoral counterpart were obtained from the pathology department, under approval of the IRB committee of the Hadassah Hospital. The tissues were sliced to thin sections of 150-400 micron; a width that reflect the average distance between adjacent blood vessel in a solid tissue. The tissues are immersed in optimized culture media, such that exchange of essential nutrients and gases to and from the solid tissue is facilitated (*Figure 1*). Viability of the tissue *ex vivo* is monitored daily by glucose uptake from the media, lactic dehydrogenase (LDH) secretion, mitochondrial dehydrogenase activity (MTT assay), tissue specific mRNA synthesis, Caspase-3 enzyme activation and by histological examination [1, 2]. Different tissues demonstrated distinct survival *ex vivo*; for example, skin could be maintained in culture for an extended period of up to 20 days, while colon carcinoma is viable for 2-4 days only. Tissues in organ culture maintain their original architecture with the cell types diversity and the extra cellular matrix unique to each solid tissue. Toward gene transfer, virus particles were either added directly to the culture medium, or else microinjected under a binocular into a selected part of the solid tissue in culture. Following vectors administration, the tissue was kept in culture for 2-6 days after which analysis of viral tropism and efficiency of reporter gene transfer were evaluated. Analysis of viral tropism in the solid tissue was carried out using both antibodies against specific cell markers to identify cell lineages and a reporter gene or antibodies against the virus to identify the transduced cells.

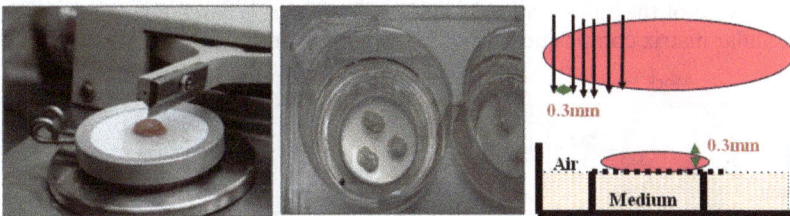

Figure 1. Preparation and maintenance of solid tissues in organ culture. Human tissues (obtained under approval of the IRB committee of the Hadassah hospital), or mouse tissues (obtained under approval of the Hebrew University Ethics Committee) were sliced to thin sections (150-400 micron) and placed in optimized medium to maintain viability for several days [1].

Viral tropism in normal colon and colon carcinoma tissues of human origin

Adenoviruses and HSV1 have been applied extensively as oncolytic viruses in both pre-clinical and clinical settings. While effective oncolytic activity was shown in animal models with several genetically modified viruses, a clear efficacy is yet to be demonstrated in controlled clinical trials. To better understand this discrepancy, we have developed an organ culture system with tumor and normal tissues derived from the same organ of the same patient and compared the tropism and oncolytic activity of wild type (WT) and genetically modified Adeno and HSV1 [3-5]. First, we compared the tissue tropism of WT Adeno-5 with that of a genetically modified Adeno, in which 7 lysine residues were inserted in the capsid (AD-PK7). This virus interacts with heparan sulfate as a cellular receptor, rather than with the CAR protein that serves as a receptor for the WT virus. While gene transfer with the capsid modified Adeno (PK7) was much more efficient than that of the WT Adeno in both human tissues, we could not demonstrate a selective transduction of the tumor over the normal colon tissue [3]. We concluded from this experiment that while some genetic modifications may affect efficiency of Adeno infection, to achieve selectivity toward the tumor requires a modification that exploits critical differences between the normal and tumor tissues.

Tropism of HSV1 to human normal colon and carcinoma tissues

HSV1 has been previously shown to preferentially infect dividing cells and furthermore, HSV1 harbours oncolytic activity against tumors, especially brain tumors, in a variety of animal models. To analyze whether HSV1 preferentially addresses human solid tumors and to decipher the mechanism of oncolysis, we applied organ cultures derived from human colon and carcinoma tissues. The results shown in *Figure 2* clearly indicate that both the WT virus (HSV-1 RSV) and the genetically modified attenuated virus (HSV-1 G47Delta) preferentially infected the human colon carcinoma over the normal colon tissue. Several factors in the solid tissue may affect efficiency of virus trafficking, including the extra-cellular components. As there are major differences in the potential structure between the normal colon and the carcinoma tissue, we investigated the potential role of two extra-cellular components in the colon, Mucin and Collagen on HSV1 infection. Both components are abundant in the normal colon but not in the carcinoma tissue (*Figure 3A*). The results in figure 3B clearly show that removal of the mucus layer by pre-treatment with DTT, which dissociates the Mucin proteins network, does indeed facilitate virus access to the normal tissue. Similarly, pretreatment of the normal colon tissue with Collagenase-2 markedly increased infection of the tissue with HSV1 [4]. Taken together, our data set from the *ex vivo* system indicate a preferential HSV-1 mediated gene transfer in favour of the human colon carcinoma tissue, that is based on differences of the extra-cellular matrix composition between the normal and carcinoma tissues.

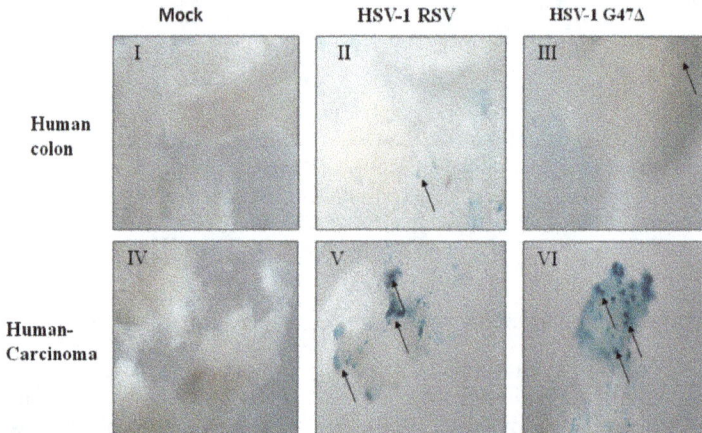

Figure 2. Herpes simplex virus type-1 (HSV-1) preferentially addresses human colon carcinoma tissues. Human colon carcinoma or normal colon mucosa tissues were prepared for organ cultures [3]. Exposure to the virus was carried out for 48 h with HSV-1RSV, or HSV-1 G47Δ (2x10⁶ IU). Both HSV-1 vectors express the β-gal gene. The β-Gal enzyme was analyzed 48 h after exposure to the virus by β-Gal staining and photographed at x40 magnification. Results of a representative experiment with tissues of one of the three patients examined are presented. Blue cells, indicated by the arrows, represent virus-modified cells. Transduction of the carcinoma tissue by the two HSV-1 vectors is higher than that of the normal colon.

Colon   Carcinoma

A. Histology

Mock   HSV-1   HSV-1 & DTT

B. HSV-1   GFP

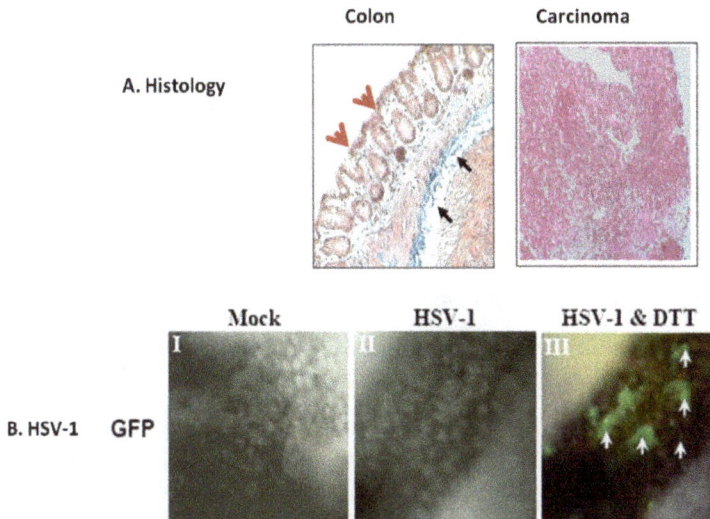

Figure 3. Mucin and collagen in the normal colon tissue interfere with HSV-1. Human normal colon and carcinoma were prepared for organ culture [3]. A. Tissues were fixed and slices of 5 micron were subjected to histological examination. Red arrows indicate the mucus layer and dark arrows show collagen deposits (blue) in the interstitial tissue. B. Human normal colon tissue was pre-treated with DTT (1 mM), washed and exposed to HSV-1 GFP for 2 days. The results indicate that removal of the mucin layer by DDT facilitated gene transfer to the colon epithelia as indicated by the white arrows.

ESTABLISHMENT OF AN ORTHOTOPIC MODEL OF MOUSE COLON CARCINOMA

We developed a new orthotopic model of colon carcinoma in mice to evaluate the oncolytic activity of HSV1 *in vivo*. Mouse colon carcinoma CT26 cells were directly injected into the rectum of Balb-C mice where the tumor developed locally [5]. As the mouse CT26 cells are transduced with the Luciferase gene, tumor growth is detected *in vivo* by exposing the mouse under a CCD camera (*Figure 4*).

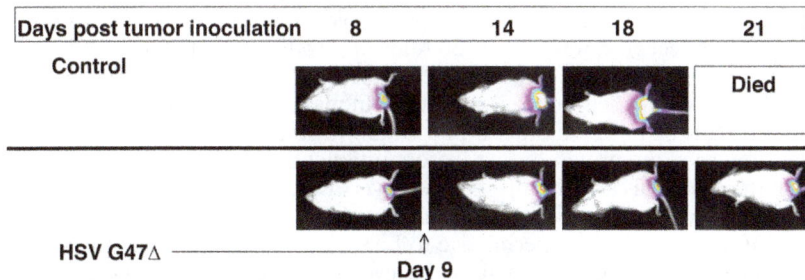

Days post tumor inoculation	8	14	18	21

Figure 4. Establishment of a new orthotropic colon-carcinoma model in mouse and the oncolytic activity of HSV-1. Mice were injected with colon carcinoma cells (CT26/Luc) to the rectum epithelia and after 8 days tumor was already noticeable by the CCD camera. On day 9 post-implantation, HSV-1G47 delta (5×10^7 IU) or PBS control was injected IT. At day 13 the mice were injected IP with Gancyclovir (GCV) 10 mg kg-1 twice daily for 14 days. At days 8, 14, 18 and 21, mice were imaged for Luciferase activity [5]. Representative mice from each group are presented.

The tumor is noticeable at 8 days post transplantation and HSV1 is injected into the tumor (IT) on day 9. The results indicated that while tumor growth was aborted following injection of the attenuated HSV-1 G47 delta, conversely the tumor continues to develop in the control group, injected with PBS. Hence, survival of the HSV1 treated group was significantly longer than that of the control group. Furthermore, in some of the treated mice the tumor altogether disappeared [5].

The *in vivo* and *ex vivo* models developed for the evaluation of oncolytic viruses therefore complement each other. Results obtained with the two colon carcinoma systems now facilitate the design of a clinical trial involing colon carcinoma patients.

Studies of Lentivirus vector tropism in solid tissues

While a wealth of information related to the capacity of lentivectors to transduce cells in culture and in animal models is available, little is known of its efficacy in clinical trials although there is growing evidence for its potential. The tropism of lentiviral vectors, pseudotyped with different glycoproteins, has been mostly studied using cultured cells while factors affecting lenti tropism and efficiency in complex solid tissue remain to be investigated. In the present study, we applied organ cultures derived from solid tissues of mouse and human origin, and in particular skin tissues, to explore other factors than cell receptors that determine lentivector transduction. Skin represents a target tissue of choice in studies related to gene based vaccination, gene therapy of skin genetic diseases and for the expression and secretion to the circulation of systemic hormones, such as erythropoietin [2]. The structure of the skin comprises differentiating keratinocytes in both the epidermal and dermal layers, as well as a variety of cells, including endothelial, neuronal and mesenchymal cells, which are specific to the dermis. The whole skin or the two separated layers can be maintained viable in organ culture, under optimal conditions, for up to 21 days [6, 7].

To analyze the contribution of the viral glycoprotein to the efficiency of skin transduction, lenti vectors were pseudotyped with two glycoproteins: VSV-G and Amphotropic. Both pseudotypes primarily transduced both the dermal and the intermediate basal layers, in both mouse and human skins (*Figure 5 A-F*). This observation indicated a specific tropism of lenti to dermal cells. Further analysis indicated that dermal mesenchymal cells and differentiating keratinocytes (Keratin 14+) were most sensitive to the virus. Interestingly, when the same multiplicity of infection was used, Lentivectors pseudotyped with the Amphotropic envelope, that utilizes the cell RAM1 protein as a receptor, was at least 50 folds more efficient in the transduction of both human and mouse skin as compared to the VSV-G pseudotype (*Figure 5 G and H*). As the two Lenti pseudotypes transduced human cells in culture equally well, we concluded that the initial interaction of virus with the solid tissue depends to a large extent on envelope protein/tissue factors interaction. To further analyze Lenti tropism in the epidermis and dermis, the two layers were separated by proteolysis and transduced in organ culture. The results indicated that while both dermis and epidermis layers of human skin were permissive to Lenti transduction, in the mouse only the dermal layer was infectable. To analyze the level of restriction to Lenti transduction in the mouse epidermis, total DNA was isolated following transduction and the reverse transcription of Lenti proviral DNA was followed. The results indicate that the block to lentivirus mediated gene transfer in the mouse epidermal cells is intracellular. While proviral DNA synthesis takes place in the mouse epidermal tissue following cell-entry, proviral DNA migration to the nucleus and subsequently its integration into the cell genome are restricted. Thus, intracellular restrictions to lentivirus transduction are present in the mouse epidermal cells; an observation that emphasizes differences between the mouse and human tissues, at least as far as tropism of Lenti vector is concerned.

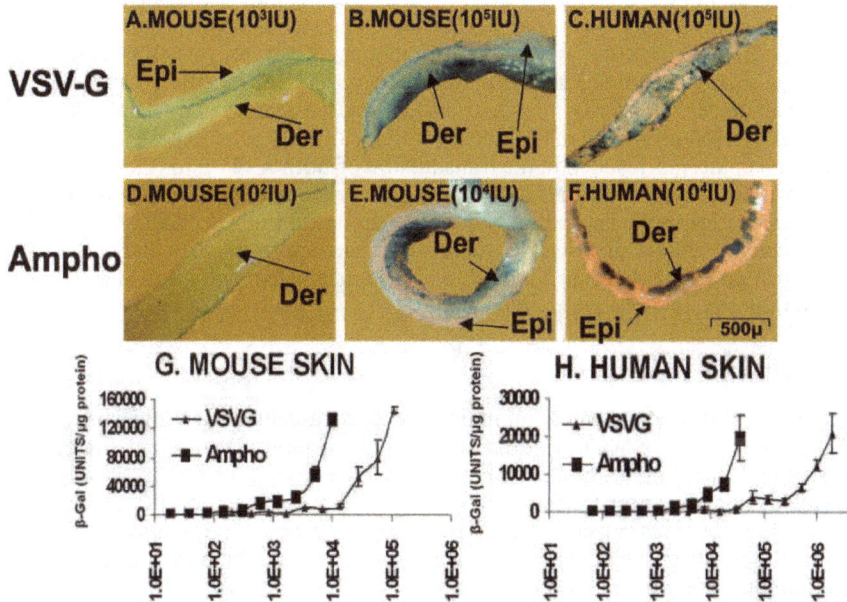

Figure 5. Transduction of murine and human skin in organ culture with lentiviral vectors pseudotype with Ampho and VSV-G. Mouse (A, B, D, and E) and human (C and F) skin organ cultures were prepared and exposed to two different Lentivector pseudotypes as described by Kunicher *et al.* [7]. Tissues were analyzed for β-gal reporter gene expression which localizes Lenti transduction primarily in the dermis and the skin basal layer. The Amphotropic pseudotype demonstrated some 50 folds higher transduction compared to the VSV-G pseudotype (G and H). The figure is reproduced with permission of *J Gene Med* (Kunicher *et al.* [6]).

Table I. Tropism of lentivectors in epidermal cells, grown in culture or in their native niche of skin tissue. Cultures of keratinocytes and organ cultures of skin were prepared from partial thickness human skin. Human tissues were obtained under the approval of the Hadassah hospital IRB committee. Skin was separated to epidermis and dermis layers by proteolysis and transduced with Lenti-GFP (VSV-G). Single cells were isolated from skin tissues after extensive trypsin treatment. Extent of gene transfer to keratinocytes was analyzed by GFP expression, using FACS [6]. The percentage of transduced cells was calculated relative to the number of Keratin marker, K14 or K15 positive cells. The results show that in cell culture and in the separated epidermis both K14+ and K15+ keratinocytes are permissive to lentivirus-mediated gene transfer In whole skin, however, the keratinocytes were excluded from virus transduction, due to physical interference with viral entry.

Cells/Tissue	K14+	K14+ infected	K15+	K15+ infected
Cultured Keratinocytes	41135	1886 (4.5%)	138	21 (15.2%)
Whole Skin	39644	33 (<0.1%)	2748	1(<0.1%)
Epidermis	33552	509 (1.5%)	121	6 (4.9%)

To further study tropism of Lenti in the human skin, we compared transduction efficiencies of human keratinocytes propagated in cell culture with keratinocytes in their "native niche", within the epidermis and dermis layers [4]. *In situ* Immuno-staining and FACS analysis of keratinocytes exposed to lenti in cell culture, indicated transduction of both differentiating keratinocytes (TA, Keratin 14+) and stem/early progenitor cells (Keratin 15+) *(Table 1)*. In comparison, transduction of keratinocytes (K14+ and K15+) in whole skin, maintained in organ culture, was very inefficient. To analyze whether physical barriers interfere with skin transduction, the epidermis was separated from the dermis by proteolysis and maintained in organ culture. Vector exposure to the separated human epidermis resulted in the transduction of both K14+ and K15+ cells, indicating that keratinocytes in the intact skin tissue are protected and exposure of the basal layer is needed for viral penetration and subsequent gene transfer *(Table 1)*. Further experiments indicate that extra-cellular matrix molecules, in particular Collagen interfere with access of the virus to the skin tissue and consequently transduction of the cells in their native niche is very inefficient [6].

DISCUSSION

Studies presented in this communication indicate that extra-cellular as well as intracellular factors determine efficiency and tropism of a variety of vectors mediated gene transfer in a three-dimensional solid tissue [1, 2, 8]. These tissue factors are distinct from the cellular receptor for viral recognition and present an additional level of restriction which deserves consideration in the design of gene therapy clinical trials. Furthermore, in several of the *ex vivo* experimental systems, transduction rates of the mouse and human tissues differ both quantitatively and qualitatively. Thus, the validation of animal experimental systems is critical, in particular when viruses of human origin are considered as vectors for gene therapy. The experiments presented here suggest that the *in vivo* mouse orthotopic carcinoma system is robust, at least in the case of oncolytic HSV1. In contrast, the observation that the mouse epidermis is not permissive to Lentivirus mediated gene transfer, while the human epidermis is emphasizes the danger of relying only on mouse-based experimental system; especially when the vector of choice was engineered from a human virus. Our studies reveal that extracellular components, such as Collagen and heparan-sulfate, act as physical barriers and a sink for the virus, thus prohibiting viral access to cell membrane receptors. These extra-cellular barriers are especially important in the case of oncolytic viruses, such as Adeno and HSV1, that are meant to specifically infect tumor cells and need to replicate and spread progenies within the solid malignant tissue to eliminate the tumor bulk. While a variety of viruses have been engineered to specifically infect tumor cells, more research is clearly required to facilitate the selective spread of virus progeny within the solid tumor. The *ex vivo* system presented here holds notable advantages in maintaining the original architecture of the investigated tissue; in addition it is important to note that blood circulation and functional immune system are missing in the organ culture and also represent key elements which can be evaluated in animal models only.

In conclusion, data presented in this paper raise several issues, related to viral tropism and spread within a solid tissue, that need to be considered in the translation and planning of a gene therapy clinical trial. Exploitation of the *ex vivo* system may interestingly address some of these issues.

ACKNOWLEDGMENTS

This work has been performed with the support of the EC-DG research through the FP6-Network of Excellence, CLINIGENE: LSHB-CT-2006-018933.

REFERENCES

1. Hasson E, Slovatizky Y, Shimoni Y, Falk H, Panet A, Mitrani E. Solid tissues can be manipulated *ex-vivo* and used as vehicles for gene therapy. *J Gene Med* 2005; 7: 261-6.

2. Brill-Almon E, Stern B, Afik D, Kaye J, Langer N, Bellomo S, *et al*. *Ex vivo* transduction of human dermal tissue structures for autologous implantation production and delivery of therapeutic proteins. *Mol Ther* 2005; 12: 274-82.

3. Kolodkin-Gal D, Zamir G, Pikarski E, Shimony N, Wu H, Haviv YS, Panet A. A novel system to study adenovirus tropism to normal and malignant colon tissues. *Virology* 2007; 357: 91-101.

4. Kolodkin-Gal D, Zamir G, Edden Y, Pikarsky E, Pikarsky A, Haim H, *et al*. A. HSV-1 preferentially targets human colon carcinoma: the role of extra-cellular matrix. *J Virol* 2008; 82: 999-1010.

5. Kolodkin-Gal D, Edden Y, Hartshtark Z, Ilan L, Khalaileh A, Pikarsky AJ, *et al*. Herpes simplex virus delivery to orthotopic rectal carcinoma results in an efficient and selective antitumor effect. *Gene Ther* 2009; 16: 905-15.

6. Kunicher N, Tzur T, Amar D, Chaouat M, Yaacov B, Panet A. Characterization of factors that determine lentiviral vector tropism in skin tissue using an *ex vivo* model. *J Gene Med* 2011; 13: 209-20.

7. Kunicher N, Falk H, Yaacov B, Tzur T, Panet A. Tropism of lentiviral vectors in skin tissue. *Hum Gene Ther* 2008; 19: 255-66.

8. Massler A, Kolodkin-Gal D, Meir K, Khalaileh A, Falk H, Izhar U, *et al*. Infant lungs are preferentially infected by adenovirus and herpes simplex virus type 1 vectors: role of the tissue mesenchymal cells. *J Gene Med* 201; 13: 101-13.

PRE-CLINICAL STUDIES, BIOSAFETY AND ANIMAL MODELS

General biosafety: immune responses, immunotoxicity and genotoxicity

COORDINATED BY
DAVID KLATZMANN
AND
CHRISTOF VON KALLE

The CliniBook: Clinical gene transfer
Edited by Odile Cohen-Haguenauer – EDK, Paris © 2012, pp. 405-419

B2-1

Assessing and taming unwanted immune responses induced by AAV gene transfer: current status, ongoing questions and future prospects

Federico Mingozzi[1]*, Anne Galy[2], David Klatzmann[3]

[1]*Center for Cellular and Molecular Therapeutics, Children's Hospital of Philadelphia, Philadelphia, PA, USA.* [2]*Inserm U951 and Généthon, Évry, France.*
[3]*Université Pierre et Marie Curie, UPMC Université Paris 6; CNRS UMR7211; Inserm U959, Hôpital de la Pitié-Salpêtrière, F-75013, Paris, France.*
mingozzi@email.chop.edu
* Corresponding author

INTRODUCTION

Recombinant gene transfer vectors derived from adeno-associated virus (rAAV) are currently tested in several phase I/II gene therapy trials to treat rare genetic diseases. In spite of being non-inflammatory and well-tolerated in animals, rAAV vectors have proven to be more immunogenic in humans than initially expected. An increasingly-large body of evidence from preclinical and clinical studies shows that immune responses to rAAV-mediated transfer depend on the context but are characterized by robust antibody responses, induction of capsid-specific T cells and involve innate immune recognition of the vector components (*Figure 1*). There is also evidence that rAAV can be used to induce transgene-specific tolerance. Better understanding the molecular and cellular bases for the immunogenicity of AAV and the mechanisms of AAV-mediated gene immunization, is therefore of great interest for the medical application of this viral vector system. More generally, understanding immune responses to AAVs should be heuristic for the entire field of gene therapy relying on the use of viral gene transfer vectors.

NATURE OF IMMUNE RESPONSES INDUCED BY AAV-MEDIATED GENE TRANSFER

Antibodies recognizing AAV vectors

Clinical gene transfer studies conducted over the past several years identified the host immune responses directed against AAV vectors as a major hindrance for the successful *in vivo* application of this platform. Humoral immunity to viral vectors is the first barrier to overcome when the vector is delivered systemically. For AAV vectors, this issue is particularly relevant, as humans are exposed early in life to the wild type virus through natural infection and develop neutralizing antibodies (NAb) cross-reacting with a wide range of capsid serotypes. Maternal anti-AAV antibodies can be found very early in life in newborns, before the direct exposure to the virus [1, 2]; these antibodies decrease in titer few months after birth before increasing again starting around 2 years of age [2].

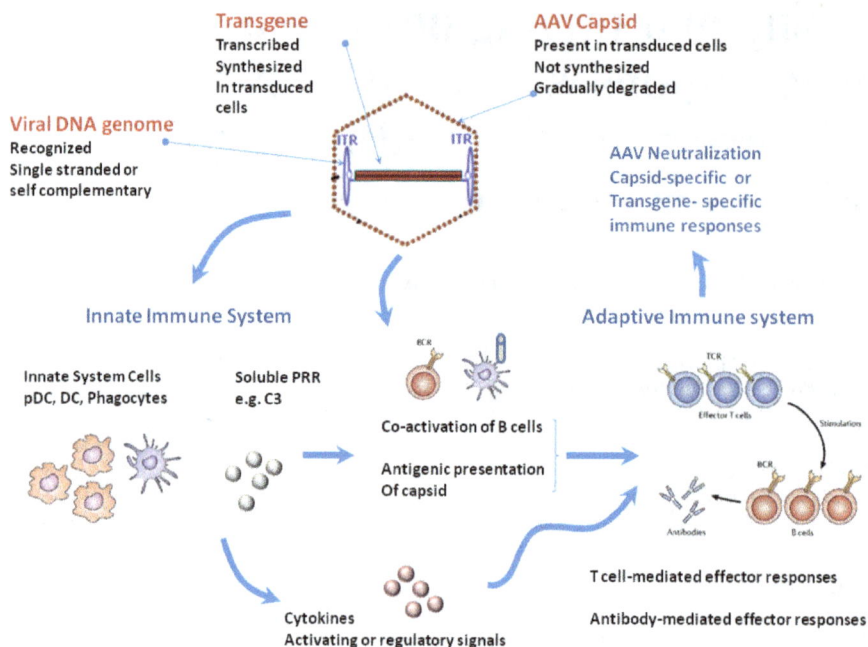

Figure 1. AAV vectors have a simple structure composed by a protein viral capsid and a single stranded DNA genome. No viral coding sequences are retained in AAV vectors, which are naturally replication deficient. Upon entering into and transducing a target cell, the viral capsid is slowly degraded and cleared. Capsid degradation involves ubiquitination and proteasomal processing, which leads to presentation of capsid epitopes onto MHC class I and class II molecules to CD8 and CD4 T cells. The transgene product, the second antigen associated with AAV vectors, is expressed for a long time after transduction. Potentially harmful immune responses directed against either the AAV capsid antigen or the transgene product can arise. Activation of capsid-specific T cells directed against the AAV capsid has been documented in several studies and was associated with loss of therapeutic efficacy. Immune responses directed against the transgene product have been documented in several animal models of gene transfer and, recently, in a handful of clinical studies. Recently, the interactions of AAV vectors with innate immune system have been the focus of several *in vivo* and *in vitro* studies. The interaction of AAV with cells of the innate system and with soluble pathogen-recognition receptors triggers cytokine responses and immune-modulatory signals that influence the development of T and B cell adaptive immune responses. The viral DNA genome is thought to be recognized by the innate immune system as a pathogen-associated motif.

Results from the first clinical trial for rAAV liver gene transfer for hemophilia B suggested a major impact of relatively low NAb titers on vector transduction [3]. Several studies were conducted with the aim of determining both the prevalence of NAb to AAV vectors in the general population and the impact of NAb on AAV transduction. Anti-AAV2 antibodies are the most prevalent (up to 70% of healthy humans), followed by less commonly prevalent serotypes like AAV5, AAV9, and AAV8 [4]. Pre-existing seropositivity to AAV has also been documented in patient cohorts [5] and it is therefore problematic to use gene therapy vectors with capsid serotypes against which the majority of patients can be immunized. Experiments in passively immunized mice [6] and naturally infected non-human primates [7] confirmed the results observed in the first clinical trials using recombinant AAV vector (rAAV) gene transfer [3] and show that NAb titers as low as 1:5 can completely block vector transduction.

It is important to note that NAb directed against AAV vectors are likely to have an impact on transduction efficiency depending on the route of delivery. Efficient vector neutralization is seen when the vector is delivered intravascularly, a strategy explored for skeletal muscle targeting to treat hemophilia and muscular dystrophy [8, 9], or when the vector is introduced into extravascular body compartments where NAb are present [10, 11]. Conversely, subretinal [12-14], intracranial [15], or intramuscular [16-18] vector administration is not majorly affected by the presence of anti-AAV NAb in serum.

Whether or not patients are seropositive for AAV, a single administration of the vector in the course of the clinical trials can induce capsid specific antibody responses [19, 20]. At the moment, without immunosuppression, the likelihood of becoming immunized against the AAV capsid following gene therapy is generally sufficient to preclude gene therapy protocols based on multiple systemic administrations of the same vector.

T cell responses specific for the AAV capsid

Early preclinical studies in mice, rats, dogs, non-human primates, and other animal models of gene transfer failed to fully appreciate the potential immunogenicity of AAV vectors. The importance of capsid T cell responses was realized in the first clinical trial in which a rAAV2 vector was introduced into the liver of human subjects as capsid T cell responses were identified as the possible cause of short-lived transgene expression [3, 21].

Following this initial observation, immunological monitoring was conducted in several other AAV gene transfer clinical studies in which the vector was administered to the muscle, to the subretinal space, to the brain, and systemically. Results are now starting to become available and are discussed further below. Meanwhile, studies in healthy donors showed that humans carry a population of antigen-specific memory CD8$^+$ T cells probably arising from wild-type AAV infections [21]. These capsid-reactive T cells are detectable early in life in humans, similarly to anti-AAV neutralizing antibodies.

Until the first evidence of capsid-specific T cell responses had been obtained in human trials, animal studies had generally overlooked and failed to specifically examine capsid-specific T cell responses following administration of rAAV. Murine epitopes from several AAV capsids have now been identified [22]. Much attention has been initially paid to capsid-specific CD8$^+$ T cells [23-25]. More recently, AAV capsid-specific CD4$^+$ T cell responses have been characterized in mice, and appear to be differentially induced according to serotypes. Yet, capsid-specific CD4$^+$ T cells play an essential role in capsid-specific CD8 T cell responses in mice as demonstrated by CD4-depleting antibody strategies [26]. In addition, the induction of specific IgG2c and IgG3 isotype subclasses in mice in response to various rAAV serotypes emphasizes the importance of underlying capsid-specific Th1 T cell responses for specific immunoglobulin switch processes (A. Galy, manuscript submitted).

Innate immune responses against AAV

During immune reactions, T cell help is influenced by innate responses that provide essential accessory signals [27, 28]. It is now clear that upon administration in organisms, rAAV encounters a system of innate defenses (recently reviewed by Rogers and colleagues [29]). While the administration of rAAV is well-tolerated in mice and triggers little inflammation compared to adenoviral vectors [30], AAV viral particles interact with proteins of the complement system that facilitate uptake of AAV by macrophages, trigger cytokine production and contribute to B cell responses to AAV2 in mice [31]. These studies provide strong evidence that innate immune recognition of AAV occurs and probably involves both the recognition of viral genome and capsid determinants. How innate recognition impacts on the development of T and B cell adaptive immune responses remains to be studied in detail.

Transgene-specific immune responses induced by AAV gene transfer. Can immune tolerance be achieved?

Gene therapy for monogenic diseases often relies on the expression of a transgene expressed from the vector, to correct the disease. While rAAV have demonstrated their advantage as non-inflammatory gene transfer vectors, transgene-specific immune responses can also be readily induced by rAAV-mediated intramuscular (IM) gene transfer [32]. The context is important and several factors are involved. Preclinical models have shown that a variety of transgenes including circulating factors such as EPO, coagulation factor VIII (F.VIII) and IX (F.IX), leptin, myostatin, or tissue proteins such as sarcoglycans can be produced at significant levels following gene transfer in skeletal muscle (as reviewed in [33]) but strong immunosuppression may be needed to maintain gene expression at high levels in non-tolerant transgene-null animals [32, 34]. The antigenic dose and route of administration are also important. It is clear that the IM route of administration is in itself immunogenic as it is possible to induce cellular and antibody-mediated immune responses to the transgene product by direct IM administration but not by vascular delivery of the same rAAV vector in murine, canine, or non-human primate models [35-38]. Thus, maintaining long-term expression of a foreign protein following rAAV-mediated gene transfer can represent a significant challenge.

Novel tissue-specific expression strategies exploiting the specific patterns of cellular micro RNAs have been developed to control transgene expression and to improve the efficacy of gene transfer [39] compared to tissue-specific promoters which may not always be tightly restricted nor effective at controlling immune responses [40]. This strategy has been essentially used with lentiviral vector-mediated gene delivery in the liver or intravenously, and has been very efficient at promoting long-term transgene expression of F.IX in F.IX-null mice [39] and enabling UGT1A1 gene transfer in the Gunn rat model [41]. At the same time, the strategy was found to be relatively inefficient in the case of hydrodynamic plasmid delivery in liver or muscle. Whether or not this strategy works with rAAV is not clear. In work presented at a Clinigene meeting in Annecy (January 2009), A. Galy's laboratory reported that they could effectively tolerize against an immmunogenic transgene by insertion of mir142.3p target sequences (which restricts expression in antigen preenting cells) in the AAV vector. This highlights that direct antigenic presentation of the transgene by antigen presenting cells is essential in this particular context. It thus emphasizes that rAAV are capable of transducing professional APCs *in vivo*, contrary to early postulates. Therefore it is important to understand interactions between the vector and APCs in organisms.

The outcome of gene transfer to the liver substantially differs from muscle-directed gene transfer in terms of transgene immunogenicity. Early experiments in hemophilia B mice receiving AAV vectors encoding for human F.IX transgene administered to the liver showed the absence of neutralizing antibody response against the transgene product in this setting [42]. This lack of responsiveness has been associated with the induction of CD4$^+$CD25$^+$FoxP3$^+$ regulatory T cells (Tregs). Actually, expansion of transgene-specific Tregs has been described in mice receiving hepatic gene transfer with a variety of vectors, including AAV, lentiviral and retroviral vectors [39, 42-44], encoding for various trans-genes like ovalbumin [45], human acid α-glucosidase [46], or α-galactosidase A [47] and the non secreted transgene cytoplasmic beta-galactosidase [48]. In addition, mice toler-ized to F.IX by means of hepatic gene transfer with AAV vectors also developed CD8$^+$ T cell tolerance, results in the absence of CTL responses following immunological chal-lenge with an adenovirus expressing F.IX given intramuscularly [49]. These data nicely recapitulate findings in hemophilia B dogs carrying a *null* mutation in the cF.IX gene, which develop antibodies against the donated wild type cF.IX transgene product follow-ing AAV gene transfer to muscle [32], but not liver [50].

The pivotal role of Tregs in tolerance induction following AAV mediated gene transfer has been confirmed by studies performed both in mice and non-human primates. The adoptive transfer of Tregs from tolerized mice render host mice tolerant while the de-pletion of Tregs with anti-CD25 antibodies breaks tolerance [51]. In non-human pri-mates, animals receiving an anti-CD25 antibody prior to AAV-F.IX gene transfer also mounted robust neutralizing antibody responses to the transgene product [52], and the administration of anti thymocite globulin has the same effect [53].

The role of liver in tolerance induction has been extensively studied. The liver is a unique immunological environment (reviewed by Thomson and Kolle [54]). It is there-fore not entirely surprising that tolerance to a transgene can be induced by expressing the latter in the liver. However, this unique liver immune environment still retains the ability to mount an immune response, mainly triggered through the activation of the innate immune system [54]. This has potentially important implication for the devel-opment of gene transfer therapeutics targeting the liver.

THE CLINICAL EXPERIENCE

As cruelly reminded by the TeGenero disaster trial [55], it is notorious that preclinical studies in animal models are not always representative of findings in humans. Therefore much of our relevant understanding of immunogenicity of rAAV will be gained from careful analysis of immune responses in clinical trials.

Liver-directed gene transfer

Hepatocytes are an attractive target tissue for the development of gene-based ther-apeutics [56]. Thus far, all the clinical efforts to develop liver-directed gene ther-apeutics with AAV vector have focused around hemophilia B, caused by the lack of circulating functional coagulation F.IX [57]. Hemophilia represents an ideal disease model for gene therapy as: a) clinical endpoints are well defined and b) these are easily measured; c) the therapeutic range is very wide; d) functional clot-ting factors can be produced by a variety of tissues, including liver, muscle, and fibroblasts [8, 58-60].

Compared to other tissues, liver presents several advantages as a target for AAV-me-diated gene transfer in hemophilia B. First, it is the natural site of biosynthesis of clot-ting factors, so the post-translational modifications take place efficiently; second, since it is a highly vascularized organ, access to the systemic circulation is efficient, thus conferring a dose advantage compared to other target tissues; third, expression of antigens in transduced hepatocytes is associated with induction of tolerance rather than immunity (this aspect of hepatic gene transfer is extensively discussed in the section on transgene immune responses) [56].

The pre-clinical work supporting AAV-mediated gene transfer to liver for hemophilia B is compelling [50, 61-63]. Long-term expression (>9 years) at therapeutic levels (6-8% of normal levels) in hemophilic dogs was achieved after infusing a single dose of $1x10^{12}$ vector genomes (vg)/kg of AAV-canine F.IX into the portal vein without production of neutralizing antibodies to the transgene product [63].

The first clinical dose-escalation study of liver gene transfer for hemophilia B used an AAV2 vector encoding for the F.IX transgene under the control of a liver-specific promoter. Vector ($8x10^{10}$, $4x10^{11}$, or $2x10^{12}$ vg/kg) was delivered through the hepatic artery [3]. The first subject from the high dose cohort ($2x10^{12}$ vg/kg), showed therapeutic levels of F.IX expression initially, in the range of 10-12%, sufficient to convert his disease phenotype from severe to mild [50]. However, beginning 4 weeks after vector infusion, F.IX levels began to fall, and gradually returned to baseline (<1%) at 10 weeks after vector infusion. Concurrently, the subject experienced a transient, self-limited, asymptomatic elevation of liver enzymes (AST and ALT). No inhibitory or non-inhibitory antibodies to the F.IX transgene product were measured in this subject. A second subject, enrolled in the study at a 5-fold lower dose than E also experienced an asymptomatic, self-limited liver enzyme elevation, with similar kinetics. ELISpot analysis of T cell responses in peripheral blood mononuclear cells (PBMC) showed IFN-γ production in response to AAV capsid peptides, but not to F.IX peptides [3]. Direct staining of subject G's PBMC with the AAV-specific MHC I pentamer showed the expansion and contraction of a population of capsid-specific CD8$^+$ T cells after vector infusion, with a time course closely matching the rise and fall of serum transaminases [21]. Even after >2 years post vector administration memory capsid-specific CD8$^+$ T cells remained detectable in peripheral blood.

The initial observations in the AAV2-F.IX trial led to an intense debate within the gene therapy community because these responses had not been predicted by preclinical work in animals and because it was now necessary to devise strategies for avoiding immune responses directed against AAV transduced cells; some of these maneuvers will be discussed later in this chapter.

Recently, investigators at St. Jude Children's Research Hospital in Memphis, TN, and University College London, UK, developed a more efficient expression cassette and vector [61, 62]. A clinical trial testing this newly developed vector has been recently initiated. Hemophilia B subjects received the AAV8-F.IX vector intravenously at doses of $2x10^{11}$vg/kg, $6x10^{11}$vg/kg, and $2x10^{12}$vg/kg [64]. No T cell responses directed against the AAV-8 capsid were seen at the low vector dose, while they could be detected at the intermediate dose. No loss of FIX transgene expression and no elevation of liver enzymes have been observed in these 4 subjects. However, activation of capsid specific CD8$^+$ T cells, with loss of transgene expression and increase in liver enzymes was detected 2 out of 2 subjects from the high-dose cohort, who received $2x10^{12}$ vg/kg of vector, ~8 to 9 weeks after vector delivery. In these subjects, a short course of steroids, administered at the time of liver enzyme elevation and loss of transgene expression, was able to at least partially rescue transgene expression [65]. Additional studies, currently undergoing, will help assessing the safety of this approach in a larger subject cohort and, in the future at higher vector doses.

Muscle gene transfer

Direct intramuscular gene transfer using AAV vectors has been explored for a number of indications, including hemophilia B [17, 66], lipoprotein lipase (LPL) deficiency [18], α_1-antitrypsin deficiency [16, 67, 68], and muscular dystrophies [69-71]. In addition, cardiac muscle has also been targeted through an intravascular approach, for cardiac failure [72].

Monitoring of capsid T cell responses was implemented in several of these clinical studies, which resulted in the generation of one of the largest dataset on capsid T cell responses in humans. With few exceptions, results accumulated suggest that the magnitude of T cell responses directed against the AAV capsid roughly correlates with the dose of vector administered, a result in agreement with the findings in AAV liver gene transfer. These studies also showed that humans can mount cytotoxic T cell responses against AAV transduced target cells.

While AAV vector administration in humans results in capsid-specific T cell activation; the open question is what is the clinical relevance of the detection of these T cells. In some of the studies discussed [19, 68, 70], detection of capsid-specific T cells has been associated with lack of evidence of target tissue transduction or loss of transgene expression to some extent. Further analysis of results of clinical gene transfer studies will help clarify this last point.

Ocular gene transfer and CNS gene transfer

The eye and central nervous system (CNS) are generally considered to be immune sanctuaries because of anatomical and biological adaptations that limit pathogen entry and subdue immune effector responses. This is probably meant to prevent tissue damage since these tissues have limited regenerative capacities. Accordingly, delivery of small doses of AAV vectors to the brain or the subretinal space is generally associated with little to no immune response to the capsid detectable in serum and PBMC. A modest increase in anti-AAV antibodies was documented following vector administration in subjects undergoing intracranial gene transfer for Parkinson's disease [15, 73-75], Canavan disease [76], and late infantile neuronal ceroid lipofuscinosis [77]. Similarly, subretinal administration of an AAV-2 vector encoding the RPE65 transgene resulted in minimal and transient anti-capsid humoral responses and no detectable capsid T cell responses in humans [13, 14].

Safety of AAV vector readministration to the contralateral eye in subjects who previously received AAV2-RPE65 gene transfer [13] is currently being tested (ClinicalTrials.gov ID# NCT01208389). Preclinical studies in RPE65-deficient dogs and non-human primates suggest that the approach is safe, and subretinal vector readministration to animals previously exposed to AAV vectors does not seem to trigger harmful immune responses against the AAV capsid [12]. Human studies confirmed these preclinical results as AAV vector readministration to the contralateral eye in subjects who previously received an AAV vector subretinally triggered minimal to no systemic antibody response to the viral vector, and no T cell responses to capsid or transgene product [78]. Thus, administering small doses of rAAV in immune sanctuaries may represent, at the moment, the most efficacious application of this vector in gene therapy for rare diseases.

ONGOING QUESTIONS IN THE FIELD AND FUTURE PROSPECTS

Pre-existing humoral immunity to AAV. Can we circumvent the problem?

Eradication of neutralizing antibodies directed against the AAV capsid is a difficult task. Despite the considerable efforts devoted to achieve this goal, only partial success has been achieved thus far. Possible strategies tested towards this end are the following:

Select less seroprevalent AAV serotypes
Studies in humans show that some AAV serotypes are less prevalent than others. Granted that serotypes with different antibody reactivity profile and similar affinity for the target tissue are available, switching AAV serotype to treat subjects otherwise untreatable because of NAb is a potentially feasible strategy. One limitation to this approach is the high level of sequence homology of different AAV capsids, which results in high levels of cross-reactivity of anti-AAV NAb.
Development of novel, artificial AAV serotypes is also a promising approach. One strategy explored is the development of a library of AAV capsids with error-prone PCR techniques [79], followed by selection of capsid mutants for both tropism directed to the target tissue (*e.g.* tropism for hepatocytes) and resistance for NAb [80].

Plasmapheresis
A recent report [81] showed that repeated cycles of plasmapheresis are effective in lowering anti-AAV NAb. Plasmapheresis is an established and safe technique used to isolate or eliminate components from blood. The approach suffers from the limitation that it is not very effective in reducing higher antibody titers [81], which may require the use of a combination of plasmapheresis and immunosuppression in a subset of subjects carrying high-titer NAb to AAV.

Immunosuppression
One potential advantage for immunosuppression used in the context of AAV gene transfer is that, unlike organ transplant or autoimmune disease, the duration of the intervention is relatively short.
In this section we will only discuss results and potential efficacy of B cell depletion using rituximab as a strategy to reduce anti-AAV NAb. However, many other drugs could be used to reduce anti-AAV antibodies, as a general approach, the choice should necessarily focus on drugs that are already licensed for clinical use.
Rituximab, a chimeric mouse-human monoclonal antibody specific to human CD20, is one of the front-line drugs available to target B cells. Rituximab was first approved in 1997 for the treatment of B-cell malignancies; more recently the drug has been approved for several other non-malignant diseases due to its efficacy and safety profile [82]. Analysis of anti-AAV2 neutralizing antibody titers in rheumatoid arthritis patients following a single course of rituximab (two intravenous administrations at a two-week interval) showed a dropped in NAb titer in subjects with titers <1:400, compared to subjects with higher titers in whom no change in NAb was noted [11]. This result is consistent with observations in acquired hemophilia patients, where B cell depletion is less effective in patients with high-titer inhibitors [83] and with recent results in non-human primates [84]. Finally, a recent example of use of immunosuppression to attenuate humoral responses to capsid following vector administration comes from the work of McIntosh and colleagues [85]. In this study, a short course of immunosup-

pression with a combination of a non-depleting anti-CD4 antibody and cyclosporine A resulted in lower anti-AAV antibody formation, which allowed for vector readministration.

Modulation of AAV capsid-specific T cell responses

Immunosuppression of AAV gene transfer-induced immune responses
Aside from the modulation of humoral immunity to the AAV capsid, a short course of immunosuppression (IS), given around the time of gene transfer, has been proposed as a strategy to create a window of time during which cytotoxic T cell responses directed against AAV capsid are blunted while capsid antigen itself is cleared from the transduced cells. This strategy is being tested in humans in a clinical trial of AAV-2 gene transfer for hemophilia B (ClinicalTrials.gov ID:NCT00515710) in which the vector is co-administered with a short course of mycophenolate mofetil and sirolimus. Another study of AAV-1 intramuscular gene transfer for lipoprotein lipase deficiency has tested the safety of MMF and cyclosporine A in the context of gene transfer. Preliminary results from both studies (Mingozzi and High, unpublished results and [19]) show that the approach is safe.
Recent data indicate that treatment of AAV-transduced cells with the proteasome inhibitor bortezumib, at doses comparable to those used in the clinic (serum levels 30-100 nmol/l), results in decreased capsid antigen presentation [86]. This may be a feasible and relatively safe intervention to reduce capsid immunogenicity. However the fate of capsid proteins after proteasome inhibition is currently unknown and remains an important question to address.
Overall, the use of immunosuppression is certainly an attractive approach to address the problem of anti-AAV NAb. However, aside from the risks related to immunosuppression itself, such as increased rate of infections, additional caution should be used when planning to use any kind of immunosuppressive drug in the context of gene transfer, especially in the setting of liver-directed gene transfer, in which $CD4^+CD25^+FoxP3^+$ Tregs homeostasis is essential to establish and maintain tolerance to the transgene product [42, 51-53, 87]. This was recently reported in two studies of liver gene transfer for hemophilia B in non-human primate models, which showed that drugs targeting the IL-2 receptor CD25, highly expressed in Tregs [52], or lymphocyte depleting drugs like antithymocyte globulin [53], can result in neutralizing antibody responses directed against the transgene product.

Immunoregulation with interleukine-2

IL-2 was identified almost 30 years ago for its capacity to stimulate T cells *in vitro* [88, 89]. It has first been used in the clinic for boosting effector immune responses in certain types of cancer and infectious diseases, although with disappointing results [90, 91]. This limited effect of IL-2 has now been explained by the fact that IL-2 also plays a major role in the peripheral survival and suppressive function of Tregs.
In agreement with these observations, others and we showed that low dose IL-2 administration leads to preferential expansion and activation of Tregs in men and mice [92, 93]. Moreover, we performed the first clinical trial aimed at inducing Tregs using IL-2 administration in patients with an autoimmune disease, in this case HCV-related vasculitis. The treatment was safe and led to a major Treg expansion and clinical improvement [94].
It thus, now appears that low dose IL-2 represents a novel class of immuno-regulatory drug, acting by a specific Treg expansion/activation. We are currently evaluating

whether the co-administration of IL-2 (by drug injection or concomitant gene transfer) can result in better tolerance to the transgene product.

CONCLUSIONS

A wide range of viruses, including AAVs, are developed simultaneously and sometimes by the same teams as recombinant vectors for gene therapy and for vaccination. Ironically, the induction of an immune response to the transgene product expressed represents a potential drawback or even hazard for a gene therapy, while being the gist of a vaccine strategy. Given the stakes, the efforts and ingeniousness developed for both applications, - and realizing that progress in one direction can immediately be exploited towards the other - it makes little doubts that the bottleneck of immune responses to either the transgene product and/or gene transfer vectors will be (at least in part) solved in the near future.

ACKNOWLEDGMENTS

This work was supported by: the Center for Cellular and Molecular Therapeutics at the Children's Hospital of Philadelphia and the National Institute of Health (RO1HL094396 and PO1HL078810); institutional grants by University Pierre and Marie Curie, INSERM and CNRS; *EC-DG research FP6-Network of Excellence, CLINIGENE: LSHB-CT-2006-018933*; Persist project (EC FP7 Health Grant Agreement no: 222878) and funds from the French Muscular Dystrophy Association (AFM).

REFERENCES

1. Li C, Narkbunnam N, Samulski RJ, Asokan A, Hu G, Jacobson LJ, *et al*. Neutralizing antibodies against adeno-associated virus examined prospectively in pediatric patients with hemophilia. *Gene Ther* 2011; June 23.

2. Calcedo R, Morizono H, Wang L, McCarter R, He J, Jones D, *et al*. Adeno-associated virus antibody profiles in newborns, children, and adolescents. *Clin Vaccine Immunol* 2011; 18: 1586-8.

3. Manno CS, Pierce GF, Arruda VR, Glader B, Ragni M, Rasko JJ, *et al*. Successful transduction of liver in hemophilia by AAV-Factor IX and limitations imposed by the host immune response. *Nat Med* 2006; 12: 342-7.

4. Boutin S, Monteilhet V, Veron P, Leborgne C, Benveniste O, Montus MF, *et al*. Prevalence of serum IgG and neutralizing factors against adeno-associated virus (AAV) types 1, 2, 5, 6, 8, and 9 in the healthy population: implications for gene therapy using AAV vectors. *Hum Gene Ther* 2010; 21: 704-12.

5. Chirmule N, Propert K, Magosin S, Qian Y, Qian R, Wilson J. Immune responses to adenovirus and adeno-associated virus in humans. *Gene Ther* 1999; 6: 1574-83.

6. Scallan CD, Jiang H, Liu T, Patarroyo-White S, Sommer JM, Zhou S, *et al*. Human immunoglobulin inhibits liver transduction by AAV vectors at low AAV2 neutralizing titers in SCID mice. *Blood* 2006; 107: 1810-7.

7. Jiang H, Couto LB, Patarroyo-White S, Liu T, Nagy D, Vargas JA, *et al*. Effects of transient immunosuppression on adenoassociated, virus-mediated, liver-directed gene transfer in rhesus macaques and implications for human gene therapy. *Blood* 2006; 108: 3321-8.

8. Arruda VR, Hagstrom JN, Deitch J, Heiman-Patterson T, Camire RM, Chu K, *et al*. Posttranslational modifications of recombinant myotube-synthesized human factor IX. *Blood* 2001; 97: 130-8.

9. Rodino-Klapac LR, Montgomery CL, Bremer WG, Shontz KM, Malik V, Davis N, *et al*. Persistent expression of FLAG-tagged micro dystrophin in nonhuman primates following intramuscular and vascular delivery. *Mol Ther* 2010; 18: 109-17.

10. Cottard V, Valvason C, Falgarone G, Lutomski D, Boissier MC, Bessis N. Immune response against gene therapy vectors: influence of synovial fluid on adeno-associated virus mediated gene transfer to chondrocytes. *J Clin Immunol* 2004; 24: 162-9.

11. Mingozzi F, Chen Y, Edmonson SC, Zhou S, Thurlings RM, Tak PP, High KA, Vervoordeldonk MJ. Prevalence and pharmacological modulation of humoral immunity to AAV vectors in gene transfer to synovial tissue. *Gene Ther* 2012; July 12 (online).

12. Amado D, Mingozzi F, Hui D, Bennicelli JL, Wei Z, Chen Y, *et al*. Safety and efficacy of subretinal readministration of a viral vector in large animals to treat congenital blindness. *Sci Transl Med* 2010; 2: 21ra16.

13. Maguire AM, High KA, Auricchio A, Wright JF, Pierce EA, Testa F, *et al*. Age-dependent effects of RPE65 gene therapy for Leber's congenital amaurosis: a phase 1 dose-escalation trial. *Lancet* 2009; 374: 1597-605.

14. Maguire AM, Simonelli F, Pierce EA, Pugh EN Jr, Mingozzi F, Bennicelli J, *et al*. Safety and efficacy of gene transfer for Leber's congenital amaurosis. *N Engl J Med* 2008; 358: 2240-8.

15. Kaplitt MG, Feigin A, Tang C, Fitzsimons HL, Mattis P, Lawlor PA, *et al*. Safety and tolerability of gene therapy with an adeno-associated virus (AAV) borne GAD gene for Parkinson's disease: an open label, phase I trial. *Lancet* 2007; 369: 2097-105.

16. Brantly ML, Chulay JD, Wang L, Mueller C, Humphries M, Spencer LT, *et al*. Sustained transgene expression despite T lymphocyte responses in a clinical trial of rAAV1-AAT gene therapy. *Proc Natl Acad Sci USA* 2009; 106: 16363-8.

17. Manno CS, Chew AJ, Hutchison S, Larson PJ, Herzog RW, Arruda VR, *et al*. AAV-mediated factor IX gene transfer to skeletal muscle in patients with severe hemophilia B. *Blood* 2003; 101: 2963-72.

18. Stroes ES, Nierman MC, Meulenberg JJ, Franssen R, Twisk J, Henny CP, *et al*. Intramuscular administration of AAV1-lipoprotein lipase S447X lowers triglycerides in lipoprotein lipase-deficient patients. *Arterioscler Thromb Vasc Biol* 2008; 28: 2303-4.

19. Mingozzi F, Meulenberg JJ, Hui DJ, Basner-Tschakarjan E, Hasbrouck NC, Edmonson SA, *et al*. AAV-1-mediated gene transfer to skeletal muscle in humans results in dose-dependent activation of capsid-specific T cells. *Blood* 2009; 114: 2077-86.

20. Murphy SL, Li H, Mingozzi F, Sabatino DE, Hui DJ, Edmonson SA, *et al*. Diverse IgG subclass responses to adeno-associated virus infection and vector administration. *J Med Virol* 2009; 81: 65-74.

21. Mingozzi F, Maus MV, Hui DJ, Sabatino DE, Murphy SL, Rasko JE, *et al*. CD8+ T-cell responses to adeno-associated virus capsid in humans. *Nat Med* 2007; 13: 419-22.

22. Sabatino DE, Mingozzi F, Hui DJ, Chen H, Colosi P, Ertl HC, *et al*. Identification of mouse AAV capsid-specific CD8+ T cell epitopes. *Mol Ther* 2005; 12: 1023-33.

23. Li C, Hirsch M, Asokan A, Zeithaml B, Ma H, Kafri T, *et al*. Adeno-associated virus type 2 (AAV2) capsid-specific cytotoxic T lymphocytes eliminate only vector-transduced cells coexpressing the AAV2 capsid *in vivo*. *J Virol* 2007; 81: 7540-7.

24. Li H, Murphy SL, Giles-Davis W, Edmonson S, Xiang Z, Li Y, *et al*. Pre-existing AAV capsid-specific CD8+ T cells are unable to eliminate AAV-transduced hepatocytes. *Mol Ther* 2007; 15: 792-800.

25. Wang L, Figueredo J, Calcedo R, Lin J, Wilson JM. Cross-presentation of adeno-associated virus serotype 2 capsids activates cytotoxic T cells but does not render hepatocytes effective cytolytic targets. *Hum Gene Ther* 2007; 18: 185-94.

26. Mays LE, Vandenberghe LH, Xiao R, Bell P, Nam HJ, Agbandje-McKenna M, *et al.* Adeno-associated virus capsid structure drives CD4-dependent CD8+ T cell response to vector encoded proteins. *J Immunol* 2009; 182: 6051-60.

27. Iwasaki A, Medzhitov R. Regulation of adaptive immunity by the innate immune system. *Science* 2010; 327: 291-5.

28. Kawai T, Akira S. The role of pattern-recognition receptors in innate immunity: update on Toll-like receptors. *Nat Immunol* 2010; 11: 373-84.

29. Rogers GL, Martino AT, Aslanidi GV, Jayandharan GR, Srivastava A, Herzog RW. Innate immune responses to AAV vectors. *Front Microbiol* 2011; 2: 194.

30. Zaiss AK, Liu Q, Bowen GP, Wong NC, Bartlett JS, Muruve DA. Differential activation of innate immune responses by adenovirus and adeno-associated virus vectors. *J Virol* 2002; 76: 4580-90.

31. Zaiss AK, Cotter MJ, White LR, Clark SA, Wong NC, Holers VM, *et al.* Complement is an essential component of the immune response to adeno-associated virus vectors. *J Virol* 2008; 82: 2727-40.

32. Herzog RW, Mount JD, Arruda VR, High KA, Lothrop CD Jr. Muscle-directed gene transfer and transient immune suppression result in sustained partial correction of canine hemophilia B caused by a null mutation. *Mol Ther* 2001; 4: 192-200.

33. Herzog RW. AAV-mediated gene transfer to skeletal muscle. *Methods Mol Biol* 2004; 246: 179-94.

34. Miao CH, Ye P, Thompson AR, Rawlings DJ, Ochs HD. Immunomodulation of transgene responses following naked DNA transfer of human factor VIII into hemophilia A mice. *Blood* 2006; 108: 19-27.

35. Cao O, Hoffman BE, Moghimi B, Nayak S, Cooper M, Zhou S, *et al.* Impact of the underlying mutation and the route of vector administration on immune responses to factor IX in gene therapy for hemophilia B. *Mol Ther* 2009; 17: 1733-42.

36. Toromanoff A, Adjali O, Larcher T, Hill M, Guigand L, Chenuaud P, *et al.* Lack of immunotoxicity after regional intravenous (RI) delivery of rAAV to nonhuman primate skeletal muscle. *Mol Ther* 2010; 18: 151-60.

37. Arruda VR, Stedman HH, Haurigot V, Buchlis G, Baila S, Favaro P, *et al.* Peripheral transvenular delivery of adeno-associated viral vectors to skeletal muscle as a novel therapy for hemophilia B. *Blood* 2010; 115: 4678-88.

38. Haurigot V, Mingozzi F, Buchlis G, Hui DJ, Chen Y, Basner-Tschakarjan E, *et al.* Safety of AAV factor IX peripheral transvenular gene delivery to muscle in hemophilia B dogs. *Mol Ther* 2010; 18: 1318-29.

39. Brown BD, Venneri MA, Zingale A, Sergi Sergi L, Naldini L. Endogenous microRNA regulation suppresses transgene expression in hematopoietic lineages and enables stable gene transfer. *Nat Med* 2006; 12: 585-91.

40. Liu YL, Mingozzi F, Rodriguez-Colon SM, Joseph S, Dobrzynski E, Suzuki T, *et al.* Therapeutic levels of factor IX expression using a muscle-specific promoter and adeno-associated virus serotype 1 vector. *Hum Gene Ther* 2004; 15: 783-92.

41. Schmitt F, Remy S, Dariel A, Flageul M, Pichard V, Boni S, *et al.* Lentiviral vectors that express UGT1A1 in liver and contain miR-142 target sequences normalize hyperbilirubinemia in Gunn rats. *Gastroenterology* 2010; 139: 999-1007.

42. Mingozzi F, Liu YL, Dobrzynski E, Kaufhold A, Liu JH, Wang Y, *et al.* Induction of immune tolerance to coagulation factor IX antigen by *in vivo* hepatic gene transfer. *J Clin Invest* 2003; 111: 1347-56.

43. Follenzi A, Battaglia M, Lombardo A, Annoni A, Roncarolo MG, Naldini L. Targeting lentiviral vector expression to hepatocytes limits transgene-specific immune response and establishes long-term expression of human antihemophilic factor IX in mice. *Blood* 2004; 103: 3700-9.

44. Xu L, Mei M, Haskins ME, Nichols TC, O'Donnell P, Cullen K, *et al.* Immune response after neonatal transfer of a human factor IX-expressing retroviral vector in dogs, cats, and mice. *Thromb Res* 2007; 120: 269-80.

45. Dobrzynski E, Mingozzi F, Liu YL, Bendo E, Cao O, Wang L, *et al.* Induction of antigen-specific CD4+ T-cell anergy and deletion by *in vivo* viral gene transfer. *Blood* 2004; 104: 969-77.

46. Franco LM, Sun B, Yang X, Bird A, Zhang H, Schneider A, *et al.* Evasion of immune responses to introduced human acid alpha-glucosidase by liver-restricted expression in glycogen storage disease type II. *Mol Ther* 2005; 12: 876-84.

47. Ziegler RJ, Lonning SM, Armentano D, Li C, Souza DW, Cherry M, *et al.* AAV2 vector harboring a liver-restricted promoter facilitates sustained expression of therapeutic levels of alpha-galactosidase A and the induction of immune tolerance in Fabry mice. *Mol Ther* 2004; 9: 231-40.

48. Martino AT, Nayak S, Hoffman BE, Cooper M, Liao G, Markusic DM, *et al.* Tolerance induction to cytoplasmic beta-galactosidase by hepatic AAV gene transfer: implications for antigen presentation and immunotoxicity. *PLoS One* 2009; 4: e6376.

49. Dobrzynski E, Fitzgerald JC, Cao O, Mingozzi F, Wang L, Herzog RW. Prevention of cytotoxic T lymphocyte responses to factor IX-expressing hepatocytes by gene transfer-induced regulatory T cells. *Proc Natl Acad Sci USA* 2006; 103: 4592-7.

50. Mount JD, Herzog RW, Tillson DM, Goodman SA, Robinson N, McCleland ML, *et al.* Sustained phenotypic correction of hemophilia B dogs with a factor IX null mutation by liver-directed gene therapy. *Blood* 2002; 99: 2670-6.

51. Cao O, Dobrzynski E, Wang L, Nayak S, Mingle B, Terhorst C, *et al.* Induction and role of regulatory CD4+CD25+ T cells in tolerance to the transgene product following hepatic *in vivo* gene transfer. *Blood* 2007; 110: 1132-40.

52. Mingozzi F, Hasbrouck NC, Basner-Tschakarjan E, Edmonson SA, Hui DJ, Sabatino DE, *et al.* Modulation of tolerance to the transgene product in a nonhuman primate model of AAV-mediated gene transfer to liver. *Blood* 2007; 110: 2334-41.

53. Finn JD, Favaro P, Wright JF, Mingozzi F, High KA, Arruda VR. Rabbit anti-thymocyte globulin (rATG) administrated concomitantly with liver delivery of AAV2-hFIX can promote inhibitor formation in Rhesus macaques. *Blood* 2010; 116: 3765 (abstract).

54. Thomson AW, Knolle PA. Antigen-presenting cell function in the tolerogenic liver environment. *Nat Rev Immunol* 2010; 10: 753-66.

55. Suntharalingam G, Perry MR, Ward S, Brett SJ, Castello-Cortes A, Brunner MD, *et al.* Cytokine storm in a phase 1 trial of the anti-CD28 monoclonal antibody TGN1412. *N Engl J Med* 2006; 355: 1018-28.

56. Mingozzi F, High KA. Therapeutic *in vivo* gene transfer for genetic disease using AAV: progress and challenges. *Nat Rev Genet* 2011; 12: 341-55.

57. Pollak ES, High KA. Hemophilia A: Factor IX deficiency. In: Scriver CR, Beaudet AL, Valle D, Sly WS, eds. *The metabolic and molecular bases of inherited disease*, 5th ed. New York: Mc-Graw Hill, 2001: 4393-413.

58. Snyder RO, Miao C, Meuse L, Tubb J, Donahue BA, Lin HF, *et al.* Correction of hemophilia B in canine and murine models using recombinant adeno-associated viral vectors. *Nat Med* 1999; 5: 64-70.

59. Palmer TD, Thompson AR, Miller AD. Production of human factor IX in animals by genetically modified skin fibroblasts: potential therapy for hemophilia B. *Blood* 1989; 73: 438-45.

60. High KA. AAV-mediated gene transfer for hemophilia. *Ann NY Acad Sci* 2001; 953: 64-74.

61. Nathwani AC, Gray JT, McIntosh J, Ng CY, Zhou J, Spence Y, *et al.* Safe and efficient transduction of the liver after peripheral vein infusion of self-complementary AAV vector results in stable therapeutic expression of human FIX in nonhuman primates. *Blood* 2007; 109: 1414-21.

62. Nathwani AC, Rosales C, McIntosh J, Rastegarlari G, Nathwani D, Raj D, *et al*. Long-term safety and efficacy following systemic administration of a self-complementary AAV vector encoding human FIX pseudotyped with serotype 5 and 8 capsid proteins. *Mol Ther* 2011; 19: 876-85.

63. Niemeyer GP, Herzog RW, Mount J, Arruda VR, Tillson DM, Hathcock J, *et al*. Long-term correction of inhibitor-prone hemophilia B dogs treated with liver-directed AAV2-mediated factor IX gene therapy. *Blood* 2009; 113: 797-806.

64. Fagone P, Wright JF, Nathwani AC, Nienhuis AW, Davidoff AM, Gray JT. Systemic errors in quantitative polymerase chain reaction titration of self-complementary adeno-associated viral vectors and improved alternative methods. *Hum Gene Ther* 2011; September 23.

65. Nathwani AC, Tuddenham EG, Rangarajan S, Rosales C, McIntosh J, Linch DC, *et al*. Adenovirus-associated virus vector-mediated gene transfer in hemophilia B. *N Engl J Med* 2011; 365: 2357-65.

66. Kay MA, Manno CS, Ragni MV, Larson PJ, Couto LB, McClelland A, *et al*. Evidence for gene transfer and expression of factor IX in haemophilia B patients treated with an AAV vector. *Nat Genet* 2000; 24: 257-61.

67. Brantly ML, Spencer LT, Humphries M, Conlon TJ, Spencer CT, Poirier A, *et al*. Phase I trial of intramuscular injection of a recombinant adeno-associated virus serotype 2 alphal-antitrypsin (AAT) vector in AAT-deficient adults. *Hum Gene Ther* 2006; 17: 1177-86.

68. Flotte TR, Trapnell BC, Humphries M, Carey B, Calcedo R, Rouhani F, *et al*. Phase 2 clinical trial of a recombinant adeno-associated viral vector expressing alpha(1)-antitrypsin: interim results. *Hum Gene Ther* 2011; 22: 1239-47.

69. Mendell JR, Campbell K, Rodino-Klapac L, Sahenk Z, Shilling C, Lewis S, *et al*. Dystrophin immunity in Duchenne's muscular dystrophy. *N Engl J Med* 2010; 363: 1429-37.

70. Mendell JR, Rodino-Klapac LR, Rosales XQ, Coley BD, Galloway G, Lewis S, *et al*. Sustained alpha-sarcoglycan gene expression after gene transfer in limb-girdle muscular dystrophy, type 2D. *Ann Neurol* 2010; 68: 629-38.

71. Mendell JR, Rodino-Klapac LR, Rosales-Quintero X, Kota J, Coley BD, Galloway G, *et al*. Limb-girdle muscular dystrophy type 2D gene therapy restores alpha-sarcoglycan and associated proteins. *Ann Neurol* 2009; 66: 290-7.

72. Jaski BE, Jessup ML, Mancini DM, Cappola TP, Pauly DF, Greenberg B, *et al*. Calcium upregulation by percutaneous administration of gene therapy in cardiac disease (CUPID trial), a first-in-human phase 1/2 clinical trial. *J Card Fail* 2009; 15: 171-81.

73. Christine CW, Starr PA, Larson PS, Eberling JL, Jagust WJ, Hawkins RA, *et al*. Safety and tolerability of putaminal AADC gene therapy for Parkinson disease. *Neurology* 2009; 73: 1662-9.

74. Marks WJ Jr, Bartus RT, Siffert J, Davis CS, Lozano A, Boulis N, *et al*. Gene delivery of AAV2-neurturin for Parkinson's disease: a double-blind, randomised, controlled trial. *Lancet Neurol* 2010; 9: 1164-72.

75. Marks WJ Jr, Ostrem JL, Verhagen L, Starr PA, Larson PS, Bakay RA, *et al*. Safety and tolerability of intraputaminal delivery of CERE-120 (adeno-associated virus serotype 2-neurturin) to patients with idiopathic Parkinson's disease: an open-label, phase I trial. *Lancet Neurol* 2008; 7: 400-8.

76. McPhee SW, Janson CG, Li C, Samulski RJ, Camp AS, Francis J, *et al*. Immune responses to AAV in a phase I study for Canavan disease. *J Gene Med* 2006; 8: 577-88.

77. Worgall S, Sondhi D, Hackett NR, Kosofsky B, Kekatpure MV, Neyzi N, *et al*. Treatment of late infantile neuronal ceroid lipofuscinosis by CNS administration of a serotype 2 adeno-associated virus expressing CLN2 cDNA. *Hum Gene Ther* 2008; 19: 463-74.

78. Bennett J, Maguire AM, Mingozzi F, Pierce EA, Chung DC, Bennicelli J, *et al*. Safety and efficacy of re-administration of AAV2.hRPE65v2 in subjects with Leber congenital blindness due to RPE65 mutations. *Mol Ther* 2011; 19: 600 (abstract).

79. Perabo L, Endell J, King S, Lux K, Goldnau D, Hallek M, *et al*. Combinatorial engineering of a gene therapy vector: directed evolution of adeno-associated virus. *J Gene Med* 2006; 8: 155-62.

80. Stone D, Koerber JT, Mingozzi F, Podsakoff GM, High KA, Schaffer DV. Associated virus variants that evade human neutralizing antibodies. *Mol Ther* 2010; 18: 8 (abstract).

81. Monteilhet V, Saheb S, Boutin S, Leborgne C, Veron P, Montus MF, *et al*. A 10 patient case report on the impact of plasmapheresis upon neutralizing factors against adeno-associated virus (AAV) types 1, 2, 6, and 8. *Mol Ther* 2011; 19: 2084-91.

82. Gurcan HM, Keskin DB, Stern JN, Nitzberg MA, Shekhani H, Ahmed AR. A review of the current use of rituximab in autoimmune diseases. *Int Immunopharmacol* 2009; 9: 10-25.

83. Stasi R, Brunetti M, Stipa E, Amadori S. Selective B-cell depletion with rituximab for the treatment of patients with acquired hemophilia. *Blood* 2004; 103: 4424-8.

84. Mingozzi F, Chen Y, Murphy SL, Edmonson SC, Tai A, Price SD, *et al*. Pharmacological modulation of humoral immunity in a nonhuman primate model of AAV gene transfer for hemophilia B. *Mol Ther* 2012; 20: 1410-6.

85. McIntosh JH, Cochrane M, Cobbold S, Waldmann H, Nathwani SA, Davidoff AM, *et al*. Successful attenuation of humoral immunity to viral capsid and transgenic protein following AAV-mediated gene transfer with a non-depleting CD4 antibody and cyclosporine. *Gene Ther* 2011; June 30.

86. Finn JD, Hui D, Downey HD, Dunn D, Pien GC, Mingozzi F, *et al*. Proteasome inhibitors decrease AAV2 capsid derived peptide epitope presentation on MHC class I following transduction. *Mol Ther* 2010; 18: 135-42.

87. Brown BD, Cantore A, Annoni A, Sergi LS, Lombardo A, Della Valle P, *et al*. A microRNA-regulated lentiviral vector mediates stable correction of hemophilia B mice. *Blood* 2007; 110: 4144-52.

88. Morgan DA, Ruscetti FW, Gallo R. Selective *in vitro* growth of T lymphocytes from normal human bone marrows. *Science* 1976; 193: 1007-8.

89. Smith KA. Interleukin-2: inception, impact, and implications. *Science* 1988; 240: 1169-76.

90. Chang AE, Rosenberg SA. Overview of interleukin-2 as an immunotherapeutic agent. *Semin Surg Oncol* 1989; 5: 385-90.

91. Giedlin MA, Zimmerman RJ. The use of recombinant human interleukin-2 in treating infectious diseases. *Curr Opin Biotechnol* 1993; 4: 722-6.

92. Lemoine FM, Cherai M, Giverne C, Dimitri D, Rosenzwajg M, Trebeden-Negre H, *et al*. Massive expansion of regulatory T-cells following interleukin 2 treatment during a phase I-II dendritic cell-based immunotherapy of metastatic renal cancer. *Int J Oncol* 2009; 35: 569-81.

93. Grinberg-Bleyer Y, Baeyens A, You S, Elhage R, Fourcade G, Gregoire S, *et al*. IL-2 reverses established type 1 diabetes in NOD mice by a local effect on pancreatic regulatory T cells. *J Exp Med* 2010; 207: 1871-8.

94. Saadoun D, Rosenzwajg M, Joly F, Six A, Carrat F, Thibault V, *et al*. Regulatory T-cell responses to low-dose interleukin-2 in HCV-induced vasculitis. *N Engl J Med* 2011; 365: 2067-77.

The CliniBook: Clinical gene transfer
Edited by Odile Cohen-Haguenauer – EDK, Paris © 2012, pp. 420-431

B2-2
Predicting immune responses to viral vectors and transgenes in gene therapy and vaccination: the coming of systems biology

BERTRAND BELLIER, ADRIEN SIX, VÉRONIQUE THOMAS-VASLIN, DAVID KLATZMANN*

UPMC Université Paris 06, UMR 7211, F-75013 Paris, France; Centre National de la Recherche Scientifique CNRS, UMR 7211, Bâtiment CERVI, Hôpital Pitié-Salpêtrière, 83 boulevard de l'Hôpital, F-75013 Paris, France; Inserm, U959, F-75013 Paris, France.
<u>*david.klatzmann@upmc.fr*</u>
* Corresponding author

INTRODUCTION

A wide range of viruses are developed simultaneously and sometimes by the same teams as recombinant vectors for gene therapy and for vaccination. Ironically, the induction of an immune response to an expressed transgene represents a potential drawback or even hazard for a gene therapy, while being essential to a vaccine strategy. Thus, understanding the global nature and the specific aspects of the immune responses to viral vectors and to transgene is crucial to optimize both gene therapy and vaccination approaches. In this respect, classical measurements of cellular and humoral immune responses to viral or transgenic antigens in experimental models or in clinical trials can provide valuable information. However, because of the complexity of the immune system that cannot be fully explored with these investigations, novel methods are required to tackle this problem. Systems biology offers a new approach to investigate immune responses on a more global scale. It recently proved efficient to better understand and even predict immune responses to vaccination with attenuated or inactivated viruses in humans. Here, we review and discuss systems vaccinology and its translation to the study of immune responses to viral vectors.

In vaccination, besides attenuated or inactivated pathogens used to induce immunity against homologous pathogens, recombinant viral vectors can deliver heterologous antigens and be used for vaccination against heterologous pathogens. Two types of immune responses are developed, one against the proteins of the viral vectors, and one against the expressed genes that can be the transgene only or a mixture of the transgene and some vector genes. The antigens are expressed directly inside host cells, as during natural infection. Antigens so expressed are made available to the intracellular antigen-processing machinery, allowing processing of the antigen and binding the resulting peptides into major histocompatibility complex (MHC) molecules, allowing their presentation to T-cells and activation of cytotoxic T lymphocytes (CTLs). In gene therapy, similar types of vectors are often used, the antigen being replaced by a transgene coding for a therapeutic protein. The immune response against viral vectors themselves is problematic for both vector purposes, while there is a conflict of interests regarding the immune responses to the transgene that are required for vaccination and feared for gene therapy.

VIRAL VECTORS IMMUNOGENICITY

Recombinant viral vectors have several features that make them excellent immunogens and vehicles for vaccine delivery. First, by nature, viruses have evolved to efficiently infect cells and express their genome. Second, as our immune system has evolved to respond and destroy harmful organisms, viral proteins are often strong immunogens that have intrinsic adjuvant properties [1, 2]. Finally, viruses can infect directly antigen-presenting cells, thereby favouring direct CTL activation. As a whole, these and other features have enabled the development of immunization protocols based on viral vector administration. Various viral vectors have been developed (*Table I*) and reached clinical use [3]. Certain types have been reported to be more efficient than others in inducing immune responses and are mainly used for vaccination purposes.

Table I. Key features of vaccine vectors.

Viral Vector	Type	Insert	Advantages	Issues
Adenovirus	Replicating or non-replicating ds DNA	5-8 kb	No integration High immunogenicity Infects dividing and non-dividing cells and DCs Many strains available	Pre-existing immunity to certain strains
Adeno-associated virus	Non-replicating ss DNA	<5 kb	Non-pathogenic Tropism for DCs	Insert size Possible integration Production uses helper virus
Alphavirus	Non-replicating +ss RNA	<8 kb	No integration No anti-vector immunity Tropic for DCs	Insert size Production
Herpesvirus	Non-replicating ds DNA	<50 kb	Broad tropism including DCs Durable immunity	Pre-existing immunity Low immunogenicity Neurotropism
Measles virus	Replicating -ss RNA	>5 kb	No integration Tropism for DCs Persistent immunity	Pre-existing immunity
Poxviruses	Replicating or non-replicating ds DNA	>10 kb	Licensed veterinary vaccine Various strains available MVA known clinical safety High immunogenicity	Pre-existing immunity
Vesicular stomatitis virus	Replicating -ss RNA	>5 kb	No integration Production No pre-existing immunity	Neurotropism

GENERAL CONSIDERATION ON VACCINE IMMUNOGENICITY AND PROTECTIVE IMMUNITY

Following vaccination, both the innate and the adaptive immune systems synergize to elicit an immune response. Indeed, after vaccine inoculation, antigen-presenting cells – notably dendritic cells (DCs) – uptake antigens and then present processed antigens to naïve T lymphocytes, including CD4$^+$ T cells that provide help to B cells to mount antibody responses, and to naïve CD8$^+$ T cells to trigger their antigen-driven clonal expansion and differentiation into CTLs.

Recently, the importance of the innate immune response has been recognized in determining the orientation of the quality and quantity of the adaptive immune response. Indeed, the discovery of *Pathogen Recognition Receptors* (PRRs) such as *Toll*-like receptor (TLR), expressed at the surface of most immune system cells and triggered in a specific manner upon ligation of various classes of *Pathogen-Associated Molecular Patterns* (PAMPs), places this initial recognition event as a key to the overall immune response. In this context, antigen-presenting cells are activated and efficiently present processed antigens to T lymphocytes and initiate the adaptive immune response. This double-step recognition system must be added to the complexity of the immune system's activation and regulation, and places the innate response and associated inflammatory processes as key actors in the immune response to vaccination [4, 5].

Most vaccines trigger both B and T cell responses, although the nature of the vaccine has a direct influence on the type of immune effectors that are predominantly elicited to mediate protective efficacy (*Table II*). The quality of the vaccine-induced immune response depends especially on the type of vaccine, the route of administration, the quality of antigen presentation, and timing between challenges.

Table II. Parameters of vaccine efficacy.

To be effective a vaccine should be capable of eliciting a number of features:
• Favourable activation of antigen-presenting cells to initiate antigen processing and presentation to T cells
• Broad activation of T and B cells to give a high yield of memory cells
• Generation of memory B cells, production of antibodies, in response to antigen-specific B cell activation that neutralize infectious agents by binding specifically to their surface. In addition, antibodies can target the invading pathogen for destruction by either complement or antibody-dependent cellular cytotoxicity
• Generation of memory CTL to limit the spread of infectious agents by recognizing and killing infected cells or secreting specific antiviral cytokines
• Generation of memory CD4+ T cells which do not prevent but participate to the reduction, control and clearance of pathogens by producing cytokines that support activation and differentiation of B cells and CTL
• Generation of memory T cells to several epitopes, to overcome MHC variations across the population and limit immune response escape of the pathogen
• Limit the recruitment/expansion of Treg, concomitant to the induction of vaccine-specific immune responses
• Long-term immune memory persistence, often related to persistent antigen presentation and chronic infection

We still have an incomplete understanding of all of the immune response's components that form a protective response, even for many licensed vaccines. Prior to the 1990s, most vaccination programs had been developed and evaluated, based on the efficacy of vaccine to induce high titres of antibodies and vaccine programs did not focus on the quality of the T cell response in relation to protection against disease. Noteworthy, most successful vaccines currently in use were developed with little understanding of cellular immune responses or memory responses.

IMMUNOLOGIC RATIONALE FOR SELECTING VECTORS FOR VACCINATION

The immunological rationale for selecting a particular viral vector for vaccination purposes includes how well the heterologous gene is expressed because the quantity of antigen may affect the extent of the immune response. In addition, the type of cells that produce the antigen following transfection by the virus vector, may affect the nature and potency of the immune response. Additionally, the capacity to generate specific type of immune responses, including CTLs, must be taken into account. Another factor influencing the choice of vector is the vector persistence, which might be useful for prolonging immunity. As many of the characteristics leading to the induction of optimal immunity are not completely understood (such as the activation of the innate immune system by various components of vectors and the effect upon the adaptive immunity), it is hard to know exactly what would be the best vector for a given target.

Understanding the immune responses that correlate with control or eradication of the infectious agent in infected individuals gives valuable information as to the type of immune responses aimed for an efficient vaccination. However, the choice of the best vector to induce these responses is often empirical or just based on proprietary know-how and/or IP of the developers.

EVALUATION OF VACCINE EFFICACY

To generate vaccine-mediated protection is a complex challenge when the rules and identity of vaccine-induced immune correlates of protection are uncertain. Vaccine protective efficacy is primarily conferred by the induction of antigen-specific antibodies. However, the peak of vaccine-induced antibody titres (*i.e.* antibody response quantity) does not solely explain antibody-mediated protection. The quality of such antibody responses (*e.g.* their avidity, epitope mapping, glycosylation, diversity...), as well as that of the associated T-cell response, have been identified as determining factors of high-affinity antibody responses and efficient immune memory. Different types of memory T cells (central-memory and effector-memory) have been identified based on their functional and migratory properties and therefore contribute differently to the long-lasting cellular immunity [6].

New methods have emerged to assess a growing number of vaccine-associated immune parameters, raising questions relative to the optimal markers to study and their correlation with vaccine induced protection. Traditionally, the primary vaccine efficacy surrogate markers were the antibody titre to vaccine antigens or the measurement of antibody function such as anti-viral neutralizing activity. More recently, the measurement of T-cell function in conjunction, with or without antibody measurements, has been used to assess vaccine efficacy (*e.g.* measurement of epitope immunoreactivity at the individual cell level using the ELISPOT, simultaneous measurement of intra-cellular cytokine production and cell phenotype using flow cytometry, binding of tetramers to cell surface receptors). New biomarkers evaluate T cell functions (*e.g.* memory, helper, effector), as well as T cell interactions with other cells of the immune system such as dendritic or antigen presenting cells. Notably, as shown by the development of multi-colour flow cytometry (see below), these methods assess vaccine efficacy at the individual immune cell level rather than measuring the total immune response.

Current ways to monitor vaccine immunogenicity provide very limited information and substantial efforts are required to propose comprehensive immunological assessments. Notably, traditional immunomonitoring methods used to depict vaccine immunogenicity are not suitable to predict vaccine efficacy. For example, assays for antibodies are often based on antigen binding, when binding antibodies do not necessarily have functions. Thus, an integrated evaluation of vaccine efficiency should consider various multi-scale and multiparametric variables, including (i) antigenicity of the vaccine preparation, (ii) cellular and humoral immunogenicity, (iii) effective immune protection of the organism and (iv) potential efficiency of the host (age-, disease- or treatment-related immunodeficiency).

Investigations should be done at the various scales of the organism response (protection) to lower levels (*i.e.* cell populations, cell, and gene). The goal is to establish correlates between protection and cellular and molecular responses: mucosal response, local antibody production, timely B-cell and T-cell responses, appropriate effector or regulatory biological pathways. Systems immunology provides new tools to concomitantly assess such responses, to investigate the dynamics and lymphocyte repertoire modifications following an immunization, to better understand the mechanisms of cell activation, and to derive models of efficient vaccine-induced immune responses.

SYSTEMS VACCINOLOGY

Finding novel methods to define the key, early correlates of vaccination would therefore be invaluable but represents a considerable challenge. To this end, the expanding knowledge on molecular mechanisms of immune responses, the availability of high throughput genomic and proteomic technologies and the development of integrative Systems Biology offer new approaches for modelling vaccine-induced immune responses and open the possibility to establish predictive signatures of effective responses. The immune system is a dynamic and responsive fluid tissue, made of a very large set of diverse, circulating, though interconnected cells with loop/circuit types of interactions. A better understanding of immune responses can benefit from global approaches aimed not only at studying the individual components involved, but also at studying and modelling (i) the complex interactions between these components and (ii) most importantly their spatial and temporal aspects [7]. Systems biology develops tools to tackle this type of complexity, based on analyzing large data sets with non-supervised methods and/or through modelling, to extract/generate statistically significant results, irrespective of pre-conceived hypotheses [8, 9]. The systems biology framework should provide novel analyses of immune responses, identifying response-specific signatures and assessing their predictive value. The principle of this approach is to integrate high-throughput data, *e.g.* any omics, and produce a model for the triggered immune response.

In this line, a wealth of complementary immunomonitoring technologies has emerged in order to follow a number of immunological parameters related to measure vaccine-induced immune responses. These include the evaluation of (i) innate immune responses, *e.g.* dendritic cell activation [10], inflammatory response, complement activation, (ii) adaptive antibody responses, *e.g.* antibody and B cell immune responses [11], neutralizing antibodies [12], non-neutralizing antibodies, antibody-dependent cell cytotoxicity (ADCC), (iii) adaptive T-cell immune responses, *e.g.* CTL activity, T-cell specificity using tetramer/peptides, cytokine production [13], (iv) lymphocyte repertoire diversity, *e.g.* Immunoscope/CDR3 spectratyping, TCR/Ig rearrangement quantification, TCR/Ig deep sequencing [14, 15]. Moreover, the rapid progress in flow cytometry implies that an increasing number of parameters can be looked at simultaneously, which is highly relevant for a more comprehensive assessment of lymphocyte characteristics, in particular their multifunctional profile. The challenge is to globally analyse these multiscale multiparametric high-throughput data in order to extract characteristic signatures of immune response and vaccine efficiency, and thus predictors of protection against further infectious challenges.

Historically, progress in vaccine development has come in waves produced by technological revolutions. Current developments translate vaccinology as a combinatorial science, which studies the diversity of pathogens and the complexity of the immune system, through screening and immunoinformatic tools. A future and more radical advance for vaccine development could arise from using a systems biology approach for the immune system, leading to the creation of a virtual or *in silico* immune system capable of complex simulations [16-18].

IMMUNOINFORMATICS MODELLING AND VACCINE DEVELOPMENT

A major goal of immunoinformatics is to develop tools for computational vaccinology and accelerate development of new vaccines. Current approaches applied to vaccinology aim at predicting vaccine immunogenicity allowing its accelerated advancement to clinical development, without the uncertainties of the current vaccine development processes.

Reverse vaccinology

Reverse vaccinology involves the *in silico* screening of a pathogen entire genome to identify genes encoding proteins with the attributes of good vaccine targets that could be included in viral vectors. This reverse approach takes advantage of the increasing availability of whole pathogen genome sequences, either single pathogenic isolate or pan-genomes (the genomic information from several isolates) of a pathogenic species. Indeed, the genome sequence provides an exhaustive catalogue of virtually all protein antigens that the pathogen can express at any time. Reverse vaccinology thus begins with bioinformatics analysis to identify antigens *in silico* that are then tested experimentally. This approach, used originally against meningococcus, allows fast identification of candidate antigen as target for vaccination and provides new solutions for those vaccines which have been difficult or impossible to develop [19, 20]. Several curated databases are now developing this comprehensive information about experimentally-validated antigens, *e.g.* Protegen [21], IEDB [22], AntigenDB [23].

Immunomics

Immunomics or Computational vaccinology makes use of modelling of antigen processing and presentation in order to support the T cell epitope mapping. Web-accessible computational methods have been developed for each different antigen processing steps including proteasome cleavage, transport by the transporter associated with antigen processing, binding of peptides to MHC molecules, and presentation on the cell surface [16, 24-26]. For example, PEPVAC (Promiscuous Epitope-based VACcine) is a tool optimized for the formulation of multi-epitope vaccines with broad population coverage, using HLA binding profile matrices coupled to filter immunoproteasome cleavage using probabilistic modelling [27]. OptiTope offers a step-by-step interface to assist immunologists in designing epitope-based vaccines. It relies on an original algorithm that maximizes the overall immunogenicity of an epitope set [28]. Using such prediction tools, novel T cell epitopes have been discovered across various targets, including pathogen antigens, cancer antigens, autoantigens and allergens.

Immunomics is now leading to vaccine informatics combining immunoinformatics algorithms and resources to predict T- and B-cell immune epitopes to *in silico* protein immunogenicity prediction, systematic transcriptomics and proteomics gene expression analyses, data and literature mining, and Vaccine Ontology formalism in order to offer computer-based strategies for automated vaccine development [29].

Vaccinomics

A new era of genomic vaccinology and computational prediction methods comes out, enabling systematic screening of multiple complete genomes of pathogens, together with analysis of the variability of pathogens and/or HLA complex. Vaccinomics, a branch of omics, encompasses the fields of immunogenetics and immunogenomics applied to understanding the mechanisms of heterogeneity in immune responses to vaccines [30, 31]. It investigates heterogeneity in host genetic markers that results in variations in vaccine-induced immune responses, with the aim of predicting and minimizing vaccine failures or adverse events.

SYSTEMS VACCINOLOGY

While genomics has been successfully used to identify new vaccine antigens, the systems biology framework is also a promising tool for evaluating vaccine-induced immune responses, identifying response-specific signatures and assessing their predictive value.
A first proof of concept was brought by Pulendran and colleagues who applied a systems biology approach to study the immune response induced by the yellow fever vaccine, one of the most successful vaccines ever developed [32]. Their strategy involved immunology, genomics and bioinformatics in order to gain a global picture of the nearly 30,000 genes, proteins and cells participating in immune responses to vaccination. Using this approach, the investigators identified gene expression signatures in blood a few days after the vaccination and could predict, with up to 90% accuracy, the strength of the immune response to the yellow fever vaccine. Sékaly *et al.* made similar observations using functional genomics coupled to polychromatic flow cytometry, showing a strong and coordinated initial response that determines the ensuing efficient polyfunctional and lasting adaptive response [33]. Both studies underline a strong correlation between the early innate immunity-related events and the protective vaccine response. The consistency of these predictive signatures across several trials, for both CD8+ T cell and antibody responses to the yellow fever vaccine, raises the possibility that these rules or their components might have broad applicability for different types of immunogens designed to protect against diverse pathogens. This systems biology-based approach helps identifying early innate response-related molecular signatures predicting immunity and bringing new insights into vaccine response mechanisms [34]. Therefore, systems biology approaches provide a global picture of vaccine-induced immune responses at an early time point after vaccination. These gene expression signatures of early innate immune activation predict the ensuing adaptive immune responses.
Thus, in addition to providing a potential tool for the forward assessment of vaccine efficacy, the findings from this systems approach provide a starting point for the development of new hypotheses aimed at elucidating the parameters that control memory T cell and antibody production. Similar studies are now extending to other available successful vaccines aiming at building a reference immunome database of vaccine-induced responses compared to baseline measurements before vaccination, as advocated by R. Germain [9]. This regards, for example, HIV [35] or adjuvant research [10, 36]. Another area in which systems biology can bring additional insight is in reinvestigating failed vaccine candidates, such as the Merck MRKAd5 HIV vaccine [37].

RATIONAL DEVELOPMENT OF NOVEL GENETIC VACCINES

The complex combinatorial nature of molecular mechanisms that regulate immune system function has, in the past, limited our ability to fully predict immune responses. By bringing together high-throughput experimental methods and information technology, our ability to decipher complex interactions that occur in the immune system has significantly improved. The current developments in computational vaccinology, including systemic models of vaccine responses, aim at establishing such immune correlates and thus at accelerating the development of effective vaccines. Considerable efforts and specific research programme are currently developed with this specific purpose. In this line, a number of research initiatives has been supported, such as VIOLIN (Vaccine Investigation and Online Information Network) integrates in a dedicated database of curated vaccine experimental data, a vaccine target prediction algorithm and a vaccine ontology. In the same line, DyNAVacS is a web-based integrative tool assisting researchers in designing and optimizing their DNA vaccine design [38].

MATHEMATICAL AND COMPUTER MODELLING

Vaccine design and evaluation should also gain from mathematical/*in silico* models for host/pathogen interactions, and from immune response modelling (see for reviews [16, 39]). For example, one can consider ImmSim, a cellular automata-based simulator of immune responses used to compare the behaviour of 64 virtual viruses with various speeds of growth, infectivity level and lethal load. Protection against infection conferred by different vaccine strategies could be tested and showed how different viruses are more susceptible to either antibody or T-cell mediated responses [40]. Recently, this has been improved to test various simulations of classical immunization experiments, investigate the role of MHC haplotype heterozygosity, thus offering a means to *in silico* better understanding the immune responses [41].

More generally, mathematical and computer modellers have developed strategies to represent immune components with the languages of statecharts [42] or to provide visual simulations of their behaviour with multi-agent technologies [43]. The proof of concept that complex mathematical modelling can be automatically generated from graphical communication medium designed by biologists [44] opens new potential for the development of efficient and predictive models in vaccinology.

COMPUVAC AND CLINIGENE CONTRIBUTION TO THE STUDY OF IMMUNE RESPONSE TO VACCINE AND GENE THERAPY VECTORS

In the past years, we have contributed to vaccine development within the scope of CompuVac (http://gevads.cs.put.poznan.pl/preview/; login: viewer; password: password), a European FP6 integrated project devoted to the rational development of a novel platform of genetic vaccines and its application to HCV vaccination [45]. We (i) assembled a platform of viral vectors and virus-like particles, all expressing the same model antigens, (ii) developed standardized protocols for immune response monitoring, and (iii) generated a database and bioinformatics tools to comparatively evaluate the different vectors. The database was then further explored under Clinigene, with the understanding that the early immune responses to vaccine vectors also speaks for the early immune response to gene therapy vectors.

Vaccine vectors were systematically evaluated for T-cell and B-cell immune response induction in parallel with the measurement of early transcriptome changes in spleen dendritic cells harvested 6 hours after vaccine inoculation. Following an analysis scheme using unsupervised and supervised algorithms [46], we have systematically extracted statistically significant molecular signatures across all vaccine vectors analyzed. We then constructed a signature-based "random forest" [47] T-cell response prediction model using a training set (*Figure 1*). This prediction model was then used to analyze an independent data set composed of vectors that are both used for vaccine and gene therapy development. We showed that spleen dendritic cell transcriptome changes as early as 6 hours after vaccine injection are predictive of antigen-specific T-cell responses measured at days 10 or 12 (manuscript in preparation).

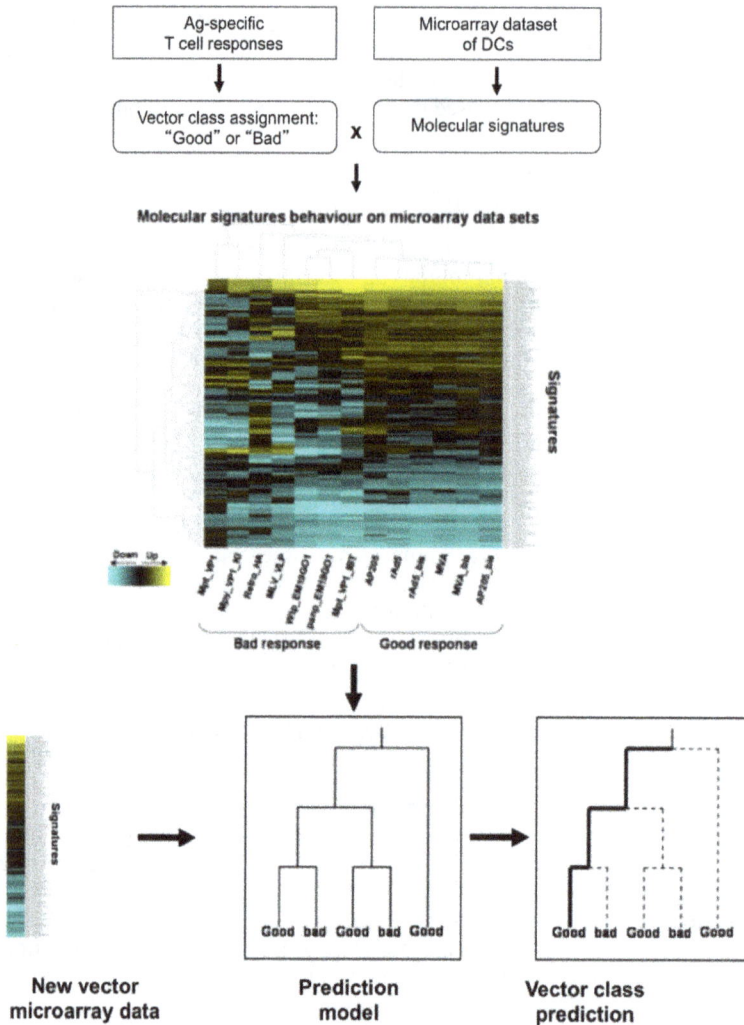

Figure 1. Strategy to predict antigen-specific T-cell responses of new candidate vaccines. Microarray datasets of dendritic cells (DCs), performed 6 hours after immunization, and antigen-specific T-cell responses induced by reference vaccines are used as prior knowledge (training set) to create a prediction model. This model is then applied to predict candidate vector immunogenicity (vector class prediction) based on the specific DCs microarray data.

CONCLUSION

Recent advances in systems biology have now broad implications for vaccinology, and likewise gene therapy. Elucidation of clusters of signatures that correlate with vaccine immunogenicity should facilitate not only the rapid screening of vaccines but also the formulation of new hypotheses on how vaccines mediate long-term protective immune responses. This could finally lead to the development of new tools, as vaccine chip including limited number of gene probe sets that can identify predictive signatures for all the correlates of immunogenicity and protection. The key to success relies on good interactions between multidisciplinary experts of immunology, vaccinology, computer science, bioinformatics, biostatistics... Systems vaccinology thus offers great hope for future translation of basic immunology research advances into successful vaccines. Complementary to the "classical" approach of vaccine development, it should speed up vaccine development and vaccine candidate selection in addition to bringing new hypotheses to the underlying mechanisms in efficient vaccine-induced immune responses. It should be emphasized that any advances in this field, aiming at improving immune responses, can immediately be translated into advances in the opposite direction, the development of less immunogenic gene therapy vectors and methods. It is not unreasonable to predict that an age will come (soon) when vaccine and gene therapy development will use *in silico* prediction of immune responses.

ACKNOWLEDGMENTS

This work has been performed with the support of the EC-DG research through the FP6-Network of Excellence, CLINIGENE: LSHB-CT-2006-018933.

REFERENCES

1. Molinier-Frenkel V, Lengagne R, Gaden F, Hong SS, Choppin J, Gahery-Segard H, *et al.* Adenovirus hexon protein is a potent adjuvant for activation of a cellular immune response. *J Virol* 2002; 76: 127-35.

2. Spohn G, Keller I, Beck M, Grest P, Jennings GT, Bachmann MF. Active immunization with IL-1 displayed on virus-like particles protects from autoimmune arthritis. *Eur J Immunol* 2008; 38: 877-87.

3. Liu MA. Immunologic basis of vaccine vectors. *Immunity* 2010; 33: 504-15.

4. Schenten D, Medzhitov R. The control of adaptive immune responses by the innate immune system. *Adv Immunol* 2011; 109: 87-124.

5. Medzhitov R. Inflammation 2010: new adventures of an old flame. *Cell* 2010; 140: 771-6.

6. Zielinski CE, Corti D, Mele F, Pinto D, Lanzavecchia A, Sallusto F. Dissecting the human immunologic memory for pathogens. *Immunol Rev* 2011; 240: 40-51.

7. Schubert C. Systems immunology: complexity captured. *Nature* 2011; 473: 113-4.

8. Benoist C, Germain RN, Mathis D. A plaidoyer for systems immunology. *Immunol Rev* 2006; 210: 229-34.

9. Germain R. Towards a grand unified theory. Interview by Amy Maxmen. *J Exp Med* 2010; 207: 266-7.

10. Pulendran B. Modulating vaccine responses with dendritic cells and Toll-like receptors. *Immunol Rev* 2004; 199: 227-50.

11. Bondada S, Robertson DA. Assays for B lymphocyte function. *Curr Protoc Immunol* 2003; Chapter 3: Unit 3.8.

12. Ochsenbauer C, Kappes JC. New virologic reagents for neutralizing antibody assays. *Curr Opin HIV AIDS* 2009; 4: 418-25.

13. Seder RA, Darrah PA, Roederer M. T-cell quality in memory and protection: implications for vaccine design. *Nat Rev Immunol* 2008; 8: 247-58.

14. Boudinot P, Marriotti-Ferrandiz ME, Pasquier LD, Benmansour A, Cazenave PA, Six A. New perspectives for large-scale repertoire analysis of immune receptors. *Mol Immunol* 2008; 45: 2437-45.

15. Boyd SD, Marshall EL, Merker JD, Maniar JM, Zhang LN, Sahaf B, *et al.* Measurement and clinical monitoring of human lymphocyte clonality by massively parallel VDJ pyrosequencing. *Sci Transl Med* 2009; 1: 12ra23.

16. Flower DR. Immunoinformatics and the *in silico* prediction of immunogenicity. An introduction. *Methods Mol Biol* 2007; 409: 1-15.

17. Coward J, Germain RN, Altan-Bonnet G. Perspectives for computer modeling in the study of T cell activation. *Cold Spring Harb Perspect Biol* 2010; 2: a005538.

18. Germain RN, Meier-Schellersheim M, Nita-Lazar A, Fraser ID. Systems biology in immunology: a computational modeling perspective. *Annu Rev Immunol* 2011; 29: 527-85.

19. Rappuoli R. Reverse vaccinology, a genome-based approach to vaccine development. *Vaccine* 2001; 19: 2688-91.

20. Sette A, Rappuoli R. Reverse vaccinology: developing vaccines in the era of genomics. *Immunity* 2010; 33: 530-41.

21. Yang B, Sayers S, Xiang Z, He Y. Protegen: a web-based protective antigen database and analysis system. *Nucleic Acids Res* 2011; 39: D1073-8.

22. Zhang Q, Wang P, Kim Y, Haste-Andersen P, Beaver J, Bourne PE, *et al.* Immune epitope database analysis resource (IEDB-AR). *Nucleic Acids Res* 2008; 36: W513-8.

23. Ansari HR, Flower DR, Raghava GP. AntigenDB: an immunoinformatics database of pathogen antigens. *Nucleic Acids Res* 2010; 38: D847-53.

24. Brusic V, Bajic VB, Petrovsky N. Computational methods for prediction of T-cell epitopes: a framework for modelling, testing, and applications. *Methods* 2004; 34: 436-43.

25. De Groot AS. Immunomics: discovering new targets for vaccines and therapeutics. *Drug Discov Today* 2006. 11: 203-9.

26. Flower DR, Macdonald IK, Ramakrishnan K, Davies MN, Doytchinova IA. Computer aided selection of candidate vaccine antigens. *Immunome Res* 2010; 6 (suppl 2): S1.

27. Reche PA, Reinherz EL. PEPVAC: a web server for multi-epitope vaccine development based on the prediction of supertypic MHC ligands. *Nucleic Acids Res* 2005; 33: W138-42.

28. Toussaint NC, Kohlbacher O. OptiTope: a web server for the selection of an optimal set of peptides for epitope-based vaccines. *Nucleic Acids Res* 2009; 37: W617-22.

29. He Y, Rappuoli R, De Groot AS, Chen RT. Emerging vaccine informatics. *J Biomed Biotechnol* 2010; 2010: 218590.

30. Poland GA, Ovsyannikova IG, Jacobson RM. Personalized vaccines: the emerging field of vaccinomics. *Exp Opin Biol Ther* 2008; 8: 1659-67.

31. Poland GA, Oberg AL. Vaccinomics and bioinformatics: accelerants for the next golden age of vaccinology. *Vaccine* 2010; 28: 3509-10.

32. Querec TD, Akondy RS, Lee EK, Cao W, Nakaya HI, Teuwen D, *et al.* Systems biology approach predicts immunogenicity of the yellow fever vaccine in humans. *Nat Immunol* 2009; 10: 116-25.

33. Gaucher D, Therrien R, Kettaf N, Angermann BR, Boucher G, Filali-Mouhim A, *et al*. Yellow fever vaccine induces integrated multilineage and polyfunctional immune responses. *J Exp Med* 2008; 205: 3119-31.

34. Nakaya HI, Wrammert J, Lee EK, Racioppi L, Marie-Kunze S, Haining WN, *et al*. Systems biology of vaccination for seasonal influenza in humans. *Nat Immunol* 2011; 12: 786-95.

35 Fonseca SG, Procopio FA, Goulet JP, Yassine-Diab B, Ancuta P, Sekaly RP. Unique features of memory T cells in HIV elite controllers: a systems biology perspective. *Curr Opin HIV AIDS* 2011; 6: 188-96.

36 Lindqvist M, Nookaew I, Brinkenberg I, Samuelson E, Thorn K, Nielsen J, Harandi AM. Unraveling molecular signatures of immunostimulatory adjuvants in the female genital tract through systems biology. *PLoS One* 2011; 6: e20448.

37 Sekaly RP. The failed HIV Merck vaccine study: a step back or a launching point for future vaccine development? *J Exp Med* 2008; 205: 7-12.

38. Harish N, Gupta R, Agarwal P, Scaria V, Pillai B. DyNAVacS: an integrative tool for optimized DNA vaccine design. *Nucleic Acids Res* 2006; 34: W264-6.

39. Cohn M, Mata J. Quantitative modeling of immune responses. *Immunol Rev* 2007; 216: 5-8.

40. Kohler B, Puzone R, Seiden PE, Celada, F. A systematic approach to vaccine complexity using an automaton model of the cellular and humoral immune system. I. Viral characteristics and polarized responses. *Vaccine* 2000; 19: 862-76.

41. Rapin N, Lund O, Bernaschi M, Castiglione F. Computational immunology meets bioinformatics: the use of prediction tools for molecular binding in the simulation of the immune system. *PLoS One* 2010; 5: e9862.

42. Vainas O, Harel D, Cohen IR, Efron S. Reactive animation: from piecemeal experimentation to reactive biological systems. *Autoimmunity* 2011; 44: 271-81.

43. Chavali AK, Gianchandani EP, Tung KS, Lawrence MB, Peirce SM, Papin JA. Characterizing emergent properties of immunological systems with multi-cellular rule-based computational modeling. *Trends Immunol* 2008; 29: 589-99.

44. McEwan CH, Bersini H, Klatzmann D, Thomas-Vaslin V, Six A. A computational technique to scale mathematical models towards complex heterogeneous systems. In: *Cosmos - Proceedings of the 2011 workshop on complex systems modelling and simulation*. Luniver Press, 2011: 162 p.

45. Garrone P, Fluckiger AC, Mangeot PE, Gauthier E, Dupeyrot-Lacas P, Mancip J, *et al*. A primeboost strategy using virus-like particles pseudotyped for HCV proteins triggers broadly neutralizing antibodies in macaques. *Sci Transl Med* 2011; 3: 94ra71.

46. Pham HP, Dérian N, Chaara W, Bellier B, Klatzmann D, Six A. Identification of biologically relevant molecular signatures from independent component analysis sources. *Int J Bioinformatics Data Mining* 2012 (in press).

47. Liaw A, Wiener M. Classification and regression by randomForest. *R News* 2002; 2: 18-22.

The CliniBook: Clinical gene transfer
Edited by Odile Cohen-Haguenauer – EDK, Paris © 2012, pp. 432-442

B2-3
Biosafety analysis in preclinical and clinical studies

MANFRED SCHMIDT[1]*,**, STEPHANIE LAUFS[1]**, ALESSANDRO AIUTI[2,3],
PATRICK AUBOURG[4], CHRISTOPHER BAUM[5], LUCA BIASCO[2,6], NATHALIE CARTIER[4],
HANSJÖRG HAUSER[7], EUGENIO MONTINI[2], PHILIPPE MOULLIER[8,9,10],
RICHARD O. SNYDER[8,9,11], DAGMAR WIRTH[7], CHRISTOF VON KALLE[1]

[1] *Department of Translational Oncology, National Center for Tumor Diseases (NCT) and German Cancer Research Center (DKFZ), Heidelberg, Germany.*
[2] *San Raffaele Telethon Institute for Gene Therapy, Milano, Italy.*
[3] *University of Rome Tor Vergata, Rome, Italy.*
[4] *Faculty of Pharmaceutical and Biological Sciences, Inserm U745 and University Paris-Descartes, Paris, France.*
[5] *Institute of Experimental Hematology, Hannover Medical School, Hannover, Germany.*
[6] *Università Vita-Salute San Raffaele, Milano, Italy.*
[7] *Helmholtz Center for Infection Research (HZI), Braunschweig, Germany.*
[8] *Department of Molecular Genetics and Microbiology, College of Medicine, University of Florida, Gainesville, FL, USA.*
[9] *Laboratoire de Thérapie Génique, Inserm UMR649, IRT UN, Nantes, France.*
[10] *Généthon, Évry, France.*
[11] *Department of Pediatrics, College of Medicine, University of Florida, FL, USA.*
*Corresponding author
**Authors contributed equally
Contributing authors are listed in alphabetic order
manfred.schmidt@nct-heidelberg.de

CLONALITY AND BIOSAFETY ANALYSIS

The concept of using retroviral vector integration sites as clonal markers for individual cells and their clonal progeny can be traced back to the 1980's. Already in 1985 several groups [1, 2] made use of such a 'clonal tracking' approach and monitored the fate of hematopoietic progenitor and stem cells in a syngenic mouse model. However, this model could not be adopted to xenogenic transplantation models due to low transduction efficiency of human CD34+ cells and the limited number of engrafted cells. In this era, clonality analyses relied on restriction fragment length polymorphisms using Southern-blot analysis most exclusively without sequencing and determination of the exact genomic integration site localization.

Over the last decades, substantial progress has been achieved in optimizing gene transfer parameters and the viral delivery systems, yielding high-level transduction efficiencies, and sustained expression of the transgene and long-term correction of the treated diseases. In line with these improvements, also efficient technologies to identify and sequence integration sites emerged, allowed to dissect the gene-corrected cell pool and gave new insights into the physiology of blood regeneration. Thereof, linear amplification-mediated (LAM) PCR shows the most convincing approach for highly sensitive comprehensive integration site analyses to assess gene therapy agents and gene modified cells. Meanwhile, integrating oncoretroviral and lentiviral vectors are successfully used in several clinical gene therapy studies. However, with increasing efficiency it became obvious that vector integration into the genome may also cause severe adverse effects: in several patients suffering from X-linked Severe Combined Immunodeficiency (X-SCID) or X-linked Chronic Granulomatous Disease (X-CGD) the treatment caused insertional activation of protooncogenes and uncontrolled clonal malignant proliferation, respectively. With the decoding of the human and other mammalian genomes together with large scale integration site assays, the original clonality studies to uncover tissue regeneration and to identify individual clonal contributions became highly important for vector biosafety assessment.

LAM-PCR meets all the requirements necessary for *in vivo* monitoring of viral vector integration sites and associated biosafety studies. It has been developed to identify the insertion site profile of different viral vector systems (oncoretro-, foamy-, lentiviral and AAV vector integration) [3] down to the single cell level [4]. The reliability and robustness of this method result from the initial preamplification of the vector-genome junctions preceding non target DNA removal *via* magnetic selection. Subsequent steps are carried out on a semisolid streptavidin phase, including synthesis of complementary double strands, restriction digest, ligation of a linker cassette to the genomic end of the DNA fragment and exponential PCR(s) with vector- and linker cassette-specific primers. LAM-PCR can be adjusted to all unknown DNA sequences adjacent to a known DNA sequence (*Figure 1*).

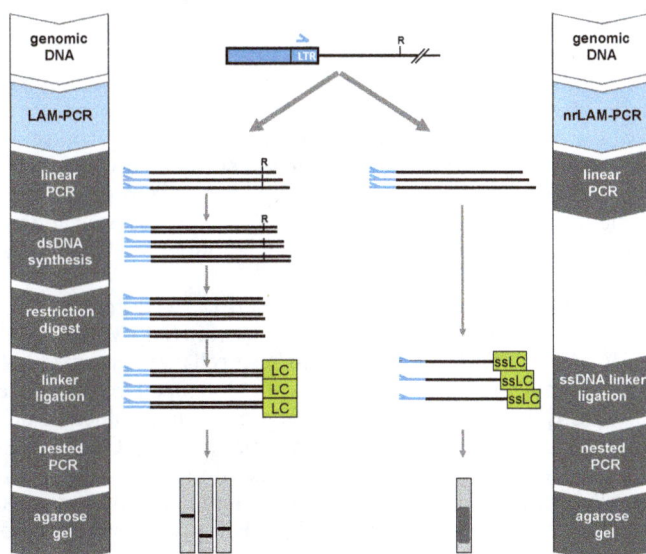

Figure 1. LAM-PCR *versus* nrLAM. Schematic comparison between standard and non-restrictive LAM-PCR (R: restriction enzyme; LC: linker cassette; ssLC: single stranded linker cassette; ssDNA: single stranded DNA).

However, integration site analyses such as LAM-PCR require a restriction digest generating unevenly small fragments of the host genome. We could show that each restriction motif allows the identification of only a fraction of all genomic integrants, hampering the understanding and prediction of biological consequences after vector insertion. To overcome these site-recovery biases introduced by the use of restriction enzymes, a model has been developed to define genomic access of the viral integration site that provides optimal restriction motif combinations and minimizes the percentage of non accessible insertion loci. A new nonrestrictive LAM-PCR (nrLAM-PCR) approach, though less sensitive compared to LAM-PCR, that has superior capabilities for comprehensive unbiased integration site retrieval in preclinical and clinical samples independent of restriction motifs and amplification inefficiency was established [5, 6]. This innovative technique has now been adapted for all common high-frequent integrating (retro, lenti, foamy) and low frequent integrating (AAV, integrase-deficient retro- and lentiviral vectors) viral vectors and cell types/tissues (*e.g.* blood, liver, muscle, eyecup, brain). The technique has proven its usefulness in *in vitro* studies and preclinical studies and clinical trials.

Our understanding of high and low frequent integrating viruses and their influence on the biology of the affected cells and potential clinical outcomes may benefit enormously of novel high throughput next generation sequencing technologies. Large scale integration site profiling to monitor the cell fate of the gene corrected cell population and to assess vector biosafety will decisively help to translate gene therapeutic approaches to the clinics. Thus, to allow for large-scale screening of integrated proviruses, a high-throughput analysis pipeline involving next-generation sequencing and data mining was developed. Massive parallel sequencing technologies (454/Roche; Solexa/Illumina) have already proven their potential for whole genome transcriptome and methylome sequencing analyses. With comparable resolution, small DNA fragments such as PCR products can be analyzed, too. With a combinatorial approach of LAM-PCR/nrLAM-PCR and next generation sequencing, time- and cost-efficiency of integration site sequence retrieval has been improved by several logs compared to standard Sanger sequencing technologies.

For further high-throughput analysis the development of automated bioinformatic data analysis tools was essential. Thus, optimized software applications were developed: *IntegrationSeq* and *IntegrationMap* [7], and others (manuscript in revision) allow large scale and standardized analysis of insertion sites of viral vectors. Furthermore, the gaining need of the scientific community for public insertion site profiling tools by implementing an advanced tool termed *QuickMap* [8] was addressed. The *QuickMap* application was made available on a public web platform at http://www.gtsg.org.

Furthermore, a database, which to date contains more than 77,334 different vector insertion sites derived from previous analyses on different vectors (ASLV, FIV, MMTV, HTLV, HIV, EIAV, FV, MLV, and SIV) and different host cells was designed. All insertion sites stored in this database were subjected to the developed analysis pipeline and characterized insertions with regard to localization on chromosomes, in or next to genes, cancer genes, fragile sites, transcription factor binding sites, CpG islands, or repetitive elements (SINE, LINE, LTR). A random insertion site set consisting of 1,000,000 sequences reliably reflects random distribution and currently serves as our reference for all analyses of experimental data. We identified specific insertion profiles of the different retroviruses that resemble genomic finger prints, which allow to distinguish between different retroviruses (*Figure 2*).

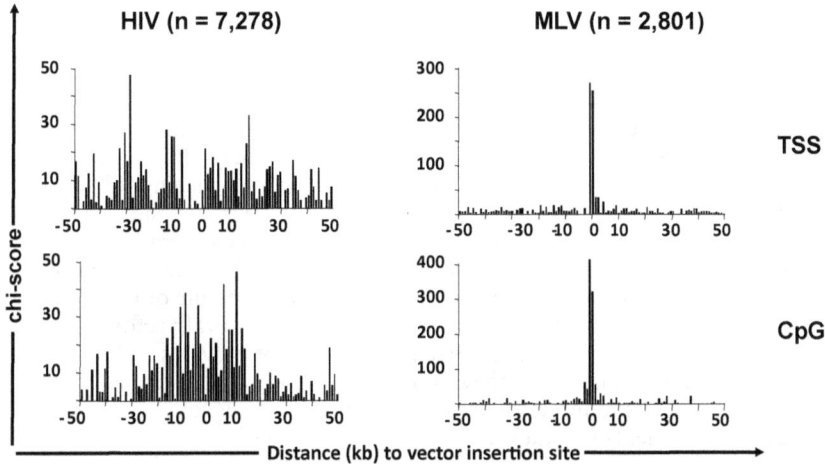

Figure 2. Genomic profiles in the vicinity of vector insertion sites of HIV and MLV. Within a ± 50 kb distance to a vector insertion site, the genomic features transcription start sites (TSS) and CpG islands (CpG) were detected and compared to data obtained from a representative random set (containing 10^6 random insertion sites). The resulting chi-square deviations are shown as vertical bars.

Following successful establishment of a retroviral insertion site database, we performed a first meta-analysis of all HIV insertion sites stored therein (n~46.000). This initial analyses resulted in the identification of 'insertional gaps' in the human genome, which resemble non favored and/or sterically inaccessible regions located ± 1 kb around the transcription start site of transcriptionally active genes, where we found significant underrepresentation of insertion.

BIOSAFETY ANALYSIS IN PRECLINICAL STUDIES

Exploitation of chromosomal integration sites for stable viral vector production

Currently, a number of distinct retroviral packaging cell lines which have been developed on the basis of either murine or human cell lines are in use. Based on stable integration of the retroviral vector into the host genome they are exploited for the production of infectious particles [9-12]. Beside the vector design, the copy number and the position effects of the vectors mediated by its chromosomal integration have a great influence on the titer of a retroviral vector. Genetic modification of these cells relies on unpredictable integration site distribution of the viral vector, making it impossible to investigate the properties of retroviral vectors independent of the variable influences of the integration site locus. Accordingly, screening of appropriate integration sites that support optimal vector expression is still the state-of-the-art for establishment of producer cell lines - a time-consuming and tedious procedure [13]. Rational design of vectors that takes advantage of beneficial effects of a given integration site on virus production became recently possible, thereby allowing to exploit the positive impact of a given integration site [13, 14].
While a number of stable retroviral producer cells have been developed so far, the establishment of lentiviral producer cells does not seem to be straight forward. The elu-

cidation of the nature of integration sites capable of supporting lentiviral vector production would accelerate the progress to develop a system for stable lentiviral vector production. The performance of several lentiviral vectors was systematically evaluated using a technology that relies on the use of packaging cell lines with predefined integration sites. For this purpose a set of independent cell clones was established with single copy integration of a lentiviral vector. Further, lentiviral vectors were integrated into two previously tagged high expressing sites of 293 cells, namely 1B2 and 293-3. Integration site analysis was performed based on next generation sequencing [13]. The results show that the promoter, viral vector orientation, and integration site are the main determinants of the titer. Furthermore, the viral production systems were exploited to evaluate read-through activity. Read-through is thought to be caused by inefficient termination of vector transcription and is inherent to the nature of retroviral vectors. The frequency of transduction of sequences flanking the viral vectors from both integration sites was assessed. The approach presented here provides a platform for systematic design and evaluation of the efficiency and safety of integrating viral vectors optimized for a given producer cell line [13]. For further details see also chapter: "Restrictions and requirements for stable lentiviral producer cells".

Analyzing recombinant AAV integration frequency in different tissues and preclinical settings by deep sequencing

Recombinant adeno-associated virus (rAAV) vectors are low-frequency integrating vectors. We have shown that in nonhuman primates (NHP), rAAV vectors integrate inefficiently into the chromosomes of myocytes and reside predominantly as episomal monomeric and concatemeric circles. Interestingly, the episomally persistent rAAV genomes assimilate into chromatin with a typical nucleosomal pattern seen for cellular chromosomes. Such a *bona fide* chromatin structure may be important for episomal maintenance and sustained transgene expression over years. These findings were obtained from primate muscles transduced with rAAV1 and rAAV8 vectors for up to 22 months after intramuscular delivery of 5×10^{12} viral genomes/kg [15].

In the context of the predominance of episomal forms, LAM-PCR has been successfully combined with next generation sequencing platforms and semi-automated bioinformatic data mining to detect rAAV proviruses and characterize complex rAAV concatemeric structures *in vivo*. Cos (an African green monkey cell line) derived single cell clones harboring a defined number of rAAV integration sites were generated and characterized. These clones serve as rAAV insertional standards (rAIS) and show varying levels of inverted terminal repeat (ITR) rearrangements as well as full ITRs, and allow assessing the relative insertion frequency of rAAV *in vivo*. Limiting dilutions of the rAIS have allowed the lower limit of sensitivity to be determined for the method. It is feasible to detect rAIS-specific integration sites and determine the efficiency for retrieving ITR with different length and varying complexity of secondary structures. Assessing the retrieval frequency of the rAIS spiked into *in vivo* muscle and liver samples having an excess of episomal rAAV genomes showed a linear relationship between the relative sequence counts and decreasing copy numbers of the rAIS. The introduction of rAIS has enabled us to semi-quantitatively measure the retrieval frequency of individual insertion sites and episomes in rAAV transduced tissues, providing a calculation of the integration frequency of rAAV in skeletal muscle and liver of large animal models. We show that integration of rAAV with therapeutically relevant vector occurs at very low frequency (between 10^{-4}-10^{-5}) both in liver and muscle of NHP but with no preference for specific genomic loci (manuscript in submission). These insights obtained from large animal models prospectively give a reliable genotoxic risk assessment of rAAV for clinical trials based on integration frequency and long-term persistence *in vivo*.

In vitro modeling of the genotoxic potential of retroviral vectors

With the background of insertional genotoxicity and in order to develop safe and predictable gene therapy guidelines for clinical trials a new assay based on *in vitro* expansion of primary murine hematopoietic cells and selection in limiting dilution was designed and validated. The authors showed that SIN (self inactivating) vectors using a strong internal retroviral enhancer/promoter may transform cells by insertional mutagenesis. Most transformed clones, including those obtained after dose escalation of SIN vectors, showed insertions upstream of the third exon of Evi1 and in reverse orientation to its transcriptional orientation. Normalizing for the vector copy number, we found the transforming capacity of SIN vectors to be significantly reduced when compared with corresponding LTR vectors [16]. Further studies investigated the insertion patters of a series of self-inactivating (SIN) vectors using a sensitive cell culture assay. It turned out that the lentiviral insertion pattern was approximately threefold less likely than the gammaretroviral to trigger transformation of primary hematopoietic cells. However, lentivirally induced mutants also showed robust replating, in line with the selection for common insertion sites (CIS) in the first intron of the Evi1 proto-oncogene. This potent proto-oncogene thus represents a CIS for both gammaretroviral vectors and lentiviral vectors, despite major differences in their integration mechanisms. Altering the vectors' enhancer-promoter elements had a greater effect on safety than the retroviral insertion pattern. Mechanistic studies support the conclusion that enhancer-mediated gene activation is the major cause for insertional transformation of hematopoietic cells, opening rational strategies for risk prevention [17].

In vivo modelling of the genotoxic potential of retroviral vectors

Lentiviruses such as HIV type 1 (HIV-1) and their derived vectors show a stronger preference for integrating within active transcription units without an obvious bias for proliferation-associated genes or transcriptional start sites. This might indicate that the potential for triggering oncogenic adverse events by insertional mutagenesis is quite low [18, 19]. It was of great scientific interest to investigate the oncogenic potential of prototypical murine leukemia virus (MLV)-derived, γ-retroviral and lentiviral vectors. As a model system an *in vivo* genotoxicity assay based on transduction and transplantation of a tumor-prone knockout mouse model with murine hematopoietic stem/progenitor cells was used. In this model the animals lack the tumor suppressor gene cyclin dependent kinase inhibitor 2A (Cdkn2a) [20]. The Cdkn2a locus has a central role in regulating senescence and preventing cell transformation caused by aberrant oncogene expression. Because Cdkn2a inactivation synergizes with several types of cancer-promoting lesions, *Cdkn2a⁻/⁻* mice have been valuable in insertional mutagenesis studies for identifying cancer genes, many of which are highly relevant in human oncogenesis. The relevance of the CDKN2A pathway in human tumor suppression is well documented because of its frequent inactivation in almost all types of human cancer [21, 22]. Moreover, two X-linked SCID (X-SCID) patients affected by γ-retrovirus induced leukemia from 2 independent clinical trials had lost expression of the CDKN2A locus as a secondary mutation [23, 24]. These findings indicate that CDKN2A plays a role also in the pathophysiology of human leukemias triggered by γ-retroviral insertions in clinical trials and further validate the choice of this model to assess vector genotoxicity. It turned out that γ-retroviral treatment triggered a dose-dependent acceleration of tumor onset in transplanted mice, whereas lentiviral did not. The lentiviral vectors differed from the γ-retroviral in the molecular design [25, 26] and the integration site selection [18, 19, 27, 28]. However, the relative contribution of these features to the lower genotoxicity of lentiviral vectors remained unknown. In another study using the same animal model the authors demonstrated that lentiviral vectors can act as insertional mutagens provided that the vectors are designed to contain strong enhancer-promoter sequences in their long terminal repeats (LTRs). Furthermore, it has been shown that the genotoxic risk of lentiviral vectors is significantly lower than that of currently used γ-retroviral vectors. Improvements in vector design, such as self-inactivating (SIN) LTRs, greatly reduce the genotoxic risk in both lentiviral and γ-retroviral vectors. These data strongly support the adoption of vectors with SIN LTRs for clinical trials of gene therapy.

BIOSAFETY ANALYSIS IN CLINICAL STUDIES

Optimisation and validation of pyrosequencing for retroviral vector integration site analyses in clinical studies

The analysis of genomic distribution of retroviral vectors is a powerful tool to monitor possible "vector-on-host" effects in gene therapy clinical trials but could also provide crucial information about "host-on-vector" influences based on target cell genetic and epigenetic state. On this issue we had the unique occasion to compare the insertional profile of the identical MLV-vector in the context of the same ADA-SCID genetic background but in two different gene therapy (GT) trials based on repeated infusions of transduced mature lymphocytes (PBL) or a single infusion of hematopoietic stem/progenitor cells (HSC). Through our collaboration between Alessandro Aiuti's group at HSR-Milan and the group of Manfred Schmidt and Christof von Kalle at NCT/DKFZ-Germany with support form the CliniGene-NoE in the context of a flexibility project, we were able to collect, both at the time of transduction and years after infusion, a total of 2198 unique insertions from 4 patients that received PBL-GT and 1959 retroviral insertion sites from 4 patients that underwent HSC-GT. In both trials the MLV-vector showed the classical preferences for gene-rich regions and TSSs. However, by the analysis of the functions of hit genes, insertions from PBL-GT significantly favoured genes involved in immune system, T cell functions and T-cell specific signalling pathways (TCR, IL-2, IL-15) differently from HSC-GT and random insertions. We also analysed the expression profile of T cells and CD34+ cells at the time of transduction showing that genes differentially expressed in the two target cells were differentially hit by insertions in the two groups of patients *in vitro* and *ex vivo*. We speculated that chromatin accessibility of target cells could have driven the insertions towards cell-specific regions. Thus, we cross-compared our integration datasets with hypersensitive sites (HSS) mapped on T cells and several histone modifications mapped both on T cells and HSC/HPC through ChIP-seq technique. We found that insertions in PBL-GT were on average two times closer to an T-cell HSS than retroviral integrations from HSC-GT. In addition the vector preferentially landed close to histone modifications associated with open chromatin like H3K4me3 both *in vitro* and *ex vivo*. Strikingly, we discovered that only H3K27me3 was cell-specifically disfavoured, thus representing a key epigenetic determinant of cell-type dependent insertion distribution. Our study showed that MLV-vector insertions are cell-specific, linked to genetic-chromatin state of target cells *in vitro* and their proximity to specific epigenetic features *in vivo* may also physiologically influence the survival of vector positive cells in absence of adverse events [29].

Additionally, we have optimized and applied high throughput integration site analyses followed by 454 pyrosequencing and bioinformatical datamining to analyze in depth the clonal inventory that is present long-term in patients undergoing ADA-SCID gene therapy. Indeed, upon retroviral mediated gene correction of HSC each transduced progenitor is univocally marked by an integration site and can be tracked by retroviral tagging. We previously showed that ADA-SCID-GT with CD34+ cells resulted in multilineage engraftment, in the absence of aberrant expansions [30, 31]. We performed a comprehensive longitudinal insertion profile of distinct bone marrow (BM) and peripheral blood (PB) cell types in 4 patients 3-6 years after GT, retrieving to date 2350 unique insertion sites by LAM-PCR and high-throughput sequencing. We could uncover in each lineage the frequency of identical integrants among different haematopoietic compartments. BM cells and PB granulocytes displayed the highest proportion of shared integrants (up to 58.1%), reflecting the real-time repopulating activity of gene-corrected progenitors. Strikingly, we detected "core integrants", shared between CD34+ cells and both lymphoid and myeloid lineages at multiple time points, stably tagging long-term multipotent progenitors overtime. Tracking two of these integrants (proximal to the MLLT3 and LRRC30 genes) by specific PCR we confirmed the multilineage contribution to haematopoiesis of these clones, showing fluctuating lineage outputs over a period of 5 years. We also retrieved 170 integrations in T cell subtypes from patients who received infusions of transduced lymphocytes, showing evidence that naive T cell clones may survive for up to 10 years after infusion. We are currently designing mathematical models whose application to our insertion datasets will potentially uncover new information on the fate and activity of haematopoietic progenitors and their differentiated progeny years after transplantation in GT patients. In conclusion, through retroviral tagging, we can now track single transduced HSC activity directly in humans. This study could provide information of reference for ongoing and future GT approaches for hematological diseases.

Vector clonality and biosafety studies in clinical gene therapy for the treatment of X-linked cerebral adrenoleukodystrophy

X-linked adrenoleukodystrophy (ALD) is a severe brain demyelinating disease in boys that is caused by a deficiency in ALD protein, an adenosine triphosphate-binding cassette transporter encoded by the *ABCD1* gene. ALD progression can be halted by allogeneic hematopoietic cell transplantation (HCT) [32]. A gene therapy trial in three ALD patients was initiated. After removing autologous CD34+ cells from the patients and transduction with a lentiviral vector expressing wild-type ABCD1, the cells were re-infused into the patients after they had received myeloablative treatment. In the follow-up (span of 24 to 30 months) polyclonal reconstitution was detected. The results strongly suggest that hematopoietic stem cells were transduced in the patients. Beginning 14 to 16 months after infusion of the genetically corrected cells, progressive cerebral demyelination in the two patients stopped a clinical outcome comparable to that achieved by allogeneic HCT. These results show that lentiviral vectors are suitable for transferring therapeutic genes to hematopoietic stem cells, and provide the first example of successful gene therapy for a severe neurodegenerative disease. However, several common insertion sites (CIS) were found in the patients' cells, suggesting that LV integrations conferred a selective advantage. High-throughput LV integration site analysis on human hematopoietic stem progenitor cells engrafted in immunodeficient mice was performed and the same CISs reported in patients with ALD were found. Conversely, cancer-triggering integrations at CISs found in tumor cells from γ-retroviral vector-based clinical trials and oncogene-tagging screenings in mice always target a single gene and are contained in narrow genomic intervals. These findings imply that LV CISs are produced by an integration bias toward specific genomic regions rather than by oncogenic selection [33].

ACKNOWLEDGMENTS

This work has been performed with the support of the EC-DG research through the FP6-Network of Excellence, CLINIGENE: LSHB-CT-2006-018933.

REFERENCES

1. Dick JE, Magli MC, Huszar D, Phillips RA, Bernstein A. Introduction of a selectable gene into primitive stem cells capable of long-term reconstitution of the hemopoietic system of W/Wv mice. *Cell* 1985; 42: 71-9.

2. Jordan CT, *Lemischka* IR. Clonal and systemic analysis of long-term hematopoiesis in the mouse. *Genes Dev* 1990; 4: 220-32.

3. Schmidt M, Schwarzwaelder K, Bartholomae C, Zaoui K, Ball C, Pilz I, *et al*. High-resolution insertion-site analysis by linear amplification-mediated PCR (LAM-PCR). *Nat Methods* 2007; 4: 1051-7.

4. Schmidt M, Zickler P, Hoffmann G, Haas S, Wissler M, Muessig A, *et al*. Polyclonal long-term repopulating stem cell clones in a primate model. *Blood* 2002; 100: 2737-43.

5. Gabriel R, Eckenberg R, Paruzynski A, Bartholomae CC, Nowrouzi A, Arens A, *et al*. Comprehensive genomic access to vector integration in clinical gene therapy. *Nat Med* 2009; 15: 1431-6.

6. Paruzynski A, Arens A, Gabriel R, Bartholomae CC, Scholz S, Wang W, *et al*. Genome-wide high-throughput integrome analyses by nrLAM-PCR and next-generation sequencing. *Nat Protoc* 2010; 5: 1379-95.

7. Giordano FA, Hotz-Wagenblatt A, Lauterborn D, Appelt JU, Fellenberg K, Nagy KZ, *et al*. New bioinformatic strategies to rapidly characterize retroviral integration sites of gene therapy vectors. *Methods Inf Med* 2007; 46: 542-7.

8. Appelt JU, Giordano FA, Ecker M, Roeder I, Grund N, Hotz-Wagenblatt A, *et al*. QuickMap: a public tool for large-scale gene therapy vector insertion site mapping and analysis. *Gene Ther* 2009; 16: 885-93.

9. Danos O, Mulligan RC. Safe and efficient generation of recombinant retroviruses with amphotropic and ecotropic host ranges. *Proc Natl Acad Sci USA* 1988; 85: 6460-4.

10. Markowitz D, Goff S, Bank A. A safe packaging line for gene transfer: separating viral genes on two different plasmids. *J Virol* 1988; 62: 1120-4.

11. Miller AD, Chen F. Retrovirus packaging cells based on 10A1 murine leukemia virus for production of vectors that use multiple receptors for cell entry. *J Virol* 1996; 70: 5564-71.

12. Ory DS, Neugeboren BA, Mulligan RC. A stable human-derived packaging cell line for production of high titer retrovirus/vesicular stomatitis virus G pseudotypes. *Proc Natl Acad Sci USA* 1996; 93: 11400-6.

13. Gama-Norton L, Herrmann S, Schucht R, Coroadinha AS, Low R, Alves PM, *et al*. Retroviral vector performance in defined chromosomal Loci of modular packaging cell lines. *Hum Gene Ther* 2010; 21: 979-91.

14. Schucht R, Coroadinha AS, Zanta-Boussif MA, Verhoeyen E, Carrondo MJ, Hauser H, Wirth D. A new generation of retroviral producer cells: predictable and stable virus production by Flp-mediated site-specific integration of retroviral vectors. *Mol Ther* 2006; 14: 285-92.

15. Penaud-Budloo M, Le Guiner C, Nowrouzi A, Toromanoff A, Cherel Y, Chenuaud P, *et al.* Adeno-associated virus vector genomes persist as episomal chromatin in primate muscle. *J Virol* 2008; 82: 7875-85.

16. Modlich U, Bohne J, Schmidt M, von Kalle C, Knoss S, Schambach A, Baum C. Cell-culture assays reveal the importance of retroviral vector design for insertional genotoxicity. *Blood* 2006 108: 2545-53.

17. Modlich U, Navarro S, Zychlinski D, Maetzig T, Knoess S, Brugman MH, *et al.* Insertional transformation of hematopoietic cells by self-inactivating lentiviral and gammaretroviral vectors. *Mol Ther* 2009; 17: 1919-28.

18. Schroder AR, Shinn P, Chen H, Berry C, Ecker JR, Bushman F. HIV-1 integration in the human genome favors active genes and local hotspots. *Cell* 2002; 110: 521-9.

19. Wu X, Li Y, Crise B, Burgess SM. Transcription start regions in the human genome are favored targets for MLV integration. *Science* 2003; 300: 1749-51.

20. Montini E, Cesana D, Schmidt M, Sanvito F, Ponzoni M, Bartholomae C, *et al.* Hematopoietic stem cell gene transfer in a tumor-prone mouse model uncovers low genotoxicity of lentiviral vector integration. *Nat Biotechnol* 2006; 24: 687-96.

21. Sherr CJ. The INK4a/ARF network in tumour suppression. *Nat Rev Mol Cell Biol* 2001; 2: 731-7.

22. Sherr CJ. Principles of tumor suppression. *Cell* 2004; 116: 235-46.

23. Hacein-Bey-Abina S, Garrigue A, Wang GP, Soulier J, Lim A, Morillon E, *et al.* Insertional oncogenesis in 4 patients after retrovirus-mediated gene therapy of SCID-X1. *J Clin Invest* 2008; 118: 3132-42.

24. Howe SJ, Mansour MR, Schwarzwaelder K, Bartholomae C, Hubank M, Kempski H, *et al.* Insertional mutagenesis combined with acquired somatic mutations causes leukemogenesis following gene therapy of SCID-X1 patients. *J Clin Invest* 2008; 118: 3143-50.

25. Follenzi A, Ailles LE, Bakovic S, Geuna M, Naldini L. Gene transfer by lentiviral vectors is limited by nuclear translocation and rescued by HIV-1 pol sequences. *Nat Genet* 2000; 25: 217-22.

26. Roberts MR, Cooke KS, Tran AC, Smith KA, Lin WY, Wang M, *et al.* Antigen-specific cytolysis by neutrophils and NK cells expressing chimeric immune receptors bearing zeta or gammasignaling domains. *J Immunol* 1998; 161: 375-84.

27. Hematti P, Hong BK, Ferguson C, Adler R, Hanawa H, Sellers S, *et al.* Distinct genomic integration of MLV and SIV vectors in primate hematopoietic stem and progenitor cells. *PLoS Biol* 2004; 2: e423.

28. Lewinski MK, Yamashita M, Emerman M, Ciuffi A, Marshall H, Crawford G, *et al.* Retroviral DNA integration: viral and cellular determinants of target-site selection. *PLoS Pathog* 2006; 2: e60.

29. Biasco L, Ambrosi A, Pellin D, Bartholomae C, Brigida I, Roncarolo MG, *et al.* Integration profile of retroviral vector in gene therapy treated patients is cell-specific according to gene expression and chromatin conformation of target cell. *EMBO Mol Med* 2011; 3: 89-101.

30. Aiuti A, Cassani B, Andolfi G, Mirolo M, Biasco L, Recchia A, *et al.* Multilineage hematopoietic reconstitution without clonal selection in ADA-SCID patients treated with stem cell gene therapy. *J Clin Invest* 2007; 117: 2233-40.

31. Aiuti A, Cattaneo F, Galimberti S, Benninghoff U, Cassani B, Callegaro, L, *et al.* Gene therapy for immunodeficiency due to adenosine deaminase deficiency. *N Engl J Med* 2009; 360: 447-58.

32. Cartier N, Hacein-Bey-Abina S, Bartholomae CC, Veres G, Schmidt M, Kutschera I, *et al.* Hematopoietic stem cell gene therapy with a lentiviral vector in X-linked adrenoleukodystrophy. *Science* 2009; 326: 818-23.

33. Biffi A, Bartolomae CC, Cesana D, Cartier N, Aubourg P, Ranzani M, *et al.* Lentiviral vector common integration sites in preclinical models and a clinical trial reflect a benign integration bias and not oncogenic selection. *Blood* 2011; 117: 5332-9.

PART II

Clinical trials and regulatory issues

COORDINATED BY
ODILE COHEN-HAGUENAUER,
NANCY M.P. KING
AND
BERND GÄNSBACHER

Clinical trials

Coordinated by
Odile Cohen-Haguenauer,
and
Bernd Gänsbacher

The CliniBook: Clinical gene transfer
Edited by Odile Cohen-Haguenauer – EDK, Paris © 2012, pp. 447-451

C1-1
A clinical trial of AAV-mediated gene therapy for Leber congenital amaurosis 2

Alexander J. Smith, Robin R. Ali*

UCL Institute of Ophthalmology, Department of Genetics, 11-43 Bath Street, London
EC1V 9EL, United Kingdom.
r.ali@ucl.ac.uk
* Corresponding author

Inherited retinal degeneration as a target for gene therapy

Inherited retinal degenerations (IRD) form a large group of genetically and pheno-typically heterogeneous diseases that are characterised by a, usually progressive, loss of photoreceptor cells and concomitant loss of vision. Approximately 1 in 3000 people in Europe and the United States is affected by IRDs. To date about 150 genes and a further 50 loci have been identified, mutations in which can lead to retinal dystrophy (see http://www.sph.uth.tmc.edu/Retnet/). The majority of these disorders are inherited in a recessive or X-linked fashion, and these loss-of-function mutations are potential targets for gene supplementation therapy [1].

While most forms of retinal dystrophy are caused by defects in the photoreceptor cells, the form of RP that was the first to be treated with gene therapy, Leber congenital amaurosis type 4 (LCA4) caused by mutations in the *RPE65* gene, is a primary RPE defect [2, 3]. A decade of gene therapy studies in animals has shown that some forms of retinal dystrophy are more amenable to treatment than others and it appears that, in general, RPE defects are easier to treat than photoreceptor defects. This is because the RPE forms a single layer of cells that are efficiently transduced by viral vectors, whereas there are many more photoreceptors arranged in multiple layers, making gene transfer to these cells less efficient. Furthermore, as the RPE cells support the neural cells of the retina, partial correction of RPE function might have significant impact on photoreceptor function and survival.

Preclinical studies of AAV gene therapy for RPE65 deficiency

A landmark study for retinal gene therapy was provided by the successful treatment of a dog model of LCA caused by mutations in the *RPE65* gene [4, 5], findings that were later confirmed in mouse studies [6, 7]. The retinal isomerohydrolase RPE65 is involved in the conversion of all-*trans*-retinoids to 11-*cis*-retinoids, regenerating the

visual pigment after exposure to light. In its absence, the visual cycle is interrupted resulting in a lack of visual pigment [8]. In the RPE65-deficient dog, rod photoreceptor
function is virtually absent even though the cells are initially healthy. Subretinal injection of an AAV2 or AAV4 vector expressing *RPE65* results in restoration of rod photoreceptor function, assessed by electroretinography, and consequently improved visual
mobility in dim light [4, 9]. The virtual absence of cell division in the mammalian eye
has meant that, despite the fact that recombinant AAV does not integrate efficiently
into the host genome, the treatment effect has persisted for at least five years in the
treated dogs [10].

AAV-MEDIATED GENE THERAPY FOR LEBER CONGENITAL AMAUROSIS 2 IN THE CLINIC

LCA2, caused by RPE65 deficiency, is characterised by impaired vision from birth
and a progressive degeneration that leads to complete blindness in early adulthood.
Despite the severity of the retinal dystrophy caused by defects in RPE65, it was the
first form of retinal dystrophy to be chosen for clinical trials, not only because of im-
pressive results following pre-clinical studies in both small and large animal models,
but also because its characteristics allow rapid assessment of efficacy. Gene replacement therapy for this disorder would be expected to improve vision due to restoration
of absent photoreceptor function whilst for many disorders, particularly adult-onset
conditions, the aim would be preservation of vision by preventing photoreceptor loss.
Furthermore, the relatively slow rate of photoreceptor cell loss in the Briard dog reflects the fact that the photoreceptor cells in RPE-derived retinal dystrophies are in-
herently healthy, suggesting that a good recovery of the photoreceptor cell function
should be feasible.

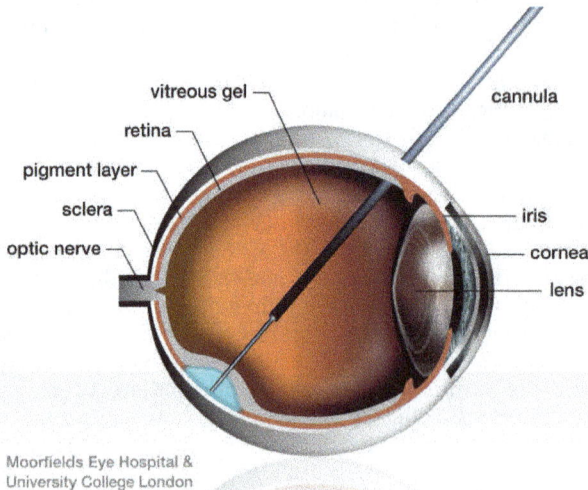

Figure 1. Schematic representation of subretinal administration of gene therapy vector in human
eyes. After three-port vitrectomy, recombinant adeno-associated virus vector can be delivered
through the retina to the subretinal space of one eye, by means of a subretinal cannula. Vector administration can involve up to one third of the total retinal area, including the macula.

In February 2007, we started the first clinical trial of gene therapy for LCA at UCL Institute of Ophthalmology and Moorfields Eye Hospital. By the end of the year, two additional trials had started in the United States - one at Scheie's Center for Hereditary Retinal Degenerations, University of Pennsylvania and the University of Florida College of Medicine in Gainesville and another at the Children's Hospital of Philadelphia and the University of Pennsylvania. The trial at UCL had a strong emphasis on safety and for its initial phase included only young adult participants with advanced disease. The AAV2 vector used, carrying the human *RPE65* cDNA under control of a human RPE65 promoter fragment, was administered subretinally using a *trans*-retinal approach (*Figure 1*). This vector had previously been shown to result in successful restoration of photoreceptor function in dogs [9, 11]. Assessments of vector safety included routine examination of the retina, evaluation of humoral or cellular immune responses to the AAV vector capsid or the transgene product, and measurement of disseminated vector genomes extraocularly. Efficacy of the gene therapy treatment was determined using a variety of objective and subjective assessments of retinal structure and function by means of clinical assessment, retinal imaging, psychophysical techniques, and electrodiagnostic methods. The end point for efficacy for each patient was defined as any improvement in visual function that was greater than the test-retest difference for each technique.

During the first 12 months following treatment, we observed no clinically significant intraocular inflammation and detected no immune responses to either AAV capsid or RPE65 in any of the patients. We found consistent evidence, on the basis of both microperimetry and dark-adapted perimetry, of improved retinal sensitivity in one patient. Microperimetry showed that in an area extending from the outer macula to a point beyond the major vascular arcade, the retinal sensitivity improved progressively in the right (study) eye by as much as 14 dB (a factor of 25). Thus, the patient could see small spots of light that were 1/25 as bright as those that could be seen before treatment. There was no improvement in the left (control) eye. Using dark-adapted perimetry, we could measure in 18 locations across the inferior retina, an improvement in sensitivity of more than 20 dB, or 100 times the sensitivity threshold observed at baseline. An assessment of vision involved the patient navigating a (continuously changing) maze under strictly controlled light conditions. The patient displayed an improvement in his visual mobility in low light (a decrease in travel time from 77 seconds to 14 seconds and a decrease in mobility errors from 8 to 0 for the study eye), which was substantially greater than the modest learning effect which was seen in the control eye, and which was consistent with the improvement in visual function established by means of perimetry [12].

It is not clear whether the improvement in visual responses in the peripheral macula is rod-mediated or cone-mediated. Neither can we be sure that the improvement in visual function is entirely due to enhanced levels of RPE65 in the retina. Evidence for this could be obtained only by biopsy of retinal material, which would be unsafe and unethical. Central macula function and visual acuity did not improve, despite exposure of this region to the vector; this may be due either to amblyopia (*i.e.* the study eye was amblyopic) or to a requirement for higher levels of RPE65 at the fovea. Visual function improved in only one patient, who had better baseline visual acuity in both the study eye and the control eye than either of the other patients. He was not the youngest patient, but he probably had less advanced retinal disease at baseline, which may explain why the improvement in this patient was not observed in the other patients. Whether further retinal degeneration is delayed in any of the patients will become apparent only after several years. The results of this study suggest that subretinal administration of recombinant AAV vector is not associated with immediate adverse events in patients with severe retinal dystrophy and that AAV-mediated RPE65 gene therapy can lead to modest improvements in visual function, even in patients with advanced degeneration.

COMPARISON WITH OTHER LCA2 GENE THERAPY TRIALS

All three clinical trials of gene supplementation therapy against LCA2 used an AAV2 vector carrying the human *RPE65* gene, although the promoter sequences driving expression varied, using either the tissue-specific human RPE65 promoter [12] or the constitutive cytomegalovirus immediate early promoter [13, 14]. Reports of preliminary and/or full results of these trials indicate that, despite differences in administered viral titres, injection volumes and assessment methods, all three studies could detect improvements in retinal light sensitivity and vision [12-16]. Where assessments allowed for distinction of rod and cone vision, for most subjects the improvements were detected in rod photoreceptor sensitivity, although in some cases there was a robust improvement detected in the cone-mediated visual function [16].

Despite these successes, the current therapies are open to improvement. *E.g.* in none of the subjects in these trials the treatment resulted in an increase in ERG responses [12, 14, 15]. This differs from the results of the pre-clinical studies in mice and dogs, where substantial electrophysiological improvements were routinely recorded. The reason behind this discrepancy has not yet been resolved, but the slow rate of rod recovery that was found in one of the trials could point towards an inadequacy in the amount of RPE65 protein produced [16], which could similarly have been responsible for the lack of detectable ERG responses.

ACKNOWLEDGMENTS

This work has been performed with the support of the EC-DG research through the FP6-Network of Excellence, CLINIGENE: LSHB-CT-2006-018933.

REFERENCES

1. Smith AJ, Bainbridge JW, Ali RR. Prospects for retinal gene replacement therapy. *Trends Genet* 2009; 25: 156-65.

2. Gu SM, Thompson DA, Srikumari CR, Lorenz B, Finckh U, Nicoletti A, *et al*. Mutations in RPE65 cause autosomal recessive childhood-onset severe retinal dystrophy. *Nat Genet* 1997; 17: 194-7.

3. Marlhens F, Bareil C, Griffoin JM, Zrenner E, Amalric P, Eliaou C, *et al*. Mutations in RPE65 cause Leber's congenital amaurosis. *Nat Genet* 1997; 17: 139-41.

4. Acland GM, Aguirre GD, Ray J, Zhang Q, Aleman TS, Cideciyan AV, *et al*. Gene therapy restores vision in a canine model of childhood blindness. *Nat Genet* 2001; 28: 92-95.

5. Narfstrom K, Katz ML, Bragadottir R, Seeliger M, Boulanger A, Redmond TM, *et al*. Functional and structural recovery of the retina after gene therapy in the RPE65 null mutation dog. *Invest Ophthalmol Vis Sci* 2003; 44: 1663-72.

6. Pang JJ, Chang B, Kumar A, Nusinowitz S, Noorwez SM, Li J, *et al*. Gene therapy restores vision-dependent behavior as well as retinal structure and function in a mouse model of RPE65 Leber congenital amaurosis. *Mol Ther* 2006; 13: 565-72.

7. Bennicelli J, Wright JF, Komaromy A, Jacobs JB, Hauck B, Zelenaia O, *et al*. Reversal of blindness in animal models of Leber congenital amaurosis using optimized AAV2-mediated gene transfer. *Mol Ther* 2008; 16: 458-65.

8. Bok D. The role of RPE65 in inherited retinal diseases. *Retina* 2005; 25: S61-2.

9. Le Meur G, Stieger K, Smith AJ, Weber M, Deschamps JY, Nivard D, *et al*. Restoration of vision in RPE65-deficient Briard dogs using an AAV serotype 4 vector that specifically targets the retinal pigmented epithelium. *Gene Ther* 2006; 14: 292-303.

10. Acland GM, Aguirre GD, Bennett J, Aleman TS, Cideciyan AV, Bennicelli J, *et al*. Long-term restoration of rod and cone vision by single dose rAAV-mediated gene transfer to the retina in a canine model of childhood blindness. *Mol Ther* 2005; 12: 1072-82.

11. Annear MJ, Bartoe JT, Barker SE, Smith AJ, Curran PG, Bainbridge JW, *et al*. Gene therapy in the second eye of RPE65-deficient dogs improves retinal function. *Gene Ther* 2011; 18: 53-61.

12. Bainbridge JWB, Smith AJ, Barker SS, Robbie S, Henderson R, Balaggan K, *et al*. Effect of gene therapy on visual function in Leber's congenital amaurosis. *N Engl J Med* 2008; 358: 2231-9.

13. Maguire AM, Simonelli F, Pierce EA, Pugh EN Jr, Mingozzi F, Bennicelli J, *et al*. Safety and efficacy of gene transfer for Leber's congenital amaurosis. *N Engl J Med* 2008; 358: 2240-8.

14. Hauswirth W, Aleman TS, Kaushal S, Cideciyan AV, Schwartz SB, Wang L, *et al*. Phase I trial of Leber congenital amaurosis due to RPE65 mutations by ocular subretinal injection of adeno-associated virus gene vector: short-term results. *Hum Gene Ther* 2008; 19: 979-90.

15. Simonelli F, Maguire AM, Testa F, Pierce EA, Mingozzi F, Bennicelli JL, *et al*. Gene therapy for Leber's congenital amaurosis is safe and effective through 1.5 years after vector administration. *Mol Ther* 2010; 18: 643-50.

16. Cideciyan AV, Aleman TS, Boye SL, Schwartz SB, Kaushal S, Roman AJ, *et al*. Human gene therapy for RPE65 isomerase deficiency activates the retinoid cycle of vision but with slow rod kinetics. *Proc Natl Acad Sci USA* 2008; 105: 15112-7.

The CliniBook: Clinical gene transfer
Edited by Odile Cohen-Haguenauer – EDK, Paris © 2012, pp. 452-458

C1-2
Gene therapy for X-linked adrenoleukodystrophy based on lentiviral correction of hematopoietic stem cells

Nathalie Cartier[1,2*], Salima Hacein-Bey-Abina[3,4,5], Cynthia C. Bartholomae[6], Manfred Schmidt[6], Christof Von Kalle[6], Pierre Bougnères[2], Alain Fischer[4], Marina Cavazzana-Calvo[3,4,5], Patrick Aubourg[1,2]

[1]*Inserm UMR745, University Paris-Descartes, 75279 Paris, France.*
[2]*Department of Pediatric Endocrinology and Neurology, Hôpital Bicêtre,*
94275 Kremlin-Bicêtre, France.
[3]*Department of Biotherapy, Hôpital Necker-Enfants Malades, 75743 Paris, France.*
[4] *Inserm UMR768, University Paris-Descartes, 75743 Paris, France.*
[5]*Clinical Investigation Center in Biotherapy, Groupe Hospitalier Universitaire Ouest,*
75743 Paris, France.
[6]*National Center for Tumor Diseases and German Cancer Research Center,*
69120 Heidelberg, Germany.
*Corresponding author : N. Cartier, MD, Inserm U745, Faculty of Pharmaceutical
Sciences, Paris Descartes University, 4 avenue de l'Observatoire, 75006 Paris, France.
nathalie.cartier@inserm.fr

X-LINKED ADRENOLEUKODYSTROPHY (X-ALD)

X-linked adrenoleukodystrophy (X-ALD) is a peroxisomal neurodegenerative disorder with a very broad clinical spectrum ranging from the most severe childhood cerebral form to late-onset spinal cord disease called adrenomyeloneuropathy (AMN). X-linked adrenoleukodystrophy (X-ALD) is caused by mutations in the ABCD1 gene that encodes a transporter (ALD protein) localized into the peroxisomal membrane and involved in the metabolism of very-long-chain fatty acids (VLCFA). Deficiency in ALD protein leads to an accumulation of VLCFA in plasma and tissues and progressive demyelination in the central nervous system (CNS). X-ALD is characterized by a marked phenotypic variation, even within the same family, which is not correlated to the levels of VLCFA or ABCD1 mutations. The cerebral form affects boys between 5 and 12 years of age and leads to a vegetative stage or death within 2 to 5 years [1, 2]. Adult ALD males develop between 20 and 30 years of age a milder form of X-ALD, called adrenomyeloneuropathy, that is characterized by progressive paraplegia due spinal cord involvement. Thirty five percent of AMN males are at risk to develop cerebral demyelination and overall, 65% of ALD males are at risk of developing fatal cerebral demyelination in childhood or adulthood [1, 2].

HEMATOPOIETIC CELL TRANSPLANTATION (HCT) IN X-ALD

When performed at an early stage of cerebral demyelination, allogeneic HCT allogeneic HCT is the only therapeutic approach that can arrest the progression of cerebral demyelination in boys with X-ALD [3-5]. Similar benefits of allogeneic HCT have been demonstrated in adults with cerebral X-ALD. However, it is not yet known whether allogeneic HCT can prevent or rescue adrenomyeloneuropathy. The absence of biological markers that can predict the evolutivity of cerebral disease is a major limitation to propose in due time allogeneic HCT to X-ALD patients who develop cerebral demyelination. HCT remained associated with significant risks of severe graft *versus* host disease and prolonged immune deficiency [6, 7] the mortality risk of HCT performed with HLA matched unrelated donor or cord blood remains close to 15% to 20% in children and 30% to 40% in adults when using full myeloablation with cyclophosphamide and busulfan, the most common conditioning regimen used up to now in ALD.

The mechanism by which HSCT arrests the neuroinflammatory demyelinating process in ALD is not known. The conditioning regimen has no effect by itself [8]. Although, yet speculative, it is possible that HCT in ALD allows to correct abnormal function of brain microglia, whether or not this deficiency is related to the accumulation of VLCFA. Microglia, the guard cells of the central nervous system (CNS), are a quite various population of non-neuronal cells that form up to 20% of all glial cells and are ubiquitously distributed throughout the CNS and are derived from bone marrow cells. The subset of bone marrow cells that are the progenitors of microglia has not been fully characterized, but microglial cells are likely to have a myelomonocytic origin, deriving from myeloid precursors in the bone marrow [9, 10]. The long-term benefits of allogeneic HCT in X-ALD are mediated by the replacement of brain microglial cells. However, the ALD protein is a transmembrane peroxisomal protein that cannot be secreted. Therefore, in constrast to CNS lysosomal storage disorders like Hurler syndrome, Globoid cell leukodystrophy or metachromatic leukodystrophy, in which normal enzyme produced by donor-derived microglia can be secreted and then recaptured by other CNS cells, this mechanism of cross-correction does not occur in X-ALD.

HSC GENE THERAPY IN X-ALD USING A LENTIVIRAL VECTOR

Since allogeneic HCT remains associated with significant morbidity and mortality risks, particularly in adults, and not all X-ALD patients have donors we hypothesized that hematopoietic stem cell (HSC) gene therapy could be an appropriate therapeutic alternative. Transplantation of autologous HSCs genetically modified to express the missing protein would circumvent the majority of the problems associated with allogeneic HCT. To correct ALD CD34$^+$ cells from the bone marrow In the absence of selective growth advantage of corrected cells in ALD, we turned to the use of a lentiviral vector. Lentiviral vectors can transduce nondividing cells and were shown, *in vitro* and *in vivo* in mice, to allow more efficient gene transfer into HSCs than murine gammaretrovirus vectors [11, 12]. Our preclinical work indicated that ALD gene transfer with lentiviral vector demonstrated efficient transduction of CD34$^+$ cells and biochemical correction of monocytes/macrophages derived from transduced ALD protein-deficient human CD34$^+$ cells [13]. *In vivo* expression of ALD protein in human monocytes and macrophages derived from engrafted human stem cells was demonstrated *in vivo*, after transplantation in nonobese diabetic/severe combined immunod-eficient (NOD/SCID) mice [14]. We showed that human bone marrow-derived cells were able to migrate into the brain of transplanted mice where they differentiated into microglia expressing the human ALD protein.

PROTOCOL DESIGN

Based on these preclinical data and safety data concerning the production and the use of HIV-1 derived lentiviral vector, approval for a HSC gene therapy trial in X-ALD was granted by the French regulatory agency in december 2005. This clinical protocol concerns boys between 5 and 15, with early progressive cerebral demyelination, who are candidates to HST but without HLA-matched donor or cord blood. CD34+ cells are selected from PBMCs after G-CSF stimulation and transduced *ex vivo*. A portion of non-transduced CD34+ cells are cryopreserved for rescue transplantation.

Peripheral blood mononuclear cells (PBMCs) are taken from the patients after stimulation by intravenous injection of granulocyte colony stimulating factor (G-CSF). CD34+ are positively selected. After prestimulation for 19 hours in the presence of cytokines (SCF, MGDF, Flt3-L, IL-3), CD34+ cells cells are transduced with the lentiviral vector for 16 hours. After transduction, a sample of transduced cells (5% of total transduced cells) is used for release testing (including in particular three replication-competent lentivirus (RCL) assays performed at Genosafe (Evry, France) and analysis of ALD protein expression and vector copy number. The remaining cells are cryopreserved in liquid nitrogen until release testing are completed.

When all release tests are completed, patients receive full myeloablative conditioning regimen with cyclophosphamide and busulfan to favor engraftment of the gene-corrected HSCs. Cryopreserved transduced CD34+ cells are then thawed and infused. Follow-up includes evaluation of efficacy and polyclonality of hematopoietic reconstitution with transduced cells, and clinical and radiological neurological outcome.

LENTIVIRAL VECTOR DESIGN

The MND-ALD lentivector used for the trial is a self-inactivating lentiviral vector in which the U3 region in the 3'LTR was deleted, and carries the expression cassette for the human ABCD1 cDNA under the expression of the MND (myeloproliferative sarcoma virus enhancer, negative control region deleted, dl587rev primer binding site substituted) promoter. The MND-ALD lentivector is pseudotyped with the vesicular stomatitis virus (VSV.G) envelope. This CG1711 hALD (MND-ALD) clinical vector was designed and produced under GMP guidelines by Cell Genesys Inc (South San Francisco, Ca, USA) (*Figure 1*). Vector was packaged using a third generation plasmid combination expressing Gag, Pol and Rev, deleted of the six other HIV-1 genes that are responsible for HIV-1 pathogenesis (*vif, vpr, vpu, nef, env, tat*). Absence of replication competent lentivirus (RCL) in the vector stock was determined.

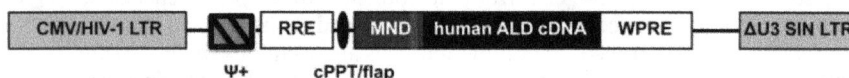

Figure 1. CG1711 hALD (MND-ALD) vector design. The CG1711 hALD (MND-ALD) vector is a self-inactivating (SIN) lentiviral vector. The U3 region in the 3'LTR was deleted (U3). This vector contains the expression cassette for the human ALD cDNA driven by the MND promoter. LTR, long terminal repeat; Ψ+, packaging signal; cPPT/flap, central polypurine tract; RRE, Rev-responsive element; WPRE, woodchuck hepatitis virus posttranscriptional regulatory element.

CLINICAL RESULTS AND FOLLOW-UP

Patients P1 and P2 were aged of 7.5 and 7 years respectively at time of gene therapy. These 2 patients had progressive cerebral neuroinflammatory demyelinating form of X-ALD determined by brain MRI, were candidate for allogeneic HCT but had no HLA–matched donor or cord blood. CD34+ cells were selected from PBMCs after G-CSF stimulation and transduced *ex vivo*. After all release tests were completed, patients received full myeloablative conditioning regimen with cyclophosphamide and busulfan. Cryopreserved transduced CD34+ cells were then thawed and infused (4.6 x 10^6 to 7.2 x 10^6 cells per kilogram, respectively in P1 and P2).

Patients were followed for adverse events and monitoring of bone marrow engraftment and neurological outcome. The procedure was clinically uneventful. Hematopoietic recovery occurred at day 13 to 15 after transplant and was sustained thereafter. Bone marrow aspirates were normal at 12 months and 24 months after gene therapy and all RCL tests were negative up to the last follow-up.

Expression of ALD protein in transduced CD34+ cells and PBMCs

Both patients had ABCD1 gene mutation that resulted in the absence of detectable ALD protein in their peripheral blood mononuclear cells (PBMCs). The efficacy of the HSC transduction was assessed by studying the percentage of hematopoietic cells expressing the lentivirally-encoded ALD protein in the peripheral blood using immunocytochemistry. ALD protein expression analysis was performed in transduced CD34+ cells before reinfusion, then at each time point of the follow-up after gene therapy, in monocytes, granulocytes, T and B lymphocytes.

Transduction efficacy of CD34+ cells (analyzed 5 days after transduction) ranged from 33% (P2) to 50% (P1). Respectively 20% and 33% of PBMCs from the 2 treated patients expressed the lentivirally-encoded ALD protein, 2 months after infusion of the transduced CD34+ cells. The percentage of corrected PBMCs decreased with time but stabilized at 10-13% around 16 months after gene therapy and remained stable up to 36 months after gene therapy.

In both patient, ALD protein was expressed at similar percentage in granulocytes, monocytes (that have short half-life) and in B and T-lymphocytes (that have longer half-life) at different time-points after gene therapy. Thirty-six months after gene therapy, this percentage ranged from 7-10% for P1 and 12-14% for P2.

In bone marrow CD34+ cells, expression of ALD protein was also stable, ranging from 18-20% (12 months) to 18% (24 months) in patients P1 and P2.

Vector copy number in transduced cells

ALD protein expression correlated with the number of integrated lentiviral copy per transduced CD34+ cell and PBMC evaluated by quantitative PCR. The mean numbers of integrated lentiviral copy per cell were 0.72 and 0.54 in transduced CD34+ cells from P1 and P2, respectively; in the PBMCs from P1 and P2, the vector copy number was respectively 0.165 and 0.2 ,16 months after gene therapy.

Integration Site (IS) characterization using 3'LTR mediated LAM-PCR, sequencing and datamining

A detailed integration site characterization was performed at the different time-points of the follow-up using linear amplification-mediated polymerase chain reaction (LAM-PCR) and high throughput 454 pyrosequencing of linear amplification mediated PCR amplicons (GS Flx; Roche Diagnostics) [15].

LAM-PCR analyses on >98% enriched $CD14^+$, $CD15^+$, $CD3^+$, $C19^+$, and bone marrow $CD34^+$ cells revealed a high number of distinct insertion sites (IS), indicating a consistently polyclonal distribution of lentivirally corrected hematopoietic cells.

We used high throughput 454 pyrosequencing of linear amplification mediated PCR amplicons to evaluate whether identical lentiviral insertion sites between lymphoid and myeloid lineages could be evidenced. Such common insertion would suggest transduction of primitive hematopoietic progenitors or hematopoietic stem cells. The observed numbers of identical lentiviral amplicons in lymphoid and myeloid cells from P1 and P2 were very significantly higher than the values expected by chance alone.

The quantitative contribution of individual clones harboring lentiviral integration to hematopoiesis is determined by ordering the abundance of distinct IS in different hematopoietic cell lineages using. This allows us to evaluate the possible emergence of individual dominant clones that could result from lentiviral integration. The retrieval frequency of a given lentiviral amplicon by high-throughput sequencing depends from the amount of DNA and therefore the number of cells harboring this IS. This method allows a good estimate of clonal contribution provided that a sufficient amount of DNA is tested and that there is no bias in the amplification of IS by LAM-PCR by choosing an optimized set of restriction enzymes. Using this methods we could conclude that no dominant clone emerged among active hematopoietic clones in the two treated patients.

NEUROLOGICAL OUTCOME OF THE 2 TREATED PATIENTS

Before gene therapy, patient #1 had normal verbal IQ (VIQ =104) and performance IQ (PIQ= 99). PIQ decreased at 74 and VIQ remained identical (104), 24 months after gene therapy. PIQ remained stable thereafter. Neurologic examination of patient #1 remained normal. This patient is in a specialized school because of attentional/executive deficits related to white matter lesions in the frontal lobes.

Patient #2 developed cuts in the lower parts of his visual field, initially without loss of visual acuity. Amputation of his visual fields started 16 months post-gene therapy and progressed up to 30 months; it was then associated with severe loss of visual acuity, without further aggravation up to 36 months after gene therapy. Patient #2 has no other neurologic deficits. His cognitive functions were normal prior to gene therapy (VIQ= 101, PIQ= 119 and total IQ = 111). Those values remained stable (103, 111 and 98) 20 months after gene therapy but declined at 102, 88 and 83, 30 months after gene therapy, reflecting significant visuo-spatial deficits. Despite his visual deficits, patient #2 follows normal school in the normal degree for his age, with help to adjust his visual problems.

Brain MRI was performed at each time point of the follow-up. In patient #1, brain MRI showed that cerebral demyelinating lesions arrested to progress 12-14 months after gene therapy. No further changes in the extent of cerebral demyelinating lesions was then observed, up to 36 months after gene therapy. A decline of cognitive functions was observed due to the progression of demyelinating lesions in the frontal white matter during the first 12-14 months post-gene therapy, a finding that that is very often observed after allogeneic HCT. In patient #2, brain MRI showed that cerebral demyelination arrested to progress 16 months after gene therapy (*Figure 2*). Up to 36 months after gene therapy, no changes in the extent of cerebral demyelinating lesions was observed.

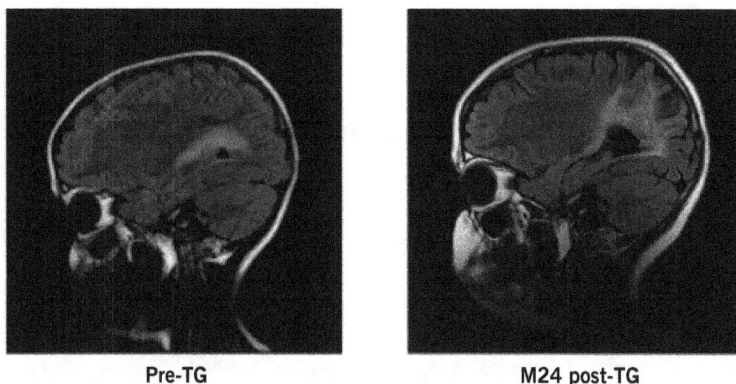

| Pre-TG | M24 post-TG |

Figure 2. Brain MRI from patient # 2 before and 24 months after gene therapy.

CONCLUSION

Two boys with progressive and lethal cerebral form of X-ALD were successfully treated with lentiviral HSC gene therapy [16]. Stable expression of the lentivirally-encoded ALD protein was demonstrated in the long term in peripheral blood monocytes, granulocytes and lymphocytes. We identified Identical lentiviral integration sites in myeloid and lymphoid cells, which argues for the transduction of HSCs. HSC-based gene therapy could thus represent a valuable therapeutic option for X-ALD patients with progressive cerebral demyelination as HSC gene therapy abrogates the morbidity and mortality risks associated with conventional allogeneic HCT. Longer follow-up of these 2 treated patients and outcome of 2 X-ALD patients treated more recently is awaited to confirm these encouraging results.

ACKNOWLEDGMENTS

A. Salzman and R. Salzman; P. Working and Cell Genesys staff (lenti-MND-ALD vector); P.A. and N.C. were supported by grants from Inserm, European Leukodystrophy Association, Association Française contre les Myopathies, La Fondation de France, the STOP-ALD foundation, La Fondation Avenir, Établissement Français des Greffes, Thermo Fisher Scientific, the 6th Framework European Economic Community (EEC) Programme (LSHM-CT2004-502987) and the Programme Hospitalier de Recherche Clinique (AOM 3043, French Health Ministry). S.H.-B.-A., L.D.-C., L.C., F.L., A.F., and M.C.-C. were supported by Inserm, Assistance Publique-Hôpitaux de Paris, Centre d'Investigation Clinique-Biotherapy, and Association Française contre les Myopathies. C.V.K. and M.S. were supported by grants from the Deutsche Forschungsgemeinschaft (SPP 1230), the German Ministry of Education and Research (TREATID), the Helmholtz Association, the EEC Programme 7th Framework CONSERT and with the support of the EC-DG research FP6-Network of Excellence, CLINIGENE: LSHB-CT-2006-018933.

REFERENCES

1. Dubois-Dalcq M, Feigenbaum V, Aubourg P. Neurobiology of X-linked adrenoleukodystrophy, a demyelinating peroxisomal disorder. *Trends Neurosci* 1999; 22: 4-122.

2. Moser HW, Mahmood A, Raymond GV. X-linked adrenoleukodystrophy, *Nat Clin Pract Neurol* 2007; 3: 140-51.

3. Aubourg P, Blanche S, Jambaque I, Rocchiccioli F, Kalifa G, Naud-Saudreau C, *et al.* Reversal of early neurologic and neuroradiologic manifestations of X-linked adrenoleukodystrophy by bone marrow transplantation. *N Engl J Med* 1990; 322: 1860-6.

4. Shapiro E, Krivit W, Lockman L, Jambaque I, Peters C, Cowan M, *et al.* Long term effect of bone marrow transplantation for childhood onset cerebral X-linked adrenoleukodystrophy. *Lancet* 2000; 356: 713-8.

5. Peters C, Charnas LR, Tan Y, Ziegler RS, Shapiro EG, De For T, *et al.* Cerebral X-linked adrenoleukodystrophy: the international hematopoietic cell transplantation experience from 1982 to 1999. *Blood* 2004; 10: 881-8.

6. Cheng FW, Lee V, To KF, Chan KC, Shing MK, Li CK. Post-transplant EBV-related lymphoproliferative disordercomplicating umbilical cord blood transplantation in patients of adrenoleukodystrophy. *Pediatr Blood Cancer* 2009; 53: 1329-31.

7. Hwang WY, Samuel M, Tan D, Koh LP, LimW, Linn YC. A meta-analysis of unrelated donor umbilical cord blood transplantation versus unrelated donor bone marrow transplantation in adult and pediatric patients. *Biol Blood MarrowTransplant* 2007; 13: 444-53.

8. Nowaczyk MJ, Saunders EF, Tein I, Blaser SI, Clarke JT. Immunoablation does not delay the neurologic progression of X-linked adrenoleukodystrophy. *J Pediatr* 1997; 131: 453-5.

9. Eglitis MA, Mezey E. Hematopoietic cells differentiate into both microglia and macroglia in the brains of adult mice. *Proc Natl Acad Sci USA* 1997; 94: 4080-5.

10. Priller J, Flügel A, Wehner T, Boentert M, Haas CA, Prinz M, *et al.* Targeting gene-modified hematopoietic cells to the central nervous system: use of green fluorescent protein uncovers microglial engraftment. *Nat Med* 2001; 7: 1356-61.

11. Naldini L, Blomer U, Gallay P, Ory D, Mulligan R, Gage FH, *et al. In vivo* gene delivery and stable transduction of nondividing cells by a lentiviral vector. *Science* 1996; 272: 263-7.

12. Miyoshi H, Smith KA, Mosier DE, Verma IM, Torbett BE. Transduction of human CD34+ cells that mediate long term engraftment of NOD/SCID mice by HIV vectors. *Science* 1999; 283: 682-6.

13. Benhamida S, Pflumio F, Dubart-Kupperschmitt A, Zhao-Emonet JC, Cavazzana-Calvo M, Rocchiccioli F, *et al.* Transduced CD34+ cells from adrenoleukodystrophy patients with HIV derived vector mediate long term engraftment of NOD/SCID mice. *Mol Ther* 2003; 7: 317-24.

14. Asheuer M, Pflumio F, Benhamida S, Dubart-Kupperschmitt A, Fouquet F, Imai Y, Aubourg P, Cartier N. Human CD34+ cells differentiate into microglia and express recombinant therapeutic protein. *Proc Natl Acad Sci USA* 2004; 101: 3557-62.

15. Schmidt M, Schwarzwaelder K, Bartholomae C, Zaoui K, Ball C, Pilz I, *et al.* High resolution insertion site analysis by linear amplification mediated PCR (LAMPCR). *Nat Methods* 2007; 4: 1051.

16. Cartier N, Hacein-Bey-Abina S, Bartholomä C, Veres G, Schmidt M, Kutschera I, *et al.* Hematopoietic stem cell gene therapy with lentiviral vector in X adrenoleukodystrophy. *Science* 2009; 326: 818-23.

The CliniBook: Clinical gene transfer
Edited by Odile Cohen-Haguenauer – EDK, Paris © 2012, pp. 459-464

C1-3

Immune reconstitution after gene therapy for adenosine deaminase severe combined immunodeficiency (ADA-SCID)

IMMACOLATA BRIGIDA[1], ALESSANDRO AIUTI[1,2]*

[1]San Raffaele Telethon Institute for Gene Therapy, Milan, Italy; [2]Department of Pediatrics, University of Rome Tor Vergata, Children's Hospital Bambino Gesù, Rome, Italy.
a.aiuti@hsr.it
* Corresponding author

ADENOSINE DEAMINASE SEVERE COMBINED IMMUNODEFICIENCY

ADA-SCID belongs to the family of Severe Combined Immunodeficiency (SCID), a group of heterogeneous genetic disorders characterized by a block of T lymphocyte differentiation and variably abnormal development of B or NK lymphocytes [1]. SCID represents a paradigm for gene therapy approaches due to the severity of the disease and the unmet medical need. Mutations in the ADA gene are responsible for approximately 15-20% of all cases of SCIDs, with an overall prevalence of 1:375.000 to 1:660.000 live births [2]. Children lacking ADA show an accumulation of ADA substrates adenosine and deoxyadenosine in the plasma and an increase of purine metabolites in lymphoid tissues and RBC. Therefore, ADA-SCID patients suffer from lymphopenia (T, B and NK), absence of both cellular and humoral immune function [3], severe opportunistic infections and failure to thrive. Non-immunological defects were described as frequently associated with organ damage, neurological and skeletal alterations [4, 5], and behavioral impairments [6]. Without treatment, the condition is fatal in the first year of life, thus necessitating early intervention [7].

Clinical management of ADA-SCID

Three therapeutic options are available to treat ADA-SCID [7, 8]. The golden standard treatment is bone marrow transplant from HLA-identical family donor without conditioning, accounting for 11% of total transplants for SCIDs performed in Europe, with an overall survival of 87% [7-10]. This procedure still remains available for a minority of patients, but ensures normalization in absolute lymphocyte and T cell numbers and metabolic reconstitution [11]. Transplant with reduced intensity conditioning has been suggested to allow faster and complete B cell reconstitution and better metabolic reconstitution due to the higher level of chimerism established [12]. In the absence of HLA-identical donors, allogeneic transplantation is associated with reduced survival, higher risk of complications and delayed/suboptimal immune reconstitution [7]. Enzyme replacement therapy was introduced as a lifesaving, noncurative treatment for patients lacking an HLA-matched donor [13, 14], aiming to decrease toxic metabolites concentrations, thereby correcting the metabolic abnormalities. The kinetics and the extent of immune recovery vary between patients, but often associated with an incomplete long-term immune recovery, a gradual decline of both mitogenic proliferative response and antigenic responses few years after treatment, lymphopenia and requirement of IVIg replacement [15-17]. Furthermore, manifestations of immune dysregulations, autoimmunity and allergy have been reported [18,19]. The major drawback for the worldwide diffusion of PEG-ADA therapy is the cost of treatment, representing a considerable burden for national health systems [2].

Gene therapy is a promising therapeutic option for genetic disorders of the immune system. In the last decades, gene therapy with retroviral vectors has been developed as a successful and safe alternative strategy for those ADA-SCID patients that could not have access to BMT or for whom ERT was not sufficient to maintain adequate immune reconstitution. The first pilot trials for ADA-SCID started in 1990s, with the infusion of genetically transduced PBL or HSC [20-22], without discharge of PEG-ADA. However, the relatively low gene transfer efficiency and engraftment levels observed in these trials, particularly in the B-cell and myeloid compartment, prevented substantial clinical benefit and patients continued to receive ERT [23]. Studies performed on patients treated with transduced PBL or HSC clearly demonstrated the need for increasing gene transfer efficiency into HSC and introducing a chemotherapeutic pre-conditioning in new clinical trials to achieve a persistent engraftment of multipotent progenitors expressing ADA.

Long term outcome of gene-therapy treated patients

Since year 2000, more than 30 ADA-SCID patients have been treated with gene therapy in different centers worldwide [8, 24, 25]. The successful outcome of the first 10 patients treated at HSR-TIGET has been recently described.

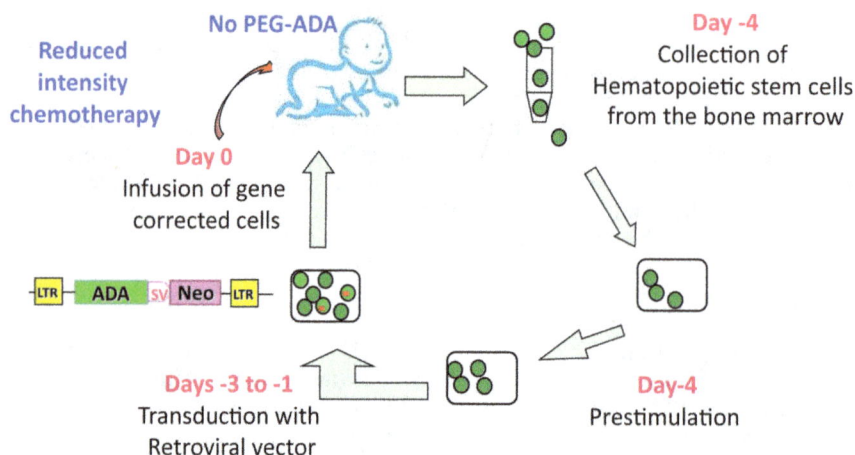

Figure 1. Schematic representation of the main phases of the gene therapy clinical protocol for ADA-SCID conducted at HSR-TIGET. Patients received autologous gene corrected bone marrow CD34+ cells combined to low dose busulfan, resulting in correction of the metabolic and immunological defect and clinical benefit.

All enrolled ADA-SCID patients lacked an HLA-identical sibling donor and were included either because they had failed ERT or did not have access to long-term PEG-ADA in the country of origin. Patients received a reduced intensity conditioning with busulfan (4 mg/kg) and PEG-ADA was discontinued before gene therapy in order to facilitate the selective advantage for gene-corrected cells [23, 25] (*Figure 1*). All patients presented with early onset form of the disease, with a median age at onset of 2 months (range 1-5 mo) and a median age at gene therapy of 1.7 years (range 0.6 - 5.6). One out of 10 patients was directly treated with HSC-GT; 4 patients failed a haploidentical BM transplant, and the other 6 patients received PEG-ADA for more than 6 months before GT, with ad inadequate response. The mean dose of CD34+ cells infused was 8.2x10^6/kg. Five additional patients were then treated with promising results (data not shown). At present, all treated children are alive, and only two patients have required ERT after gene therapy ([25] and A. Aiuti, unpublished data). Our cumulative data showed that vector transduced cells can sustain ADA enzymatic activity and efficient systemic detoxification. Gene corrected cells were detected in all myeloid and lymphoid subsets, the latter being more represented due to their survival advantage. High levels of transduction were detected long-term in peripheral blood T and B lymphocytes and natural killer (NK) cells (50-90% on average), whereas one log lower gene-corrected cells were detected in the bone marrow cells in CD34+ cells, granulocytic, megakaryocytic, and erythroid cells (3-9% on average) [23]. The reconstitution of the immune system was also documented by the recovery of polyclonal thymopoiesis in the majority of patients, with normalization of the Vbeta repertoire, increase of T cell counts and improvement of their TREC levels during follow up. An in depth analysis of patients at early and late F.U. showed an improvement of absolute counts of lymphocytes and CD4+ cells at late time points, even though the numbers of CD4+ and naive CD4+ cell counts were lower as compared to data from HLA-identical BMT patients (*Figure 2*). This clearly demonstrated that the recovery of the peripheral T-cell compartment is driven by both naïve and memory cells, to an extent comparable to what is observed in patients undergoing allogeneic BMT, although occurring at a slower pace compared with that of the control BMT group. Indeed, in the early phase post-transplant, the percentage of naive CD4 and CD8 cells was higher after GT [26].

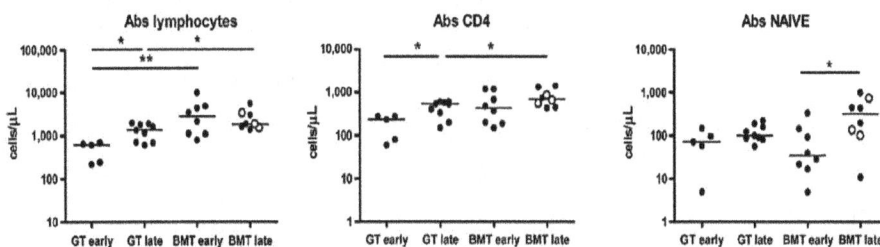

Figure 2. Absolute lymphocyte counts of GT and BMT-treated patients at early and late follow-up. Total lymphocyte, total CD4+, and naive CD4+ T-cell subsets are reported. Patients with ADA-SCID undergoing BMT are represented as empty circles in the BMT group. Counts are reported as absolute number of cells/μl. (Adapted from [26] with permission).

Moreover, gene corrected cells were found in both naïve and memory cells, coexisting with a population of untransduced cells, that decreased at later time. This result underlies the stronger selective advantage for vector-positive memory T cells over untransduced cells possibly occurring during peripheral expansion and/or antigen-specific stimulation (*Figure 3*) [26].

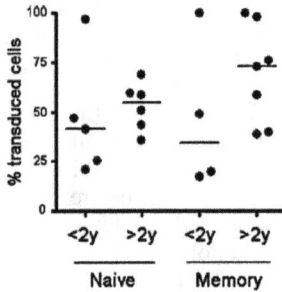

Figure 3. Quantification of transduced cells in naïve or memory T cells from GT patients at early and late follow up. The percentage of transduced cells is calculated by quantitative PCR for vector specific sequences. (Adapted from [26] with permission).

Thymus activity improved, even slowly, also in one of the oldest patients treated (5.6 years of age) who had not shown any sign of thymic function during the previous long course of PEG-ADA treatment. However, the increase in TREC was slower than those observed after allogeneic transplant during follow up, in line with the fact that patients received highly purified CD34$^+$ cells. Overall, it reached levels comparable to those of transplanted patients or healthy donors at more than 3 years of treatment. The reduction in TREC content in the naïve compartment is in agreement with an increased percentage of cycling cells at early time points of FU (<2 years). This would indicate that homeostatic proliferation has occurred in the earliest phases of T cell repopulation after treatment, resulting in dilution of TREC content, with a tendency to normalize at later time points [26]. The presence of vector-transduced cells after more than 5 years of treatment indicates long-term maintenance of genetically corrected cells. However, non-transduced cells coexisted with transduced T, B and NK cells in the periphery, suggesting a possible rescue of non-transduced cells by the detoxification provided from gene corrected cells. T-cell functions, including susceptibility to apoptosis [27], normalized after GT. Proliferative response to mitogens (*Figure 4*) and antigens fell in the range of healthy controls after 1 year of therapy, with evidence of antibody production to specific antigens in 7 patients following vaccination ([25] and unpublished observations). The progressive restoration of immune and metabolic functions led to significant improvement of patients' development and protection from severe infections, without adverse events related to gene therapy.

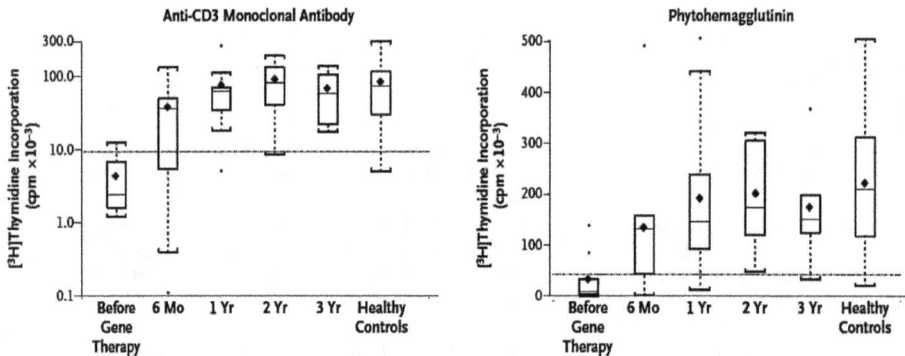

Figure 4. Proliferative response to mitogens. *In vitro* proliferative responses to bound anti-CD3 (on a log10 scale, left side) and to PHA (on a linear scale, right side) after 3 days of stimulation, assessed by thymidine incorporation assay. The dashed horizontal line represents the 5th percentile for healthy controls. (Adapted from [25] with permission).

CONCLUSIONS

Our cumulative data show that a single infusion of bone marrow CD34$^+$ cells combined with low dose busulfan conditioning, results in the correction of the metabolic defect in all lineages of the hematopoietic system, including myeloid cells. Moreover, the presence of shared vector integrations among multiple hematopoietic lineages demonstrated stable engraftment of multipotent HSC. Integrations were also found within and/or near potentially oncogenic loci, but did not result in selection or expansion of malignant cell clones *in vivo* [28, 29], underlining the importance of a continuous monitoring of the safety of this treatment. If gene therapy for ADA-SCID will become a standard treatment, the choice between different treatment options should be based on the risk/ benefit ratio, the availability and costs of the different options [23]. The future development of innovative vector technology, such as lentiviral vectors, might further improve its efficacy and safety profile.

ACKNOWLEDGEMENTS

This work was supported by Fondazione TELETHON and grants from the European Commission. EC-DG research through the FP6-Network of Excellence, CLINIGENE: LSHB-CT-2006-018933.

REFERENCES

1. Fischer A, De Saint Basile G, Disanto JP, Hacein-Bey S, Sharara L, Cavazzana-Calvo M. Gene therapy of primary immunodeficiencies. *Adv Nephrol Necker Hosp* 1997; 26: 107-20.

2. Aiuti A, Brigida I, Ferrua F, Cappelli B, Chiesa R, Marktel S, Roncarolo MG. Hematopoietic stem cell gene therapy for adenosine deaminase deficient-SCID. *Immunol Res* 2009; 44: 150-9.

3. Hirschhorn RCF. Immunodeficiency due to defects of purine metabolism. In: *Primary immunodeficiency diseases: a molecular and genetic approach*, chapter 12, 2nd ed. Oxford: Oxford University Press, 2006: 169-96.

4. Honig M, Albert MH, Schulz A, Sparber-Sauer M, Schutz C, Belohradsky B, *et al*. Patients with adenosine deaminase deficiency surviving after hematopoietic stem cell transplantation are at high risk of CNS complications. *Blood* 2007; 109: 3595-602.

5. Sauer AV, Mrak E, Hernandez RJ, Zacchi E, Cavani F, Casiraghi M, *et al*. ADA-deficient SCID is associated with a specific microenvironment and bone phenotype characterized by RANKL/OPG imbalance and osteoblast insufficiency. *Blood* 2009; 114: 3216-26.

6. Rogers MH, Lwin R, Fairbanks L, Gerritsen B, Gaspar HB. Cognitive and behavioral abnormalities in adenosine deaminase deficient severe combined immunodeficiency. *J Pediatr* 2001; 139: 44-50.

7. Gaspar HB, Aiuti A, Porta F, Candotti F, Hershfield MS, Notarangelo LD. How I treat ADA deficiency. *Blood* 2009; 114: 3524-32.

8. Cappelli B, Aiuti A. Gene therapy for adenosine deaminase deficiency. *Immunol Allergy Clin North Am* 2010; 30: 249-60.

9. Antoine C, Muller S, Cant A, Cavazzana-Calvo M, Veys P, Vossen J, *et al*. Long-term survival and transplantation of haemopoietic stem cells for immunodeficiencies: report of the European experience 1968-99. *Lancet* 2003; 361: 553-60.

10. Gennery AR, Slatter MA, Grandin L, Taupin P, Cant AJ, Veys P, *et al*. Transplantation of hematopoietic stem cells and long-term survival for primary immunodeficiencies in Europe: entering a new century, do we do better? *J Allergy Clin Immunol* 2010; 126: 602-610/e601-611.

11. Buckley RH, Schiff SE, Schiff RI, Markert L, Williams LW, Roberts JL, *et al*. Hematopoietic stem-cell transplantation for the treatment of severe combined immunodeficiency. *N Engl J Med* 1999; 340: 508-16.

12. Cancrini C, Ferrua F, Scarselli A, Brigida I, Romiti ML, Barera G, *et al*. Role of reduced intensity conditioning in T-cell and B-cell immune reconstitution after HLA-identical bone marrow transplantation in ADA-SCID. *Haematologica* 2010; 95: 1778-82.

13. Hershfield MS. PEG-ADA replacement therapy for adenosine deaminase deficiency: an update after 8.5 years. *Clin Immunol Immunopathol* 1995; 76: S228-232.

14. Hershfield MS, Buckley RH, Greenberg ML, Melton AL, Schiff R, Hatem C, *et al*. Treatment of adenosine deaminase deficiency with polyethylene glycol-modified adenosine deaminase. *N Engl J Med* 1987; 316: 589-96.

15. Booth C, Gaspar HB. Pegademase bovine (PEG-ADA) for the treatment of infants and children with severe combined immunodeficiency (SCID). *Biologics* 2009; 3: 349-58.

16. Weinberg K, Hershfield MS, Bastian J, Kohn D, Sender L, Parkman R, Lenarsky C. T lymphocyte ontogeny in adenosine deaminase-deficient severe combined immune deficiency after treatment with polyethylene glycol-modified adenosine deaminase. *J Clin Invest* 1993; 92: 596-602.

17. Hershfield MS. Adenosine deaminase deficiency: clinical expression, molecular basis, and therapy. *Semin Hematol* 1998; 35: 291-8.

18. Ozsahin H, Arredondo-Vega FX, Santisteban I, Fuhrer H, Tuchschmid P, Jochum W, *et al*. Adenosine deaminase deficiency in adults. *Blood* 1997; 89: 2849-55.

19. Notarangelo LD, Stoppoloni G, Toraldo R, Mazzolari E, Coletta A, Airo P, et al. Insulin-dependent diabetes mellitus and severe atopic dermatitis in a child with adenosine deaminase deficiency. *Eur J Pediatr* 1992; 151: 811-4.

20. Onodera M, Ariga T, Kawamura N, Kobayashi I, Ohtsu M, Yamada M, *et al*. Successful peripheral T-lymphocyte-directed gene transfer for a patient with severe combined immune deficiency caused by adenosine deaminase deficiency. *Blood* 1998; 91: 30-6.

21. Bordignon C, Notarangelo LD, Nobili N, Ferrari G, Casorati G, Panina P, *et al*. Gene therapy in peripheral blood lymphocytes and bone marrow for ADA-immunodeficient patients. *Science* 1995; 270: 470-5.

22. Blaese RM, Culver KW, Miller AD, Carter CS, Fleisher T, Clerici M, *et al*. T lymphocyte-directed gene therapy for ADA-SCID: initial trial results after 4 years. *Science* 1995; 270: 475-80.

23. Ferrua F, Brigida I, Aiuti A. Update on gene therapy for adenosine deaminase-deficient severe combined immunodeficiency. *Curr Opin Allergy Clin Immunol* 2010; 10: 551-6.

24. Aiuti A, Roncarolo MG. Ten years of gene therapy for primary immune deficiencies. *Hematology Am Soc Hematol Educ Program* 2009, 682-9.

25. Aiuti A, Cattaneo F, Galimberti S, Benninghoff U, Cassani B, Callegaro L, *et al*. Gene therapy for immunodeficiency due to adenosine deaminase deficiency. *N Engl J Med* 2009; 360: 447-58.

26. Selleri S, Brigida I, Casiraghi M, Scaramuzza S, Cappelli B, Cassani B, *et al*. *In vivo* T-cell dynamics during immune reconstitution after hematopoietic stem cell gene therapy in adenosine deaminase severe combined immune deficiency. *J Allergy Clin Immunol* 2011; 127: 1368-75.

27. Cassani B, Mirolo M, Cattaneo F, Benninghoff U, Hershfield M, Carlucci F, *et al*. Altered intracellular and extracellular signaling leads to impaired T-cell functions in ADA-SCID patients. *Blood* 2008; 111: 4209-19.

28. Aiuti A, Cassani B, Andolfi G, Mirolo M, Biasco L, Recchia A, *et al*. Multilineage hematopoietic reconstitution without clonal selection in ADA-SCID patients treated with stem cell gene therapy. *J Clin Invest* 2007; 117: 2233-40.

29. Biasco L, Ambrosi A, Pellin D, Bartholomae C, Brigida I, Roncarolo MG, *et al*. Integration profile of retroviral vector in gene therapy treated patients is cell-specific according to gene expression and chromatin conformation of target cell. *EMBO Mol Med* 2011; 3: 89-101.

The CliniBook: Clinical gene transfer
Edited by Odile Cohen-Haguenauer – EDK, Paris © 2012, pp. 465-474

C1-4

Gene therapy in Alzheimer disease patients

MARIA ERIKSDOTTER-JÖNHAGEN[1,3]*, BENGT LINDEROTH[2,4], PER ALMQVIST[2,4], GÖRAN LIND[2,4],
HELGA EYJOLFSDOTTIR[1,3], ERIK SUNDSTRÖM[1,5], ÅKE SEIGER[1,3,5], LARS WAHLBERG[1,6]

[1] Department of Neurobiology, Caring Sciences and Society, Division of Clinical Geriatrics,
Karolinska Institutet, Sweden. [2] Department of Clinical Neuroscience, Karolinska Institutet,
Stockholm, Sweden. [3] Department of Geriatrics. [4] Department of Neurosurgery, Karolinska
University Hospital, Stockholm, Sweden. [5] Stockholms Sjukhem, Stockholm, Sweden.
[6] NsGene A/S, Ballerup, Denmark.
* Corresponding author: Pr Maria Eriksdotter-Jönhagen, Department of Neurobiology,
Caring Sciences and Society, Division of Clinical Geriatrics, Karolinska Institutet and
Karolinska University Hospital, Huddinge, Novum, Plan 5, SE-141 86 Stockholm, Sweden.
maria.eriksdotter.jonhagen@ki.se

BACKGROUND

The population in the western world gets increasingly older. Disorders with cognitive disturbances increase with age and dementia diseases are among the most common. In Sweden approximately 90 000 patients are afflicted by the most common dementia disorder, Alzheimer´s disease (AD) and 36 millions worldwide [1]. AD is progressive with a successive decline in cognitive functions. One early symptom is episodic memory loss as well attention and planning difficulties. There is no cure and the effects of the symptomatic treatment available today, cholinesterase inhibitors and memantine are transient and moderate. Although many treatment trials have been carried out, there has as yet been no breakthrough concerning treatment of AD and new therapies are thus badly needed.

The central cholinergic system

The central cholinergic system is known to play an important role in AD. Cognitive decline in AD has been associated with central cholinergic dysfunction and neu-rodegenerative changes in the basal forebrain, where the cholinergic circuitry projects to the cerebral cortex and hippocampus [2-4]. Indeed, neurotoxic lesions of the cholinergic system in experimental animals induce performance deficits, including memory and spatial disturbances as evaluated with the Morris swim maze. Marked reductions of cholinergic markers have been found in the cerebral cortex even at an early disease stage in Alzheimer´s patients [4]. Moreover, reduced number of neurons containing choline acetyltransferase (ChAT) and the declining presence of vesicular acetylcholine transporter correlate very well with the severity of dementia, as determined by the Mini-Mental State Examination. Treatment with cholinesterase-inhibitors have shown to stabilize cognition and memory function in patients with early AD for up to 12 months, but the therapeutic effects are transient [5].

Rational for nerve growth factor (NGF) in Alzheimer's disease

NGF belongs to the family of neurotrophins and mediates its effects *via* tropomyosin receptor kinase TrkA and p75[NTR] receptors [4-6]. In normal subjects, endogenous NGF is synthesized by post-synaptic cortical and hippocampal neurons, and signals through the TrkA and p75 receptors located on the cholinergic terminals. The activated receptor complex is then retrogradely transported from the target areas, *i.e.* cortex and hippocampus to the cholinergic nuclei in the basal forebrain [7]. NGF has demonstrated regenerative and neuroprotective effects on basal forebrain cholinergic neuron in animals [8] and prevents cholinergic degeneration induced by injury, excitotoxicity, aging or amyloid overexpression [4, 9]. Several studies have reported decreased levels of NGF and NGF receptors in the basal forebrain in patients with AD, while NGF levels in hippocampus and cortex are unchanged or increased supporting the hypothesis that the normal NGF signalling and/or transport in AD is impaired [4]. Positive effects of NGF on cell survival and neurological functionality have been demonstrated in several animal studies which indicate that sustained local delivery of NGF to the cholinergic basal forebrain can arrest and even reverse the degeneration of the basal forebrain cholinergic neurons that are involved in the cognitive decline in AD [5].

The cholinergic nerve cells in the basal forebrain have been shown to undergo trophic changes in the earliest stages of AD, such as a loss of TrkA receptor expression [4, 10]. A leading hypothesis concerning the decline in cholinergic function therefore states that a loss of trophic support to cholinergic neurons precedes the loss of cholinergic phenotype seen in late AD [5]. The mechanisms behind the reduced neurotrophic support in AD are not completely understood, but deficits in this transport and/or signaling of NGF as well as imbalance in the ratio of NGF and its precursor pro-NGF may play a role [4, 9, 10]. Interestingy, pro-NGF, which is increased in AD brains [11] has been shown to bind to the p75 receptor resulting in pro-apoptotic signalling, while studies of NGF binding to the TrkA receptor have shown enhanced survival signalling. Thus, an imbalance between the ratio of pro-NGF and NGF could then suggest a shift towards pro-apoptotic signalling [4, 10]. Furthermore, NGF has been shown to inhibit the amyloidogenic processing of APP, mediated by a complex series of molecular events and by interactions among NGF receptors [12] linking NGF also to amyloid pathology in AD. For example, TrkA reduces and p75 activates BACE (β-secretase) cleavage of the amyloid precursor protein to Aβ [4].

Thus, NGF is emerging as a potential disease modifying therapeutic agent, *i.e.* counteracting the cholinergic dysfunction and attenuating the rate of degeneration of basal forebrain neurons in AD. Since NGF does not pass the blood brain barrier, it is a challenge to find a suitable administration route. Several techniques have been developed for the delivery of therapeutic compounds to the CNS, including intrathecal and intracerebroventricular drug delivery by infusion pump systems and gene therapy [13].

Clinical studies

Intracerebroventricular delivery
Our research group has previously performed a small clinical study in 3 AD patients infusing mouse 2.5S NGF into the cerebral lateral ventricle [14, 15] (*Table I*). In this study, nicotinic receptors and regional cerebral blood flow were both increased in the neocortex following NGF-infusion, as analysed by positron emission tomography (PET) imaging. This effect was maintained for several months after the NGF infusion was stopped. In addition, EEG activity showed signs of normalised activity in these patients. However, due to adverse events, including centrally induced neuropathic pain and weight loss, the intracerebroventricular NGF infusion study was stopped prematurely [15]. It was later shown in animal studies, that when NGF was infused directly into the brain parenchyma no pain-related effects were found [16].

Table I. Previous studies in Alzheimer patients treated with intracerebral NGF infusion.

Clinical studies investigating intracerebral NGF administration in (AD)				
Reference	Type of study	Duration of treatment	Dosage, route of adm	Number of subjects
Olson *et al.* 1992 [14], Eriksdotter-Jönhagen *et al.* 1998 [15]	Open-label, Phase I exploratory study to assess efficacy and safety of intra-cerebroventricular infusion of NGF in AD	Continuous infusion of NGF for 3 months	A total of 6,6 mg beta-NGF purified from male mouse submandibular glands administered into the lateral cerebral ventricles months in the first 2 patients; A total of 0.55 mg NGF for 3 shorter periods in the 3rd patient	3 (2 females, 1 male) Age: 69, 57, 61 years
Tuszynski *et al.* 2005 [18]	Open-label, Phase I, exploratory study with the ojective to assess effect and safety of *ex vivo* NGF gene delivery in AD	Autologous fibroblasts genetically modified to express human NGF were injected into the basal forebrain. Follow-up of patients at several stages during a 2-year period post treatment	NGF production was 25-75 ng NGF/10^6 cells/day. Subjects 1 and 2 received unilateral injections of 2.5×10^6 cells. Subjects 3-6 were injected bilaterally with a total of 5.0×10^6 cells. Subjects 7-8 were injected bilaterally with 10.0×10^6 cells. Injections were done into the cholinergic nucleus basalis of Meynert	8 subjects (5 females, 3 males), mean age 67 ± 2.6 years, range 54-76 years

Gene therapy with local delivery of NGF

Based on the findings described above, it was clear, that local NGF delivery directly to the cholinergic basal forebrain would be preferred, but poses a clinical and technical challenge. It has been shown, that long-term intraparenchymal NGF lentiviral-mediated gene delivery reverses age-related cholinergic decline patterns in primates with no side effects [17]. The first study using gene therapy in patients with AD was published in 2005 [18]. Data from from this 2-year, open-label, phase I study in alzheimer patients, following *in vivo* NGF gene-delivery by using retroviral vectors encoding NGF in autologous fibroblasts (*Table I*), showed a significant increase of glucose uptake in several cortical regions and cognitive tests showed scores that were stabilised or declined at a slower rate than expected [18]. A phase II clinical trial using Adeno-associated viral (AAV) vectors expressing human NGF is currently ongoing (ClinicalTrials.gov Identifier: NCT00876863).

Viral vector-mediated gene transfer is able to express a therapeutic gene and deliver regional doses of potent biologics long-term without the need for refilling or replacement. However, there are certain limitations with *in vivo* gene therapy, particularly the permanent genetic modification of the patients brain cells and the obvious inability to control and stop the targeted release. In order to circumvent these problems, we have worked with an encapsulated cell technology (EC biodelivery), developed by NsGene A/S, a Danish biotechnology company. The implant is a catheter-like device containing a genetically engineered NGF secreting human cell line housed behind a semi-permeable hollow fibre membrane at its tip which can be implanted, removed and exchanged at demand. Encapsulation provides immunoisolation and protects foreign cells from the host immune system while nutrients, oxygen and therapeutic products can diffuse freely across the capsule walls [19, 20].

A great advantage over traditional *ex vivo* or in *vivo gene* therapy approaches is that the NGF-delivery can be stopped by removing the device with the genetically modified NGF-producing cells from the brain.

Encapsulated cell delivery of NGF

First clinical trial to Alzheimer patients

We have recently performed the first clinical trial in AD patients using encapsulated NGF-producing cells with safety and tolerability as primary outcome measures. This was a 12-month, open label, single center, phase I, dose-escalation study of EC biodelivery of NGF to the cholinergic basal forebrain of six patients with mild to moderate AD (*Table II*) [21, 22]. The NGF biodelivery device, NsG202, is a gene therapy medicinal product. It consists of cells expressing human NGF (but no pro-NGF) housed in an implantable device. For a detailed description of the technical platform see [23]. In brief, a spontaneously immortalized retinal pigmental epithelial cell line was grown *in vitro* and transfected and stably modified with the human NGF gene under control of a modified CMV promoter containing an intron. A clone producing high levels of NGF was selected releasing $1,7 \pm 0,7$ ng/24 h NGF per capsule. A 150 mm long and 1 mm wide, hollow, polyurethane tether was attached to an 11 mm long polyether sulphone hollow fiber (the active part). The hollow fiber was filled with the NGF releasing cells attached to a polyvinyl alcohol foam scaffolding. Filled devices were kept in sealed, sterile containers and were tested for sterility, mycoplasma, cell leakage, and NGF production before released. A shelf life of 5 weeks after release was validated for the study [23]. At implantation the active part was placed in the basal forebrain (*Figure 1*).

Table II. Demographic data on included alzheimer patients I-VI in the first study using encapsulated cellbiodelivery of NGF to the basal forebrain.

	I	II	III	IV	V	VI
Age (y)	63	55	65	57	60	73
Gender (F/M)	F	F	M	M	F	F
AD diagnosis (y)	2	2	1	1	2	1
AD stage	mild	moderate	mild	mild	mild	mild

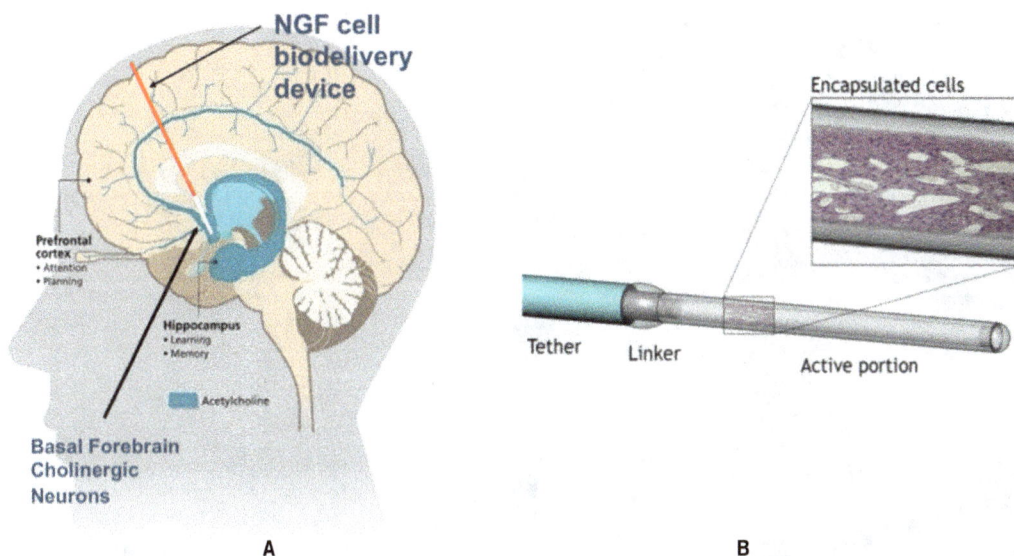

A   B

Figure 1. Schematic drawing of the device implanted in the basal forebrain (A). In the enlarged picture and cut-out view of the tip, the encapsulated genetically modified cells are growing on the polyvinol alcohol foam within the membrane allowing for influx of nutrients and efflux of NGF. The membrane is linked to a tether which at the other end is attached to the skull bone (B).

The delivered daily dose of NGF was low in this initial safety study, but at a level anticipated to yield therapeutic effects, as experimental devices tested in the rat striatum positively affected the size of the surrounding normal cholinergic neurons. In addition, the NsG0202 implant released similar levels of NGF previously shown to be effective in animal models with cholinergic dysfunction [24].

Surgical implantation

Prior to surgery, patients had undergone clinical and cognitive evaluations as well as lumbar puncture, magnetic resonance imaging (MRI) and PET scans of brain and EEG. Patients were anesthetized prior to surgery, attached to a Leksell stereotactic frame and a stereotactic planning MRI study was performed to identify the target areas and the trajectories. A custom-made frame adapter was attached to the arch of the Leksell stereotactic frame and used for the implantation of the EC Biodelivery device (*Figure 1*). The first three patients received implants in nucleus Meynert (Ch4 region) bilaterally and the latter three patients also received bilateral implants in the vertical limb of the diagonal band (Ch2 region, *Figure 2*). The Ch4 contains most of the cholinergic cell bodies that project to cortical targets and to the amygdala. Its cortical projections are involved in attention and planning. This site was also the target of one of the previous clinical studies [18]. However, since also memory impairment is a major early deficit in AD and the hippocampus is affected by large numbers of plaques and tangles, we also targeted the nucleus of the vertical limb of the diagonal band of Broca (Ch2) to treat the cholinergic projections to the hippocampal areas in the second cohort of patients.

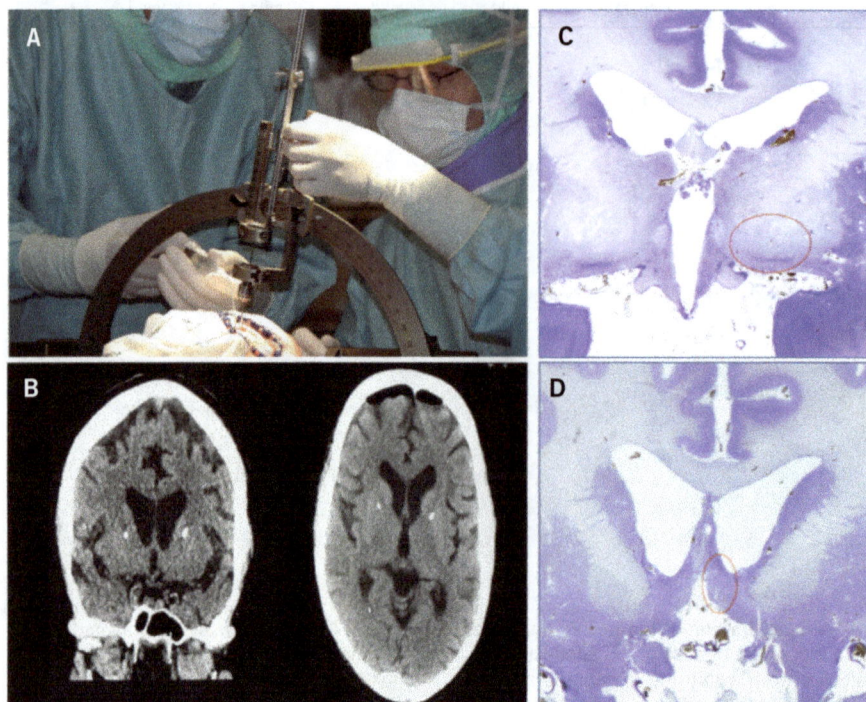

Figure 2. A photograph showing the stereotactic insertion of the NGF biodelivery device by the neurosurgeon (A). B shows the CT scans directly after surgery showing the trajectories of the barium impregnated tether seen as a white dot bilaterally. The tip of the tether with the active part is not radiologically visible. Note the marked atrophy of the Alzheimer brain. The black area in front of frontal cortex in the sagittal CT scan is air from surgery, which disappears within days (B). In C and D the coronal sections show the cholinergic Nissl stained cell bodies in the Ch4 region (encircled in C) and the Ch2 region (encircled in D) in the basal forebrain.

Postoperative care and monitoring

Patients were in postoperative care for 5-7 days and then discharged. As expected, there was a few days of transient headache postoperatively for the majority of the patients and one patient had an episode of transient confusion. After discharge from hospital, patients were carefully monitored for 12 months and the same tests performed at baseline were repeated at 3 and 12 months postoperatively.

Twelve months after implantation, the NsG0202 devices were safely explanted under general anesthesia in all 6 patients without complications. NGF release from each implant was sampled and cell morphology analyzed.

All patients tolerated the procedures well and many variables of this advanced product were validated [21, 23]. In two of the six treated patients, significant cognitive improvement associated with improvements on nicotinic receptor binding assessed with PET (*Figure 3*) and EEG biomarkers was found [21, 22]. This study has shown for the first time that it is feasible to implant encapsulated cells using a catheterlike device into the basal forebrain of AD patients and that the procedure is well tolerated. Moreover, we have shown that it is technically possible using stereotactic neurosurgery to place implants in the Ch2 region of the brain of man, which has never been done before.

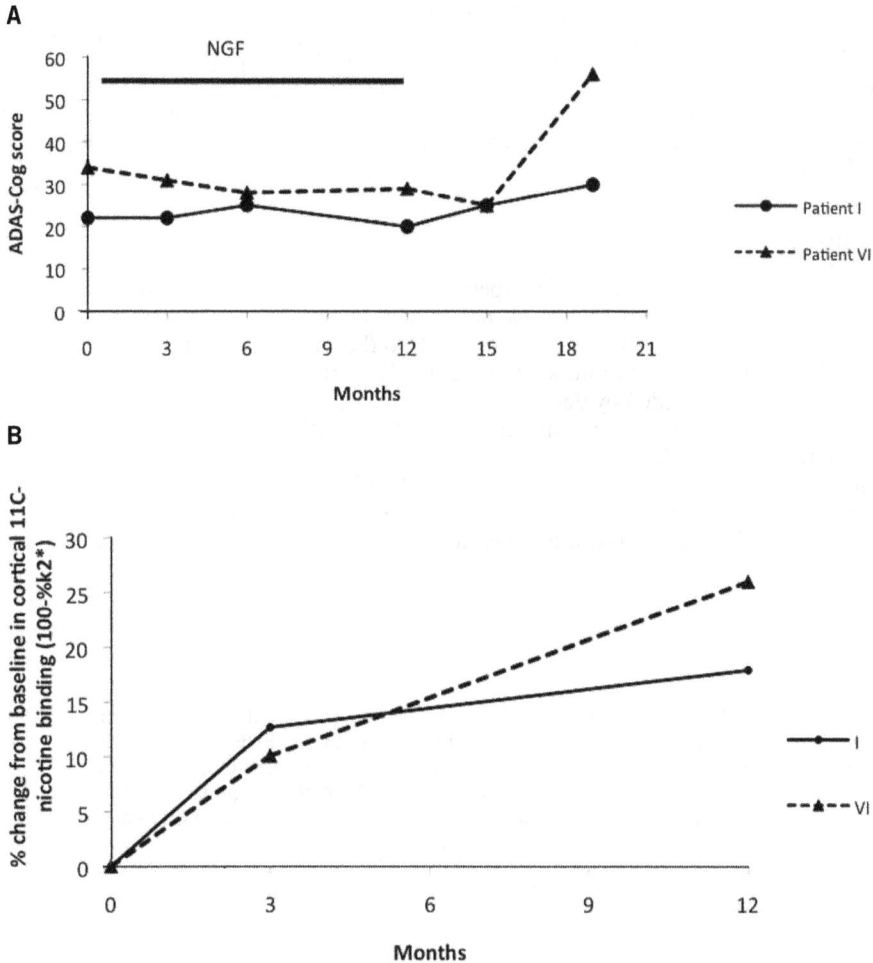

Figure 3. ADAS-Cog scores (A) and percentage change in ^{11}C-nicotine binding from baseline assessed with PET in patient #I and #VI (B). Please note that the scores from the cognitive test ADAS-Cog improved during treatment at 12 months (reduced scores as compared to baseline scores) in A. When the NGF treatment stopped after 12 months the cognitive function worsened (increasing scores) at 19 months. The ^{11}C-nicotine binding in mean cortical areas increased in both patient #I and #VI at 3 and 12 months compared to baseline, at 12 months with 18 and 26 % respectively (B).

The successful removal of the devices gave us a unique opportunity to study cell release and cell survival among the encapsulated cells after being kept for 12 months in the human basal forebrain. Analyses of viability and NGF content after 12 months showed that removed devices released NGF at about 10% of the rate at implantation with few viable cells remaining. Results from a previous 12-month mini-pig toxicology study showed however essentially intact cell viability and function of similar implants during a 12-month period [24]. This discrepancy between the mini-pig and patient studies may be related to the difference in implantation instrumentation used between the species or differences in the diffusion of nutrients and/or waste products through the semi-permeable capsule wall in the AD *versus* the mini-pig brain. Immunological host-*versus*-graft reaction is a less likely explanation of poor cell survival in the AD study, as the NGF secreting human cell line was well protected from immune rejection in the xenogeneic milieu of the mini-pig brain. The polyvinyl alcohol scaffolding used to support the attachment and the cells also tended to degenerate and mineralize over time. To improve efficacy in future studies, cell survival and NGF release from the encapsulated cells require amelioration.

CONCLUSIONS

The first steps towards a possibly new therapeutic strategy for AD based on local delivery of a bioactive molecule to cholinergic neurons in the basal forebrain have been taken. It has been shown, that local delivery of NGF to the basal forebrain in AD patients is possible and safe. With more work to define the optimal dose and long-term function of new cell lines, aided by device improvement, EC biodelivery of NGF has the potential to become a new treatment strategy for AD, which combines the advantages of gene therapy with the simplicity and safety of an implantable and retrievable device. This strategy is probably not suitable for all AD patients but may be a treatment option for younger AD patients in otherwise relatively good medical condition rendering them eligible for neurosurgical intervention.

ACKNOWLEDGEMENTS

This study was supported by grants from Clinigene (European network for the Advancement of Clinical Gene Transfer and Therapy), FP6-Network of Excellence, CLINIGENE: LSHB-CT-2006-018933 from the Regional agreement on medical training and clinical research (ALF) between Stockholm County Council and the Karolinska Institutet, the Swedish Alzheimer Foundation, Gustaf V and Queen Victorias Freemason foundation, the Swedish Brain Power Consortium and NsGene A/S.

REFERENCES

1. Alzheimer's disease International. *World Alzheimer Report*, 2010.

2. Bartus RT. On neurodegenerative diseases, models, and treatment strategies: lessons learned and lessons forgotten a generation following the cholinergic hypothesis. *Exp Neurol* 2000; 163: 495-529.

3. Mesulam M. The cholinergic lesion of Alzheimer's disease: pivotal factor or sideshow? *Learn Mem* 2004; 11 : 43-9.

4. Mufson EJ, Counts S, Perez SE, Ginsberg SD. Cholinergic system during the progression of Alzheimer's disease: therapeutic implications. *Exp Rev Neurother* 2008; 8: 1703-18.

5. Williams B, Eriksdotter-Jonhagen M, Granholm L. Nerve growth factor in treatment and pathogenesis of Alzheimer's disease. *Progr Neurobiol Aging* 2006; 80: 114-28.

6. Eriksdotter-Jonhagen M. NGF treatment in dementia. *Alz Dis Ass Disord* 2000; 14: S31-8.

7. Seiler M, Schwab ME. Specific retrograde transport of nerve growth factor (NGF) from neocortex to nucleus basalis in the rat. *Brain Res* 1984; 300: 33-6.

8. Hefti F. Nerve growth factor (NGF) promotes survival of septal cholinergic after fimbrial transections. *J Neurosci* 1986; 6: 2166-72.

9. Cattaneo A, Capsoni S, Paoletti F. Towards non invasive nerve growth factor therapies for Alzheimer's disease. *J Alzheimer Dis* 2008; 15: 255-83.

10. Cuello AC, Bruno MA, Allard S, Leon W, Julita MF. Cholinergic involvement in Alzheimer's disease. A link with NGF maturation and degradation. *J Mol Neurosci* 2010; 40: 230-5.

11. Fahnestock M, Michalski B, Xu B, Coughlin MD. The precursor pro-nerve growth factor is the predominant form of nerve growth factor in the brain and is increased in Alzheimer's disease. *Mol Cell Neurosci* 2001; 18: 210-20.

12. Calissano P, Amaduro G, Matrone C, Ciafre S, Marolda R, Corsetti V, *et al*. Does the term trophic actually mean anti-amyloidogenic? The case of NGF. *Cell Death Differ* 2010; 17: 1126-33.

13. Tuszynski MH. Growth factor gene therapy for neurodegenerative disorders. *Lancet Neurol* 2002; 1 : 51-7.

14. Olson I, Nordberg A, von Holst H, Bäckman L, Ebendal T, Alafuzoff I, *et al*. Nerve growth factor affects 11C-nicotine binding, blood flow, EEG and verbal episodic memory in an Alzheimer patient (case report). *J Neural Transm* 1992; 4: 79-95.

15. Eriksdotter-Jönhagen M, Nordberg A, Amberla K, Bäckman L, Ebendal T, Meyerson B, *et al*. Intracerebroventricular infusion of nerve growth factor in three patients with Alzheimer's disease. *Dement Geriatr Cogn Disord* 1998; 9: 246-57.

16. Hao JX, Ebendal T, Xu XJ, Wiesenfeld-Hallin Z, Eriksdotter Jönhagen M. Intracerebroventricular infusion of nerve growth factor induces pain-like responses in rats. *Neurosci Lett* 2000; 286: 208-12.

17. Nagahara AH, Bernot T, Moseanko R, Brignolo L, Blesch A, Conner JM, *et al*. Long-term reversal of cholinergic neuronal decline in aged non-human primates by lentiviral NGF gene delivery. *Exp Neurol* 2009; 215: 153-9.

18. Tuszynski MH, Thal L, Pay M, Salmon DP, Sang UH, Bakay R, *et al*. A phase 1 clinical trial of nerve growth factor gene therapy for Alzheimers disease. *Nat Med* 2005; 11: 551-5.

19. Lindvall O, Wahlberg L. Encapsulated cell biodelivery of GDNF: a novel clinical strategy for neuroprotection and neuroregeneration in Parkinson's disease? *Exp Neurol* 2008; 209: 82-8.

20. Winn SR, Lindner MD, Lee A, Haggett G, Francis JM, Emerich DF. Polymer-encapsulated genetically modified cells continue to secrete human NGF for over one year in rat ventricles: behavioral and anatomical consequences. *Exp Neurol* 1996; 140: 126-38.

21. Eriksdotter-Jonhagen M, Linderoth B, Almqvist P, Aladellie L, Lind G, Nordberg A, *et al.* Therapy of Alzheimer´s disease with NGF. *Neurobiol Aging* 2010; 31S: S9.

22. Eriksdotter-Jönhagen M, Linderoth B, Lind G, Aladellie L, Almkvist O, Andreasen N, *et al.* Encapsulated cell biodelivery of NGF to the basal forebrain in patients with Alzheimer´s disease. *Dement Geriatr Cogn Disord* 2012; 33: 18-28.

23. Wahlberg LU, Lind G, Almqvist PM, Kusk P, Tornøe J, Juliusson B, *et al.* Targeted therapy of NGF in Alzheimer's disease with EC Biodelivery™: a technology platform for restorative neurosurgery. *J Neurosurg* 2012; 117: 340-7.

24. Fjord-Larsen L, Kusk P, Tornøe J, Juliusson J, Torp M, Bjarkam CR, *et al.* Long-term delivery of nerve growth factor by encapsulated cell biodelivery in the Göttingen minipig basal forebrain. *Mol Ther* 2010; 18: 2164-72.

The CliniBook: Clinical gene transfer
Edited by Odile Cohen-Haguenauer – EDK, Paris © 2012, pp. 475-478

C1-5
Cardiovascular gene therapy trials

SEPPO YLÄ-HERTTUALA

A.I. Virtanen Institute, University of Eastern Finland, P.O. Box 1627, FI-70211 Kuopio, Finland.
seppo.ylaherttuala@uef.fi

INTRODUCTION

Cardiovascular diseases are the leading cause of mortality and morbidity in Western world in spite of improved management of risk factors and availability of significantly improved medical therapies and invasive treatments for coronary heart disease (CHD). Also, peripheral arterial disease is increasingly common in elderly patients and causes significant clinical problems with claudication, delayed ulcer healing and risk of amputations.

In cardiovascular diseases, basic pathological change is atherosclerosis which occludes main arteries bringing blood to heart and peripheral tissues. However, it is well known that if occlusion of arteries develops slowly, many patients can develop collateral arteries that bypass occluded original arteries and maintain adequate tissue perfusion. Therefore, it has been logical to assume that it might be possible to treat severe vascular diseases with therapeutic angiogenesis which aims to grow new capillaries and larger arteries in ischemic tissues [1]. Several growth factors are available to induce therapeutic vascular growth, and phase I/II clinical trials have been conducted in this area [2].

MECHANISMS OF THERAPEUTIC VASCULAR GROWTH

Vascular endothelial growth factors (VEGFs) and fibroblast growth factors (FGFs) are the most commonly used growth factors in therapeutic angiogenesis trials. Other growth factors used for the induction of therapeutic angiogenesis include hepatocyte growth factor and hypoxia-inducible factor-1α. Early experience with injection of recombinant growth factor proteins, however, has clearly shown that recombinant proteins cannot induce any beneficial effects in patients [3]. Growth factors can induce both sprouting angiogenesis and enlargement of existing capillaries and collateral networks. However, it remains unclear how long stimulation in ischemic muscles is needed to induce durable functional new collateral vessels and capillary networks. Currently it is assumed that transient expression for a few weeks should be enough for a useful therapeutic effect. This opinion is based on numerous animal experiments, which have demonstrated safety and efficacy of this treatment approach both in CHD and peripheral vascular disease [3].

Table I. Vascular gene therapy trials.

Trial	Therapeutic [target] application	Therapeutic agent	Administration	Control treatment	n	Primary endpoint	[a]Results
Peripheral arterial disease							
VEGF peripheral vascular disease trial	Therapeutic angiogenesis in PAD (claudication)	AdVEGF$_{165}$ or Plasmid/ liposome VEGF$_{165}$	Intraarterial injection at the angioplasty site	Ringer's lactate	54	Increased vascularity in angiography at 3 months	Positive
RAVE trial	Therapeutic angiogenesis in PAD (claudication)	AdVEGF$_{121}$	Intramuscular injections	Vehicle (no virus)	105	PWT at 12 weeks	Negative
Tamaris	Therapeutic angiogenesis in PAD (CLI)	Naked FGF-1 plasmid	Intramuscular injections	Vehicle	525	Time to major amputation or death at 1 yr	Negative
Coronary heart disease							
KAT	Therapeutic angiogenesis in CAD (CCS class II-III)	AdVEGF$_{165}$ or plasmid/ liposome VEGF$_{165}$	Intracoronary injection at the angioplasty site	Ringer's lactate	103	Improved myocardial perfusion at 6 months	Positive (adenovirus group only)
REVASC trial	Therapeutic angiogenesis in CAD (CCS II-IV)	AdVEGF$_{121}$	Intramyocardial injection via mini thoracotomy	Best medical treatment (no placebo treatment)	67	Time to 1 mm ST-segment depression on ETT at 26 weeks	Positive
Euroinject one trial	Therapeutic angiogenesis in CAD (CCS III-IV) Naked	VEGF$_{165}$	Plasmid Percutaneous Intramyocardial injections	Placebo plasmid	74	Improved myocardial perfusion at 3 months	Negative
AGENT-3	Therapeutic angiogenesis in CAD (CCS II-IV)	AdFGF-4	Intracoronary injection	Vehicle	416	ETT at 12 weeks	Negative (subgroup of >55 yr with CCS III-IV positive)
AGENT-4	Therapeutic angiogenesis in CAD (CCS II-IV)	AdFGF-4	Intracoronary injection	Vehicle	116	ETT at 12 weeks	Negative

Abbreviations: ABI, ankle brachial index; Ad, adenovirus; CLI, critical limb ischemic; FGF, fibroblast growth factor; HIF-1α, hypoxia inducible factor-1α; HGF, hepatocyte growth factor; PAD, peripheral arterial disease; PWT, peak walking time; VEGF, vascular endothelial growth factor.

[a] A measure of the efficacy in relation to the study protocol-defined primary or secondary endpoint.

Abbreviations: Ad, adenovirus; apoB, apolipoprotein B; CAD, coronary artery disease; CCS, Canadian cardiovascular society; ETT, exercise tolerance testing; FGF, fibroblast growth factor; HIF-1α, hypoxia inducible factor-1α; LDL, low density lipoprotein; SPECT, single-photon emission computed tomography; VEGF, vascular endothelial growth factor.

[a] A measure of the efficacy in relation to the study protocol-defined primary or secondary endpoint α.

CLINICAL GENE THERAPY TRIALS FOR THERAPEUTIC ANGIOGENESIS

Angiogenic VEGF gene therapy was initially tested with naked plasmids both in peripheral vascular disease and CHD, but current experience seems to justify conclusion that plasmid vectors may not be efficient enough to prominently increase myocardial perfusion, collateral growth, or improve clinical status of the patients. Most commonly used vector in vascular applications is adenovirus. Some vascular gene therapy trials are listed in *Table I*.

For the peripheral vascular disease adenoviral delivery of VEGF has produced increased vascularity in angiography at 3 months in patients with severe peripheral vascular disease after intra-arterial catheter-mediated injection [4]. However, RAVE trial [5] and Tamaris [6] trial produced negative primary endpoints. Therefore, it is currently unclear what is the efficacy of direct gene transfer to peripheral muscles in human patients. Most likely, low gene transfer efficiency and inefficient delivery route may have compromised clinical outcomes of trials in peripheral vascular disease.

In CHD intracoronary injection of adenovirus expressing VEGF has produced positive endpoint as improved myocardial perfusion at 6 month timepoint [7] in patients with moderate to severe CHD. However, Revasc [8] and Euroinject trial [9] with direct intramuscular injection of plasmid-driven VEGF expression and AGENT-4 trial [10] with intracoronary injection of adenovirus FGF-4 produced negative results, although a subgroup in AGENT-3 [10] trial showed a positive endpoint in exercise tolerance test.

Current conclusion about the experience from cardiovascular gene therapy trials is that inefficient delivery systems and too low gene transfer efficiency have probably resulted in less than optimal clinical outcomes. Improving efficiency of the gene delivery and time of expression of the growth factors are factors that need to be optimized in further clinical trials. Also, more long-term expression with AAV and lentiviral vectors might be an option although it is clear that unregulated long-term expression of angiogenic growth factors does not produce useful physiological changes in large animal models [11].

Safety of gene therapy trials with adenoviral and plasmid vectors has been very good and recently two long-term follow-up studies have confirmed that there is no increased risk of cancer or other adverse effects in patients treated with both plasmid and adenoviral delivered VEGFs [12, 13].

ACKNOWLEDGEMENTS

This study was supported by grants from the Academy of Finland, Tekes (the Finnish Funding Agency for Technology and Innovation).
This work has been performed with the support of the EC-DG research through the FP6-Network of Excellence, CLINIGENE: LSHB-CT-2006-018933.

REFERENCES

1. Ylä-Herttuala S, Alitalo K. Gene transfer as a tool to induce therapeutic vascular growth. *Nat Med* 2003; 9: 694-701.

2. Ylä-Herttuala S, Rissanen TT, Vajanto I, Hartikainen J. Vascular endothelial growth factors. Biology and current status of clinical applications in cardiovascular medicine. *J Am Coll Cardiol* 2007; 49: 1015-26.

3. Rissanen TT, Ylä-Herttuala, S. Current status of cardiovascular gene therapy. *Mol Ther* 2007; 15: 1233-47.

4. Mäkinen K, Manninen H, Hedman M, Matsi P, Mussalo H, Alhava, E, Ylä-Herttuala S. Increased vascularity detected by digital subtraction angiography after VEGF gene transfer to human lower limb artery. A randomized, placebo- controlled, double-blinded phase II study. *Mol Ther* 2002; 6: 127-33.

5. Rajagopalan S, Mohler ER 3rd, Lederman RJ, Mendelsohn FO, Saucedo JF, Goldman, CK, *et al.* Regional angiogenesis with vascular endothelial growth factor in peripheral arterial disease: a phase II randomized, double-blind, controlled study of adenoviral delivery of vascular endothelial growth factor 121 in patients with disabling intermittent claudication. *Circulation* 2003; 108: 1933-8.

6. Belch J, Hiatt WR, Baumgartner I, Driver IV, Nikol S, Norgren L, Van Belle E, on behalf of the TAMARIS Committees and Investigators. Effect of fibroblast growth factor NV1FGF on amputation and death: a randomised placebo-controlled trial of gene therapy in critical limb ischaemia. *Lancet* 2011; 377: 1929-37.

7. Hedman M, Hartikainen J, Syvänne M, Stjernvall J, Hedman A, Kivelä A, *et al.* Safety and feasibility of catheter-based local intracoronary vascular endothelial growth factor gene transfer in the prevention of postangioplasty and in-stent restenosis and in the treatment of chronic myocardial ischemia. *Circulation* 2003; 107: 2677-83.

8. Stewart DJ, Hilton JD, Arnold JM, Gregoire J, Rivard A, Archer SL, *et al.* Angiogenic gene therapy in patients with nonrevascularizable ischemic heart disease: a phase 2 randomized, controlled trial of AdVEGF(121) (AdVEGF121) versus maximum medical treatment. *Gene Ther* 2006; 13: 1503-11.

9. Kastrup J, Jorgensen E, Ruck A, Tagil K, Glogar D, Ruzyllo, W, *et al.* Direct intramyocardial plasmid vascular endothelial growth factor-A165 gene therapy in patients with stable severe angina pectoris. A randomized double-blind placebo-controlled study: the Euroinject One trial. *J Am Coll Cardiol* 2005; 45: 982-8.

10. Barbeau G, Beatt K, Betriu A, Janssens S, Martinez-Rios M, Mautner B, *et al.* Adenoviral fibroblast growth factor-4 gene therapy in patients with stable angina. 12-month results of a double blind randomized multicenter trial. *J Am Coll Cardiol* 2006; 47 (suppl 1): 305A.

11. Karvinen H, Pasanen E, Rissanen TT, Korpisalo P, Vähäkangas E, Jazwa A, *et al.* Long-term VEGF-A expression promotes aberrant angiogenesis and fibrosis in skeletal muscle. *Gene Ther* 2011; 18: 1180.

12. Muona K, Mäkinen K, Hedman M, Manninen H, Ylä-Herttuala S. 10-year safety follow-up in patients with local VEGF gene transfer to ischaemic lower limb. *Gene Ther* 2011, July 21 (online). doi: 10.1038/gt.2011.109.

13. Hedman M, Muona K, Hedman A, Kivelä A, Syvänne M, Eränen J, *et al.* Eight-year safety follow-up of coronary artery disease patients after local intracoronary VEGF gene transfer. *Gene Ther* 2009; 16: 629-34.

The CliniBook: Clinical gene transfer
Edited by Odile Cohen-Haguenauer – EDK, Paris © 2012, pp. 479-485

C1-6
AAV-mediated gene therapy for haemophilia B

DEEPAK RAJ[1,3], EDWARD G.D. TUDDENHAM[1,2], ARTHUR W. NIENHUIS[4], ULRIKE REISS[4], ANDREW M. DAVIDOFF[5], AMIT C. NATHWANI[1,2,3*]

[1]*Department of Haematology, UCL Cancer Institute,* [2]*Katharine Dormandy Haemophilia Centre and Thrombosis Unit, Royal Free NHS Trust,* [3]*National Health Services Blood and Transplant, United Kingdom and* [4]*Department of Hematology,* [5]*Department of Surgery, St. Jude Children's Research Hospital, Memphis, TN, USA.*
amit.nathwani@ucl.ac.uk
*Corresponding author

INTRODUCTION

Haemophilia B, an X-linked bleeding condition has long been recognised as an ideal target for gene therapy approaches. It is a monogenetic disorder that arises because of mutations in the *Factor 9 (FIX)* gene, which codes for the FIX protein, a serine protease that is essential for normal blood clot formation [1]. Therefore, haemophilia B patients suffer from recurrent, often life threatening, bleeding episodes that occur without any apparent injury. What makes haemophilia B a good target for gene therapy is that a small increase in blood FIX levels, to above 1% of its normal values in the blood, is sufficient to reduce the severity of the bleeding episodes and risk of death [2]. Additionally the *FIX* cDNA is small enough to fit into most vector systems. Current treatment consisting of FIX protein concentrate infusion is effective at arresting bleeding episodes but it is not curative. Prophylaxis with FIX protein concentrates has been shown to reduce the frequency of spontaneous bleeding but entails injections of FIX protein every two to three days (due to the short half life of the protein) for the lifetime of patients, which is invasive, inconvenient and expensive (£100,000/year/patient). Consequently this is available to only about 20% of the world's haemophilia patients who live in affluent countries [3].

Many different vector systems have been evaluated for haemophilia gene therapy, each having strengths and weaknesses [4-6]. Because FIX replacement is safe and effective, gene therapy must also offer a high potential for benefit with only a minimal risk. Therefore, we and others have focused on vectors based on adeno-associated virus (AAV) since these vectors have an excellent safety profile [7-10]. AAV is endemic in the human population but does not cause disease. It mediates expression mainly from episomal copies and has a low propensity to integrate into chromosomal DNA, thus reducing the risk of insertional oncogenesis [11]. Importantly, a single administration of AAV vector encoding FIX has resulted in long-term expression of FIX at therapeutic levels in murine and canine models of haemophilia B resulting in lifetime correction of the bleeding tendency without toxicity [12-15]. It has proven harder to get similar results in patients with severe haemophilia B. Intramuscular administration of AAV2 vectors encoding hFIX was safe [16]. Muscle biopsy showed evidence of expression of hFIX at the site of administration but this did not result in sustained plasma FIX levels at >1% of physiologic values [17]. A subsequent trial with AAV2 vectors administered into the hepatic artery was briefly effective in one subject of seven treated. This subject was treated at the highest dose of 2×10^{12} vg/kg and showed an increase in plasma hFIX levels to peak values of 12% of normal at approximately 4 weeks after gene transfer. Unfortunately, the transduced liver cells were subsequently eliminated by a T-cell mediated immune response to vector capsid peptide expressed on the surface of transduced hepatocytes. Consequently the plasma FIX level fell to base line values of <1% within 8 weeks of vector infusion [18].

PRECLINICAL EVALUATION OF A NOVEL APPROACH FOR GENE THERAPY OF HAEMOPHILIA B

We developed an approach for gene therapy of haemophilia B with the aim of overcoming some of the obstacles faced by the previous AAV-based haemophilia B clinical trials. A codon optimised version of the *hFIX* (*hFIXco*) gene was synthesized and cloned downstream of a compact synthetic liver-specific promoter (*LP1*) to enable packaging into self-complementary AAV vectors (scAAV-LP1-hFIXco), which have a packaging capacity of only 2.3kb [19]. Our preclinical studies in mice and non-human primates (NHP) showed that scAAV vectors were more potent than comparable single stranded AAV (ssAAV) vectors, raising the possibility of achieving therapeutic levels of hFIX using lower and potentially safer doses of vector [20, 21]. Finally, the scAAV-LP1-hFIXco vector was pseudotyped with AAV serotype 8 capsid. This offered several potential advantages over strategies using AAV2 vectors, including the following:

(i) The lower seroprevalence in humans (~25% compared with over 70% for AAV2) [22], thus providing an greater likelihood of potential participants being naïve to the study vector serotype.

(ii) More rapid uncoating and transduction of host cells, resulting in higher transgene expression following administration of AAV8 vectors when compared to AAV2 vectors.[24]

(iii) Efficient transduction of hepatocytes following vector administration by the peripheral venous route due to the unique tropism of AAV8 for the liver [25]. This simple non-invasive route of vector administration made vector administration safer for patients with a bleeding diathesis than when vector was administered using more invasive procedures.

The safety and efficacy of peripheral vein administration of scAAV-LP1-hFIXco was assessed in non-human primates (NHP) prior to initiating the clinical trial. The NHP model enabled us to establish that:

(i) AAV vectors pseudotyped with AAV8 capsid could mediate efficient gene transfer in animals with pre-existing immunity to an alternative serotype of AAV due to wild-type infection or prior vector [23].

(ii) Biodistribution of scAAV2/8-LP1-hFIXco following peripheral vein administration was comparable to that observed after administration of the same dose of vector into the mesenteric vein [26].

(iii) Expression of transgenic FIX protein was maintained at therapeutic levels for over 8 years following administration of a single dose of vector, and expression levels remain within the therapeutic range [27].

(iv) Liver tumours were not observed following gene transfer with scAAV2/8-LP1-hFIXco in NHP (n=23) as assessed by annual ultrasound scan and regular survey of the liver following laparotomy and serial liver biopsies. Molecular studies confirmed that most of the AAV genomes were maintained in an episomal form [26, 27]. Integration of vector into the host cell genome was detected at low frequency and seemed to occur randomly within coding and non-coding regions with no evidence of activation of oncogenes or disruption of tumour suppressor genes (unpublished data).

THE ENROLMENT PROCESS FOR A PHASE I TRIAL USING SCAAV2/8-LP1-HFIXCO FOR GENE THERAPY OF HAEMOPHILIA B

The first 6 patients to enter the trial were recruited in London and treated over a 12 month period at minimum intervals of 6 weeks between patients. Subjects had to be over the age of 18 years with severe haemophilia B with no evidence of inhibitors, negative for hepatitis C RNA and HIV, and with normal liver function. Subjects also took part in an extensive informed consent process at two levels. At the first level (screening consent), the trial process was outlined and likely risks explained so that informed consent for tests to determine eligibility could be given. Following these tests about a third of the volunteers were found eligible to proceed. Common reason for ineligibility were presence of pre-existing antibodies to AAV serotype 8, evidence of on-going infection with hepatitis B or C virus or HIV or a higher risk of developing neutralising antibody to FIX protein. A second level of more detailed informed consent was carried out for the subjects eligible to proceed, with independent assessment of the subjects' grasp of the risk involved and willingness to enter the trial.

THE MAIN OBSERVATIONS OF THE PHASE I CLINICAL TRIAL

The recruited subjects were divided into 3 cohorts of 2 participants each and received scAAV2/8-LP1-hFIXco vector by peripheral vein at vector doses of $2x10^{11}$ vg/kg, $6x10^{11}$ vg/kg and $2x10^{12}$ vg/kg respectively.

The low dose subjects who consented did so in the full knowledge that the vector dose they would receive was unlikely to benefit them, and would also preclude their having a further dose of the same vector as their immune system would reject subsequently administered AAV particles of the same serotype. Both low-dose subjects achieved hFIX levels of approximately 2% of normal as assessed by a bioactivity assay (one-stage clotting assay) following vector infusion. This level was significantly higher than their baseline FIX activity of <1% of normal and was consistent with endogenous synthesis of FIX. The first subject was able to discontinue prophylaxis and has remained free of spontaneous bleeds, though he has required on-demand FIX treatment on 8 occasions over a period of 2 years to cover accidental injuries and elective surgery. The second patient has needed to continue on prophylaxis, albeit with decreased frequency of dosing, due to much more severe pre-existing joint damage which further increased his risk of bleeding.

As both subjects had attained levels of less than 3%, which was below our therapeutic endpoint, the next two subjects were treated at the intermediate dose level of $6x10^{11}$ vg/kg. Subject 3 attained a stable base line of 2%, but due to pre-existing joint damage has needed to continue prophylaxis, but at increased intervals of once every 2 weeks compared to twice weekly before gene transfer. Subject 4 attained a baseline level of approximately 3% and has not required prophylaxis for over a year.

At the highest dose level of $2x10^{12}$vg/kg, peak hFIX levels of 8% and 12% were achieved in subjects 5 and 6 respectively. Subject 5 appeared to develop a cellular immune response to transduced hepatocytes, which resulted in a 10-fold increase in liver enzymes and a drop in hFIX levels to 3% of normal at around 7 weeks after therapy. A course of prednisolone was administered, leading to resolution of liver inflammation without complete loss of transgene expression. This subject has not required prophylaxis for over 12 months following gene transfer. Subject 6 also developed a slight increase in liver enzyme levels over baseline at around 9 weeks following therapy. Although liver enzymes levels were still within the normal range the subject was started on a course of prednisolone to avert a full-blown T cell response against the transduced hepatocytes. His liver enzyme levels promptly returned to baseline values and he has not required any treatment with FIX concentrates despite living a very active life.

None of the subjects developed neutralizing antibodies to hFIX, though all 6 participants did develop a humoral immune response to AAV8 capsid. More crucial was the development of a T cell mediated immune response to the viral capsid, as assessed by ELISpot assay. This response appeared to be dose dependent, as it did not appear in the low dose cohort, but was detectable above baseline values in the subjects in the intermediate and high dose cohorts. It is unclear why a transminitis was not observed in the intermediate dose cohort. One possibility is that the capsid antigen load in these subjects may have been lower than the threshold required to trigger a "full-blown" immunological response resulting in loss of hepatocytes and a rise in liver enzymes.

SUMMARY AND FUTURE CHALLENGES

A single peripheral vein administration of our novel scAAV2/8-LP1-hFIXco vector was sufficient to mediate hFIX synthesis in all the patients in the study, even at the lowest vector dose. Expression of transgenic hFIX has been maintained at levels >1% of normal for at least 12 months. Four of the six patients enrolled have been able to discontinue prophylaxis without suffering spontaneous bleeding episodes even when they undertook activity that had previously triggered a bleed.

A cellular immune response directed against transduced hepatocytes was clearly observed in one of the patients in the high dose cohort at about 7 weeks following gene transfer. This resolved following commencement of a course of glucocorticoids. The other patient developed a smaller increase of liver enzymes, though this occurred after a period of intense physical activity, and may therefore not represent vector-mediated toxicity.

Further studies which involve expansion of the high dose cohort are underway to address the following questions:

(i) Will vector induced transaminitis occur in all subjects treated at the highest dose level?

(ii) Will prophylactic use of glucocorticoids at the first sign of increase in liver enzymes abrogate the cellular T cell response without compromising transgene expression?

(iii) What will be the effect of removing empty particles, which accounted for about 90% of the capsid protein load infused, on transgene expression and cellular immunity [29]?

As the vector genome is maintained in an episomal form, it is expected that the transgene expression may decrease over time. All of our subjects remain under observation so that we can define the total duration of expression following scAAV-mediated gene transfer.

Our study, aside from demonstrating the potential of scAAV vectors to mediate expression of transgenic hFIX at therapeutic levels, has highlighted the need for more reliable assays for quantification of biologically active viral particles and contaminants within clinical grade vector preparations, as well as the need for more efficient scalable methods for vector production so that sufficient vector can be made to support the wider availability of this approach.

An important factor that undoubtedly contributed to the success of the trial was the willingness of several groups to work together towards a common goal of successful and safe gene transfer for haemophilia B. This goal appears to have been accomplished in part but longer follow-up and a larger cohort of patients is now required to establish the duration of transgene expression and the absence of long-term toxicity.

ACKNOWLEDGMENTS

This work was supported by Medical Research Council, UK, The Katharine Dormandy Trust, UK, Department of Health, UK, NHSBT, UK Department of Health's NIHR Biomedical Research Centres funding award to UCLH/UCL, UK, NIHR Programme Grant A for Molecular and Tissue Engineering, UK, as well as The ASSISI Foundation of Memphis, the American Lebanese Syrian Associated Charities (ALSAC), The National Heart, Lung, and Blood Institute grant HL094396 in the United States, The Royal Free Hospital Charity Special Trustees Fund 35, The Royal Free Hospital NHS Trust. This article presents independent research commissioned by the National Institute for Health Research (NIHR) under its Programme Grants scheme (RP-PG-0310-1001). The views expressed in this publication are those of the author(s) and not necessarily those of the NHS, the NIHR or the Department of Health in the UK.

We thank Anja Griffioen, Paul Eddlemon, Alison Evans, and Paul Lloyd-Evans for their help with trial related activities including vector importation and qualification, data entry as well as regulatory affairs.

We are deeply indebted to all the study subjects for their interest and participation in this study.

REFERENCES

1. Nathwani AC, Tuddenham EG. Epidemiology of coagulation disorders. *Baillieres Clin Haematol* 1992; 5: 383-439.

2. White GC 2nd, Rosendaal F, Aledort LM, Lusher JM, Rothschild C, Ingerslev J. Definitions in hemophilia. Recommendation of the scientific subcommittee on factor VIII and factor IX of the scientific and standardization committee of the international society on thrombosis and haemostasis. *Thromb Haemost* 2001; 85: 560.

3. Ponder KP, Srivastava A. Walk a mile in the moccasins of people with haemophilia. *Haemophilia* 2008; 14: 618-20.

4. Roth DA, Tawa NE Jr, O'Brien JM, Treco DA, Selden RF. Nonviral transfer of the gene encoding coagulation factor VIII in patients with severe hemophilia A. *N Engl J Med* 2001; 344: 1735-42.

5. Powell JS, Ragni MV, White GC 2nd, Lusher JM, Hillman-Wiseman C, Moon TE, Cole V, Ramanathan-Girish S, *et al.* Phase 1 trial of fviii gene transfer for severe hemophilia a using a retroviral construct administered by peripheral intravenous infusion. *Blood* 2003; 102: 2038-45.

6. Chuah MK, Collen D, VandenDriessche T. Clinical gene transfer studies for hemophilia A. *Semin Thromb Hemost* 2004; 30: 249-56.

7. Brantly ML, Chulay JD, Wang L, Mueller C, Humphries M, Spencer LT, Rouhani F, Conlon TJ, *et al.* Sustained transgene expression despite T lymphocyte responses in a clinical trial of rAAV1-AAT gene therapy. *Proc Natl Acad Sci USA* 2009; 106: 16363-8.

8. Mendell JR, Rodino-Klapac LR, Rosales XQ, Coley BD, Galloway G, Lewis S, Malik V, Shilling C, *et al.* Sustained alpha-sarcoglycan gene expression after gene transfer in limb-girdle muscular dystrophy, type 2d. *Ann Neurol* 2010; 68: 629-38.

9. Simonelli F, Maguire AM, Testa F, Pierce EA, Mingozzi F, Bennicelli JL, Rossi S, Marshall K, *et al.* Gene therapy for Leber's congenital amaurosis is safe and effective through 1.5 years after vector administration. *Mol Ther* 2010; 18: 643-50.

10. Maguire AM, High KA, Auricchio A, Wright JF, Pierce EA, Testa F, Mingozzi F, Bennicelli JL, *et al.* Age-dependent effects of RPE65 gene therapy for Leber's congenital amaurosis: a phase 1 dose-escalation trial. *Lancet* 2009; 374: 1597-605.

11. Nakai H, Yant SR, Storm TA, Fuess S, Meuse L, Kay MA. Extrachromosomal recombinant adeno-associated virus vector genomes are primarily responsible for stable liver transduction *in vivo*. *J Virol* 2001; 75: 6969-76.

12. Chao H, Samulski R, Bellinger D, Monahan P, Nichols T, Walsh C. Persistent expression of canine factor IX in hemophilia B canines. *Gene Ther* 1999; 6: 1695-704.

13. Chao H, Monahan PE, Liu Y, Samulski RJ, Walsh CE. Sustained and complete phenotype correction of hemophilia B mice following intramuscular injection of AAV1 serotype vectors. *Mol Ther* 2001; 4: 217-22.

14. Mount JD, Herzog RW, Tillson DM, Goodman SA, Robinson N, McCleland ML, Bellinger D, Nichols TC, *et al.* Sustained phenotypic correction of hemophilia B dogs with a factor IX null mutation by liver-directed gene therapy. *Blood* 2002; 99: 2670-6.

15. Harding TC, Koprivnikar KE, Tu GH, Zayek N, Lew S, Subramanian A, Sivakumaran A, Frey D, *et al.* Intravenous administration of an AAV-2 vector for the expression of factor IX in mice and a dog model of hemophilia B. *Gene Ther* 2004; 11: 204-13.

16. Kay MA, Manno CS, Ragni MV, Larson PJ, Couto LB, McClelland A, Glader B, Chew AJ, *et al.* Evidence for gene transfer and expression of factor IX in haemophilia B patients treated with an AAV vector. *Nat Genet* 2000; 24: 257-61.

17. Manno CS, Chew AJ, Hutchison S, Larson PJ, Herzog RW, Arruda VR, Tai SJ, Ragni MV, *et al.* Aav-mediated factor IX gene transfer to skeletal muscle in patients with severe hemophilia B. *Blood* 2003; 101: 2963-72.

18. Manno CS, Pierce GF, Arruda VR, Glader B, Ragni M, Rasko JJ, Ozelo MC, Hoots K, *et al.* Successful transduction of liver in hemophilia by aav-factor ix and limitations imposed by the host immune response. *Nat Med* 2006; 12: 342-7.

19. Nathwani AC, Gray JT, Ng CY, Zhou J, Spence Y, Waddington SN, Tuddenham EG, Kemball-Cook G, *et al.* Self-complementary adeno-associated virus vectors containing a novel liver-specific human factor IX expression cassette enable highly efficient transduction of murine and nonhuman primate liver. *Blood* 2006; 107: 2653-61.

20. Wang Z, Ma HI, Li J, Sun L, Zhang J, Xiao X. Rapid and highly efficient transduction by double-stranded adeno-associated virus vectors *in vitro* and *in vivo. Gene Ther* 2003; 10: 2105-11.

21. McCarty DM, Fu H, Monahan PE, Toulson CE, Naik P, Samulski RJ. Adeno-associated virus terminal repeat (TR) mutant generates self-complementary vectors to overcome the rate-limiting step to transduction *in vivo. Gene Ther* 2003; 10: 2112-8.

22. Gao GP, Alvira MR, Wang L, Calcedo R, Johnston J, Wilson JM. Novel adeno-associated viruses from Rhesus monkeys as vectors for human gene therapy. *Proc Natl Acad Sci USA* 2002; 99: 11854-9.

23. Davidoff AM, Gray JT, Ng CY, Zhang Y, Zhou J, Spence Y, Bakar Y, Nathwani AC. Comparison of the ability of adeno-associated viral vectors pseudotyped with serotype 2, 5, and 8 capsid proteins to mediate efficient transduction of the liver in murine and nonhuman primate models. *Mol Ther* 2005; 11: 875-88.

24. Thomas CE, Storm TA, Huang Z, Kay MA. Rapid uncoating of vector genomes is the key to efficient liver transduction with pseudotyped adeno-associated virus vectors. *J Virol* 2004; 78: 3110-22.

25. Nakai H, Fuess S, Storm TA, Muramatsu S, Nara Y, Kay MA. Unrestricted hepatocyte transduction with adeno-associated virus serotype 8 vectors in mice. *J Virol* 2005; 79: 214-24.

26. Nathwani AC, Gray JT, McIntosh J, Ng CY, Zhou J, Spence Y, Cochrane M, Gray E, *et al.* Safe and efficient transduction of the liver after peripheral vein infusion of self-complementary aav vector results in stable therapeutic expression of human fix in nonhuman primates. *Blood* 2007; 109: 1414-21.

27. Nathwani AC, Rosales C, McIntosh J, Rastegarlari G, Nathwani D, Raj D, Nawathe S, Waddington SN, *et al.* Long-term safety and efficacy following systemic administration of a self-complementary aav vector encoding human fix pseudotyped with serotype 5 and 8 capsid proteins. *Mol Ther* 2011; 19: 876-85.

28. Nathwani AC, Tuddenham EG, Rangarajan S, Rosales C, McIntosh J, Linch DC, Chowdary P, Riddell A, *et al.* Adenovirus-associated virus vector-mediated gene transfer in hemophilia B. *N Engl J Med* 2011; 365: 2357-65.

29. Allay JA, Sleep S, Long S, Tillman DM, Clark R, Carney G, Fagone P, McIntosh JH, *et al.* Good manufacturing practice production of self-complementary serotype 8 adeno-associated viral vector for a hemophilia B clinical trial. *Hum Gene Ther* 2011; 22: 595-604.

The CliniBook: Clinical gene transfer
Edited by Odile Cohen-Haguenauer – EDK, Paris © 2012, pp. 486-491

C1-7
ProSavin®: a lentiviral vector approach for the treatment of Parkinson's disease

STÉPHANE PALFI[1*], R. SCOTT RALPH[2], KYRIACOS MITROPHANOUS[2]

[1]*Service de neurochirurgie, APHP, Hôpital Henri Mondor, 51, avenue du Maréchal de Lattre de Tassigny, UPEC, Faculté de médecine, 94010 Créteil Cedex, France.*
[2]*Oxford BioMedica plc, The Oxford Science Park, Medawar Centre, Oxford OX4 4GA, United Kingdom.*
stéphane.palfi@hmn.aphp.fr
*Corresponding author

Parkinson's disease is a progressive disorder of the central nervous system (CNS) that affects over two million people in Europe and the United States [1-3]. Clinically, the disease is characterized by a decrease in spontaneous movements, gait difficulty, postural instability, rigidity and tremor leading to significant disability 10 to 15 years after the onset of the disease [4]. Parkinson's disease is commonly characterised by a degeneration of numerous neuronal pathways within the CNS. The most important being the loss of pigmented neurons within the substantia nigra that project afferences to the striatum, resulting in decreased dopamine availability. The clinical symptomatology manifests when the loss of dopamine in the striatum is in excess of 60% [4].

The quality of life for PD patients has significantly improved since the widespread use of the dopamine precursor L-dihydroxyphenylalanine (L-DOPA) and there is likely to be an improvement on survival from using this treatment (reviewed in [5]). However, the association of the progression of dopamine depletion and the prolonged intake of intermittent oral L-DOPA is associated with irregular involuntary movements known as dyskinesias (reviewed in [6]). Symptoms called motor fluctuations can also occur with the progression of the disease and reflect the decreased efficiency of L-DOPA conversion to dopamine. Dyskinesias and motor fluctuations are associated with a hyperactive response to dopamine replacement [7] coupled with an increased loss of dopaminergic neurons. As the disease advances there is an increased requirement for higher doses of L-DOPA to manage the PD symptoms, but this in turn leads to increased motor fluctuations. These fluctuations in motor function are described as the "ON/OFF" phenomena in which L-DOPA provides periods of benefit ("ON") and periods where the benefit is wearing off ("OFF") prior to the next dose. Such fluctuations are correlated with the highest and lowest plasma concentrations of dopamine [8], where peak plasma levels produce dyskinesias and the trough between doses results in an akinetic state. Motor fluctuations are also linked to decreased L-DOPA absorption in the proximal small intestine and disrupted gastric emptying [9], thereby implicating a real clinical need for continual delivery of dopamine to the striatum. A number of studies have assessed L-DOPA infusions *via* intravenous and enteric routes. Improvements in clinical motor fluctuation have been demonstrated and stability of plasma concentrations observed, in addition to being safe and well tolerated [10]. It is estimated that less than one percent of orally administered L-DOPA penetrates the brain and despite advances to increase its availability in the CNS and reduce peripheral side effects, with various metabolic enzyme inhibitors, only five to 10% reaches the brain. It should however be recognised that with advancing severity of PD the link between plasma levels of L-DOPA and the motor responses become less definite, such that patients experience sudden "OFF" periods and have variable delays in response to subsequent L-DOPA doses. In addition to disruptions in motor function, systemic administration of L-DOPA, either *via* oral or infusion formulations is associated with neuropsychological adverse reactions and peripheral side effects such as nausea and vomiting, hypotension, cardiac arrhythmias and gastric disturbances.

All these therapeutic issues and discomfort highlight the need to develop novel methods to induce a continuous and local release of dopamine in the striatum.

Thus, the rationale for a dopamine gene therapy approach in Parkinson's disease is to provide sufficient dopamine locally to the striatum to restore beneficial movements but in the absence of central and peripheral side effects, by delivering a continual supply of dopamine. This is potentially beneficial by 'smoothing out' the dopamine stimulation and hence reducing the motor function side effects associated with the pulsatile delivery of exogenous L-DOPA. This finding would have a significant impact on the management of PD as it is thought that the chronic exposure to exogenous L-DOPA is part of an as yet poorly defined mechanism for creating predisposition to dyskinesia and reducing the sensitivity to L-DOPA.

There are two types of gene delivery systems currently being explored as gene therapy approaches to the treatment of PD. One is based on Adeno-Associated Virus (AAV) and the other on lentiviruses, which have been considered to be appropriate vectors for the delivery and long-term expression of the genes required for therapy. While the absolute merits of the two vector systems will emerge over time, the lentiviruses appear to be well-suited for this type of therapy. Lentiviral vectors derived from non human primates (NHP) are promising gene therapy delivery systems as they are capable of transducing non-dividing cells such as neurons and are able to maintain long term expression [11, 12].

ProSavin® is made using a lentiviral vector based on the equine infections anaemia virus (EIAV). It has been modified such that it no longer carries any of the original viral genes and has had all extraneous viral nucleic acids removed so that approximately 10% of the original virus remains [13-15]. ProSavin® delivers three human genes critical to the dopamine biosynthetic pathway. The vector inserts these genes permanently into the chromosomes by a process referred to as integration. The proteins encoded by ProSavin® vector are, a truncated form of the human tyrosine hydroxylase (TH) gene (which lacks the N-terminal 160 amino acids involved in feedback regulation of TH [16]), the human aromatic L-amino-acid decarboxylase (AADC), and the human GTP-cyclohydrolase 1 (CH1) gene.

ProSavin® integrates into human chromosomes and assays have been developed to determine the site preference for EIAV vectors, including ProSavin®. In studies where the integration site of vector was mapped to chromosomal position, no integration hot spots, as defined as more than one integration site located within a 100kb region, were observed in a total of more than 500 sites analysed. These studies also demonstrated that there was no obvious preference for integration within specific chromosomes. ProSavin® demonstrates a similar preference for gene-rich regions of the chromosome, as has been identified for other lentiviruses and lentiviral vector systems [17].

Dopamine is synthesized in a pathway that involves the enzymes TH, that catalyses the synthesis of L-DOPA from tyrosine, and AADC, that converts L-DOPA to dopamine. Additionally, TH has a requirement for a cofactor, tetrahydrobiopterin (BH4), the biosynthesis of which is rate-limited by CH1 (*Figure 1*). The human genes for each of these enzymes have been inserted into the ProSavin® lentiviral vector in such a way as to allow coordinated expression in the target cell. In experimental studies, non-dopaminergic cell lines and primary rat embryonic striatal neurons were engineered to secrete dopamine by treatment with this vector. It is important to note that even cells that do not have the specialised secretory vesicles for releasing dopamine at presynaptic terminals, and this includes striatal neurons, will release dopamine. Furthermore the production of dopamine in non-dopaminergic primary striatal neurons did not affect the GABAergic phenotype of these cells, as assessed by GABA release assays.

The mechanism of action of ProSavin® is therefore to enable striatal neurons to produce and secrete dopamine. The dopamine diffuses throughout the putamen and it is assumed that it interacts with the dopamine receptors on the surface of the striatal neurons and initiates a dopaminergic signalling pathway that is evidently therapeutic. This model for the mechanism of action is supported by nonclinical studies that show efficacy at the level of whole animal behaviour, at the level of brain metabolism and single neuronal electrophysiology.

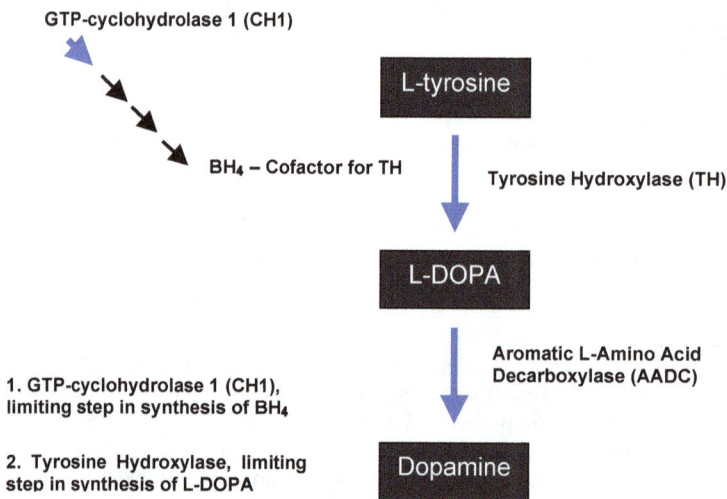

Figure 1. Dopamine biosynthetic pathway.

The effects of ProSavin® have been studied both *in vivo* and *in vitro* using appropriate animal models and cell based assays to assess the potential clinical risks and benefits of ProSavin®. Early studies used prototype vectors and some changes have been made during development. All of the pivotal toxicology and biodistribution studies have used the exact manufacturing process. Nonclinical pharmacology studies have been performed with ProSavin® in two well established and commonly used animal models of PD, the 6-Hydroxydopamine (6-OHDA) lesioned rat model and the MPTP lesioned Cynomolgus macaque model.

Pharmacology studies conducted in the 6-OHDA lesioned rat model with ProSavin® demonstrated sustained expression of TH, AADC, CH1 and effective production of dopamine resulting in a significant reduction in the apomorphine-induced contra-lateral rotations in ProSavin® treated rats compared to control animals [18].

The MPTP lesioned Cynomolgus macaque model has been utilised in a short term and a long term pharmacology study using similar clinical configuration of ProSavin® [19].

Video Movement Analysis (VMA) indicated an improvement in total distance moved (TDM), maximum velocity (MV) and rearing behaviour frequency (RE) in ProSavin® treated animals during the video-recording period which measured akinesia, bradykinesia and posture respectively. Furthermore these effects were sustained for the duration of the study which was eight weeks in the short term study and for 12 months in the long term study. One animal remained on study and showed behavioural correction at 44 months the last time point assessed. Three animals treated identically but with a vector expressing a control non-therapeutic gene and three untreated MPTP lesioned control animals did not demonstrate significant behavioural correction. The possibility that the ProSavin® treated animals might have been less severely Parkinsonian was excluded by *post-mortem* analysis of the lesion. The extent of MPTP lesioning was assessed in the short term study using antibodies against TH. Immunohistochemical analysis indicated severe depletion of TH-positive neurons in the SNc indicating near complete lesioning of the nigroputamenal dopaminergic tract [19].

Analysis of the ProSavin® treated animals was consistent with the hypothesis that the therapeutic effect was due to ProSavin® treatment. ProSavin® treated animals in the short term study showed increased expression of TH, AADC and CH1 in the putamen, compared to control animals. In addition microdialysis studies were also performed in 3 ProSavin® treated NHP, 3 MPTP lesioned NHP, 3 LacZ MPTP NHP and 3 unlesioned control NHP to assess extracellular dopamine levels in the putamen. Baseline dopamine levels in the putamen of the unlesioned animal were similar to published data [20-22]. The data demonstrated a significant decrease in dopamine levels in the MPTP lesioned animal compared to control animal levels and in the ProSavin® treated animal levels were increased to 50% of the normal levels [19].

A formal dose ranging study evaluating ProSavin® was undertaken. Four cohorts of four animals were matched for random blinded treatment. One cohort received ProSavin® at the vector titre previously demonstrated as efficacious and the number of tracts per putamen, location of tracts and number and volume of deposits per tract also replicated those previously demonstrated as efficacious. In two cohorts the array of deposits of ProSavin® remained unchanged but the vector titre was reduced to 1/10th or 1/100th of that previously demonstrated as efficacious. The cohort treated at the highest dose showed clear evidence of efficacy. No evidence of efficacy was observed when the lower (1/10th, 1/100th) vector titres were used.

All preclinical and nonclinical data performed in two different species indicate that the medical challenge of developing gene transfer therapies capable of local and continuous stimulation of dopamine receptors has now been met suggesting that this gene therapy strategy is now ready for clinical application in human disease. Thus, these preclinical studies are now being translated into a phase I/II clinical trial in PD patients that investigates the safety and efficacy of this gene therapy.

S. *Palfi* et al.

Acknowledgments

Oxford BioMedica plc has been an acting industry partner of the EC-DG research through the FP6-Network of Excellence, CLINIGENE: LSHB-CT-2006-018933.

References

1. Lang AE, Lozano AM. Parkinson's disease. First of two parts. *N Engl J Med* 1998; 339: 1044-53.

2. Lang AE, Lozano AM. Parkinson's disease. Second of two parts. *N Engl J Med* 1998; 339: 1130-43.

3. Young R. Update on Parkinson's disease. *Am Fam Physician* 1999; 59: 2155-2167, 2169-2170.

4. Bennett DA, Beckett LA, Murray AM, Shannon KM, Goetz CG, Pilgrim DM, Evans DA. Prevalence of Parkinsonian signs and associated mortality in a community population of older people. *N Engl J Med* 1996; 334: 71-6.

5. Fox SH, Katzenschlager R, Lim SY, Ravina B, Seppi K, Coelho M, *et al*. The movement disorder society evidence-based medicine review update treatments for the motor symptoms of Parkinson's disease. *Mov Disord* 2011; 26 (suppl 3): S2-41.

6. Prashanth LK, Fox S, Meissner WG. L-Dopa-induced dyskinesia-clinical presentation, genetics, and treatment. *Int Rev Neurobiol* 2011; 98: 31-54.

7. Widnell MD. Pathophysiology of motor fluctuations in Parkinson's disease. *Mov Disord* 2005; 20 (suppl 11): S17-22.

8. Blanchet PJ, Allard P, Gregoire L, Tradif F, Bedard PJ. Risk factors for peak dose dyskinesia in 100 levodopa-treated Parkinsonian patients. *Can J Neurol Sci* 1996; 23: 189-98.

9. Hardoff R, Sula M, Tamir A, Soil A, Front A, Badarna S, Honigman S, Giladi N. Gastric emptying time and gastric motility in patients with Parkinson's disease. *Mov Disord* 2001; 16: 1041-7.

10. Nyholm D, Aquilonius S. Levodopa infusion therapy in Parkinson's disease. *Clin Neuropharmacol* 2004; 27: 245-56.

11. Saenz DT, Poeschla EM. FIV: from lentivirus to lentivector. *J Gene Med* 2004; 6: S95-104.

12. Miskin J, Chiplase D, Roh II J, Beard G, Wardell T, Angell D, *et al*. A replication competent lentivirus (RCL) assay for equine infectious anaemia virus (EIAV)-based lentiviral vector. *Gene Ther* 2006; 13: 196-205.

13. Mitrophanous K, Yoon S, Roh II J, Patil D, Wilkes FJ, Kim VN, *et al*. Stable gene transfer to the nervous system using a non-primate lentiviral vector. *Gene Ther* 1999; 6: 1808-18.

14. Rohll JB, Mitrophanous KA, Martin-Rendon E, Ellard FM, Radcliffe PA, Mazarakis ND, Kingsman SM. Design, production, safety, evaluation, and clinical applications of nonprimate lentiviral vectors. *Methods Enzymol* 2002; 346: 466-500.

15. Bienemann AS, Martin-Rendon E, Cosgrave AS, Glover CP, Wong LF, Kingsman SM, et al. Long-term replacement of a mutated nonfunctional CNS gene: reversal of hypothalamic diabetes insipidus using an EIAV-based lentiviral vector expressing arginine vasopressin. *Mol Ther* 2003; 7: 588-96.

16. Moffat, M, Harmon S, Haycock J, O'Malley KL. L-DOPA and dopamine-producing gene cassettes for gene therapy approaches to Parkinson's disease. *Exp Neurol* 1997; 144: 69-73.

17. Hacker CV, Vink CA, Wardell TW, Lee S, Treasure P, Kingsman SM, Mitrophanous KA, Miskin JE. The integration profile of EIAV-based vectors. *Mol Ther* 2006 ;14: 536-45.

18. Azzouz M, Martin-Rendon E, Barber RD, Mitrophanous KA, Carter EE, Rohll JB, *et al.* Multicistronic lentiviral vector-mediated striatal gene transfer of aromatic L-amino acid decorboxylase, thyrosine hydroxylase and GTP cyclohydrolase I induces sustained transgene expression, dopamine production and functional improvements in a rat model of Parkinson's disease. *J Neurosci* 2002; 22: 10302-12.

19. Jarraya B, Boulet S, Ralph GS, Jan C, Bonvento G, Azzouz M, *et al.* Dopamine gene therapy for Parkinson's disease in a nonhuman primate without associated dyskinesia. *Sci Transl Med* 2009; 1: 2ra4.

20. Bradberry CW, Barrett-Larimore RL, Jatlow P, Rubino SR. Impact of self-administered cocaine and cocaine cues on extracellular dopamine in mesolimbic and sensorimotor striatum in rhesus monkeys. *J Neurosci* 2000; 10: 3874-83.

21. Cass WA, Grondin R, Andersen AH, Zhang Z, Hardy PA, Hussey-Andersen LK, *et al.* Iron accumulation in the striatum predicts aging-related decline in motor function in rhesus monkeys. *Neurobiol Aging* 2007; 2: 258-71.

22. Skirboll S, Wang J, Mefford I, Hsiao J, Bankiewicz KS. *In vivo* changes of catecholamines in hemiparkinsonian monkeys measured by microdialysis. *Exp Neurol* 1990; 2: 187-93.

Ethical and Regulatory Issues

COORDINATED BY
ODILE COHEN-HAGUENAUER,
ALASTAIR KENT
AND
NANCY M.P. KING

The CliniBook: Clinical gene transfer
Edited by Odile Cohen-Haguenauer – EDK, Paris © 2012, pp. 495-503

C2-1
Ethics in translation from research to therapy

NANCY M.P. KING[1], ODILE COHEN-HAGUENAUER[2]*, ALASTAIR KENT[3]

[1] JD, Professor, Department of Social Sciences and Health Policy, Wake Forest
University School of Medicine, Co-Director, WFU Center for Bioethics, Health, and
Society, Wells Fargo 14, Medical Center Boulevard, Winston-Salem, NC 27157, USA.
[2] Clinigene-NoE Coordinator, École Normale Supérieure de Cachan, CNRS UMR 8113, 61,
avenue du Président Wilson, F-94235 Cachan Cedex, France, and Oncogénétique, Department
of Medical Oncology, Hospital Saint-Louis, AP-HP; Faculté de Médecine, Université
Paris-Diderot, Sorbonne Paris-Cité, 75475 Paris Cedex 10, France.
[3] Director, Genetic Alliance UK, Unit 4D, Leroy House, 436 Essex Road, London N1 3QP,
United Kingdom.
* Corresponding author. odile.cohen@lbpa.ens-cachan.fr

Gene transfer research has moved in recent years from great uncertainty to great promise in at least some areas, as a result of coordinated effort by scientists around the
world. At the same time, scholarship on the ethics of research with translational
biotechnologies has matured considerably, in order to keep up with the questions arising from these scientific developments and the prospect of including gene therapies in
the therapeutic armamentarium for at least some patients.

There are three important general areas in which gene transfer research has significantly
influenced the development and application of research ethics, policy, and practice:

1. ethical issues in translational and first-in-humans trials (including design questions and research priorities);
2. decision-making in light of risks and alternatives (with XSCID at the forefront);
3. patient advocacy and informed consent.

This chapter highlights key ethical issues in research involving translational biotechnologies, and shows how gene transfer research has led the way in addressing these issues in practice, policy, and scholarship.

THE RESEARCH TRAJECTORY

Gene transfer research catapulted into the public consciousness little more than 20
years ago, as a type of research using novel, promising, and for some, highly concerning
biologic interventions to address some of the rarest and most serious of human genetic
diseases. Like many other new fields in medical science, it is heterogeneous in many
ways, using a diversity of materials and methods on a wide variety of diseases, encompassing an extremely broad range of scientific and medical disciplines, and requiring
a great deal of collaboration, coordination, and sharing of data and expertise. When
the first human gene transfer trials began, they were conducted in parallel with plat-

form studies, vector development and refinement, basic explorations of immunology and immunotoxicity, gene-finding, animal model development, etc. The combination of rapid progress and gaps in basic research resulted in a high degree of uncertainty and the early recognition that what we think we know can change over time [1].

The scope of human gene transfer research expanded quickly; it has been viewed as highly promising for a wide range of diseases, both rare inherited conditions and more common complex disorders, including neurodegenerative diseases like Parkinson's and the development of angiogenic interventions for diabetic neuropathies and cardiovascular disorders. Demonstrations of at least some success in clinical research has been demonstrated in rare disorders – not only in X-SCID but also in *e.g.* adrenoleukodystrophy using a lentiviral vector, ADA-SCID, and Leber's congenital amaurosis. In addition, much gene transfer research is now – and has been for some time – oncology research, including so-called cancer vaccine trials and other means of attacking tumors without the extreme toxicity of standard chemotherapies. The picture of translational progress across the field is thus extremely complex, although separable generally into two strategies: *ex vivo* genetic manipulation of cells (including adult stem cells) to be infused into patient-subjects, and direct *in vivo* administration of transgene and vector, as with AAV vectors and anti-cancer approaches.

FIRST-IN-HUMAN TRIALS

As the traditional study phase designations (I, II, and III before marketing in Phase IV) continue to become more fluid and less informative outside the context of standard pharmaceutical research, the first time an agent is tried in humans has become an important focus of study design and research ethics [8]. The field of gene transfer research is one of the first among novel biologics to thoroughly consider the ethical issues that arise in first-in-human (FIH) trials. Key issues include determining how much and what type of preclinical information supports moving to human studies, and determining who should be the first subjects. These issues raise questions of both research design and research ethics. It is essential to bear in mind that the primary objective of FIH trials is to establish safety, despite sometimes excessive expectations attached to this early stage of research, and to the field of gene transfer research in particular.

When is it ethically appropriate to move to FIH trials

Decisions about what lines of research to pursue using gene transfer are based on many factors, both scientific and social. Determining when it is ethically appropriate to move into human trials requires assessing the preclinical information available and asking three closely related questions:

1. Has the point been reached when it is reasonable to conclude that no additional meaningful information can be obtained without using human subjects? Are laboratory and animal data sufficient, and adequately informative? Gene transfer research has highlighted gaps and difficulties in the use of animal models, particularly large animal models. In addition, the field is still developing basic understanding of mechanisms, working to develop *in vitro* assays to predict safety, and creating both platform studies and disease-specific modeling. Thus, determining when it is appropriate to move from preclinical to clinical research is by no means an easy judgment. Ultimately, the information essential to determining the safety and efficacy of a novel intervention in humans can be gathered only from clinical trials enrolling humans as subjects; nonetheless, moving to clinical trials prematurely because of scientific excitement or impatience may fail both to protect patient-subjects and to provide adequate evaluable data.

2. Has the amount of uncertainty (about not only risks of harm but also the potential for direct benefit from the line of research) been reduced as far as possible? The answer to this question depends on what preclinical information is currently available or can and should still be obtained. It thus depends upon the state of the art at the time. And it must be acknowledged that some degree of irreducible uncertainty will always remain. However, lack of information cannot, in a given instance, justify moving into clinical trials if the gap is too big and uncertainty is too great. Hence the third question:

3. Is the remaining amount of irreducible uncertainty small enough that it is fair to patient-subjects to offer them participation in a clinical gene transfer trial? Answering this question requires careful consideration and justification of the implications of research involving humans. It is basic that risks of harm to research subjects should be minimized as far as possible, and that the balance of risks of harm and potential benefits from the research be reasonable [2]. The primary goal of research is knowledge production, and research that is poorly conceived, designed, or conducted is unethical not only if harm results, but anytime it exposes subjects to risks of harm without producing generalizable knowledge [3].

Evolving knowledge, risks of harm and potential benefit

As we have noted, in gene transfer research, knowledge advances so rapidly that different generations of vectors and new refinements of assays, delivery methods, and the like are often being tested at the same time. This makes data transparency especially important, so that knowledge can be effectively shared. CliniGene has provided an essential cooperative network mechanism to maximize the efficiency of research in this complex field, and to promote knowledge-sharing without unduly impairing the ability to bring products to market.

How much uncertainty is too much? How much risk is too great? These questions may at times appear to be matters of autonomy and informed consent alone. That is, when the risks of harm appear significant but little is known about the anticipated effects in humans, investigators may be tempted to allow patients themselves to determine whether they wish to become research subjects. However, investigators have the duty to make only fair and reasonable offers, based on the available science. There may be times when it is more morally prudent, as well as more scientifically reasonable, to return to preclinical research than to enroll human subjects and expose them to unknown risks [4]. Indeed, the need to return to preclinical research might easily be the conclusion of a FIH trial. Obviously, not all interventions studied in FIH research will be shown to be safe enough to move forward into phase II trials enrolling additional patients as subjects. This reality underscores the tentative nature of research, and should be emphasized as a part of informed consent.

Thus, it is not paternalistic to refrain from prematurely moving to FIH trials, since the warrant for research is scientific. This is true even when potential subjects are eager to enroll, because the potential for direct benefit to the subjects, while often suggestive, always represents a significant uncertainty in FIH research. Delaying an offer of trial participation, especially for a FIH trial, is very different from denying a patient access to a proven treatment [5]. In this context, the role of the Research Ethics Committee/Institutional Review Board is crucial in identifying and evaluating the potential benefits and risks of harm posed by experimental interventions. Given the highly specialized nature of gene transfer research, it is essential that the REC/IRB have access to adequate expertise. It is necessary to evaluate accurately what is proposed scientifically in order to understand the ethical implications of the proposed research.

Even so, it is undoubtedly true that the determination to move into humans is necessarily affected by the nature of the disease, the available alternatives, the scientific context, and many other factors that may be better understood by patient-subjects than by investigators or even treating physicians. Gene transfer research has helped to highlight the importance of these factors and the complexities of the decision to move into the clinic by virtue of the unprecedented scrutiny given to it worldwide, both as a result of the public deliberations of oversight bodies like the Recombinant DNA Advisory Committee (RAC) of the National Institutes of Health in the US and the Gene Therapy Advisory Committee in the UK, and because of some highly publicized deaths and severe adverse events in trials around the world and the resulting media attention.

DECISIONS IN AN IMPERFECT WORLD

A tentative stratification scheme

The biggest ethical challenge for gene transfer research lies in moving forward with this logical, scientifically promising, and highly complex technology, with the hope of ultimately developing interventions with the capacity to reduce or relieve symptoms, prolong life, or perhaps even cure, but without waiting for certainty. The primary duties of investigators toward their research subjects are (1) to protect them from undue harm and (2) to avoid disadvantaging them by depriving them of the chance to benefit from established treatments. With the safety of patient-subjects foremost, then, determining how best to move forward means deciding when to go forward and which patient-subjects should go first. From whom may the most be learned at the least risk to them? Very sick subjects may be at greater risk of harm, but may value the chance of benefit highly. However, the effects of the disease, of the intervention, and of prior treatment may be difficult to disentangle in very sick subjects. Yet healthier subjects may sometimes be too well to provide the data needed to move to later-phase trials. And balancing harms and benefits is greatly complicated when direct benefits begin to materialize but significant harms are seen as well.

Important insights into the consideration of ethical issues in research design may be gained by an analysis of the conditions and characteristics of proposed research, including the severity and stage of the potential subjects' disease, the availability and effectiveness of existing treatments, what is known about the risks of harm, and whether the experimental intervention offers a reasonable likelihood of potential benefit [1]. For example, gene transfer research testing an experimental intervention for a life-threatening condition might proceed quite differently when there is an established treatment and when there is none. When no effective treatment exists, the safety of research subjects is, as always, of paramount importance, but it may be appropriate to test technologies that offer lesser potential for direct benefit. When established treatments are available to patient-subjects, the rationale for developing an experimental intervention must be that it is reasonably likely to prove superior to existing treatment – more effective, safer, longer-lasting, less burdensome, and the like. Protecting patients from the loss of the chance to benefit from existing treatments, when available, is paramount (*Figure 1*).

The X-SCID and SCID-ADA primary immunodeficiencies paradox

The story of X-linked severe combined immunodeficiency provides an important example of a complex and ongoing effort to address ethical challenges and improve both basic and clinical science in a rapidly changing field. The only reasonably effective established treatment for X-SCID is a bone marrow or hematopoietic stem cell transplant from a matched or at least a haploidentical donor. However, many patients have no matches available to them. The success of gene transfer in X-SCID began to improve when younger patients were enrolled as research subjects, and the majority of subjects have enjoyed persistent correction of their immune deficiency. Unfortunately, it was soon discovered that insertional mutagenesis was responsible for the development of leukemias in a high percentage of subjects [10]. Most of these leukemias were successfully treated, but at least one subject has died.

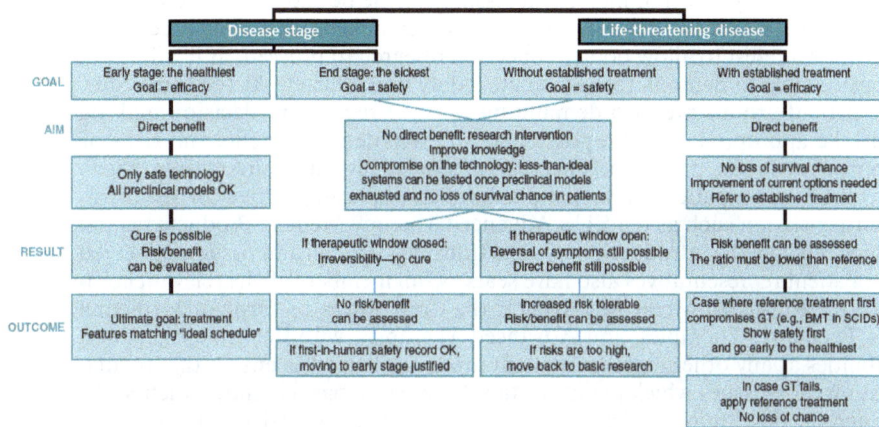

	Disease stage		Life-threatening disease	
GOAL	Early stage: the healthiest Goal = efficacy	End stage: the sickest Goal = safety	Without established treatment Goal = safety	With established treatment Goal = efficacy
AIM	Direct benefit	No direct benefit: research intervention Improve knowledge		Direct benefit
	Only safe technology All preclinical models OK	Compromise on the technology: less-than-ideal systems can be tested once preclinical models exhausted and no loss of survival chance in patients		No loss of survival chance Improvement of current options needed Refer to established treatment
RESULT	Cure is possible Risk/benefit can be evaluated	If therapeutic window closed: Irreversibility—no cure	If therapeutic window open: Reversal of symptoms still possible Direct benefit still possible	Risk benefit can be assessed The ratio must be lower than reference
OUTCOME	Ultimate goal: treatment Features matching "ideal schedule"	No risk/benefit can be assessed	Increased risk tolerable Risk/benefit can be assessed	Case where reference treatment first compromises GT (e.g., BMT in SCIDs) Show safety first and go early to the healthiest
		If first-in-human safety record OK, moving to early stage justified	If risks are too high, move back to basic research	In case GT fails, apply reference treatment No loss of chance

Figure 1. Model stratification scheme for planning first-in-human GT clinical trials*.
*Reprinted from King NMP, Cohen-Haguenauer O. En route to ethical recommendations for gene transfer clinical trials. Mol Ther 2008; 16: 432-8.

Thus, younger patient-subjects get a better response but are at risk of insertional mutagenesis. The US NIH Recombinant DNA Advisory Committee has therefore recommended that X-SCID patients not be enrolled as research subjects unless they lack transplant matches, at least until more is learned that can reduce this risk. Ongoing efforts to understand, predict, and control gene insertion and to develop vectors that protect against oncogenesis have made progress, but no one has argued that clinical trials should halt while awaiting experimental interventions likely to pose lower risks. Indeed, it could be argued that it is preferable to try gene transfer first before transplantation, even when a transplant match is available for a patient-subject, for two reasons: the correction afforded by successful gene transfer may be superior, but if the gene transfer is not successful, or if insertional mutagenesis results, transplant is indicated and still available. Despite the major side-effects directly linked to gene insertion in X-SCIDs, the decision was made to continue clinical trials in ADA-SCID in Milan without any case of leukemia showing so far in the long-term follow-up of patient-subjects [11]. Gene transfer for ADA-SCID is currently the main example of safety and efficacy in this research, with an optimal risk/benefit ratio and potential for marketing authorization approval. This is a remarkable illustration of success, despite the use of imperfect technology. In ADA-SCID, gene transfer is likely to replace two standard treatments: enzyme replacement therapy, which is less efficacious and more costly, and haplo-identical bone marrow transplant, which has significant morbidity and even mortality. As this example shows, the decisions involved in determining whether and how clinical gene transfer research should go forward are complex and challenging, especially when patients face uncertainty and risk whether they become research subjects or not. The viewpoints of researchers, regulators and oversight bodies, sponsors, policymakers, ethics scholars, and other stakeholders all contribute to improving not only the research itself, but also our understanding of it. Some of the most important voices in this ongoing conversation are those of patients and families.

PATIENT ADVOCACY

Patient advocacy groups around the world are increasingly demanding a role in the ethical and regulatory decision making necessary for the development and conduct of gene transfer research [9]. Patient groups, like other stakeholders, fully accept that it is in no one's interest to allow poorly conceived research to proceed, as it will result in products unable to demonstrate adequate safety and efficacy. At the same time, however, patient groups are also demanding that the regulatory decision making framework be appropriate and proportionate to the potential benefits and risks of harm from gene transfer, particularly in comparison with available alternatives (where any exist). In Europe, patient organizations have actively campaigned for the introduction of legislation such as the EU's Advanced Therapy Medical Products regulations, which regulate the introduction of gene transfer, stem cell and tissue engineered products. Patient representatives also have seats as full members of the relevant committees of the European Medicines Agency, the Committees on Orphan Medicinal Products, Paediatric Therapies, and Advanced Therapies, with the same rights and responsibilities as any other member. Patient input has helped to ensure that regulators focus on those issues which are important to research participants, patients and families, and the development of clinically relevant science. In particular they seek to ensure that oversight bodies do not impose unreasonable hurdles in the way of promising developments.

However, patients are not pushovers who will say yes to anything. They know they have more to lose than anyone if poor quality products are allowed on to the market. For this reason, patient organizations are also increasingly becoming involved in post marketing surveillance and the appraisal procedures undertaken by bodies such as the National Institute for Health and Clinical Excellence in the UK, and its sister bodies in other jurisdictions.

INFORMED CONSENT

The consent form and the process of informed decisionmaking by potential subjects is especially challenging in FIH trials and in research involving scientifically complex novel biotechnologies like gene transfer. Gene transfer research has pioneered an important reconsideration of informed consent, through the RAC's development of an informed consent guidance document specifically designed to assist gene transfer investigators [6]. Of critical importance are: how to define and describe gene transfer and what it means to add new genes to the body; clear description of the risks of harm that have been identified in pre-clinical studies and/or in prior similar research, including their possible severity and their probability; discussion of what is uncertain and unknown; and clear identification of plans for monitoring and long-term follow-up, as well as an explanation of the importance of long-term monitoring, both for the health of subjects themselves and for knowledge production.

Information on FIH primary endpoint: to establish safety

Because gene transfer research, like much research involving novel biotechnologies, may often be viewed as a scientific breakthrough with great therapeutic promise even in its early stages, informed consent discussion of the potential for direct benefit is particularly critical. Patients who are potential subjects may have high expectations for direct benefit; investigators may as well. Yet defining what should count as a reasonable expectation of direct benefit, and describing it in the consent form, is not straightforward, especially in the case of FIH trials in particular, where the primary objective remains to establish safety. Therefore, the consent form and process should make clear that the primary goal of all research is to contribute to generalizable knowledge – that is, to learn something that can benefit science and future patients (usually called "societal benefit"). Research involving adults able to make their own decisions need not directly benefit the subjects as long as it benefits society and risks of harm are minimized as far as possible. Adult patient-subjects must be informed that direct benefit is not anticipated, so that they may decide about participation with this awareness. Research involving children, who are often unable to take a decision-making role, raises additional ethical concerns and may be subject to special regulatory requirements. In particular, in the US and at least some other jurisdictions, research involving children must offer the prospect of direct benefit if the risks of harm are more than minimal – which is usually the case in gene transfer research. Such a limitation is significant for gene transfer research involving disorders that primarily affect children or interventions that may be best studied by beginning with child participants, as has been shown in the X-SCID trials and may also be the case for many serious genetic disorders.

Exploring the unknown and anticipated outcome
Direct benefit is defined as benefit resulting from the receipt of the experimental intervention (as opposed to "inclusion benefits" which flow from being enrolled in the trial, such as free medical goods or services). They must be described with some specificity in order to provide patient-subjects with meaningful information. It is especially important to emphasize that in FIH trials, any conceivable direct benefits are both unlikely and represent at best only a secondary objective [5]. For example, the nature of the benefit must be described. "Your tumors may shrink if you join this study" is a better description than "You may or may not benefit if you join this study". However, tumor response is not always a direct clinical benefit that a patient-subject can experience, as it does not always correlate with feeling better or improved survival. Thus, the nature of a direct benefit often requires more than minimal explanation. This is particularly true in FIH gene transfer trials, where limited experience may limit the ability to connect surrogate efficacy endpoints, like tumor shrinkage, improved immune response, or increased levels of missing amino acids, proteins, or blood components, with clinical endpoints like longer progression-free survival and fewer infections, bleeds, or other disease episodes.

In some disorders, for example, relatively small improvements in immune system function, or percentage of circulating factor in hemophilia, may result in significant clinical improvement without fully reaching normal levels. In other disorders, small improvements will not have dramatic effects. And of course, long-term or even permanent gene correction is most desirable. In a few instances of successful gene transfer, namely the severe combined immune deficiencies, long-term correction appears to have been achieved. In early hemophilias trials, however, correction, while clinically significant in some patient-subjects, has remained transient. The likelihood that correction will not be permanent must be disclosed. Thus, the expected magnitude (size and duration) of a potential direct benefit is also significant, and in many cases closely links the nature of the benefit to the nature of the disease under consideration.

Perhaps the most difficult consent challenge in early-phase gene transfer research is probability itself. This is in part because the likelihood of success of any proven therapeutic intervention is largely unaddressed in clinical medicine; thus, when an intervention is recommended, it is rarely accompanied by a prediction of the likelihood that it will be effective. Most people assume that recommended interventions are effective. Patients with serious conditions learn that many proven treatments have a surprisingly low likelihood of success; yet most consent forms say no more than "you may or may not benefit" – a universally true statement. The inability to provide extensive and precise data about the nature, magnitude, and likelihood of both risks of harm and potential direct benefits in FIH research does not excuse investigators from attempting to give potential subjects a clear picture of the anticipated outcomes. A consent form that describes a small possibility of a specific outcome, which could have clinical significance but might not, and which could be temporary but might be long-lasting, is more informative than "you may or may not benefit" [7]. Helping potential subjects to grasp the meaning and significance of the available data for them, and to understand how the research seeks to contribute to knowledge that could help future patients, is the aim of the informed consent process. An obvious implication here is that the consent form and process should evolve over time as the study progresses and more is learned that could help facilitate the decision-making process of both current and potential subjects.

Research is not treatment: the pitfalls of false hope

Importantly, this means several things that patient advocates know well. First, research is not treatment, even when potential direct benefit is sought. Research involves a partnership between investigators and patient-subjects to produce generalizable knowledge. Second, researchers' *expectations* for the study and patient-subjects' *hopes* for themselves can diverge, for example when the investigator knows that the likelihood of direct benefit is very low, but a patient-subject joins a study because the gene transfer intervention might work, when nothing else has. This divergence is perfectly acceptable, so long as the risks of harm have been minimized and clear information has been shared in the consent form and process.

Finally, especially in FIH and other early-phase clinical trials, the information provided in the Patient Information Leaflet supporting the consent process needs to be scrutinized carefully to ensure that there is no accidental implication of therapeutic benefit. For example, gene transfer interventions may be described as "treatments" – which may be an appropriate term from the investigator's perspective but which may well lead to an expectation of clinical benefits by patients and families and also by clinicians sharing these with potential research participants. Given that gene transfer clinical trials often involve inheritable diseases, the understanding of carers and other (related) family members of the implications of participation should also be secured, especially in the case of childhood onset diseases where hope for a cure may be running at a high level.

CONCLUSIONS AND RECOMMENDATIONS

1. A balanced assessment of the potential benefits and risks of harm from gene transfer is essential. Both unrealistic promises and exaggerated threats and risks distort expectations and derail research progress.
2. The best way to secure full and informed engagement is by getting patient support organizations and patients and families involved as early as possible and keeping them in the loop as things develop. This involvement requires time and effort to develop, but the investment at an early stage will reap dividends later.
3. Creative, collaborative research contributes to scientific knowledge at the level of both laboratory and clinic. Knowledge-sharing and the parallel development of basic and clinical research have helped to build a solid foundation on which gene transfer has begun to build real success. Ongoing, transparent public discussion of the ethical issues arising in this unique field has helped to create an open decision-making climate that serves as a model for other novel biotechnologies.

4. Consolidation of state-of-the-art knowledge is essential, even while it evolves in a rapidly moving field involving cutting-edge technologies.

5. There is no substitute for FIH trials, which provide unique and essential information about safety, as primary objective, and preliminary evidence about potential benefit, as a secondary objective. Moving from the laboratory to FIH trials must continue to be encouraged and facilitated in gene transfer research.

6. Remember the timescale for sustainable development. With gene transfer we can see the goal, and the concept is beguilingly simple, but the journey is proving to be a longer one that many initially thought, with more blind alleys and setbacks along the way than we might have hoped for. There may be little doubt that gene transfer will be successful in the long run; nonetheless, for the investment to be sustained we must be as clear and as realistic as possible about the road ahead.

ACKNOWLEDGMENTS

This work has been performed with the support of the EC-DG research through the FP6-Network of Excellence, CLINIGENE: LSHB-CT-2006-018933

REFERENCES

1. King NMP, Cohen-Haguenauer O. En route to ethical recommendations for gene transfer clinical trials. *Mol Ther* 2008; 16: 432-8.

2. National Commission for the Protection of human subjects of biomedical and behavioral research. *The Belmont report: ethical principles and guidelines for the protection of human subjects of research.* Bethesda, Maryland: National Institutes of Health, 1979. http://www.hhs.gov/ohrp/humansubjects/guidance/belmont.htm

3. Emanuel E, Wendler D, Grady C. What makes clinical research ethical? *JAMA* 2000; 283: 2701-11.

4. Kimmelman J. *Gene transfer and the ethics of first-in-human trials: lost in translation.* Cambridge: Cambridge University Press, 2009.

5. King NMP. Defining and describing benefit appropriately in clinical trials. *J Law Med Ethics* 2000; 28: 332-43.

6. National Institutes of Health. *NIH guidance on informed consent for gene transfer research.* http://oba.od.nih.gov/oba/rac/ic/index.html

7. King NMP, Henderson GE, Churchill LR, Davis AM, Hull SC, Nelson DK, *et al.* Consent forms and the therapeutic misconception: the example of gene transfer research. *IRB* 2005; 27: 1-8.

8. Dresser R. First-in-human trial participants: not a vulnerable population, but vulnerable nonetheless. *J Law Med Ethics* 2009; 37: 38-50.

9. Kent A, King NMP, Cohen-Haguenauer O. Toward a proportionate regulatory framework for gene transfer: a patient group-led initiative. *Hum Gene Ther* 2011; 22: 126-34.

10. Hacein-Bey-Abina S, Von Kalle C, Schmidt M, McCormack MP, Wulffraat N, Leboulch P, *et al.* LMO2-associated clonal T cell proliferation in two patients after gene therapy for SCID-X1. *Science* 2003; 302: 415-9.

11. Aiuti A, Cattaneo F, Galimberti S, Benninghoff U, Cassani B, Callegaro L, *et al.* Gene therapy for immunodeficiency due to adenosine deaminase deficiency. *N Engl J Med* 2009; 360 : 447-58.

The CliniBook: Clinical gene transfer
Edited by Odile Cohen-Haguenauer – EDK, Paris © 2012, pp. 504-516

C2-2
Centralised regulation of gene therapy in Europe

ODILE COHEN-HAGUENAUER

CliniGene, École Normale Supérieure de Cachan, CNRS UMR 8113, 94235 Cachan, France and Department of Medical Oncology, Hôpital Saint-Louis and University Paris-Diderot, Sorbonne-Paris-Cité, 75475 Paris Cedex 10, France.
odile.cohen@lbpa.ens-cachan.fr

Gene and cell therapy medicinal products are new and innovative medicinal products. They are biological medicinal products according to Regulation (EC) No 1394/2007 within the meaning of Annex I to Directive 2001/83/EC. In addition, Part IV, Annex I to Directive 2001/83/EC as regard to the specificity of advanced therapy medicinal products (ATMPs) was revised. ATMPs are defined as gene and cell-therapy medicinal products and tissue-engineered products (*Table I*). Because of the novelty, complexity and technical specificity of advanced therapy medicinal products, specially tailored and harmonised rules were thought to be needed with view to ensuring the free movement of those products within the Community and the effective operation of the internal market in the biotechnology sector. They are subject to a centralised authorisation procedure, involving a single scientific evaluation of the quality, safety and efficacy of the product at the European Medicines Agency. ATMPs require specific expertise, which goes beyond the traditional pharmaceutical field and covers areas bordering on other sectors such as biotechnology and medical devices.

FOR THIS REASON THE COMMITTEE FOR ADVANCED THERAPIES (CAT) WAS CREATED

(http://www.ema.europa.eu/ema/index.jsp?curl=pages/special_topics/general/general_content_000504.jsp&mid=WC0b01ac058050f347), CAT is responsible for preparing a draft opinion on the quality, safety and efficacy of each advanced therapy medicinal product for final approval by the CHMP. All ATMPs intended for marketing in more than one EU-member state benefit from a single centralised evaluation and be it the case, successful autorisation via the European Medicines Agency. According to the assessment procedure, the CAT prepares a draft opinion on the quality, safety and efficacy of an ATMP which is being forwarded to the Committee for Medicinal Products for Human Use (CHMP; http://www.ema.europa.eu/ema/index.jsp?curl=pages/aboutus/general/general_content_000094.jsp&mid=WC0b01ac0580028c79). CHMP adopts in turn a recommendation for the European Commission which may either grant or refuse

Table I. Advanced Therapies Medicinal Products (ATMPs): Definitions under EU-Regulation: Directive 2009/120/EC of 14 September 2009 amending Directive 2001/83/EC: http://ec.europa.eu/health/documents/eudralex/vol-1/index_en.htm

Advanced Therapies Medicinal Products (ATMPs) means any of the following medical product for human use: a Gene Therapy Medicinal Product, a Somatic Cell Therapy Medicinal Product or a Tissue engineered product

Gene Therapy Medicinal Product
defined in Part IV of Annex I to Directive 2001/83/EC

A biology medicinal product which has the following characteristics:
(a) it contains and active substance which contains or consists of a recombinant nucleic acid used in or administered to human beings with a view to regulating, replacing, adding or deleting a genetic sequence;
(b) its therapeutic, prophylactic or diagnostic effect relates directly to the recombinant nucleic acid sequence it contains, or to the product of genetic expression of this sequence. Gene Therapy medicinal products shall not include vaccines against infectious diseases.

Somatic Cell Therapy Medicinal Product
defined in Part IV of Annex I to Directive 2001/83/EC

A biology medicinal product which has the following characteristics:
(a) contains or consists of cells or tissues that have been subject to substantial manipulation so that biological characteristics, physiological functions or structural properties relevant for the intended clinical use have been altered, or of cells or tissues that are not intended to be used for the same essential function(s) in the recipient and the donor;
(b) is presented or having properties for, or is used in or administered to human beings with a view to treating, preventing or diagnosing a disease through the pharmacological, immunological or metabolic action of its cells or tissues.
For the purpose of point (a) the manipulation listed in Annex I to Regulation (EC) N° 1394/2007, in particular, shall not be considered as substantial manipulations [*1]

Tissue engineered product
defined in Article 2.1.b of Regulation EC 1394/2007

A product that
(a) contains or consists of engineered cells or tissues, and
(b) is presented as having properties for, or is used in or administered to human beings with a view to regenerating, repairing or replacing a human tissue

A tissue engineered product main contain cells or tissues of human or animal origin, or both. The cells or tissues may be viable or non-viable. It may also contain additional substances, such as cellular products, bio-molecules, biomaterials, chemical substances, scaffolds or matrices. Products containing or consisting exclusively of non-viable human or animal cells and/or tissues, which do not contain any viable cells or tissues and which do not act principally by either pharmacological, immunological or metabolic action, shall be excluded from the definition.

Cells or tissues shall be considered "engineered" if they fulfil at least one of the following conditions (*defined in Article 2.1.c of Regulation EC 1394/2007*):

  i. The cells or tissues have been subject to substantial manipulations, so that biological characteristics, physiological functions or structural properties relevant for the intended regeneration, repair or replcament are achieved. The manipulations listed in Annex I, in particular, shall not be considered as substantial manipulations [*1]
  ii. The cells or tissues are not intended to be used for the same essential function or functions in the recipient as in the donor

---

Prominent definition applying to ATMPs in combination

Where a product contains viable cells or tissues, the pharmacological, immunological or metabolic action of those cells or tissues shall be considered as the principal mode of action of the product (*defined in Article 2.3 of Regulation EC 1394/2007*).

A product which may fall within the definition of a tissue engineered product and within the definition of a somatic cell therapy medicinal product shall be considered as a tissue engineered product (*defined in Article 2.4 of Regulation EC 1394/2007*).

A product which may fall within the definition of a somatic cell therapy medicinal product or a tissue engineered product, and a gene therapy medicinal product, shall be considered as a gene therapy medicinal product (*defined in Article 2.5 of Regulation EC 1394/2007*).

Combined ATMPs
defined in Article 2.2 of Regulation EC 1394/2007

Means a product that fulfils the following conditions: it must incorporate, as an integral part of the product, one or more medical devices within the meaning of Article 1(2)(a) of Directive 93/42/EEC or one or more active implantable medical devices within the meaning of Article 1(2)(c) of Directive 90/385/EEC, **and** (i) its cellular or tissue part must contain viable cells or tissues, **or** (ii) its cellular or tissue part containing non-viable cells or tissues must be liable to act upon the human body with action that can be considered as primary to that of the devices referred to.

[*1] **Manipulation listed in Annex I to Regulation (EC) N° 1394/2007**
http://ec.europa.eu/health/documents/eudralex/vol-1/index_en.htm: first indent of Article 2.1.c

- Cutting
- Grinding
- Shaping
- Centrifugation
- Soaking in antibiotic or antimicrobial solutions
- Sterilization
- Irradiation
- Cell separation, concentration or purification,
- Filtering
- Lyophilization
- Freezing
- Cryopreservation
- Vitrification

---

a marketing authorisation on the basis of the Agency's recommendation. CAT thus plays a central role in the assessment of ATMPs and mobilises the required expertise to do so at the EU-level, through its Working Parties: the Gene Therapy Working Party and the Cell-based Products Working Party, the case-by-case sollicitation of ad-hoc experts and Stake-holders with the organisation of consultations during 2011, of Focus Groups of Interested Parties (FGIPs). In January 2012, a one-day workshop was organised by the CAT at the European Medicines Agency, London as part of its effort to strengthen the dialogue with its stakeholders. The main aim of the workshop was to communicate the outcome of individual focus group meetings held in 2011 and consolidate views and future actions to be undertaken. Attendees were given the opportunity to send questions to the organising committee in advance: intensive interaction proved extremely fruitful and a report has been issued.

Now is a pivotal timepoint for sustained attention to and information on Gene Therapy regulatory framework, due to the:

1. Revision of the "Clinical Trials Directive", a subject which has been open for public comments to DG-Enterprise in 2010. CliniGene has contributed comments. A new revised concept paper has been submitted for public consultation until May 2011, by DG Sanco under the authority of which EMA is now being placed (no longer DG Enterprise) RE: SANCO/C/8/PB/SF D(2011) 143488. A revision under a EU-Regulation has just been brought to the European Parliament (see *Table II*).
2. Revision of The Note For Guidance On The Quality, Pre-Clinical And Clinical Aspects Of The Gene Transfer Medicinal Products, which is the main guideline. As a unique consolidated and cross-indexed reference document it is by far the most mature in the EU gene therapy field and internationally recognised as such. The original guideline was drafted over a decade ago; the revision-process will thus take into account the new framework implementing the CAT.
3. EMA-CAT based implementation of advanced therapy medicinal products regulation; besides its advisory role in the European Commission decision-making process on marketing authorisation, CAT also:
   • Gives recommendations on ATMPs classification;
   • Reviews data on the manufacture and testing of medicines developed by SMEs;
   • Contributes to scientific advice provided by the Agency on ATMPs;
   • Helps to establish an environment that encourages ATMPs development;
   • At the request of the European Commission, provides scientific expertise and advice for any initiatives related to the development of innovative medicines and therapies.

From the Clinical Trials Directive to the Clinical Trials Regulation

To guarantee the highest possible level of Public Health and to secure the availability of medicinal products to citizens across the European Union, all medicinal products for human use have to be authorised either at Member State or Community level before they can be placed on the EU market. Special rules exist for the authorisation of medicinal products for paediatric use, orphan medicines, traditional herbal medicines, vaccines and clinical trials.

Multiple and divergent assessments of clinical trials

Few clinical trials are performed in one single Member State. Rules for clinical trial authorisation should be identical in theory. But as always theory and practice are divergent. Investigators and sponsors cannot prepare as many files as there are official bodies in each member state of the European Union, in particular in the case of rare disorders and non-commercial clinical trials. A step forward towards EU-wide harmonisation of first-in-man studies application dossier has long been a request from users under the form of a comprehensive dossier which should encompass all requirements including GMOs-related aspects (see *Table III* and chapter C2-3, *ibid.*).

The EU Directive on clinical trials was published at the end of 2001 with the ambitious goal of both harmonising and facilitating EU procedures for the process of clinical trials authorization. Unfortunately, over 10 years after, many National procedures are still in place, which may jeopardise the main objective of the Directive. EU countries lost almost 20% of global trials within the past two years. In order for EU countries to continue to play an important role in the clinical research arena, both procedures

Table II. DG-Sanco : European Commission DIrectorate General Health and Consumers in charge of Medicinal products for human use : http://ec.europa.eu/health/index_en.htm

In order to help the European Union ensure the highest possible level of public health protection, in 1994 the EU established the European Medicines Agency (EMA).

a. Clinical trials: http://ec.europa.eu/health/human-use/clinical-trials/index_en.htm

Clinical trials are investigations in humans intended to discover or verify the effects of one or more investigational medicinal products ("IMPs").

The " Clinical Trials Directive " Directive 2001/20/EC,	Requirements for the conduct of clinical trials in the EU are provided for: relating to the implementation of good clinical practice in the conduct of clinical trials on medicinal products for human use
The " Good Clinical Practice (GCP) Directive" Commission Directive 2005/28/EC of 8 April 2005	Further concretises the Clinical Trials Directive, laying down principles and detailed guidelines for good clinical practice as regards investigational medicinal products for human use, as well as the requirements for authorisation of the manufacturing or importation of such products.
Guidelines further specifying various aspects of clinical trial	• The information to be submitted to the competent authorities and to the ethics committees • The requirements on safety monitoring and the reporting of adverse reactions • The requirements regarding Good Clinical Practice, including the documentation, of the clinical trials • The specific requirements regarding the products and the clinical trials • The inspections of competent authorities and the applicable procedures
These guidelines are being published and available from different sources	• The European Commission: published in Volume 10 of "EudraLex - The rules governing medicinal products in the European Union" http://ec.europa.eu/health/documents/eudralex/vol-10/index_en.htm • The European Medicines Agency: Requirements relating to the quality, safety and efficacy of products, as well as specific types of products published in Volume 3 of EudraLex http://ec.europa.eu/health/documents/eudralex/vol-3/index_en.htm • In addition, the Heads of Medicines Agencies have established a Clinical Trials Facilitation Group ("CTFG") (in which the Commission and EMA are observers), in order to discuss ongoing technical issues.

b. Revision of the Clinical trial Directive: Adoption of a Clinical Trials Regulation

On 17 July 2012, the Commission has adopted a "Proposal for a Regulation of the European Parliament and of the Council on clinical trials on medicinal products for human use, and repealing Directive 2001/20/EC (767 KB). The proposal has been submitted to the European Parliament and the Council who engage in ordinary legislative procedure.

and standards of their studies need to be improved. The foundation of the "Clinical Trials Facilitation Group" (see *Table II*) and the "Voluntary Harmonised Procedure (VHP) which involves concerted evaluation by up to three Member States Agencies have been enforced which are meant at accelerating progress with few evidence of practical success at present.

c. EudraCT	
The European database - EudraCT -	This database gives the competent authorities of the Member States, the EMA and the Commission the necessary information to communicate on clinical trials and to maintain oversight of clinical trials and IMP development: contains all ongoing or completed clinical trials falling within the scope of Directive 2001/20/EC
User manual for EudraCT	Document available on the EudraCT Supporting Documentation web page.

d. Good Manufacturing Practice

To ensure that medicinal products are consistently produced and controlled against the quality standards appropriate to their intended use, the European Union has set quality standards known as ' good manufacturing practice'. Compliance with these principles and guidelines is mandatory within the European Economic Area.

e. Pharmacovigilance : http://ec.europa.eu/health/human-use/pharmacovigilance/developments/index_en.htm

Once a medicinal product has been authorised in the Community and placed on the market, its safety is monitored throughout its entire lifespan through the EU system of pharmacovigilance.

New EU-Regulation N°520/2012 of 19 June 2012 on performance of pharmacovigilance	Provided for in Regulation (EC) No 726/2004 of the European Parliament and of the Council and Directive 2001/83/EC of the European Parliament and of the Council. Official Journal of the European Union L 159/5 (EU) No 520/201.
Complements the 2010 pharmacovigilance legislation, which starts to apply in July 2012	Providing more technical details to be observed by marketing authorisation holders, national competent authorities and EMA in the daily practice. Important piece in the new framework by strengthening the European system for monitoring the safety and use of medicines.

f. Advanced Therapies : http://ec.europa.eu/health/human-use/advanced-therapies/developments/index_en.htm

New technologies, therapies and medicines are emerging; this includes regenerative medicine, more personalised treatments, as well as the development of nanomedicines. The Commission is committed to monitoring scientific progress and to constantly review Community legislation in the light of new developments so as to make safe, novel treatments available to patients as early as possible.

Inconsistent implementation of the Clinical Trial Directive

Gene- and cell-therapy clinical trials sponsored by either academic or non-profit organisations are not necessarily performed with the intention to generate data to support an application for a marketing authorisation of a medicinal product. Therefore the CliniGene-NoE proposed to design a specific track for the evaluation/approval of these studies, especially when they are not aiming at marketing authorisation. The model of the clinical trial which seems to underpin the current legislation is that of the big Pharma driven multi-centre, large scale study. Whilst this model may be appropriate when considering the development of small molecules for common diseases, it is not relevant to new knowledge in genetics and biotechnology. In addition, when considering ATMPs in rare diseases or early development phases of innovative treatment given the reduced number of patients and the multinational accrual, within an Academic setting in many cases, the legislation should be a community legislation,

O. Cohen-Haguenauer

to facilitate international cooperation in clinical research in this field. Because accurate expertise on ATMPS can be found at the EU-wide level only, the Commission should take in consideration to centralise clinical trials authorisation for these innovative products.

Revision of the Clinical trial Directive: Adoption of a Clinical Trials Regulation

The new EU Clinical Trial Regulation, the process of which is in advanced stage of finalization, will represent an important step towards our future scenario. The proposal adopted on 17 July 2012 by the Commission has been submitted to the European Parliament and the Council who engage in ordinary legislative procedure [follow-up at the «legislative observatory» of the European Parliament or PreLex, the EU-database on interinstitutional procedures].

THE STAKEHOLDER VIEWPOINT: COMMENTING GUIDELINES AND REFLECTION PAPERS

A wonderful opportunity for improvement: the Revision of the Note For Guidance On The Quality, Pre-Clinical And Clinical Aspects Of Gene Transfer Medicinal Products

According to multiple comments communicated by the CliniGene-NoE and formerly by the Euregenethy-network, the Note For Guidance On The Quality, Pre-Clinical And Clinical Aspects Of Gene Transfer Medicinal Products, (GT-NfG) - the update of which is foreseen 10 years after entering into force - is the most mature and the best reference so far in the EU gene therapy field. While the Agency had to produce additional guidance documents according to companies' requests, the CliniGene-NoE has always viewed the so-called «mother» GT-NfG as a major reference internationally recognised since:

(i) it is user-friendly and comprehensive;
(ii) it is adequately organised: the overall hierarchy fits the case of GT-medicinal products, from vector cloning to quality, safety and clinical implementation;
(iii) it is cross-indexed from one section to the next: which makes it both accurate and user-friendly;
(iv) so far, there has been no essential issue found to be missing in this mother GT-NfG document when proceeding with side to side comparison with additional – appearing to be minor and mostly redundant – guidelines. In addition, the overall organisation of new documents was found to be missing to follow the hierarchy of the GT-NfG.

The CliniGene-NoE anticipated that the revision should not be too complicated, given the quality of the existing document, but for the definition of gene therapy, which has been modified, as newly defined in Part IV of Annex I to Directive 2001/83/EC (see *Table I*).

The regulatory framework currently enforced at the EU-centralised level is detailed in *Table III*, which length reflects on the maze of regulatory documents, which currently needs to be referred to.

Scientific novelty should be covered by reflection papers

As mentioned in many occasions, the CliniGene-NoE recommended that scientific novelty will continue to be covered not by novel guidelines but instead, by excellent reflection papers, like in the case of AAV. Guidelines revision would be required only in

Table III. EU regulatory framework applying to ATMPs/ Gene Therapy and GM-cells.

Main Legislation and Guidelines concerning ATMPs in general
1. The European Parliament and the Council of the European Union. Regulation (EC) No 1394/2007 of the European Parliament and of the Council of 13 November 2007 on advanced therapy medicinal products and amending Directive 2001/83/EC and Regulation (EC) No 726/2004. Official J. Eur. Union 10.12.2007, L324/121–L324/137 (2007).
The regulatory framework for ATMPs is established by Regulation (EC) No 1394/2007 on advanced therapy medicinal products which is designed to ensure the free movement of these medicines within the European Union (EU), to facilitate their access to the EU market, and to foster the competitiveness of European pharmaceutical companies in the field, while guaranteeing the highest level of health protection for patients. Regulation (EC) no 1394/2007 also establishes the new expert Committee on Advanced Therapies (CAT).
2. The European Parliament and the Council of the European Union. Commission Directive 2009/120/EC of 14 September 2009 amending Directive 2001/83/ EC of the European Parliament and of the Council on the Community code relating to medicinal products for human use as regards advanced therapy medicinal products. Official J. Europ. Union 15.9.2009, L242/3–L242/12 (2009)
3. European Medicines Agency Guidance on risk-based approach
3a. Committee for Medicinal Products for Human Use (CHMP): **Concept paper** on the development of a guideline on the risk-based approach according to Annex I, Part IV of Dir. 2001/83/EC applied to ATMPs; EMA/CHMP/CPWP/708420/2009: www.ema.europa.eu/pdfs/human/cpwp/70842009en.pdf
3b. Updating 3a : Committee for Advanced Therapies (CAT) and CPWP: **Draft Guideline** on the development of a guideline on the risk-based approach according to Annex I, Part IV of Dir. 2001/83/EC applied to ATMPs; EMA/CAT/CPWP/686637/2011. *Released for consultation January 2012-end of consultation 30 June 2012*
4. EC–Entreprise & Industry Directorate General - Detailed Guidelines on Good Clinical Practice specific to advanced therapy medicinal products. ENTR/F/2/SF/dn D(2009) 35810
5. Directive 2006/17/EC implementing Directive 2004/23/EC as regards certain technical requirements for the donation, procurement and testing of human tissues and cells
6. Directive 2006/86/EC implementing Directive 2004/23/EC as regards traceability requirements, notification of serious adverse reactions and events and certain technical requirements for the coding, processing, preservation, storage and distribution of human tissues and cells
7. EMA guidance documents on Biological drugs 7a. biological drug substances are available at: http://www.ema.europa.eu/ema/index.jsp?curl=pages/regulation/general/general_content_000330.jsp&mid=WC0b01ac058002956b
7b. biological drug products are available at: http://www.ema.europa.eu/ema/index.jsp?curl=pages/regulation/general/general_content_000351.jsp&mid=WC0b01ac058002956c
8. GMO Regulation :
• European Medicines Agency, Committee for Medical Products for Human use : Environmental Risk Assessments for Medicinal Products containing, or consisting of, Genetically Modified Organisms (GMOs) (Module 1.6.2) EMEA/CHMP/473191/06 Corr. Enforced July 2007 • Directive 90/219/EEC of 23 April 1990 on the contained use of genetically modified micro-organisms. • Directive 98/81/EC of 26 October 1998 amending Directive 90/219/EEC on the contained use of genetically modified micro-organisms • Directive 2001/18/EC of the European Parliament and of the Council of 12 March 2001 on the deliberate release into the environment of genetically modified organisms and repealing Council Directive 90/220/EEC. • Regulation (EC) No 1946/2003 of the European Parliament and of the Council of 15 July 2003 on transboundary movements of genetically modified organisms (Text with EEA relevance) • Regulation (EC) No 65/2004 of 14 January 2004 establishing a system for the development and assignment of unique identifiers for genetically modified organisms • Directive 2000/54/EC of the European Parliament and of the Council of 18 September 2000 on the protection of workers from the risks related to exposure to biological agents at work (7th individual directive within the meaning of Article 16(1) of Directive 89/391/EC)

EMA-CAT Guidelines on ATMPs Classification, Evaluation and Certification	
EMEA/630043/2008 (draft)	Procedural advice on the evaluation of ATMPs in accordance with article 8 of regulation (EC) N° 1394/2007 http://www.emea.europa.eu/pdfs/human/cat/63004308en.pdf
EMA/CAT/99623/2009	Procedural advice on the provision of scientific recommendation on classification of ATMPs in accordance with Article 17 of regulation (EC) N° 1394/2007 *(final January 2010)* http://www.emea.europa.eu/pdfs/human/cat/992309en.pdf
EMA/CAT/600280/2010	Reflection paper on classification of advanced therapy medicinal products www.ema.europa.eu/docs/en_GB/document_library/Regulatory_and_procedural_guideline/2012/04/WC500126681.pdf *Released for consultation April 2012-end of consultation 31 july 2012*
EMEA/CAT/418458/2008/corr	Procedural Advice on the certification of quality and non-clinical data for small and medium sized enterprises developing ATMPs. *Adopted by CAT and coming into effect: 15 October 2010* http://www.emea.europa.eu/pdfs/human/cat/41845808en.pdf
EMEA/CAT/486831/2008/corr	Scientific Guideline on the minimum quality and non-clinical data for certification of ATMPs *Adopted by CAT and coming into effect: 15 October 2010* http://www.emea.europa.eu/pdfs/human/cat/48683108en.pdf
EMA Guideline on Pharmacovigilance applying to ATMPs	
EMEA/149995/2008	Guideline on safety and efficacy follow-up - risk Management of ATMPs (GTWP, CPWP, PHVWP, BWP in common) *Adopted CHMP November 2008; coming into effect 31 December 2008* http://www.ema.europa.eu/pdfs/human/advancedtherapies/14999508enfin.pdf

EMA Scientific Guidelines on Gene Therapy	
All Guidelines, Q1A document and reflection papers are available at : http://www.ema.europa.eu/htms/human/humanguidelines/multidiscipline.htm: select «Gene Therapy» or direct link to the Gene Therapy Multidisciplinary page: http://www.ema.europa.eu/ema/index.jsp?curl=pages/regulation/general/general_content_000410.jsp&mid=WC0b01ac058002958d Direct links to individual documents are indicated when available	
General	
EMEA/CPMP/BWP/3088/99	Note for Guidance on the Quality, Preclinical and Clinical Aspects of Gene Transfer Medicinal Products (BWP, SWP, EWP in common) *Adopted by CHMP (CPMP at that time) and coming into effect: October 2001*
EMA/CHMP/GTWP/BWP /234523/2009	Concept paper on the revision of the note for guidance on the quality, pre-clinical and clinical aspects of gene transfer medicinal products www.ema.europa.eu/pdfs/human/genetherapy/23452309en.pdf *End of consultation 31 March 2010*
EMEA/CHMP/GTWP/125491/2006	Guideline on Scientific Requirements for the Environmental Risk Assessment of Gene Therapy Medicinal Products (GTWP, SWP, BWP) *Adopted by CHMP May 2008; coming into effect November 2008*
EMA/CHMP/GTWP/212377/2008	Questions and Answers document on Gene therapy (GTWP) www.ema.europa.eu/pdfs/human/genetherapy/21237708en.pdf *Adopted by CHMP 17 December 2009*
3AB1A based on Directive 75/318/EEC as amended	Guideline on the production and quality control of medicinal products derived from recombinant DNA technology *First adopted June 1987 ; Last revised December 1994*
Links to EMA Guidance documents on biological drug product or substance are indicated above	

EMA Scientific Guidelines on Gene Therapy	*(continued)*
Product-specific	
CPMP/BWP/2458/2003	Guideline on Development and manufacture of lentiviral vectors (BWP, SWP, GTWP, Biologics WP, ICH) *Adopted by CHMP May 2005; coming into operation November 2005*
CHMP/GTWP/607698/200 8 (2009)	ICH Considerations on Oncolytic Viruses (CHMP, ICH) www.ema.europa.eu/pdfs/human/genetherapy/60769808enfin.pdf *Revised version October 2009*
CHMP/GTWP/587488/200 7 (2009)	Reflection Paper on Quality, non-clinical and clinical issues relating specifically to recombinant Adeno-Associated viral vectors www.ema.europa.eu/pdfs/human/genetherapy/58748807en.pdf *End of consultation September 2009*
Non-clinical	
EMEA/273974/2005	Guideline on Non-Clinical testing for Inadvertent Germline transmission of Gene Transfer Vectors (SWP, GTWP) *Adopted by CHMP November 2006; coming into effect May 2007*
EMEA/CHMP/GTWP/125 459/2006	Guideline on Non-Clinical Studies required before first Clinical Use of Gene Therapy Medicinal Products (GTWP, SWP) *Adopted by CHMP May 2008; coming into effect November 2008*
Clinical	
EMEA/CHMP/GTWP/604 36/07 (Updated 11/13/2009)	Guideline on Follow up of patients administered with gene therapy medicinal products (GTWP, Pharmacovigilance and CAT) *Adopted by CHMP October 2009; coming into effect May 2010*
EMEA/CHMP/ICH/44903 5/2009	ICH Considerations on General Principles to Address Virus and Vector Shedding (CHMP, ICH) www.ema.europa.eu/pdfs/human/genetherapy/58748807en.pdf *Transmission to Interested Parties July 2009*
EMA/CAT/GTWP/44236/ 2009	Refection paper on design modifications of gene therapy medicinal products during development *Adopted by CAT December 2011*

EMA Scientific Guidelines on Genetically modified cells and Cell Therapy	
Genetically modified cells	
EMA/CHMP/GTWP/6716 39/2008 (2012)	Guideline on quality, non-clinical and clinical aspects of medicinal products containing genetically modified cells (GTWP, CPWP, BWP, CAT, SWP, EWP) The adopted guideline can be downloaded from EMA Gene Therapy multidisciplinary page: http://www.ema.europa.eu/ema/index.jsp?curl=pages/regulation/general/general_content_000410.jsp&mid=WC0b01ac058002958d *Adopted by CAT April 2012; coming into effect November 2012*
Cell Therapy and Tissue engineering	
Further documents can be downloaded from EMA Cell Therapy and tissue Engineering multidisciplinary page: http://www.ema.europa.eu/ema/index.jsp?curl=pages/regulation/general/general_content_000405.jsp&mid=WC0b0	
EMEA/CHMP/410869/200 6	Guideline on human cell-based medicinal products (CPWP, BWP) www.ema.europa.eu/pdfs/human/ cpwp/41086906enfin.pdf *Adopted by CHMP May 2008 ; coming into effect September 2008*
EMA/CAT/571134/2009 (revised December 2010)	Reflection paper on stem cell-based medicinal products (BWP, SWP, CPWP, CAT) *Adopted by CAT January 2011*
EMA/CAT/CPWP/573420/ 2009	Draft reflection paper on clinical aspects related to tissue-engineered products (CPWP, BWP, SWP, Guideline consistency group, CAT) *End of consultation 31 July 2012*
EMEA/CHMP/BWP/2714 75/2006	Guideline on Potency testing of cell based immunotherapy medicinal products for the treatment of cancer (BWP) *Adopted by CHMP November 2007 ; coming into effect May 2008*
EMEA/CHMP/CPWP/835 08/09	Guideline on xenogeneic cell-based medicinal products (BWP, CPWP, CAT) *Replaces and revises the Point to Consider on Xenogeneic Cell-therapy medicinal products, (CPMP/1199/02)* *Adopted by CAT & CHMP October 2009 ; coming into effect January 2010*

EC & EMA Guidance on Medical Device
Documents on Ancillary medicinal substances: Regulatory and procedural guidance can be downloaded from EMA page: http://www.ema.europa.eu/ema/index.jsp?curl=pages/regulation/general/general_content_000523.jsp&mid=WC0b01ac05800267b9

the event where conceptual issues of concern had not been considered or even deemed conceivable. For instance, there is no requirement for a specific change into the current NfG when considering the transposon-related technology. Points to be considered and issues at stake are likely to have been covered already. The same rationale applies for genetically-modified stem cell based therapy and iPS: there is no essential scientific ground for guideline revision. The CliniGene contribution to commenting Guidelines and GT-related centralised regulation is summarized in *Table IV*. This reflects on the deep and sustained commitment towards improvement which also substantiates the opinions expressed therein.

Table IV. List of EU-centralised Guidelines commented by CliniGene from March 2009 on. CliniGene has provided a forum where regulatory compliance issues can be discussed, and scientifically-based solutions are proposed, thereby facilitating the dialogue with the regulatory authorities and streamlining the development of centralized procedures. In addition, several parameters that address vector quality and safety have been actively investigated in pre-clinical models inside the Network, contributing useful and sometimes unique expertise.

Oncolytic viruses	EMEA/CHMP/GTWP/607698
Quality, non-clinical and clinical issues relating specifically to recombinant AAV	EMEA/CHMP/GTWP/587488/2007
Scientific recommendation on classification of ATMPs in accordance with article 17 of regulation (EC) N°1394/2007	EMEA/99623/2009
The EMEA Transparency policy	EMEA/232037/2009
General principles to address virus and vector shedding	EMEA/CHMP/ICH/449035/2009
Scientific Guideline on the minimum quality and non-clinical data for ATMPs certification	EMEA/CAT/486831/2008
Information on benefit-risk of medicines: patients', consumers' and healthcare professionals expectations	EMA/40926/2009
Assessment of the "Clinical Trials Directive" 2001/20/EC	ENTR/F/2/SF D(2009) 32674
Concept paper on the revision of the NfG on the quality, pre-clinical and clinical aspects of GT medicinal products	EMA/CHMP/GTWP/BWP/234523/2009
Questions and Answers document on Gene therapy	EMA/CHMP/GTWP/212377/2008
Concept paper on the development of a guideline on the risk-based approach : Annex I, Part IV of Dir. 2001/83/EC	EMA/CHMP/CPWP/708420/ 2009
Draft paper for the strategic development of EMA for 5 years	EMA/299895/2009
Detailed guidelines on GCP specific to ATMPs	ENTR/F/2/SF/dn D(2009) 35810
Reflection paper on stem cell-based medicinal products	EMA/CAT/571134/2009
Guideline on quality, non-clinical and clinical aspects of medicinal products containing genetically modified cells	EMA/CHMP/ GTWP/ 671639/2008
Concept paper submitted for public consultation: The European Commission is planning to put forward, in 2012, a legislative proposal to revise the Clinical Trials Directive 2001/20/EC	Clinical trials directive 2001/20/ec (SANCO/C/8/PB/SF D(2011) 143488)

CONCLUSION: INTEGRATING ETHICS AND REGULATION WITH SCIENCE AND CLINICAL TRANSLATION: THE CLINIGENE-NOE EXPERIENCE

An important ethical, legal and regulatory component made the CliniGene-NoE a central European Medicines Agency (EMA) stake-holder with expert advisory potential to CAT in the Gene Therapy field while in operation. The quality of interaction, which has been established with Regulatory Authorities would not have been possible at the level of individual institutions.

O. Cohen-Haguenauer

Education, policy development, advisory ethical review, information-sharing through conferences, publications, and public education that combines ethics and science and involves all relevant stakeholders in a comprehensive advisory role, as developed *via* CliniGene, holds a potential for complementing that of the regulatory authorities: this is to ensure early dialogue, robust accountability, high levels of transparency, open, clear, and timely flow of communications, and clarity of decision making roles, all of which represent key values for safe clinical trials and, ultimately, effective Gene and Cell Therapy Medicinal Products (ATMPs). Indeed, research on ATMPs must be translational – that is, coordinated across the development of technologies, assays and materials, and from preclinical through clinical trials, rather than simply focusing on research involving human subjects towards their best benefit and protection.

ACKNOWLEDGMENTS

This work has been performed with the support of the EC-DG research through the FP6-Network of Excellence, CLINIGENE: LSHB-CT-2006-018933.

REFERENCES

(most EU-Regulation, Directives, Guidelines and Reflection Papers and accurate web-links are already referenced in Tables)

1. Committee for Advanced Therapies (CAT); CAT Scientific Secretariat, Schneider CK, Salmikangas P, Jilma B, Flamion B, Todorova LR, Paphitou A, Haunerova I, Maimets T, Trouvin JH, Flory E, Tsiftsoglou A, Sarkadi B, Gudmundsson K, O'Donovan M, Migliaccio G, Ancāns J, Maciulaitis R, Robert JL, Samuel A, Ovelgönne JH, Hystad M, Fal AM, Lima BS, Moraru AS, Turcáni P, Zorec R, Ruiz S, Akerblom L, Narayanan G, Kent A, Bignami F, Dickson JG, Niederwieser D, Figuerola-Santos MA, Reischl IG, Beuneu C, Georgiev R, Vassiliou M, Pychova A, Clausen M, Methuen T, Lucas S, Schüssler-Lenz M, Kokkas V, Buzás Z, MacAleenan N, Galli MC, Linē A, Gulbinovic J, Berchem G, Fraczek M, Menezes-Ferreira M, Vilceanu N, Hrubisko M, Marinko P, Timón M, Cheng W, Crosbie GA, Meade N, di Paola ML, VandenDriessche T, Ljungman P, D'Apote L, Oliver-Diaz O, Büttel I, Celis P. Challenges with advanced therapy medicinal products and how to meet them. *Nat Rev Drug Discov* 2010; 9: 195-201.

2. Kent A, King NM, Cohen-Haguenauer O. Toward a proportionate regulatory framework for gene transfer: a patient group-led initiative. *Hum Gene Ther* 2011; 22: 126-34.

3. King NM, Cohen-Haguenauer O. En route to ethical recommendations for gene transfer clinical trials. *Mol Ther* 2008; 16: 432-8.

4. Jacqueline Corrigan-Curay, Odile Cohen-Haguenauer, Marina O'Reilly, Susan R. Ross, Hung Fan, Naomi Rosenberg, Nikunj Somia, Nancy King, Ted Friedmann, Cynthia Dunbar, Alessandro Aiuti, Luigi Naldini, Christopher Baum, Christof von Kalle, Hans-Peter Kiem, Eugenio Montini, Frederic Bushman, Brian P. Sorrentino, Manuel Carrondo, Harry Malech, Gösta Gahrton, Robyn Shapiro, Linda Wolff, Eugene Rosenthal, Robert Jambou, John Zaia, Donald B. Kohn. Challenges in vector and trial design using retroviral vectors for long-term gene correction in hematopoietic stem cell gene therapy: summary of a Symposium sponsored by the NIH Office of Biotechnology Activities and the EC DG-research NoE for the Advancement of Clinical Gene Transfer and Therapy. *Mol Ther* 2012; 20: 1084-94.

The CliniBook: Clinical gene transfer
Edited by Odile Cohen-Haguenauer – EDK, Paris © 2012, pp. 517-527

C2-3
The necessity for data sharing towards advancement of clinical translation
Building up sample IMPD* and substantiating master files

ODILE COHEN-HAGUENAUER

CliniGene, École Normale Supérieure de Cachan, CNRS UMR 8113, 94235 Cachan, France and Department of Clinical Oncology, Hôpital Saint-Louis and Université Paris-Diderot, Sorbonne Paris-Cité, 75475 Paris Cedex 10, France.
odile.cohen@lbpa.ens-cachan.fr

The CliniGene consortium has integrated its effort and skills in order to: (i) progress from gene discovery, through pre-clinical research to clinical approaches and (ii) decipher the key elements which could be drivers to clinical success so that reference standards and requisites implementing relevant good practices can be established, if possible. In order to foster safe and high quality clinical gene transfer treatments, the European Network for the advancement of gene transfer and therapy approached the definition of key-criteria resulting from interesting pre-clinical results which enable the decision as to whether it is a "go" or a "no go to the clinic" with a reasonable enough margin of confidence towards both minimized risk for harm and foreseeable success. The Clinigene-NoE has aimed to: (i) avoid the reproduction of Phase I trials asking the same questions and (ii) to prevent predictable failures to enter the clinical phase, which besides the deleterious consequences on the patients entering the study, would also penalise the field as a whole (iii) deliver practical results opening new opportunities for funding research and clinical development in this field, and thereby favour the expansion of the high-tech industry sector. So far, over 20 clinical trials have been accompanied by CliniGene.

With the prospect of building up a sample IMPD addressing gene therapy, our purpose is to accelerate regulatory approval of new clinical trials, based on systems which have been used by other teams with different genes addressing distinct conditions.

*Investigational Medicinal Product Dossier

Gene and cell therapy medicinal products are new and innovative medicinal products. They are biological medicinal products according to Regulation (EC) No 1394/2007 within the meaning of *Annex I* to Directive 2001/83/EC (see section C2-2 for details, *ibid.*). The Committee for Advanced Therapies (CAT) was created and entered into force on January 1st, 2009, which is responsible for preparing draft opinions on the quality, safety and efficacy of each advanced therapy medicinal product (ATMP) for final approval by EMA. In addition, Part IV, *Annex I* to Directive 2001/83/EC was revised as regard to the specificity of ATMPs.

As part of the centralised regulatory framework, the CTD was created for new chemical entities (NCE). These products were the first medicinal products which were globally developed and the harmonisation according to the CTD was very useful. At that time, there was no plan for products like ATMPs to use the CTD structure. There now is a need to reconsider the CTD according to ATMP requirements (new part IV, *Annex I* to Directive 2001/83/EC as regard to the specifities of ATMPs) and generate a specific format to be used in all member states, also covering GMOs related aspects and which will reduce related work and costs Europewide.

1. THE INVESTIGATIONAL MEDICINAL PRODUCTS DOSSIER (IMPD)

1.1. What is an IMPD?

The IMP dossier (IMPD) provides summary information related to the following items (definition according to EC communication March 2010):

Table I. The IMPD Contents.

1.	Quality, manufacture and control details of the IMP (CTD format) for reference medication and comparator, placebo
2.	Data from preclinical toxicology/biodistribution and pharmacology studies
3.	Data from previous clinical use (if applicable): summaries of studies (not study report)
4.	Overall risk-benefit assessment of the intended use
5.	Copies of manufacturing / import authorisations
6.	Examples of the drug product labels in national language

The Content of the dossier is thus adapted to the level of knowledge (and phase of development).

1.2. What is an Investigational Medicinal Product (IMP)?

According to the Definition in Directive 2001/20/EC (article 2 d), an Investigational Medicinal Product is either:
- a pharmaceutical form of an active substance or placebo being tested or used as a reference in a clinical trial;
- or including products already with a marketing authorisation: (i) but used or assembled (formulated or packaged) in a way different from the authorised form; or (ii) used for an unauthorised indication; or (iii) used to gain further information about the authorised form.

1.3. Clinical Trials in Europe (Detailed Regulation is provided in chapter C2-2, *ibid.*)

The conduct of Clinical Trials in Europe is placed under provisions of the Directive 2001/20/EC - (currently under revision) as the Clinical Trials Regulation.

Initial aims of the Clinical Trials Directive
- The prominent goal of the Directive was to simplify and harmonise clinical trial procedures across EU in order to: (i) protect trial subjects; (ii) help and accompany the process leading to authorisation of trials; (iii) require and secure ethical approval of all protocols; (iv) scrutinise and define the quality of study drug; (v) establish requirements for standards and inspections; (vi) frame and facilitate pharmacovigilance; (vii) encourage and streamline exchange of information between Member States; (viii) reduce duplication of paperwork for submission; (ix) overall improve the quality of research · standard operating procedures · training · monitoring · inspections · audit · use of GMP and GLP.
- Nevertheless, up until the Marketing authorisation phase, approval of clinical trials is being granted at the national level and each country has a slightly different interpretation of the Directive and related Guidelines.

Overview
- **Scope (Articles 1 and 2)**
  - Covers all trials of Medicinal Products except non-interventional trials (marketed products used for their licensed indication).
  - Includes all Phase I Studies and Investigator led studies.
  - Investigator does not need to be an MD but patient care must be placed under the supervision of an MD.

- **Commencement of Clinical Trial (Article 9)**
  - The Study can only start when: (i) ad hoc ethics committee has issued 'favourable opinion'. (ii) The Member State 'has not informed the Sponsor of any grounds for non-acceptance'.
  - The submission to Regulatory Authority and Ethics Committee can be pursued in parallel.

The need to revise Directive 2001/20/EC was unanimously accepted during the course of year 2011 and the process in underway. With respect to gene- and cell-therapy clinical trials and in particular, those sponsored by academic/non-profit organisations, they are not necessarily performed with the intention to generate data to support an application for the marketing authorisation of a medicinal product. Therefore a specific track for the evaluation/approval of these studies might deserve consideration. Whilst the model of big pharma driven multi-centre large scale study may be appropriate when considering the development of small molecules for common diseases, it is increasingly inappropriate when addressing a majority of rare disorders: indeed, the development model from phase I to phase IV does not seem accurate, given the reduced number of patients and the multinational accrual, within an Academic setting in many cases at least in early phases of the clinical studies.

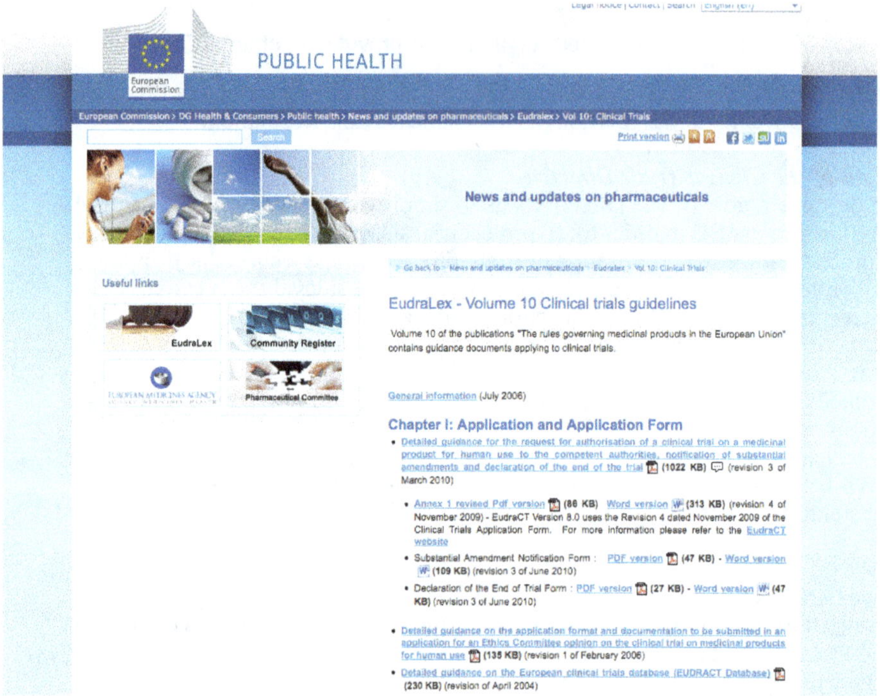

Figure 1. Clinical Trial application form: Eudralex-Volume 10. Commission Communication-revision 3. Detailed Guidance for the request for authorisation of a clinical trial on a medicinal product for human use to the competent authorities. Notification of substantial amendments and declaration of the end of the trial (March 2010). http://ec.europa.eu/health/documents/eudralex/vol10/index_en.htm

2. IMPD

The sponsor of a clinical trial must seek a Clinical Trials Authorisation (CTA) by submitting various clinical trial related documents and an Investigational Medicinal Products Dossier (IMPD): these provisions also apply for ATMPs.
According to guidance documents on the structure of both the CTA and IMPD, there are two types of IMPD:
  • Full IMPD.
  • Simplified IMPD – based on whether the product has previously been described in a CTA or an MAA.

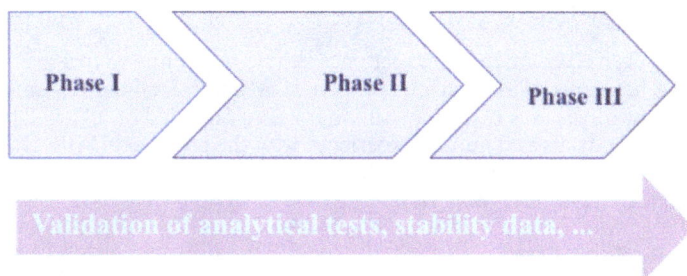

Figure 2. Quality requirements change with the phase of the clinical development.

2.1. Building the IMPD: why it is important?

This document is essential as it will form the foundation for all future regulatory documents and be used for communications to regulators about the product as well as the basis of support for Scientific Advice, Protocol Assistance, Orphan Drug Applications, etc. The IMPD gathers information generated from many sources while all documents need to be consistent. In particular, it provides comprehensive information used to determine the Risk/Benefit profile of the IMP. Therefore, the establishment of the IMPD is a team work which requires coordination and consolidation from many prospectives and complementary expertise.

2.2 Structure and Content of a CTA and IMPD

The documentation to be provided to the National Competent Authority of the Member State are the CTA and Investigational Medicinal Products Dossier, the content of which is detailed in the *Table II* below:

Table II. The Contents of CTA and IMPD.

Cover letter	draw attention to special issues in the study, unusual trial designs, F-I-H administrations, unusual products
EudraCT Number	details as applied for (European Union Drug Regulating Authorities Clinical Trials)
Clinical trial application form	contact details for Sponsor and Investigator - download from EudraCT site
Protocol	written to comply with GCP Guidelines: describes the objective(s), design, methodology, statistical considerations and organisation of a trial
Investigational Brochure	written to comply with Directive 2005/28/EC and GCP Guidelines
Investigational Medicinal Products Dossier (IMPD)	written to comply with Guidelines
Additional pieces of documentation	*e.g.*: opinion of the Ethics Committee, summary of scientific advice from any MS or EMA, PIP

2.3. IMPD Clinical Section Outline

Clinical trial and data derived from human experience should be submitted in a logical structure such as the headings of the current version of Module 5 of the Common Technical Document, or of the eCTD format. Summaries are provided of all available data from previous clinical trials and human experience with the proposed IMPs. Data must comply with the GCP directive and the Guideline: General considerations for clinical trials (CPMP/ICH/291/95) (*Table III*).

Table III. IMPD Clinical Section Outline.

Clinical Pharmacology	• Summary · Mechanism of Action · Secondary Pharmacological Effects • Pharmacodynamic Interactions
Clinical Pharmacokinetics	• Summary · Absorption · Distribution · Elimination · Pk of Metabolites • Concentration · Effect Relationships · Dose Time Dependencies • Special Populations · Interactions
Human Exposure	• Summary · Overview of Safety and Efficacy · Healthy Subject Studies • Patient Studies · Previous Human Experience · Benefits and Risks
For a First-in-Human (F-I-H) study	• Many sections have no data = 'Not Applicable'

However there are points to consider which are specific to ATMPs and gene therapy trials, which are being considered and detailed in Annex I at the end of the chapter.

2.4. IMPD – Overall Risk Benefit Assessment

In this section, the non-clinical and clinical data shall be critically analysed in relation to the potential risks and benefits of the proposed trial. The sponsor should discuss safety margins in terms of relative systematic exposure to the IMP and the clinical relevance of any findings in the non-clinical and clinical studies along with any recommendations for further monitoring of effects and safety in the clinical trials. Therefore the following issues shall be covered:
• Provide a brief summary of the non-clinical and clinical data (if any) in relation to the potential risks and benefits of the proposed trial.
• Identify any studies that were stopped early with reasons.
• Give any additional risks that might occur in special populations if relevant.
• Use all the data available to extrapolate risks in humans.
• Discuss safety margins in relation to possible exposure.
• Identify any additional monitoring that will be necessary if any.

2.5. IMPD requirements to the chemical and Pharmaceutical documentation concerning IMPs in clinical trials: the eCTD does not fit the case of ATMP

Eudralex Volume 10
Chemical and pharmaceutical documentation

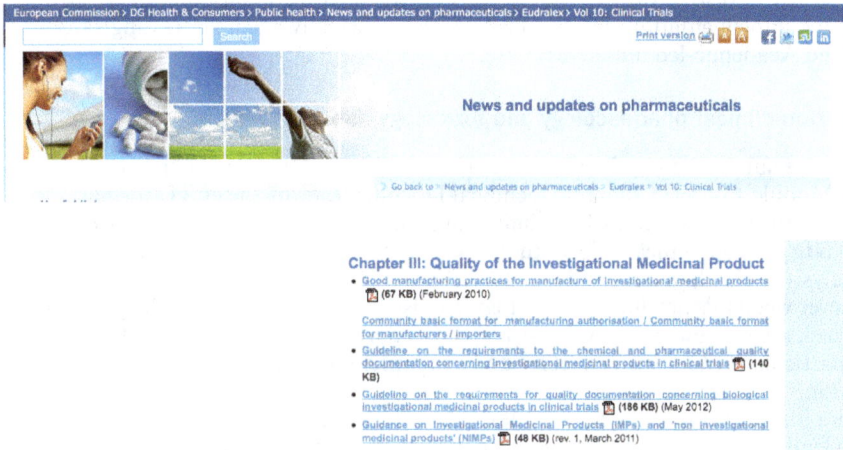

Figure 3. Guideline on the requirements to the chemical and Pharmaceutical documentation concerning IMPs in clinical trials as of Eudralex Volume 10.

As it is, the guideline on the requirements to the chemical and pharmaceutical documentation concerning IMPs in clinical trials does not fit the case of ATMPS nor that of Gene Therapy vectors and products in particular, as shown on *Figure 4*.

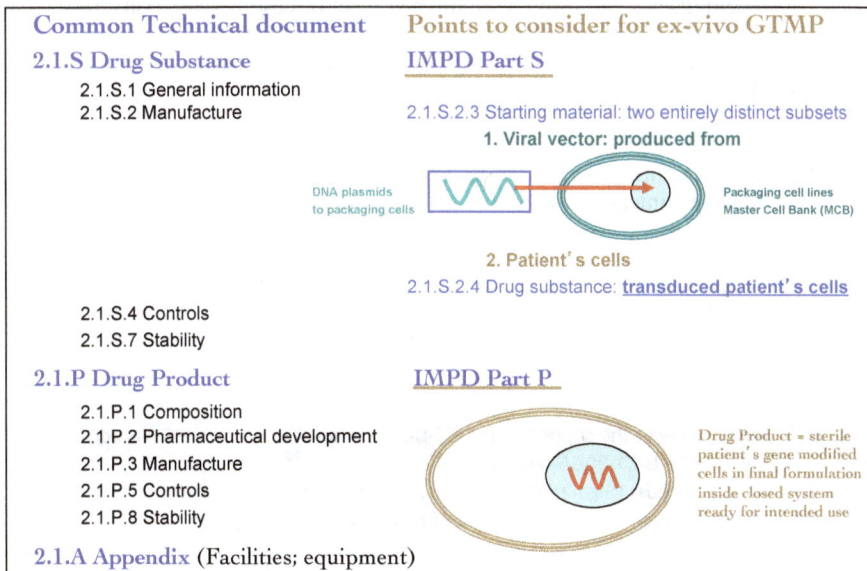

Figure 4. Example of ATMP specifics: IMPD for *ex vivo* GTMP.

O. Cohen-Haguenauer

As a first step, a frame could be established which addresses *"Lentis for ex-vivo GM-cells"* on the one hand and *"AAV in vivo"*, on the other. *"Lentis in vivo"* could be considered as the next target (*see chapter C1-7, ibid.*). The next step could consist in substantiating the IMPD with data that might be inferred from already acquired knowledge sourcing from both: (i) the literature and (ii) the clinical experience of CliniGene-related or other investigators willing to participate into an endaveour likely to streamline the implementation of new clinical trials, especially when addressing rare disorders and Academic-led initiatives.

2.6. IMPD Non-clinical pharmacology and toxicology data

Data should be submitted in a logical structure, such as the headings of the current version of Module 4 of the Common Technical Document, or of the eCTD format. Reference is made to the specific Community guidelines contained in Volume 3 of Eudralex *e.g.* Nfg on non-clinical safety studies which include the need to proceed to a critical analysis of the data and implement GLP provisions in all experiments performed. However when this preclinical toxicology/biodistribution and pharmacology data are concerned, the framework needs to be adapted to the case of ATMPs as mentioned above; in particular gene transfer vectors and gene-manipulated cells deserve further consideration.

Efforts were initiated inside the CliniGene-NoE in order to establish master-files in parallel on lentivirus vectors and AAVs, as a first priority. These vector profiles generic data-base should ideally consist of a compilation of safety and quality issues, biodistribution profiles and pharmacotoxicology, building up "master files", which will need constant update as data will show. Information gathered will vary according to the vector system. Lentivectors are being used for both *ex-vivo* transduction of gene-manipulated cells and via direct *in-vivo* administration routes while AAV-derived vectors are mostly used *in-vivo*. The data-set which need to be assembled prior to clinical authorisation follow rigorous common frames, as tentatively formulated as of *Annex II*. Specifics to the gene and disease of concern remain a subject of case-by-case consideration and testing. Indeed, we need to decipher at best how processes that are customised to each patient individually can be described in a CTD addressing individualised products like ATMPs.

When considering the next steps downstream of the CliniGene-NoE, the building up of sample IMPD and substantiating master files appears as a priority towards advancement of and facilitating clinical translation in gene therapy.

REFERENCES

References on Directives and Guidelines are indicated inside the text.

ACKNOWLEDGMENTS

This work has been performed with the support of the EC-DG research through the FP6-Network of Excellence, CLINIGENE: LSHB-CT-2006-018933.
The author thanks Christa Schroeder (Sigmaringen), Alan Boyd (Manchester) and Didier Caizergues (Généthon-Évry) for their participation into ESGCT and CliniGene meetings.

ANNEX I - DESCRIPTION OF A GENE TRANSFER CLINICAL TRIAL AND STUDY DESIGN

Beside Flow-chart and information on the study protocol

a) Sponsor (Name, address)
b) Official title of the study
c) Clinical phase if other than Pilot or Phase I) and type (randomised/non-randomised; type of making; type of controls and group assignment)
d) Principal Investigator Coordinating the clinical study (Name, mail)
e) Monocentric / Multicentric; if multicentric, National or International other centres involved (name of the centre, name of principal investigator, address);
f) Has the trial been submitted to an appropriate research ethics committee; if yes, date of approval (or review) by appropriate Research ethics committee
g) Has the trial been submitted to a relevant Health competent Authority; if yes, date of approval by regulatory authorities
h) Estimated study period
• *Inclusion period (anticipated start date)*
• *From the first patient in to the last patient out*
i) Short summary and rationale of the study including (i) name of the intervention; (ii) the condition being studied; (iii) preclinical studies, and (iv) expected outcome (*e.g.* 10 lines)
j) Condition under consideration
k) Objectives (primary and secondary)
l) Include flow-chart, trial design at the end if possible
m) Target sample size: number of patients expected in this trial
n) Key inclusion criteria
o) Key exclusion criteria
p) Gene and cell therapy specifics
• *Cell-target*
• *Gene of interest*
• *Vector system: entry according to menu/ key words*
• *Promotor/regulated transcription*
• *Targeted cell entry*
• Ex vivo/in vivo *procedure*
• *Route of administration*
• *Dose*
q) Primary outcome
r) Key secondary outcomes and time of measurement
• *Efficacy evaluation*
• *Safety evaluation and criteria selected thereof*
s) EudraCT registration number
t) Abstracts and Publications
u) Source of detailed protocol information
v) Contacts of person filling in the questionnaire
w) Contact for further information (if different from #v)

ANNEX II - GENERIC MATRIX FOR A VECTOR SYSTEM COMMON PROFILE DATA-BASE

Objectives

To establish and extract knowledge pertaining to, whenever possible, generic vector system profiles: biodistribution, pharmacokinetics and pharmacotoxicology data concerning a vector system of concern that will have to be taken into consideration whatever the gene of interest included in the final combination product.

I. Pharmacological data on the vector
1. Biodistribution and diffusion of the vector
2. Tissue targeting (transduction, transcription)
3. Gene expression: (i) Regulatory sequences: tissue or cell specific promoters, (ii) Protein coding sequences: expression of viral proteins

II. Pharmacological data on the administered product

a. Efficacy of gene transfer and expression
1. Molecular evaluation: (i) Status of transferred gene (degree of integration, number of copies, etc.); (ii) Random or targeted integration; (iii) Genetic stability of transferred sequences; (iv) Short- and long-term stability; (v) Frequency of rearrangements
2. Biological evaluation: (i) Level of expression, genotype/phenotype correlation: percentage of transferred cells; (ii) Identity and activity of the product(s) expressed; (iii) Stability of expression; (iv) Duration of expression, of the detection of the transgene, and of the detection of the vector; (v) Magnitude of the three previous items
3. Phenotypic modifications induced in the target cells: (i) Lifespan of genetically modified cells; (ii) Modifications sought (phenotypic modifications): (iii) Collateral modifications (phenotypic modifications, dose-effect relation, differentiation, change in immunogenicity...)
4. Animal studies: (i) Nude animal models; (ii) Transgenic animals; (iii) Other models
5. Satellite animals (Vector shedding)

b. Justification of the dose and route administration
(i) Routes of administration used in animal studies
(ii) Recommended doses employed: dose-ranging, repeated doses, etc.
(iii) Recommended time lapse between two administrations (knowledge acquired from the duration of expression)

III. Pharmacokinetics of the product administered
(i) Biodistribution of the administered product;
(ii) Kinetics and route of elimination;
(iii) Are the pharmacokinetic profiles altered after repeated administrations?

IV. Toxicological data on the vector
1. For all vectors: (i) Immunological reaction against the vector: immediate, or future (if re-exposure); (ii) Pathogenicity of the vector; (iii) Reactivation of integrated viruses (CMV, Herpes).

---

2. For all viral vectors: (i) Toxicity related to viremia (*e.g.* toxic shock); (ii) Cyto-toxicity of the known vector (species specificity, cell type where replication occurs); (iii) Risk of virus overproduction; (iv) Vector-related risk; (v) Recombination or complementation of the defective vector: *e.g.*, case of a retrovirus vector: lesions described with RCR emergence
3. For transgenic cells: (i) Phenotypic data; (ii) Complement-dependent destruction.

V. Toxicological data of the product administered
1. Single dose toxicity: (i) Toxic dose-ranging; (ii) Proof of non-toxicity at the recommended effective dose: maximal dose(s) without toxic effect
2. Repeated doses toxicity
3. Long-term studies: (i) Definition of long term, based on the chosen animal model; (ii) How long has the follow-up been in this animal model?
4. Potential for release of the gene: (i) Analysis performed on animal model intended to predict potential efficacy; (ii) Distribution outside of targeted cells: (a) Local pathogenicity; (b) Likelihood for dissemination in germ line; (c) Status of the germ cells; (iii) Sentinel animals
5. Toxicology for the reproductive functions: (i) Information on transfer to the germ cells; (ii) Effect on the embryo and/or foetus
6. Mutagenesis: (i) Tests of gene mutation and clastogenesis done; (ii) Insertional mutagenesis
7. Carcinogenesis
8. Immunological data
9. Other toxicological effects: (i) Linked to the expression of proteins other than that of the gene of interest; (ii) Related to impurities: (a) Reagents (e.g. cesium chloride); (b) Culture medium; (c) Excipients
10. Local tolerance

INTEGRATION
AND DISSEMINATION

The CliniBook: Clinical gene transfer
Edited by Odile Cohen-Haguenauer – EDK, Paris © 2012, pp. 531-532

C3-1
European Union support to gene transfer and gene therapy

RUXANDRA DRAGHIA-AKLI

*MD, PhD, RTD – Director Health, Research and Innovation DG European Commission,
B-1049 Brussels, Belgium.*
ruxandra.draghia-akli@ec.europa.eu

Over the years and through its Framework Programmes for Research and Technological Development, the European Union has played an important role in supporting collaborative efforts in gene transfer and gene therapy research in Europe. It has aimed to develop tools, methods and models with the ultimate goal of bringing to the clinic and the market treatments for debilitating, deadly and rare diseases. During the Fifth (1998-2002) and Sixth (2002-2006) Framework Programmes, the EU invested more than €148 million in 56 collaborative projects in this area. In particular, €12 million were allocated to a network of excellence for the advancement of clinical gene transfer and therapy, CliniGene, with a particular focus on quality and safety standards. The network gathered 41 partners of which 11 industrial partners. The topics covered by the network and described in the CliniBook speak for themselves in terms of excellence, progress in the field and critical mass of knowledge. In short timelines for medical sciences, we have moved from the empirical to products ready to enter clinical trials and to benefit patients. CliniGene was structured around platforms focussing on the various gene delivery tools, training and interactions between the participants, and the specific ethical and regulatory aspects of gene therapy. After years of questions, the field is now at the stage of translational research and clinical trials in humans and European teams are leading the field of rare disease treatment. The network can be considered as a European success story. CliniGene has also sponsored the annual meetings of the European Society of Gene and Cell Therapy and organized trainings and scientific exchanges in order to spread expertise in Europe and beyond.

During FP7, specific calls for projects involving clinical trials or targeting small and medium size enterprises and industry partners have been issued in order to further structure the field and to promote the translation phase of promising products to patients. Moreover, several partners of the CliniGene consortium have been awarded grants from FP7 for collaborative projects or from the European Research Council, demonstrating the dynamism and the excellence in the field. Additional gains in competitiveness and knowledge in ethical, safety, toxicity and regulatory aspects of the

R. Draghia-Akli

research are essential to further develop the whole field in a reinforced European regulatory context for advanced therapy medicinal products.

Recently, the first gene therapy product (Glybera®) in Europe has been approved for
the treatment of patients suffering from lipoprotein lipase deficiency with severe or
multiple pancreatitis attacks. This constitutes a major progress since 2007 when the
regulation 1394/2007 on authorisation, supervision and pharmacovigilance of advanced therapy medicinal products was published and might pave the way for future applications.

This book summarizes the achievements and perspectives of more than five years of
support to the consortium from the European Union.

The CliniBook: Clinical gene transfer
Edited by Odile Cohen-Haguenauer – EDK, Paris © 2012, pp. 533-535

C3-2
Database of clinical trials

BERND GÄNSBACHER

Institute of Experimental Oncology and Therapy Research, Klinikum rechts der Isar der Technischen Universität München, Munich, Germany.
bernd.gansbacher@lrz.tum.de

INTRODUCTION

The main reason medical databases have been established is not only the reduction of rate and impact of medical errors; also informing the public about therapeutic options, progress in respective fields and helping in the decision making process. These objectives require to be influenced by practical considerations, such as costs associated with collecting, analyzing, and interpreting the information collected and ensuring helpful and appropriate dissemination of findings.

The Clinigene Consortium decided that the value of such a database was worth the effort and decided to establish a database of European clinical gene therapy trials.

A SIMPLE STRUCTURE

Experts in the field had been contacted initially with the primary aim to establish a clinical gene transfer data base, with a direct link foreseen through the network website in order to make a publicly available list of relevant past and ongoing clinical trials in the EU. The implementation of the project started in October 2006 with the identification of appropriate IT specialists. Several proposals of database structure and application modes were evaluated and one of them selected. The database (DB) includes the following fields: 1. ID; 2. Disease; 3. Study Title; 4. Vector system; 5. Gene of interest; 6. Route of Administration; 7. Publications (specific to the CliniGene-DB); 8. Status: Open/Closed/Suspended; 9. Institution or Hospital; 10. Sponsor; 11. Contact (open a new window to send an e-mail); 12; More information (link to publicly available source: *e.g.* Orphanet) (*Table I*).

DATA SOURCING

Data from the GTAC (UK), the Swiss data base, the Spanish one and the already established Euregenethy data base, including all published gene therapy trials up until 2006 were initially used. Since then, the CliniGene communication manager is retrieving monthly data from PubMed in order to keep the DB updated and live. Data from the Orphanet database have been included and are revised at regular interval. The database was set up and started running during the course of 2009.

An especially difficult task was the integration of minimal but non-confidential information from the EMA EudraC. It is an optimal asset and productive collaboration benefitting all parties and stake-holders involved. Negotiations with EMA started in 2007. A letter had been sent to the Executive Director of EMA, Dr Thomas Lönngren to which he nicely replied. Insofar as therapies addressing pediatric patients are concerned, the Pediatric regulation 1901/2006, Art 41 introduced derogation to Art 11 of the GCP Directive 2001/20/EC whereby the information gathered through EudraCT will be made publicly available by EMA. The available data were included in the Clinigene database as well.

In general clinical registers have not generally been used in assessing the effectiveness of one technology against another, largely because they tend to be confined to single technologies. Our database includes information on different gene transfer systems. The scope for intertechnology comparisons is growing in every field, we have anticipated these demands.

CONFIDENTIALITY, PROTECTION OF INTELLECTUAL PROPERTY AND LEGAL IMMUNITY

Research in the USA has suggested that one barrier to clinicians participating in exercises of this sort stems from concerns regarding lack of confidentiality, loss of intellectual property rights and perceived increased risk of negligence suits. In many databases guarantees have been made to ensure that material submitted or unearthed during any subsequent investigations, cannot be divulged to a third party. In the UK, aggregated data compiled anonymously would be unlikely to be relevant to the facts of a particular case.

In the case of the CliniGene database a minimum of essential information was selected to minimize those risks and to foster collaborations.

Table I. Structure of essential information included into the EU-clinical trials DB. CliniGene EU-GT trials Database fields (in blue: first layer).

ID
Disease
Title
Vector
Gene of interest
Route of Administration to the Database
Publications (specific to the CliniGene Database)
Open/Closed/Suspended
Institution or Hospital
Sponsor
Contact (open a new window to send an e-mail without display of the e-mail contact)
More information (link to publicly available source: *e.g.* orphanet)

The CliniGene EU-Gene Therapy trials Database can be accessed from the CliniGene web-site: www.clinigene.eu [1].

MANDATORY OR VOLUNTARY REPORTING

Both mandatory and voluntary schemes have been shown to suffer from problems of under-reporting, an important finding in the context of studies.

Voluntary, confidential reporting schemes are more suited to promoting safety improvement since they are more likely to bring to light incidents – whether or not patients have been harmed – and to include information about latent errors. Experience suggests voluntary databases are viewed with less suspicion by prospective contributors and, if accompanied by guarantees of confidentiality, are likely to offer fuller and richer appreciations of medical error for the purposes of clinical governance than would information gained from mandatory reporting schemes.

Clinigene does not have the means for demanding mandatory reporting and choose voluntary reporting and collection of published information as the means to establish this database.

TRANSPARENCY IN DISSEMINATING KNOWLEDGE AND OUTREACH

To optimize its performance, any healthcare system requires valid and reliable routine data even at a very early stage. Routine data have a crucial role given the large and growing number of health technologies whose effectiveness, risks and costs require to be monitored. Moreover, routine data can assess the diffusion and equity of delivery of efficacious technologies in addition to the withdrawal of less efficacious ones.

Very few databases will in the foreseeable future be capable of meeting these requirements for health technology assessment. These barriers apply particularly to assessing effectiveness, with few databases matching the required criteria. In the Gene Therapy field, the GeMCRIS database represents an extremely sophisticated and comprenhesive system which encompasses all technologies and includes all NIH funded US Clinical trials [2]. Institutional arrangements for progress are generally lacking. No overall strategy exists for all healthcare databases. Concerns over confidentiality and consent are working to reduce access and perhaps to restrict the scope of clinical databases.

Against this, the continuing advances in IT and the policy requirements for improved data will lead to fundamental changes. Over time, more routine databases will meet the standards of the clinical registers.

CliniGene with its database was several steps ahead of the general field in Europe and laid the ground for an information tool which Society needs. Progress in the field of gene therapy is visible on a monthly basis and successes are already showing in patients affected with some rare disorders. To keep the public informed, databases are essential.

ACKNOWLEDGMENTS

This work has been performed with the support of the EC-DG research through the FP6-Network of Excellence, CLINIGENE: LSHB-CT-2006-018933.

REFERENCES

1. EU Inventory of clinical trials: http://141.39.175.7/eutrials/

2. NIH Genetic modification clinical research information system (GeMCRIS®): http://www.gem-cris.od.nih.gov/Contents/GC_HOME.asp

The CliniBook: Clinical gene transfer
Edited by Odile Cohen-Haguenauer – EDK, Paris © 2012, pp. 536-540

C3-3

CliniGene and ESGCT shared vision for gene therapy in Europe: past, present and future prospects

Thierry VandenDriessche[1]*, Bernd Gänsbacher[2], George Dickson[3],
David Klatzmann[4], Seppo Ylä-Herttuala[5], Luigi Naldini[6], Alastair Kent[7],
Odile Cohen-Haguenauer[8]*

[1]*Department of Gene Therapy and Regenerative Medicine, Free University of Brussels (VUB), Faculty of Medicine and Pharmacy, University Medical Center - Jette, Laarbeeklaan 103, B-1090 Brussels, Belgium.*
thierry.vandendriessche@vub.ac.be
[2]*Institute of Experimental Oncology and Therapy Research, Klinikum rechts der Isar der Technischen Universität München, Munich, Germany.*
[3]*School of Biological Sciences, Royal Holloway, University of London, Egham Hill, Egham, Surrey, TW20 0EX, United Kingdom.*
[4]*Université Pierre et Marie Curie, UPMC Université Paris 06, CNRS UMR7211, Inserm U959, Hôpital Pitié-Salpêtrière, 83, boulevard de l'Hôpital, 75013 Paris, France.*
[5]*A.I. Virtanen Institute, University of Eastern Finland, P.O. Box 1627, FI-70211 Kuopio, Finland.*
[6]*San Raffaele Telethon Institute for Gene Therapy, Department of Regenerative Medicine, Stem Cells and Gene Therapy, San Raffaele Institute Milan, Via Olgettina-58, 20132 Milan, Italy Italy.*
[7]*Genetic Alliance UK, 436 Essex Road, London, United Kingdom.*
[8]*École Normale Supérieure de Cachan, ClinGene, CNRS UMR 8113, 94235 Cachan and Department of Medical Oncology, Hôpital Saint-Louis, AP-HP; Faculté de Médecine, Université Paris-Diderot, Sorbonne-Paris-Cité, 75475 Paris Cedex 10, France.*
odile.cohen@lbpa.ens-cachan.fr
* Corresponding authors

Gene therapy becoming a clinical reality

Gene therapy offers unprecedented opportunities to treat or cure disease and alleviate human suffering. EU researchers have played key and pioneering roles in this field to demonstrate that gene therapy works effectively in patients with life-threatening diseases. A majority of infants and young patients afflicted by a range of devastating inborn diseases and that have been treated by gene therapy can now lead essentially normal lives. These remarkable and historical achievements formally prove that gene therapy, indeed stands as a realistic and successful medical intervention. Most importantly to clinicians, these successes offer new therapeutic options for patients who are currently untreatable. Since the early days, convincing evidence of the power and potential of gene therapy continues to emerge, mainly thanks to the efforts of EU researchers, and in patients suffering from a wide range of diseases, including severe combined immunodeficiencies, adrenoleukodystrophies, beta-thalassemia, congenital amaurosis, graft-versus-host disease, Parkinson's, etc. Even patients (including children) suffering from an inborn genetic disease that is not life-threatening but causes blindness experience improvement of vision – and even start to see when treated early enough in the course of the disease – following gene therapy. Selected recent examples of clinical advances in gene therapy as described in details in previous chapters of this book, clearly indicate that the momentum in this field is building up and underscore that the EU has not only taken the lead but has so far maintained a premier competitive position in this field. This situation justifies, and would be consistent with stimulating renewed EU-wide interest from biotech industry stakeholders. Given the current global economic challenges it is even more important than ever to find sustainable solutions to treat diseases of high unmet medical need. Ultimately, gene therapy may provide long-term therapies or cures not only for rare hereditary diseases but also for more common acquired disorders such as cancer – as recently shown in B-cells lymphoma –, cardiovascular disease and neurodegeneration. In the absence of effective drugs or alternative therapies, the advances in gene therapy technology represent the best hope for the many patients and families that are blighted by these various diseases.

THE CRITICAL PATH TO CLINICAL TRANSLATION: A LONG AND DIFFICULT ROAD

Despite considerable advances in gene therapy at the clinical and pre-clinical front, clinical progress has been slower than originally anticipated. Technical obstacles have been compounded with some safety concerns. However, significant progress has recently been made to improve safety profiles and risk-benefit ratios in gene therapy. It is particularly reassuring that the gene therapy vectors used today are much safer that the vectors used in the first successful gene therapy trials. Clearly, there are stringent criteria that need to be met before any advanced therapeutic medicinal product (ATMP), including gene and cell therapy products, will eventually obtain marketing authorization approval. In Europe, the Committee of Advanced Therapeutics of the European Medicines Agency, EMA-CAT, was established in 2009 in order to facilitate this process. This again is consistent with the recognition that momentum in the field is building up and the necessity to move the field forward – including the development of much larger and significant clinical trials – while maintaining the high standards of regulatory scrutiny. Several gene therapy stakeholders, including representatives for the European Society of Gene and Cell Therapy (ESGCT) are *de facto* members of the EMA-CAT. Some of the challenges faced by gene therapists are not unique to the field but are inherent to translational research at the forefront of medical innovation. Though the high hopes for gene therapy in the early 1990s did not immediately translate into clinical success it is important to recognise that these initial expectations were not realistic, and created the false impression of slow progress. In many ways, the development of gene therapy mirrors that of therapeutic monoclonal antibodies or clinical bone marrow transplantation. These biomedical and biotechnological innovations took over 25 years to perfect and have now become life-saving therapies for hundreds of thousands patients suffering from many different diseases, largely thanks to the perseverance and commitment of many academic, medical and industrial stakeholders. The road to clinical trials and product registration takes 10-15 years with conventional drug development, gene and cell therapeutics are no exception and represent the most complicated of all, thus expected to be spanning several EC framework programmes. As former emerging technologies now are becoming real options, the time has come for clinical translation making use of cutting edge technology providing preclinical steps will confirm that implementation into patients can both be safe and efficacious. It is important to take these realistic timelines into consideration when assessing the overall progress in the field. Nevertheless, as clinical experience accumulates, more basic science still will be required. Sustained funding of both high-quality science and clinical trials as a continuum – as well as a back-and-forth indication of where to go next with pivotal improvements – are necessary to guarantee successful clinical developments and the expansion of the pharmaceutical sector, based on genuine innovation and technology transfer securing further phases of clinical development.

BEYOND GENE THERAPY: DISSEMINATING KNOWLEDGE TO A BROAD SCIENTIFIC COMMUNITY

At the same token, several biomedical disciplines are harvesting the fruits of the technologies that gene therapists continue to perfect from the clinical standpoint of safety and efficacy. Indeed, gene therapy has fueled the fields of biology and medicine with technologies that are now appearing routinely in a huge number of top rank bioscience publications to address hypothesis-driven research questions of biological and medical relevance. Furthermore, there are also key emerging fields where insights and technologies from the gene therapy community are playing central and increasingly important roles. In particular, the emerging fields of RNA interference, micro-RNA and antisense therapies benefit from advances in gene therapy, since safe and efficient delivery of these RNA-based therapeutics is once again the key issue. Moreover, the recent development of induced pluripotent stem cells (iPS) for regenerative medicine by "genetic reprogramming" is intimately linked to the transfer of genes encoding reprogramming factors into somatic cells and can be considered as a *bona fide* spin-off of the gene therapy field.

THE EUROPEAN LEARNED SOCIETY FOR GENE AND CELL THERAPY (ESGCT): FIRST ESTABLISHED WORLDWIDE

The leadership position of EU researchers in gene therapy and their pioneering efforts also prompted the establishment of the first "learned society" in gene therapy, leading up to the current European Society of Gene and Cell Therapy (www.esgct.eu). ESGCT also interfaces effectively with other national and international societies with a vested interest in gene and cell therapy. The continued success of the Annual ESGCT Gene Therapy Congress, with increasing number of attendees, parallels the advances in this field and provides an attractive forum to interact with all the relevant stakeholders in this dynamic field at the forefront of biomedical research and clinical development. Though the ESGCT (and its annual congress) provides a platform for the various EU consortia to help achieve their dissemination and educational objectives, it can obviously not substitute for the EU funded consortia such as CliniGene, the EU Network of Excellence (NoE), Integrated Project (IP) or Strategic Research Project (STREP) initiatives. In particular, ESGCT does not provide financial support for experimental research activities or for clinical trials in this area and does not support collaborative networks directly other than providing a forum for discussion, education and dissemination. Conversely, there are more stakeholders in this field than there are EU-sponsored consortia. The role of the ESGCT and the various EU-sponsored consortia is therefore complementary though they share a common goal of making gene therapy a clinical reality for rare, orphan and common diseases.

MULTIDISCIPLINARY TEAM UP: THE EU-SPECIFICS TO SUCCESS

The continued interactions of gene therapy stakeholders from academia, industry, patient organisations and regulatory authorities are essential to move this field forward and work together towards a proportionate regulatory framework: if the clinical development of monoclonal antibodies and bone marrow transplantation would have undergone the same level of regulatory scrutiny as gene therapy, it is unlikely that these treatments would ever have become available to the broader patient community. The format of experimental collaboration and interactive networks supported so far by EC-DG research is ideally suited to address the different challenges of the multi-facetted field of gene therapy. These interactions have been consolidated largely thanks to EC support, through various past and ongoing NoE, IP or STREPs initiatives. In particular, EC support has enabled leading EU researchers that are active in gene and cell therapy, to collaborate, acquire and so far maintain a global leadership position in this field, by integrating rather than by fragmenting and/or duplicating research efforts. This approach is much more cost-effective and distinguishes itself fundamentally from the fragmented and often disunited approach that characterizes gene therapy efforts in the US. The complexity of issues at stakes – both at the technological and translational medicine level – requires expertise, which can be found only at the European level. Hence, these various EC funding schemes have fostered the development of EU Centers of Excellence in the gene therapy field allowing the EU to acquire and maintain a competitive edge over the US. This has been made possible through consolidated collaborative networks that effectively combine complementary expertise and know-how. Indirectly, these EC-sponsored initiatives also enhanced EU economic competitiveness resulting in academic spin-offs. The potential for a one-time curative treatment by gene therapy should be offset against the high costs of continuous therapeutic interventions for the treatment of chronic diseases. The current demographic trends in EU will only worsen the overall burden on our already overstretched health care system. To reduce the economic burden it is absolutely essential to further consolidate this vision and to take into account the mid-and long-term sustainable benefits of gene therapy relative to the initial investments made.

IN CONCLUSION: A PROMINENT REQUIREMENT TO MAINTAIN INTEGRATION BETWEEN BASIC RESEARCH AND CLINICAL TRANSLATION AT THE EU-LEVEL WITH SUPPORT OF EC-DG RESEARCH

It is absolutely pivotal that various forms of new EU-supported initiatives be continued for several reasons:
  (i) To foster excellence in gene therapy research in academia and clinical centers;
  (ii) To streamline sustained refinement of technology to warrant both safety and efficacy improvement;
  (iii) To consolidate Europe's competitive edge at the international level;
  (iv) To develop the pharmaceutical sector in this field;
  (v) To expedite and facilitate clinical translation;
  (vi) To expand the scope of target diseases treatable by gene therapy.

As highlighted in a 2010 commentary in Nature entitled "Gene therapy deserves a fresh chance": *"It is time for researchers and industry to refresh their perspective on gene therapy and to consider successes with as much intensity as its setbacks... Both scientists and clinicians now have a battery of extraordinary refined tools for preclinical and clinical studies of gene therapy. The field is ripe for further successes".*

Finally, given the recent encouraging developments in gene therapy pre-clinical studies and clinical trials, it is therefore essential to continue to invest in gene and cell therapy to address some of the outstanding questions and overcome the remaining challenges. Indeed, referring again to the field of therapy based on monoclonal antibodies, the oncology community had to wait until ASCO 2012 to witness the formidable progress obtained in metastatic breast cancer with the combination of trastuzumab and emtansine (T-DM1): T-DM1 is an antibody-drug conjugate delivering a one-two punch – trastuzumab, an antibody against HER2 attached to a chemotherapy agent, emtansine, through a linker, delivering the cell-killing agent specifically to cancer cells that express the HER2 receptor on their surface, allowing the cytotoxic agent to kill the cancer cell once internalized. The concept is not new though, as it was formulated back in the late eighties and required over 30 years to materialise. When considering cutting edge, rapidly evolving technologies that gene therapy entails and the requirement to release products which match criteria for clinical translation, there is no doubt that Molecular Therapies will continue to develop and require that visionary policy-makers grant the field with trust, patience and mandatory funding, including basic science.

Thierry VandenDriessche	President, European Society of Gene and Cell Therapy (ESGCT): 2008-2010; Member Committee of Advanced Therapies (CAT) - European Medicines Agency (EMA) - Clinicians representative: 2009-2012
Bernd Gänsbacher	ESGCT President (1998-2004)
George Dickson	ESGCT President (2006-2008); Member Committee of Advanced Therapies (CAT) - European Medicines Agency (EMA) - Clinicians representative: 2009-2012
David Klatzmann	ESGCT President (2004-2006)
Seppo Ylä-Herttuala	ESGCT President 2010-2012
Luigi Naldini	ESGCT President-Elect; Coordinator PERSIST - EU Integrated Project
Alastair Kent	Director Genetic Alliance UK; Member Committee of Advanced Therapies (CAT) - European Medicines Agency (EMA) - Patients representative: 2009-2011
Odile Cohen-Haguenauer	ESGCT Founder (1992), Coordinator CLINIGENE - EU Network of Excellence Chair ESGCT Ethics and Regulatory Committee since 2004

ACKNOWLEDGMENTS

This work has been performed with the support of the EC-DG research through the FP6-Network of Excellence, CLINIGENE: LSHB-CT-2006-018933.

AUTHOR INDEX

A

B

C

D

E

F

G

www.ingramcontent.com/pod-product-compliance
Lightning Source LLC
Chambersburg PA
CBHW081214220326
41598CB00037B/6775